.... Ph.D. CCC-SLP
Department of Communication
Sciences and Disorders
Towson University

Stuttering Therapy
An Integrated Approach to Theory and Practice

Richard Culatta
Appalachian State University

Stanley A. Goldberg
San Francisco State University

Allyn and Bacon
Boston   London   Toronto   Sydney   Tokyo   Singapore

Copyright © 1995 by Allyn & Bacon
A Simon & Schuster Company
Needham Heights, Mass. 02194

Series editor: Kris Farnsworth
Editorial Assistant: Christine M. Shaw
Production Administrator: Joe Sweeney
Cover Administrator: Suzanne Harbison
Composition Buyer: Linda Cox
Manufacturing Buyer: Louise Richardson

Library of Congress Cataloging-in-Publication Data

Culatta, Richard.
   Stuttering therapy : an integrated approach to theory and practice
/ Richard Culatta, Stanley A. Goldberg.
    p. cm.
   Includes bibliographical references and index.
   ISBN 0-02-326311-3
   1. Stuttering—Treatment. 2. Stuttering—Bibliography.
I. Goldberg, Stanley A. II. Title.
RC424.C85 1994
616.85′54—dc20   94-33140
                                       CIP

Printed in the United States of America

10 9 8 7 6 5 4 3   99

This book is dedicated to

Herbert Rubin
Source, mentor, role model, and friend

Our Parents, for their caring and love
Mary and Salvatore
Helen and Irving

Our Families, for their patience and understanding
Janet, Richard, Elizabeth, and Katherine
Wendy, Jessica, and Justin

And the many clients
who have contributed to our knowledge of stuttering

The known is finite, the unknown infinite; intellectually we stand on an islet in the midst of an illimitable ocean of inexplicability. Our business in every generation is to reclaim a little more land, to add something to the extent and solidity of our possessions.

Thomas Henry Huxley
on the reception of the *"Origin of Species"* (1887).

Contents

Preface   ix

Acknowledgments   xi

Section

I An Introduction to Stuttering   1

Chapter **1** Introduction   3
Four-Factor Definition of Stuttering, A Historical
Review of Modern Stuttering Research, Summary,
Study Questions

Chapter **2** Different Types of Disfluency   23
Normal Developmental Disfluencies, Stuttering,
Neurogenic Disfluency, Psychogenic Disfluency,
Language Disorders, Mixed Disfluencies,
Summary, Study Questions

Section

II

Diagnosis   47

Chapter **3**   ### The Diagnostic Interview   49

Measurement, Client Observations, Guidelines for
Constructing Interviews with Stutterers and Their
Families, The Diagnostic Interview, Resistive
Clients, Summary, Study Questions

Chapter **4**   ### Assessment Techniques   69

Overt Characteristics of Stuttering, Covert
Characteristics of Stuttering, A Comprehensive
Testing Procedure, Summary, Study Questions

Section

III

Treatment   109

Chapter **5**   ### Culture and Stuttering   111

Incidence and Occurrence, Speech Behaviors,
How Cultural Differences May Affect Therapy,
Evaluation and Intervention, Summary, Study
Questions

Chapter **6**   ### Variables Affecting Stuttering Therapy   131

The Informed Client, Work Settings, Therapeutic
Approaches, Age-Related Characteristics, Parents
and Parental Counselling, Genetic Counselling
and Stuttering, Prevention Through Early
Intervention, Clinical Efficacy, Explanations for
Clinical Failures, Summary, Study Questions

Chapter **7**   ### Intervention and Transfer
Strategies-PROLAM-GM   165

Physiological Adjustments, Rate of Speech
Manipulations, Operant Controls, Length and

Complexity of Utterance, Attitude, Monitoring,
Generalization, Maintenance, Summary, Study
Questions

Chapter **8** Synopsis of Approaches to the
Treatment of Stuttering   209

Comprehensive Alberta Stuttering Program,
Two-Factor Behavior Therapy, Cooper
Personalized Fluency Control Therapy Revised,
Extended Length of Utterance, A Program for the
Initial Stages of Fluency Therapy, Preschool
Fluency Development Program, Conversational
Rate Control Therapy, Freedom of Fluency,
Treating the School-Aged Stutterer,
Computer-Aided Fluency Establishment Trainer
(CAFET™), Behavioral Cognitive Stuttering
Therapy, Edinburgh Masking Device,
Environmental Manipulation and Family
Counselling, Techniques for Maintaining Fluency,
An Operational Approach for Stuttering Therapy,
A Program to Establish Fluent Speech, Integration
of Approaches, Stuttering Intervention Program,
Managing Stuttering, A Component Model for
Treating Stuttering in Children, Monterey Fluency
Programs, A Modeling Approach to Stuttering
Therapy for Children, Vocaltech Feedback Device,
Stutter-Free Speech, Role Therapy, Systematic
Fluency Training for Young Children, Airflow
Therapy, Multiprocess Behavioral Approach,
Symptom Modification Therapy, Clinical
Management of Childhood Stuttering, Precision
Fluency Shaping Program, Vocal Control Therapy,
Study Questions

Chapter **9** A Strategy for Constructing
Intervention Protocols   259

The Decision-Making Process, Case History
Models, Summary, Study Questions

Epilogue Challenge for the Future   275

Appendices

Appendix **A** Research Bibliography   277

Appendix **B** Self Help and Professional
Interest Groups   399

Bibliography   401

Author Index   425

Subject Index   431

Preface

Over the past 15 years, more than 1,400 articles and 30 books have been written about stuttering. Some contain precise data relating to stuttering behaviors; others transform data into intervention strategies; still others espouse particular clinical philosophies. As academicians and clinical educators, we have continually attempted to organize the information into a gestalt that will allow not only us, but also our students, to understand the disorder, to assess it, and to develop empirically verifiable intervention approaches. The purpose of this book is to present a unique way of determining how we, as clinical scientists, can develop and implement the best form of therapy for our clients. Matthews (1986) wrote that current knowledge is based on the work of our predecessors. We concur with this concept. Although we present some new and different ways of looking at stuttering therapy, we gratefully acknowledge the work of our predecessors and our contemporaries. We have tried to understand the thinking of our colleagues and to filter their contributions through our own experiences. When possible, we have consulted with them, and when not, we used our best judgments.

The first step toward eventually providing therapy is to understand some of the basics of the disorder. What is stuttering? How do we define it? How does it differ from other forms of disfluency? These issues are covered in Section 1. Without an understanding of the basic concepts on which therapy is based, clinicians are in danger of developing intervention protocols that might be ineffective or inefficient.

With an understanding of the defining parameters of stuttering, it is then possible to begin the diagnostic process. Effective assessment involves not only appropriate application of specific protocols, but also understanding how to conduct the diagnostic process. We have therefore chosen to present (in Section

2) not only specific techniques, but also interviewing principles that may help clinicians gather needed data.

Section 3 is devoted to therapy, both an understanding of what is available, and a method for constructing individualized intervention protocols. We have come to understand that communication is not free of culture. As a result, we attempted to highlight how in a multilingual and culturally diverse society speech-language pathologists must be sensitive to the beliefs and values that stutterers bring into the therapy process. In this section, we also summarize 32 intervention programs and compare them using PROLAM-GM, a methodology developed by the authors that allows clinicians to identify behaviors and attitudes that should be treated.

Appendix A, the research bibliography, is a compilation of more than 1400 articles summarized by Psychological Abstracts since 1973. We have categorized these citations by content into 29 categories. In addition, we have highlighted the efforts of scholars from outside of the United States by presenting citations for research published in 10 global regions. It is our hope that the research bibliography will be of interest and assistance to students, research scholars, and those interested in a comprehensive viewing of the last two decades of scholarly activity, both in the United States and the rest of the world.

Throughout this text, we attempted to tackle problematic issues head on. If we have not provided information as complete or concise as readers would like, we apologize. Sometimes it is more important to ask the right questions than it is to supply the wrong answers. We believe that the most certain way to ensure the failure of a treatment is to ignore these problematic issues that clinicians must face, and to reduce therapy to blindly following the iron clad "rules" of an intervention protocol. Successful therapy is done by thinking clinicians who apply valid strategies to problems in meaningful ways.

A note about gender references. When it was appropriate every attempt was made to keep the text gender-neutral. On those occasions when that was not possible, people who stuttered where identified as *he* and speech-language pathologists as *she*. Our rationale is that the field of speech-language pathology is more than 90% female and stutterers are most often men.

Acknowledgments

The authors have not and do not work in a vacuum. We are taught by our mentors, colleagues, clients, and students. We are grateful to them for helping us take the steps needed to solve the problems standing between our clients and normal speech. Our mentors who helped in our initial understanding of stuttering were Oliver Bloodstein, Herbert Rubin, George Shames, Gene Brutten, Joseph Sheehan, Hugo Gregory, Dean Williams, William Perkins, and George Wischner. Our contemporaries have argued with us, shaped our thinking, and judged our contributions. We are most grateful to Gene Brutton, Richard Curlee, William Perkins, Hugo Gregory, Theodore Peters, Roger Ingham, Janis Costello Ingham, Herbert Seltzer, Bruce Ryan, Barbara Van Kirk Ryan, Barry Guitar, Linda Leeper, Rich Shine, Charles Healey, Charles Runyan, Rebekah Pindzola, Eugene Cooper, David Daly, Peter Ramig, Ronald Webster, Daniel Zwitman, Einer Boberg, Carl Dell, Martha Goebel, Harold Luper, Robert Mulder, Donald Mowrer, David Prins, Glyndon Riley, Jeanna Riley, Vivian Sheehan, Martin Schwartz, C. Woodruff Starkweather, Meryl Wall, Florence Meyers, The National Stuttering Project, and others that we have unintentionally left unnamed. Given this wealth of intellect to draw upon, we feel fortunate to be allowed to somehow synthesize our thinking and their work into this book. We have, of course, been as meticulous as is humanly possible in attributing thoughts, concepts, and techniques to their originators. If we have slighted anyone, it was not only unintentional, but also a function of the incorporation of their truths into our lives. Stanford University psychologist Julius E. Heuscher (*Newsweek*, 1991) explains that borrowing occurs because "Some ideas become so true that they become your own." We like to think that all the researchers and clinicians we have been fortunate enough to know are part of us.

We are deeply in debt to our students, who have continually forced us to clarify and simplify our thoughts. Their editorial guidance has been most helpful. We also must not ignore the contributions of our clients. The men, women, boys, and girls we have treated for nearly three decades provided the motivation to do a better job, and they are a constant reminder that we must do more, faster, and more effectively in helping them achieve their potential.

The final copy of this manuscript is a result of the valiant efforts of our Editor Ann Davis, who allowed us the freedom to attempt the best possible contribution we could make and the reviewers, Michael Moran, Auburn University; David Maxwell, Emerson College; Howard D. Schwartz, Northern Illinois University; Peter Ramig, University of Colorado; Robert Harris, Trenton State College; and Judith B. King, Northern Arizona University, who saved us from the embarrassment of oversights, unrecognized errors, and unfounded assumptions.

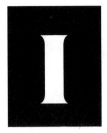

An Introduction to Stuttering

To study stuttering assessment and intervention, one must understand the terminology, the historical development of the field, and the role of clinicians. In Chapter 1, the various terms associated with the study of stuttering are presented, followed by a chronology of developments in the field of stuttering during the last 50 years. Disfluencies can take many forms, and they can result from different causes. Six types of disfluencies are discussed in Chapter 2.

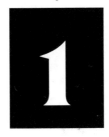

Introduction

A logical first step in exploring a topic is to define the subject of concern. There are various ways a definition can be constructed. We use an approach that is behaviorally inclusive, and operationally useful. To be behaviorally inclusive, the definition should account for all instances of a particular phenomenon, and it should simultaneously provide boundaries that differentiate that phenomenon from all others of a similar nature (Shames, 1990). To be operationally useful, the definition should provide researchers or readers with a method of clearly identifying the phenomenon to be investigated (McReynolds and Kearns, 1983).

FOUR-FACTOR DEFINITION OF STUTTERING

Our purpose in this section is to provide readers with a definition of stuttering that will help them organize and understand the information that follows. Definitions are like relationships; they can range from simple to complex. Although simple relationships are straightforward, they may lack the richness of more complex ones. Complex relationships can be very fulfilling, but they are fraught with many problems not encountered in simple relationships.

Historical Perspective

Controversies regarding how to define stuttering have existed throughout the history of our profession. In this section, four definitions of stuttering, ranging from simple to complex, are presented. These four definitions were chosen because they are historically significant, and they contributed in varying degrees to our four-factor definition presented at the end of this section. Table 1–1 shows a comparison of the definitions in terms of their major components.

Van Riper. Van Riper's (1939) early definition of stuttering has been used by generations of speech-language pathologists as an entry port to understanding the nature of stuttering. For Van Riper, stuttering occurs when the forward flow of speech is interrupted abnormally by repetitions or prolongations of a sound, a syllable, or an articulatory posture, or by avoidance and struggle behaviors. The usefulness of the definition is derived from its simplicity. Its simplicity, however, limits its applicability.

Wingate. A definition that expands on Van Riper's was provided by Wingate (1964). His attempt at defining stuttering categorizes the disorder as a disruption in the fluency of speech that is characterized by involuntary, audible, or silent repetitions or prolongations of sounds and syllables. These disruptions occur frequently or they are noticeable in character, are not readily controllable, and are sometimes accompanied by unusual movements of the speech mechanism or other body parts. Stutterers also report emotional reactions to their abnormal speech.

This definition is not only more specific than the one developed by Van Riper, but also it introduces the notion of "lack of control," a concept that expands the definition beyond identification of specific observable behaviors into the realm of feeling states.

Nicolosi and Colleagues. Nicolosi and colleagues' definition (1978) not only expands on the behavioral components of Wingate's definition, but also introduces a reference to etiology in the form of a "timing disturbance." They define stuttering as a "disturbance in the normal fluency and time patterning of speech characterized by one or more of the following: (1) audible or silent blocking; (2) sound and syllable repetitions; (3) sound prolongations; (4) interjections; (5) broken words; (6) circumlocutions; or (7) words produced with an

Table 1–1.
Comparison of Definitions of Stuttering

	Overt Behaviors	Avoidance Behaviors	Issues of Control	Emotional/ Attitudinal Reactions	Timing	Associated Behaviors	Etiology	Onset Related to Age
Van Riper	X	X						
Wingate	X		X	X				
Nicolosi	X	X			X	X	X	
Perkins	X		X		X		X	
Culatta and Goldberg	X	X	X	X		X	X	X

excess of tension. These primary characteristics may be accompanied by associated behaviors or secondary characteristics. These disturbances may be at the level of neuromuscular, respiratory, phonatory, or articulatory mechanisms. Dysfluencies are so numerous that they exceed the normal number or degree for the individual's age, sex, or the speaking situation" (p. 197).

Although Nicolosi and colleagues' definition is largely descriptive, its reference to "time patterning of speech" introduces etiology into the definition, a development that both enhances a definition and makes it more controversial. The concept that stuttering is a disorder of timing was elaborated on in a classic article by Perkins and associates (1991), in which the definition of stuttering now includes reference to specific behaviors, "lack of control," and timing.

Perkins and Associates. Perkins and associates (1991) describe stuttering as a multifaceted disorder culminating in an individual's inability to control the neuromotor timing of syllables caused by yet undetected abnormal neurolinguistic problems that cause discoordination between various systems involved in speech. The discoordination results in the various types of disfluencies heard in a stutterer's speech. This complex but elegant definition of stuttering goes beyond any that have been presented to date: It includes not only specific behaviors and etiological factors, but also elements that are related to the continuation of the behavior. However, it posits physiological, neurological, and anatomical relationships that still require verification.

Collectively, these four definitions capture the basic elements of the stuttering response, and they provide theories about its cause and possible maintenance. However, as insightful as these definitions may be, they fail to provide some of the critical features necessary for effective clinical intervention. The definition of stuttering presented in the next section not only draws from the works of these authors and other researchers, but also expands their boundaries to provide a behaviorally inclusive definition of stuttering that is operationally useful.

Four-Factor Definition of Stuttering

A definition is more than a descriptive statement that lists the critical features of an entity or a phenomenon. It usually becomes the basis on which a more global understanding of the subject develops. In the preceding definitions, each of the authors did not merely provide an objective description of the behavior, they also alluded to related concepts, such as control and etiology. We believe this approach to be both proper and clinically useful. We chose to make our definition both behaviorally operational and inclusive. The inclusive nature of a definition of necessity results in making the definition more general. However, although our definition may lack the specificity found in, for example, Nicolosi and colleagues' description of overt behaviors, it provides a framework for understanding the phenomenon of stuttering that is either not present in the other definitions or only alluded to. The proposed definition of stuttering provides information about causality, onset, development, belief systems, and behaviors.

Factor One: Stuttering is a Developmental Disorder of Childhood. If untreated, stuttering follows a predictable developmental path (Bloodstein, 1987). People who become stutterers are most often identified between the ages of 2.5 to 4 years of age (Yairi, 1983). No one becomes a stutterer much after the age of 6 (Shames and Beams, 1956). The spontaneous disfluencies of young adults and older adults that often seem to spring up "overnight" with little developmental history are usually a sign of disorders of fluency other than stuttering.

Factor Two: The Cause of Stuttering is Unknown. This point is critical in the eventual treatment of stuttering, and it demands explanation. Even though the early literature is replete with tales of stuttering caused by barking dogs and falls from high places, none of these tales has ever been substantiated (Ingham, 1984a). More reasonable explanations suggest that temporary bouts of disfluency in children can be initiated by events, such as family break-ups due to death or divorce. Their displays of disfluency, although not stuttering, are often cries for help or an indication of stress. Once the specific precipitating factor is dealt with, the disfluency usually disappears. At this point in our attempt to delineate the components of a working definition of stuttering, it is sufficient to say that stuttering is a developmental disorder of childhood, and that the cause of the stuttering is unknown by clients, parents, teachers, social workers, or speech-language pathologists.

Factor Three: Clients View Communication Differently From Normal Speakers. At some point in their lives, people who stutter learn to view speaking in a different way than normal speakers. Whether they learned to stutter is an argument considered later. They have, however, through their experiences with talking learned to expect different consequences from their attempts at speech than normal speakers. They report beliefs and internal "feelings" that differ from those of normal speakers (Bloodstein, 1984). Whether these beliefs are newly learned, as in the case of a preschooler, or are a way of life, as with an adult, any definition of stuttering must consider the clients' perceptions of the disorder. Stuttering is therefore a developmental disorder of unknown origin that changes a person's expectations about the communication process.

Factor Four: Clients Have Abnormal Overt or Covert Communication Behaviors. A viable definition must include the "something the client does" that is considered stuttering. If a client demonstrates overt symptomatology, as most do, this factor is merely an individualized descriptor of the stutterer's presenting behaviors. Examples of overt stuttering behaviors include hesitations, broken words, repetitions, interjections, prolongations, dysrhythmic phonations, visible tension, revisions, and incompleted phrases. A complete description of these behaviors and others that result in the differential diagnosis of stuttering is detailed in Chapter 2. However, not all stutterers have to demonstrate all the characteristics of disfluency to be considered stutterers. They may not have to display any of the overt symptoms with which we have come to identify stuttering to merit the label stutterer. Douglas and Quarrington (1952) labeled symptom-free stutterers as "interiorized" in terms of obvious outward characteristics, as compared to the "exteriorized" clients most often encountered. The covert internal behaviors of stuttering may be identified as avoidance, expectation of stuttering, expectation of fluency, motivation, starter devices, circumlocutions, and self-perception. These behaviors and the other components of stuttering described in the literature do not require outward symptoms to disrupt successful communication. These behaviors are also described in Chapter 2.

Summary. The four-factor definition of stuttering is as follows: Stuttering is (1) a developmental communication disorder beginning in childhood of (2) unknown origin that (3) results in a person viewing the communication process differently from a normal speaker (4) due to experiences with overt or covert factors that disrupt normal communication.

To give this definition life and to turn it into an operational definition that is of practical value, clients must be inserted into it. One example is a 4-year-old child from an essentially normal household who is moderately upset because of the number of hesitations, prolongations, or repetitions that characterize his disfluent speech. Another is a 19-year-old high school senior with a history of overt disfluencies, now under control, who refuses to speak in class because he is afraid that his disfluent behavior may return and cause him social pain. Both individuals described are stutterers: both are in pain; both share the same global features of the disorder that link them as "stutterers." However, they have little in common in terms of visible symptoms, life experiences, or conceptualization of their problem. We must be able to describe them both within our definition for it to be of value. Perhaps what we are dealing with are disorders of stuttering rather than a single disorder. In any event, the suggested operational definition and its specific application to individuals should enable us to describe our clients and to evolve treatment programs.

What was purposely omitted from this definition was the initial biasing statement that says "stuttering is a learned disorder which . . ." or "stuttering is an emotional disorder which . . ." or "stuttering is a neurologically based disorder which. . . ." These definitions that have an etiological bias tend to limit speech-language pathologists' powers of observation and perhaps lead them to force clients into categories into which they do not belong. As clinicians, we all bring our own beliefs into the study and treatment of stuttering. Speech-language pathologists cannot and perhaps should not escape from their beliefs; however, attempts should be made to restrain prejudgments as much as possible.

The proposed definition is probably not as specific as some readers would like. Critical readers perhaps can uncover some facet of stuttering that it does not cover. The task then becomes one of incorporating the new information into the proposed outline and making it even stronger. We are fond of the theory that hypothesizes if 10 speech-language pathologists were put in a room, 11 definitions of stuttering would emerge. Each would be valid in some aspects, and all would begin with "In my opinion. . . ."

A HISTORICAL REVIEW OF MODERN STUTTERING RESEARCH

Once the behavior has been defined, the next step in understanding stuttering is to trace the evolution of its study. Why do we view stutterers and stuttering as we do? How has this view changed over time? And, most importantly, do the past and the present lead to future study?

The journey from the past to the present can be an instructive one. Although the transition from one research epoch to the next is not as direct as will be suggested in this condensed overview, we do learn from each other. This is perhaps the most encouraging lesson in the still unsolved search for the cause of stuttering. Although today's approaches are certainly not totally inclusive of what has been proposed previously, neither are they independent of the past. We refine and improve the conceptualizations of our predecessors, discarding the ideas that have not stood the test of time and incorporating those that have into ever more meaningful attempts at solutions. Currently, we are at a juncture where several forces are in motion. The search for the cause of stuttering continues primarily in the work of the researchers committed to the physiological and neurological aspects of stuttering. The emotional aspects of the disorder are currently being debated in terms of stutterers' attitudes toward themselves and the communication process. Learning theory has evolved into the application of fluency-based approaches for the elimination of stuttering. The following attempt to superimpose order onto a process that resists streamlined orderly growth can help trace a pathway from the past to today.

Speech-language pathology, like other fields that deal directly with human behavior, is not isolated from its place in society at any given moment in time. As a result, the theories explaining the cause of stuttering and the treatments suggested to cure stuttering are often a result of current scientific and social thinking at the time a given piece of research is attempted. The following review of some of the pertinent landmarks in stuttering research is an attempt not only to describe the literature that has had an impact on current therapeutic strategies, but also to place it within an historical framework. The goal is both to make readers aware of significant research and to highlight the roots of some divergent views that have arisen between schools of research.

This section does not provide a totally in-depth analysis of all the research done on stuttering during the past 80 years. Readers are directed to Appendix A for a listing of most of the research in stuttering published between 1973 and 1994. In an attempt to superimpose some order on these approximately 1,400 sources, we listed them by categories. Thus, 26 separate categories ranging from "Assessment" to "Voicing" are presented, with the appropriate scholarly works cited under each category. This approach provides not only a comprehensive listing of the research for the last two decades, but also a beginning for researchers, clinicians, and students who wish to do in-depth readings in any given area. In addition, two excellent review texts by Bloodstein (1987) and Ingham (1984a) for in-depth literature analysis are available. Our purpose in this chapter is to outline how we think current treatment of stutterers and understanding of stuttering evolved.

Medical Model

It appears that early Medical Model adherents opened the door to the modern study of stuttering in their search for a simple physical cause-and-effect explanation for stuttering. They brought the prestige of a recognized researcher to an area that had previously been the domain of carnival side-show, snake-oil salespersons. Their exploration of the most obvious questions in the best scientifically available manner of the time aroused an interest in the process of communication that can be traced to current attempts at understanding the process of using fluent speech. Their attempts to answer basic questions using state-of-the-art methods legitimized stuttering research. Their findings led most researchers to leave the medical model in search of other routes to help stutterers.

However, medical researchers continue to ask questions that challenge the current belief in self-control and fluency development. It is perhaps the role of these scientists to search continually for physical causation, using the newest and best diagnostic equipment in their quest. The absence of unequivocal proof from these researchers provides the impetus for others to continue to refine differing approaches to eliminating stuttering. Regardless of our own philosophy, we must never be so arrogant that we dismiss unproved assertions simply because they are not popular with current social trends. To do so places us in danger of living on a flat planet where the sun revolves around the earth and ideas that challenge the status quo are unwelcome.

Matthews (1986); Travis (1978); and others detailed how the initial searches for causality during the 1920s and the 1930s followed the medical model with its search for physical cause and effect. Two views developed. One was essentially that stuttering must be caused by some physical or chemical breakdown in the same way that other diseases are the result of a systemic failure. The second was that inherited characteristics somehow contributed to the breakdown of at least one of the systems involved in speech production. Some of the more popular medical models appear below.

Theory of Cerebral Dominance. Because it was thought that the ability to produce and coordinate speech was controlled by the hemispheres of the cerebral cortex, a logical theory that evolved was that there had to be a failure in the workings of these cortical hemispheres. Stutterers were thought to have defective "motor lead control" or incomplete cerebral dominance. Orton and Travis (1929), in what came to be known as the "Theory of Cerebral Dominance," were able to explain theoretically the physical causation for stuttering and to suggest therapy strategies for its control. As Bloodstein (1987) reports, despite the favorable reception accorded this theory, the intervening years have not seen it gain acceptance.

Laryngeal Dynamics.   Another more recent physiologically based research endeavor attempted to pair laryngeal dynamics and stuttering behavior. Although the concept of faulty laryngeal functioning is not new (Kenyon, 1943), it has re-emerged as an area of study due to technological advances. New and more sophisticated devices have become available to measure the larynx and how it functions (Adams, 1981). These new measurement devices have raised the possibility that stutterers' voice onset times (VOT), speech initiation times (SIT), and voice initiation times (VIT), which are apparently longer under certain circumstances than those of nonstutterers, might in some way point to the larynx as a causative agent. Excellent reviews of these studies can be found by Bloodstein (1987) and Ingham (1984a). Bloodstein (1987) concludes there is little evidence that abnormal function of the larynx has any sort of primacy in stuttering behavior. Ingham (1984a) believes that the laryngeal activity studies are useful in providing another way of describing stuttering, but that they do not identify "causal components of the disorder" (p. 318).

Heredity Model.   Interest in the relationship between genetics and stuttering has existed throughout the history of our profession. As early as the 1930s, various authors hypothesized that stuttering was genetically based (Nelson, 1939; Seeman, 1937; West et al., 1939; Wepman, 1935, 1939). The role of genetics in stuttering received scant interest until Kidd, in the late 1970s, began documenting the occurrence of stuttering in the families of stutterers (Kidd, 1977, 1983; Kidd et al., 1981; Kidd et al., 1978; Kidd and Records, 1978). With each subsequent study by Kidd and colleagues, the role of heredity in stuttering became more difficult to refute. The findings were related to the occurrence of stuttering in families of stutterers and the occurrence of stuttering in twins.

Stuttering is three times more likely to occur in families with first-degree relatives who stutter when compared with the general population (Andrews, 1984). Bloodstein (1987), summarizing familial incidence, reported that a family history of stuttering ranged from 8 to 15% with stutterers, whereas nonstutterers have a significantly lower percent of occurrence in their families. Nelson (1939) reported that 68% of the families with stutterers had stuttering relatives as compared with 15.6% of nonstuttering families having stuttering relatives. Wepman (1939) reported that 71% of stutterers had other family members who stuttered, as compared with 13% of a control group used in the study. More recent research by Poulos and Webster (1991) reconfirms the older research. Their data reveal a 66% familial link, which is comparable to early studies.

Studies that examined twins showed significant differences in the occurrence of stuttering in monozygotic and dizygotic pairs (Howie, 1981). There are significantly more occurrences of stuttering in monozygotic twins who have identical genetic make-up than in dizygotic twins who share only approximately half the same genes. Howie (1981) found that the risk of stuttering in the monozygotic co-twin of a stutterer was 77%, whereas it was only 32% in the dizygotic co-twin of a stutterer.

These data suggest that stuttering is a polygenic inheritance of a common dominant gene with a multifactorial background and a sex-limitation mechanism (Goldberg, 1992). Simply put: (1) the behavior is determined by many factors, (2) the factors are both hereditary and environmental, and (3) it affects the sexes differently. If stuttering is a multifactorial polygenic inherited behavior, how do heredity and environment interact to cause the behavior to appear? The explanation involves reference to a threshold model originally presented by Falconer (1965), who maintained that the threshold at which a behavior appears may be related to genetic factors. In individuals at risk, the threshold is lower, and the behavior will appear when certain environmental factors are present. This relationship would explain why individuals who, although they would appear to be at risk for stuttering based on a pedigree, may in fact not stutter. This theory is compatible with numerous authors' beliefs that people are born with a predisposition to stutter.

Neurological Functioning. An interesting model to examine stuttering involves the use of positron emission tomography (PET) scans to determine if the neurological functioning of stutterers differs from the neurological functioning of nonstutterers. On-going research involves use of a PET scan device that is able to produce thousands of computer-generated images of the brain while the subject is performing a speech act (Ingham and Ingham, 1992). It appears that the technology is currently available to determine if there are any neurological differences between stutterers and fluent speakers. Results of these experiments have not been published. The search for physiological, hereditary, or chemical links to stuttering continues with exploration of new areas. Although some try to bridge theoretical models and clinical application (Perkins et al., 1976), much of this work is of little immediate use to current service providers. A notable exception is in the area of genetics. As a result of the on-going accumulation of information on the probability of stuttering in the progeny of individuals with a family history of stuttering, genetic counseling may soon have a place in stuttering therapy.

Psychological Model

The belief in subconscious motivation and the idea that stuttering might only be a symptom of some deeper emotional dysfunction followed medical model inquiries, and these ideas were the next major influences on modern speech-language pathology. Was the pain that stutterers' felt emotionally based? Was stuttering a sign of mental illness? These questions were asked using the Psychological Model, which emphasized the relationship between mental health and communication disorders. Years of research passed, and it appeared that group data could not differentiate stutterers from other people purely on the basis of psychological profiles. Although stutterers are not excused from emotional problems, they do not seem to be any more mentally ill than the rest of the world (Bloodstein, 1987). However, we did learn that people who are stutterers have some very different attitudes about communication and a world that demands rapid relatively flawless speech. Are stutterers born with these attitudes? Although there may be a predisposition toward disfluency, it is hardly likely that stutterers or anyone else is born with predetermined attitudes, positive or negative, about speaking. We have a need to communicate with our fellows, and we also accept the consequences of our communication attempts.

Thus, a global view of the contributions of the adherents to the Psychological Model reveals several lasting contributions. Thanks to these researchers, we are free of the constraints that dealing with emotionally disturbed people bring to therapeutic intervention. We have also learned counseling skills and therapeutic techniques that enable us to uncover information that lies beyond physical measurement. However, the most important link to the present is the idea that perhaps the behaviors and the attitudes of stutterers are not solely a reaction to deep-seated emotional differences, but rather can be learned behaviors.

The psychological model offered speech-language pathologists two significant concepts to examine. One was the view that stuttering was a neurotic behavior, and the other was a counseling approach known as nondirective therapy or client-centered therapy.

Neurotic Behavior. With the emergence of psychoanalysis, stuttering was seen as a neurotic act performed unconsciously by those with deep-rooted emotional needs. Definitions of stuttering such as the following were fairly typical of the conceptualizations of the era. "Stuttering as a psychosomatic disturbance is only a symptom of neurotic conflict. A child rendered basically helpless, insecure, and afraid, is driven toward safety and some degree of pseudo-harmony by developing neurotic trends. Since these same neurotic trends are compulsive, inappropriate and contradictory in nature, they are bound to fail in the face of the slightest threatening situation" (Barbara, 1954, p. 94).

Stuttering was identified as being the result of a number of neuroses; an expression of an infantile need for oral erotic gratification; an attempt to satisfy anal erotic needs; a covert expression of hostility; and even an unconscious desire to suppress speech. Travis (1957) developed this later concept by reporting case histories detailing the suppressed speech that clients were afraid might come uncontrollably to the surface. Guilt, anxiety, conflict, toil, and struggle were all a part of the syndrome. Simple "symptom-based" approaches to the disorder were doomed to fail and at best could only result in "symptom substitution" of other deviant behaviors. The treatment of choice was psychoanalysis, which could help the client delve into the unconscious factors causing the problem.

Because of these speculations, much of the research of individuals supporting this model has been focused on attempts to verify the existence of deep-seated, unconscious motivations that result in stuttering. Stutterers endured personality assessments of all types, including broad-based projective personality tests such as the Rorschach ink blot test (Rorschach, 1937) and the Thematic Apperception Test (Murray, 1943). More specific studies attempted to find evidence of psychosexual fixation, oral and anal eroticism, passive dependency, obsessive-compulsive traits, hostility, and aggression. Stutterers' self-conceptualizations, levels of aspiration, anxiety levels, rigidity, suggestibility, and guilt were also pondered.

Bloodstein (1987) provides a lucid and comprehensive description of these studies and their outcomes. In general, the results suggested that although stutterers as a group are not excused from emotional problems, they are no more likely than their contemporaries to have emotional disturbances. As Bloodstein reports, the evidence does not appear to indicate that the average stutterer is a distinctly neurotic or a severely maladjusted person. As might be expected with any heterogeneous population, some stutterers are better adjusted than some fluent speakers, and some stutterers are less well adjusted than their fluently speaking controls. The research does seem to indicate that stutterers as a group are not as socially well adjusted as their fluent counterparts. However, these differences may be a consequence and not a causative factor of the disorder. People who avoid normal speaking situations and who have unusual concerns about their abilities to communicate effectively are by definition maladjusted in our society. However, this is hardly a description of anxiety-plagued neurotics who are slaves to subconscious motivation.

Non-directive or Client-centered Therapy. Even the most cursory descriptions of the role of psychology in relation to stuttering must mention the contributions of Carl Rogers (1942, 1951). Although classic psychoanalysis and its questionable impact on the communication patterns of stutterers remains far removed from most speech-language pathologists, nondirective counseling techniques, or client-centered therapy, as developed by Rogers, have had a lasting effect on the treatment of stutterers. In contrast to the bubbling cauldron of repressed feelings and anxieties of classic psychoanalysis, Rogers believed that human beings are positive in character. Clients are viewed and treated as realistic, forward-moving, and rational. As a result, the therapeutic philosophy stresses that counselors should clarify client beliefs rather than prescribe courses of action. Rogers stresses "insightful" learning by clients rather than therapist-ordered activities. Many clinical techniques currently in use, regardless of underlying philosophy, can be traced in part to the formulations of Rogers. Seeman (1986), in a highly informative chapter in *Stuttering: Then and Now,* analyzes Rogerian approaches in terms of their applicability to stuttering therapy. Particularly interesting is a retrospective analysis of the impact of nondirective counseling since its inception.

As a result of the work of Rogers, current treatment of stuttering is in debt to psychology more for therapeutic technique than for theoretical substance. However, the effects of the psychoanalytic search for serious emotional dysfunction as a component of stuttering may still color clinical thinking. Cooper (1975) sampled the legacy of these beliefs in his study on clinical attitudes toward stuttering. Fifty-six percent of his population of practicing speech-language pathologists accepted the statement that most stutterers have psychological problems. Only 14% of the speech-language pathologists sampled rejected the statement that stutterers display a distorted perception of their own social relationships. Among his other findings, Cooper also reported that 82% of the clinicians believed that they must be more understanding of the feelings of stuttering clients than nonstuttering clients. Perhaps the empathy and the sympathy that has developed for stuttering clients has its roots in the psychoanalytic speculation of stutterers as emotionally different people.

There is little current research interest in differentiating stutterers as a group from nonstutterers in terms of emotional factors. Aside from periodic statements concerning the need for appropriate counseling techniques and the role of clinicians in client progress (Shames and Florance, 1980), there does not appear to be a great deal of interest in the United States in the application of psychotherapeutically oriented strategies toward the treatment of stuttering.

Manipulable Behavior Model

In the 1960s, the conceptualization of stuttering was once again modified. The belief that stuttering was a learned behavior that could be manipulated by the same conditions that affected other learned behaviors gained acceptance. The idea developed that learned behavior can be changed. Researchers freed from the diagnosis of physical or mental illness were able to study disfluency as more objective professionals. These professionals and their students began to suggest and implement approaches that would make a stutterer's communicative life more bearable. Perhaps their goals were not sufficiently lofty at first, but their highly practical approach resulted in stutterers beginning to believe that they could manipulate their speech. Shame and embarrassment were replaced with determination and willingness to change. Although theoretical concerns remained vital, these researchers, many of them stutterers, personally felt the pain of stuttering and wished to do something about the behavior immediately. From a current perspective, it is not difficult to understand why they emphasized emotional adjustment of the stutterer rather than aspiring to develop normal fluency. Yet they did show generations of stutterers and future generations of researchers that behavioral change was possible.

Researchers and clinicians who understand and treat stuttering as a disorder regulated by learning principles are a diverse group. Some believe that stuttering may be an anxiety-based disorder (Wischner, 1950; Brutten and Shoemaker, 1967), or that it can be controlled by the systematic desensitization techniques successful with phobics of all types (Wolpe, 1958). Others believe that initiation and maintenance of the disorder are learned phenomena that result from environmental influences (Johnson, 1955; Bloodstein, 1958; Shames and Sherrick, 1963). Another group believes that the disorder can be a result of heredity and learning and that each aspect contributes to the disorder in its own way (Eisenson, 1958; Ingham, 1984a).

Intervention strategies vary from parental counseling and symptom modification, to application of various operant techniques designed to facilitate the development of fluent speech. This is a mixed and at times confusing area of research and clinical application. However, it is the one area out of which the most practical treatment approaches for stuttering have developed. Regardless of theoretical beliefs, the one thread that links the following group of researchers and clinicians is their unshakable belief that stuttering, regardless of its initial form, can be modified. The degree of modification sought and the manner in which it is sought might differ, but the underlying optimism is consistent. Stuttering, whether totally or partially learned, can be changed, shaped, modified, unlearned, replaced, controlled, and monitored.

The contributions outlined are not consistent or complementary of each other. In fact, the greatest controversies exist within this area of study. Much of the confusion experienced by treatment providers probably can be traced to the various theoreticians and their suggestions for treatment that have evolved from the learning framework group. It is the goal of this section to lead readers to the present conceptualizations by tracing the research efforts of those we have categorized as being affiliated with the learning model.

Stuttering as a Learned Anxiety Response. Initial efforts to explain stuttering as a learned behavior attempted to link stuttering and anxiety. In essence, stuttering was seen as a learned anxiety reaction. Wischner (1950) postulated that stuttering was a way that some people learned to deal with anxiety. The stuttering act reduced anxiety, thereby enabling the stutterer to better cope with the environment. Sheehan (1953) hypothesized that people who stuttered were caught in an "approach-avoidance" situation, during which they wish to speak but, for a variety of reasons, they were afraid to do so. As a result, they learned the hesitations and the repetitions that are characteristic of stuttering. Bloodstein (1958) discusses stuttering as an "anticipatory-struggle reaction" that is responsive to environmental pressures. A person is anxious about his ability to communicate, and, as a result, changes his speaking behavior. It is this change that develops into stuttering. Although different in detail, each of these illustrative examples stress that stuttering is in part learned and in part a fear or an anxiety reaction.

A seemingly natural outgrowth of these theories would be therapeutic attempts to control anxiety reactions and thereby decrease or eliminate stuttering. The most direct of the approaches that evolved was that of Wolpe (1958). Known as "reciprocal inhibition therapy," the intervention strategy consisted of combining the concepts of "progressive relaxation" (Jacobson, 1938) and "systematic desensitization." Brutten and Shoemaker (1967) developed a viewpoint of stuttering that was a combination of two theories: (1) Stuttering is a classically conditioned fear response maintained by environmental stress, and (2) the stutterer's reaction to the stuttering was operantly conditioned. In practice, clients learned techniques to deal with anxiety by learning to consciously apply relaxation strategies to anxiety-producing situations. Hierarchies of feared communication situations were imagined and anticipated in therapy sessions and hopefully applied in experiences outside of therapy. Ingham (1984a) reports that these early attempts at changing behavior were neither well documented nor apparently very successful. However, they did signal a change in direction. It was now permissible and in fact preferable to work on the behavior of stuttering without fear of further complicating the underlying emotional factors that might be causative.

Diagnosogenic Theory. But what of this fear or anxiety? From where did it come initially? Perhaps the most influential theory for initiation and maintenance of stuttering ever espoused attempted to explain this initial fear. Johnson (1955) proposed the Diagnosogenic Theory, which proposed that parental reaction to a child's normal disfluencies instilled the initial anxiety. Thus, the parents' initial diagnosing of normal behavior as "stuttering" and their emotional reaction to the behavior either caused or maintained the behavior in the child. Stuttering was "not in the child's mouth but in the parents' ear." Parents were not necessarily evil people intent on injuring their children, but rather, overanxious, misinformed, and perhaps a bit too perfectionistic. Although subsequent studies have raised grave doubts about the validity of the Diagnosogenic Theory (Andrews et al., 1983; Yairi and Lewis, 1984), it set the tone for decades of intervention strategy. Even currently, despite mounting evidence that the speech of children who become stutterers is distinguishably different from those who become normally fluent (Saskia et al., 1992), much time and effort is spent attempting to uncover what parents may have done to cause their children to stutter. This is often not a productive line of inquiry, and it has led to clinician frustration and unnecessary parental guilt.

Johnson and colleagues comprised the Iowa School. This group of highly dedicated people set the tone for understanding and treatment of stuttering for the past five decades. As we attempt to trace their contributions, readers should note how many of their own beliefs can be traced to the principles espoused by these clinically oriented researchers.

Stuttering Modification. Lee Edward Travis was the first trained doctoral-level speech-language pathologist and the first director of the speech clinic at the University of Iowa. As such, he led what has been come to be called "the Iowa School." Under his leadership, Bryng Bryngleson, Wendell Johnson, Charles Van Riper, Oliver Bloodstein, and later Dean Williams brought clinical intervention for stuttering from side show trickery to the beginnings of responsible treatment. Johnson, Bryngelson, Van Riper, and Williams, who were stutterers, brought an understanding of client vulnerability and desperation to their work. The understanding and mandated empathy that they and their students brought to research and treatment were, and continue to be, legacies of stuttering intervention strategies based on their influential work.

The two most lasting contributions of Bryngelson are the therapeutic techniques based on the concepts of "objective attitude" and "voluntary stuttering." Bloodstein (1987) reports that to Bryngelson, an objective attitude meant that the stutterers would be willing to discuss their stuttering without guilt or shame. Stutterers also would be willing to enter speaking situations they feared and to communicate, stuttering if they had to, without relying on substitutions, avoidances, circumlocutions, or any other devices used to avoid stuttering. In general, this initial phase of therapy was designed to allow stutterers to display disfluencies without the usual accompanying fear. Situational or "field work" grew out of this phase, as stutterers, accompanied by clinicians and other stuttering group members, spoke and were observed in speaking situations outside the confines of the clinic. Once again, the goal was not necessarily to speak fluently, but to demonstrate mastery of the objective attitude in the face of feared situations. This healthy mind set or "mental hygiene" aspect of treatment was to become a structural underpinning of the Iowa School. It is one of the shared goals of its members. Although gaining and maintaining an "objective attitude" might lessen the stutterers' fear of any given situation, it did little to reduce or eliminate stuttering.

For therapy to improve the stutterer's life, behavior change was needed along with attitude change. In an attempt to help stutterers gain a measure of control over their speech, Bryngelson initiated "voluntary stuttering," which was a modification of Dunlap's (1932) concept of "negative practice." Dunlap hypothesized that by practicing an unwanted behavior on a conscious and purposeful level, a person could bring that behavior under control. By engaging in "voluntary stuttering," the stutterer attempted conscious control of stuttering episodes. Control was critical. Stutterers practiced their stuttering patterns and then used them in contrived situations. If a person "lost control" of his stuttering, he was to continue stuttering until control returned. A practical result of this technique was that clients often produced simple repetitions rather than the complicated patterns that characterized their stuttered speech. Johnson and Van Riper both utilized and expanded these concepts in their work.

Johnson and associates (1959), however, modified the concept of voluntary stuttering in his own distinctive way. As the originator of the Diagnosogenic Theory, Johnson firmly believed that stuttering was a disorder based on faulty perceptions of the communication process. First, there was the inaccurate diagnosis by the parents, and next, there was the stutterers' acceptance and reaction to these misdiagnoses. The difference between stutterers and normal speakers was that the stutterers reacted emotionally to their hesitations (Bloodstein, 1987). What prevented stutterers from speaking normally were the things they did to avoid stuttering. If attitudes and assumptions could be changed, then so would the behavior. Johnson utilized voluntary stuttering not to show control, but rather to allow stutterers to be disfluent on purpose so that they would cease to avoid disfluency and, as a result, lessen the fear of stuttering. Freed of the fear and tension that characterized the avoidances that were often the major components of stuttering, it would be possible for clients to stutter simply and easily. Ultimately, this simplification would evolve into essentially normal disfluencies. Much of the therapeutic process was spent reorienting the client so that their view of "normal" speech and "normal" speakers was more realistic. The language used to describe the process of stuttering and stutterers came under scrutiny. All too often, stutterers saw stuttering as something that happened to them rather than a behavior they initiated. Later, Williams further developed these concepts and influenced not only the Iowa School, but many current theorists. We discuss Williams and his critical contributions later.

It was left to Van Riper to pull the work of his colleagues together and to evolve the therapeutic rationale that has become known as "symptomatic therapy for stuttering" (Van Riper, 1973). His views are a delineation and an extension of the concepts of the Iowa School. Van Riper's programs stress reduction of anxiety about stuttering coupled with specific modification techniques based on a knowledgeable client analysis of speech behavior. During a "mental hygiene" period, the stutterer attempts to lessen fear and to prevent the negative attitudes that result from being afraid to talk. Specific speech modification techniques aimed at simplification of stuttering are then learned. The four best known techniques are "cancellation," "bounce," "pull-out," and "preparatory-set."

The goal of "cancellation" was for the stutterer to repeat the word that he stuttered on and to make some change for the better on the second attempt. The goal was not to say the word fluently, but to acknowledge the stuttering and to show control by simplification of the stuttering behavior. The stutterer was then taught a less effortful way of stuttering, which consisted of easy repetition of the initial syllables of stuttered words. This so called "bouncing" significantly simplified the stuttering moment for the stutterer. The client then learned how to "pull-out" of stuttering blocks. Once the stuttering block was started, the speaker would end the word by switching to a smooth prolongation. This easily articulated, prolonged version of the word replaced the habitual struggle for control, and it enabled the client to "pull-out" of the block in a more stable manner than usual. As clients became more facile at this approach, the "pull-out" could be initiated earlier and earlier in the sequence, with a resulting speech pattern that more closely approximated normal speech. The final tool was control of the clients' "preparatory-set." Van Riper believed that before initiation of a stuttered word, clients often assumed an articulatory posture that made it impossible to say a particular word. A client who clamped her lips together and held her breath while struggling could hardly say "Susan" or anything else for that matter. The goal of an appropriate "preparatory-set" was for the speaker to assume the physically normal articulatory settings needed to speak. Clients learned these techniques in the order described, but they applied them in the reverse order beginning with "preparatory-sets." If clients failed to assume the appropriate "preparatory-set," they would then initiate a "pull-out" to terminate the stuttering. If this approach failed, "bouncing" and finally "cancellation" of the stuttering block was performed. Thus, clients were never totally defeated. The worst that was possible was simplification of symptoms in a controlled manner.

Satisfaction of speech clinicians with less-than-fluent speech from clients was shared by all members of the Iowa School. Van Riper's term *fluent stuttering* sums up the therapeutic goals of this group.

. . . one could learn to stutter with a minimum of abnormality. It was necessary to substitute for the habitual stuttering reactions a smooth, simple pattern of interruptions without struggle and free from the devices for avoidance, post-ponement, starting and release that frequently complicated them. The goal in short, was not to speak without stuttering, but to stutter "fluently" (Bloodstein, 1981, p. 350).

This clinical goal of "better stuttering" characterized the work of ensuing generations of speech-language pathologists.

Fluency Enhancement. Williams (1957) signaled the beginnings of change when he began to write of stuttering as a behavior clients perform and not the result of an external force inflicted on them. "A person's behavior can be described. 'Stuttering' mystically conceived as an undemonstrable something, cannot be. Each person's behavior varies in observable ways under recogniz-able conditions" (1957). Stuttering is something the client is doing and as such it can be changed. Williams even went as far as suggesting that these changes should be in the positive direction of what normal speakers do when they talk. Using stuttering as a point of reference, therapy techniques at the time were attempting to control stuttering. Williams suggested that this focus did little to clarify the problem for clients and perhaps led them from taking responsibility for their speaking behavior. Williams accurately foresaw "a trend away from animism, from separation of mind and body, from special entities within a person over which he has no control . . . toward a more scientific, more de-scriptive, process-like manner of talking about . . . stuttering" (1957).

Within months of publication of Williams' article, Flanagan and colleagues (1958) published the first work that viewed stuttering as a class of behaviors that could be manipulated by response-contingent consequences. When their subjects were punished immediately after stuttering, they reported that stut-tering was reduced or eliminated. This initial work and the flood of research that followed ushered in a period of pairing operant technology and stuttering behavior. Stuttering research left the clinic and entered the laboratory.

Stuttering was then seen as a response to the environment that could be controlled with proper application of consequences by clinicians. Punishment of stuttering, reinforcement of fluency, successive approximation, time out, and delayed auditory feedback (DAF) became part of the language of re-searchers. Shames and Sherrick (1963) published a highly influential article that suggested both stuttering and normal disfluency might be considered operant behaviors. Their terminology was clearly defined. Stuttering was seen as an observable event, a response that could be manipulated in very precise ways.

The purpose of these manipulations was to increase or strengthen desired behaviors and decrease or remove unwanted behaviors. Any stimulus pre-sented immediately after a response that increased the occurrence of the re-sponse was a positive reinforcer. Punishment was by definition presentation of an aversive stimulus that decreased the occurrence of a behavior. Extinction was seen as removal of a reinforcer. Negative reinforcement occurred when an ongoing aversive situation was terminated by a desired response. Positive and negative reinforcement increased responses, whereas extinction and punishment decreased responses. Shames and Sherrick maintained that systematic and measured application of these procedures on a predetermined schedule was responsible for changing behavior. The only way to determine if a procedure was effective was to measure its results. This reliance on defining the behavior of both clinicians and clients and measuring results may have been the greatest contribution of the operant years. Objectivity was now injected into the clinical procedure, because failure could be seen as the application of improper contingencies. Also, measurement techniques enabled clinicians to evaluate the results of their therapy in replicable, quantifiable ways.

Researchers were now able to apply theoretical concepts to stuttering behavior. Martin and Siegel (1966a, 1966b) applied operant techniques to subjects who stuttered in a series of experiments. They found that stuttering could be manipulated and eliminated by application of appropriate contingent responses. The behavior, stuttering, returned when these contingencies were removed. Bloodstein (1987) reports that, "a large amount of further research has been done on the question of whether stuttering may be modified by its contingent consequences, and almost invariably the answer has been that it can" (p. 304). An excellent and comprehensive review of these and other operant studies was done by Ingham (1984a).

During this same period, Goldiamond (1965) began to study the effects DAF might have on stuttering. Essentially a modified magnetic-tape recorder, the DAF device allowed researchers to play back a subject's speech through earphones with a momentary delay. Initially, Goldiamond attempted to use DAF as a punisher. However, when he analyzed the performance data of his stuttering subjects, he found that some subjects reduced rather than increased their rate of disfluency in association with DAF. Speech was produced fluently in a slow, prolonged manner while under the influence of DAF. From these experiments, he conceived the idea of instilling a new stutter-free speech pattern to replace the stuttered speech of stuttering subjects. This work developed into the first program designed to establish normal-sounding, stutter-free speech (Goldiamond, 1965). Using decreasing amounts of DAF, he established and shaped a new pattern of normal-sounding speech with stutterers. Clients initially used slow prolonged speech while experiencing DAF. This prolonged speech helped them "beat" the usual DAF effect. The delay was systematically reduced and finally eliminated while the new speech rate was increased to approximate normal speaking. Goldiamond's work led to a shift from emphasizing reduction of stuttering to establishment of fluency.

The question then became, if stuttering can be replaced by fluent speech, is it necessary to modify stuttering at all? This question, previously unthinkable, was inspired by the researchers who resisted it most. The work of "modification of stuttering" researchers sustained the interest of other researchers and brought relief to patients while newer theories and therapies evolved. The research efforts switched from modification of stuttering to experimentally instilling fluency. In the laboratory, it was possible to replace stuttering with fluent speech; however, behavior brought about in the controlled environment of the laboratory is by no means comparable to the chaotic circumstances of the everyday world in which we live. Was it possible to take this laboratory-derived fluency produced by stutterers and translate the procedures for obtaining it into therapeutic strategies?

Stuttering research and therapy had entered a new phase: the quest for fluency. Rubin and Culatta (1971) articulated the belief that the appropriate goal for stutterers and speech-language pathologists was fluency. They believed that the stutterer's basic ability to be fluent is not in question, rather only what he says and how he says it at any moment. Complete fluency was a feasible goal of therapy for stutterers and could be directly obtained. Culatta (1976) reported that the "goal is to demonstrate to the client that he or she can speak fluently. Fluency must be acknowledged and understood. There is no secret. A client is fluent when doing the things normal speakers do."

Helping clients use fluent speech required a radical shift in the attitudes of both clients and clinicians. Modification of stuttering into a more socially acceptable form was no longer appropriate. Instead, the aim of therapy was fluency and normal speech. Perkins (1973) attempted to redefine the problem in terms of fluency when he stated that "we now view fluency as a relatively gross clinical dimension involving judgments of normal versus abnormal disfluency. When an instance of stuttering, which is abnormal disfluency, occurs it reflects a failure to achieve . . . normal speech." Shames and Egolf (1976), speaking about the goals of those committed to operant technology and behavior modification techniques, perhaps summed up the feelings of many current researchers when they stated that " . . . we feel that stutterers should not be asked to accept their stuttering, to learn to live with their stuttering and to modify it to more socially acceptable forms. The goal is . . . speech that is free of stuttering" (p. 145).

Current service provision has grown from two divergent learning theory groups, and it is split into at least two camps. The goal of the "stuttering modification" group is for clients to learn to control their stuttering behavior. The goal of the "fluency enhancement" group is for clients to use ever-increasing amounts of fluent speech until normal communication is achieved. The first group articulates the belief that stuttering can be controlled at best, whereas the second group believes that stuttering can be eliminated. The philosophical differences between the "stuttering modification" adherents and the "fluency enhancement" advocates throughout the 1970s were a major stumbling block in provision of a unified service delivery model. However, recent evidence shows that clinicians are increasingly embracing both techniques in their intervention protocols (Goldberg and Culatta, 1991).

Generalization and Maintenance

The most current thrust of research is in the area of generalization and maintenance of the gains achieved in therapy. Boberg and co-workers (1979) highlight the current need for maintenance programs as a part of treatment. The immediate and often dramatic increases in fluency achieved often fail to stand the test of time. We are just beginning to understand why post-treatment maintenance programs are needed and the causes for relapse. The major questions that need to be answered by current researchers are why maintenance programs are needed, and what are the causes of relapse by clients who have achieved fluent speech? The long and winding road continues to bend just beyond the sight of contemporary scholars.

SUMMARY

We grow as a profession by learning to understand our problems and by asking questions about their solutions. It is not always easy to determine what is the obvious question, and it is often harder still to answer it. This introduction is an attempt to outline how speech-language pathologists have asked and answered questions about stuttering. Theories and therapies do not bloom full grown without roots in fertile soil. We can effectively and efficiently map out plans for the future only if we understand our heritage as service providers to the communicatively handicapped and only if we are aware of where we have been in our search to erase stuttering.

STUDY QUESTIONS

1. Describe each of the five definitions of stuttering presented in this chapter, and indicate how they differ from each other.
2. What are the strengths and weaknesses of each model?
3. Describe the variations of the medical model.
4. Describe the variations of the psychological model.
5. Describe the variations of the manipulable behavior model.
6. Compare the research findings of the medical, psychological, and manipulable behavior models.
7. What would be the clinical implications of using each of these models?

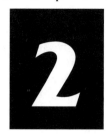

Different Types of Disfluency

Disfluencies take many forms, and they can result from different causes. Six types of disfluency have been identified.

1. Normal developmental disfluency
2. Stuttering
3. Neurogenic disfluency
4. Psychogenic disfluency
5. Language-based disfluency
6. Mixed fluency failures*

The current literature often confuses the different types of disfluency by using the generic term *stuttering* for any speech disfluency. The term is used to describe the disfluent speech of individuals with no known etiology, who are neurologically involved, emotionally disturbed, or linguistically delayed. Use of the term is based on similarities in presenting behaviors. The generic use of the term *stuttering* can obscure important differences, despite shared symptoms. Not all headaches are the result of brain tumors; not all neoplasms are carcinogenic; and not all disfluencies are stuttering. Although it is true that a side effect of some neurological and degenerative diseases is disfluent behavior, these disfluencies are not considered stuttering. Stuttering does not de-

*The concepts discussed in this chapter were originally discussed in the following works listed in the bibliography: Culatta and Leeper (1989a), Culatta and Leeper (1988), Culatta and Leeper (1987), and Leeper and Culatta (Unpublished observations).

scribe the temporary bouts of stress-induced disfluency we all experience. Although we are all "normally disfluent" some of the time, we do not all stutter sometimes. This is an important distinction for both speech-language pathologists and clients to understand. Regardless of whether it is an attempt to gain rapport with clients through shared experiences or a simple misunderstanding of the disorder, it is neither accurate nor fair for the clinician to tell a client that the temporary slips and bobbles normal speakers experience are a form of stuttering. These transitory moments, whether due to content or situation, are not the result of the same belief system and history that stutterers bring to their communication attempts. Stuttering is also not "stage fright," "elective mutism," or any of a host of emotional- or situational-specific events that may lead to a temporary inability to communicate, with either complete silence or highly disfluent speech.

Normally fluent speech is not perfect speech. All speakers pause, hesitate, repeat, and mis-speak in a variety of ways that are well within the limits of normal communication. Even the most polished and professional speaker will be disfluent at times. Under stress, most speakers may exhibit disfluencies when using unfamiliar vocabulary or when they are made to speak in unfamiliar speaking situations. These disfluencies are not abnormal, nor are they stuttering. However, once speakers cross the boundary from these normal nonfluencies to abnormal disfluencies, they are evaluated differently by their listeners.

We each have within ourselves a model of exactly what is acceptable and unacceptable in terms of fluent and nonfluent speech. However, even though the idea of fluency is easily understood, it resists a straightforward and unambiguous definition (Finn and Ingham, 1989). Often there are no stringent guidelines we may use to judge fluency other than our own judgment. A justice of the United States Supreme Court once stated that he could not define pornography, but he knew it when he saw it. Similarly, we may not be able to define normal speech in terms of its inherent disfluencies, but we know whether the speech we hear meets our standards of expected fluency. As speech-language pathologists responsible for judging the adequacy of communication, identification of disfluencies in the speech of our clients is not a terribly difficult task. Unfortunately, our work does not end with simple identification. Distinguishing normal, developmentally disfluent children from incipient stutterers, or neurologically impaired disfluent speakers from true stutterers, is a far more complex task than simply possessing the knowledge that there are different types of disfluency. Accurate identification of the source of disfluencies may determine whether our treatment approaches will be successful.

This chapter explains, compares, and contrasts the different types of disfluencies that disrupt normally fluent speech. The goal is to develop an understanding of the differential diagnosis of disfluency and how it can affect treatment strategy.

Table 2–1 outlines the types of fluency failures discussed in this chapter. The first type of disfluent speech discussed is the result of a normal developmental

Table 2–1.
Types of Fluency Failures

Normal disfluencies

Developmental

Abnormal disfluencies

Stuttering
Neurogenic dysfunction
  Motor speech disfluencies
  Neurolinguistic disfluencies
  Chemical reaction disfluencies
Psychogenic
  Emotionally based disfluency
  Manipulative disfluency
  Malingering
Language delay
Mixed fluency failure

process, and the rest are the result of different abnormalities. A child may be disfluent as a result of passing through the necessary but stressful stages of language learning. These developmental disfluencies are a routine part of the acquisition of normal language. A person may be disfluent because he or she is a stutterer. A speaker may produce disfluent speech as a result of a neurogenic dysfunction that may affect communication. There are disfluencies that are psychogenic in origin, and there are disfluencies that are the result of language delay. Each type of disfluency presents its own identifiable set of conditions that speech-language pathologists must recognize and understand prior to developing a treatment plan.

NORMAL DEVELOPMENTAL DISFLUENCIES

As children pass through the developmental stages of language learning, they will be more disfluent at certain times than others. These developmental periods of disfluency are a normal occurrence. In mastering spoken language, we become more fluent as we become more proficient. Normally communicating children hit a peak of disfluency usually between 2.5 to 4 years of age. The normal disfluencies children produce are characterized by the repetition of whole words and phrases, with occasional interjections of "uhs," "ers," and "ahs" (Perkins, 1971; Yairi and Lewis, 1984). This is a transitional stage most children leave behind as they master oral communication, and there is no need for therapeutic intervention. Worried parents need to be informed of the existence of normal developmental disfluency as a stage of development. They need to be assured of the normalcy of this phenomenon and its transitory

Name _____

Address _____

Date of birth _____

Age _____ Sex _____

Date of Test _____

Clinician _____

I. AUDITORY BEHAVIORS

- TYPE OF DISFLUENCY (mark the most typical)

Interjections	Hesitations/Gaps- Repetitions-	Prolongations- Coexisting Struggle
Probably Normal	Questionable	Probably Abnormal

- SIZE OF SPEECH UNIT AFFECTED (mark the typical level at which disfluencies occur)

Sentence/phrase-	Word-	Syllable-Sound
Probably Normal	Questionable	Probably Abnormal

- FREQUENCY OF DISFLUENCIES (compute from speech sample and mark values on continua)

- Frequency of Repetitions

```
                        2%                      5%
<-----------------------|-----------------------|----------------------->
```

Probably Normal	Questionable	Probably Abnormal

Figure 2–1
Protocol for Differentiating the Incipient Stutterer

nature. The task for speech-language pathologists is to differentiate normal developmentally disfluent children from those evidencing other disfluency patterns, especially stuttering.

It appears that the disfluencies of incipient stuttering children are markedly different from those of their normally disfluent counterparts. Children who go beyond simple repetitions and interjections to forced prolongations of sounds (Yairi and Lewis, 1984) accompanied by signs of physical struggle in producing speech (Ryan, 1984) may be "incipient stutterers" (Pindzola and White, 1986).

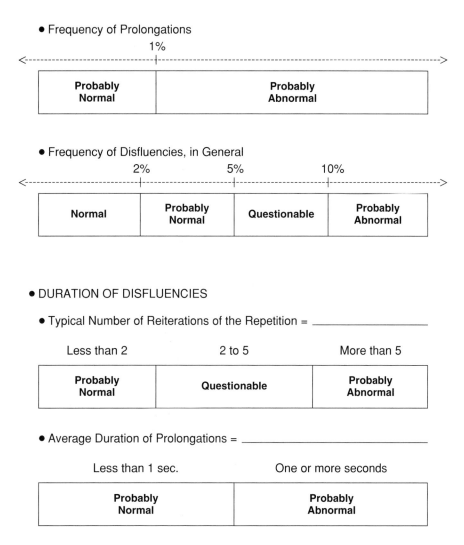

Figure 2–1
Continued next page

These children begin to repeat parts of words rather than whole words, and the frequency and duration of these episodes increase past normal expectations. Pindzola and White (1986), summarizing current beliefs, suggest that if more than 5% of a child's speech is characterized by repetitions of sounds or words and more than 1% is abnormally prolonged, the child has left the boundaries of normal developmental disfluency.

Normally fluent speech is not effortful for a speaker, and rhythm and rate should not call attention to themselves. Signs of unusual struggle or concern about the process of talking are also negative signs. The Protocol for Differen-

- AUDIBLE EFFORT (mark those that apply)

Lack of the following: Presence of the following:

Probably Normal	Probably Abnormal

_____ hard glottal attacks
_____ disrupted airflow
_____ vocal tension
_____ pitch rise
_____ others

- RHYTHM/TEMPO/SPEED OF DISFLUENCIES

Slow/normal, evenly paced   Fast, perhaps irregular

Probably Normal	Probably Abnormal

- INTRUSION OF SCHWA VOWEL DURING REPETITIONS

Schwa not heard   Presence of Schwa

Probably Normal	Probably Abnormal

- AUDIBLE LEARNED BEHAVIORS (mark those that apply)

Lack of the following: Presence of the following:

Probably Normal	Probably Abnormal

_____ word/phrase substitutions
_____ circumlocutions
_____ avoidance tactics (starters, postponers, and the like)

Figure 2–1
Continued

tiating the Incipient Stutterer (Pindzola and White, 1986) (Fig. 2–1) provides speech-language pathologists with an instrument that synthesizes much of what is known about incipient stuttering. It allows clinicians to place disfluent behaviors on a continuum and to evaluate the cumulative impact of 21 possible

II. VISUAL EVIDENCE (list behaviors observed)

● FACIAL GRIMACES/ARTICULATORY POSTURING:

● HEAD MOVEMENTS:

● BODY INVOLVEMENT:

III. HISTORICAL/PSYCHOLOGICAL INDICATORS (comment on the following based on client and/or parent interviews, observations, and supplemental tests or questionnaires, if any.)

● AWARENESS AND CONCERN (of child, of parents):

● LENGTH OF TIME FLUENCY PROBLEM HAS EXISTED:

● CONSISTENT VERSUS EPISODIC NATURE OF PROBLEM:

● REACTION TO STRESS:

● PHONEME/WORD/SITUATION FEARS AND AVOIDANCES:

● FAMILIAL HISTORY:

● OTHER COVERT FACTORS:

IV. SUMMARY OF CLINICAL EVIDENCE AND IMPRESSIONS

Reprinted from Pindzola R. and White D. T. (1986). A protocol for differentiating the incipient stutterer. *Speech and Hearing Services in the Schools* 17: 2–15.

Figure 2–1
Continued

behaviors in three major categories. This systematic compilation of observed data and clinical and parental interpretations is very helpful in determining whether the childhood disfluencies should be labeled as normal developmental disfluency or stuttering.

STUTTERING

Stuttering is the most common classification of disfluency. However, for a person to be considered a stutterer, many of the following signs and experiences must be part of the case history. First and foremost, stuttering is a disorder of childhood. It is developmental in nature, and it follows a fairly predictable path. Parents of stutterers report that, at first, the disfluency pattern is highly episodic; periods of days, weeks, or even months pass between episodes of disfluency. Gradually, the intervals shrink, and the problem becomes chronic and consistent.

Bloodstein (1960) proposed the most widely accepted schemata for the development of stuttering. At first, the disfluency pattern tends to be episodic and displayed under conditions of communicative stress or pressure. Relatively simple whole word and sound repetitions dominate early stuttering, followed by more complicated patterns as the disorder evolves. The disfluencies shift from the beginnings of sentences or phrases to all positions in utterances. Initially, they tend to be located primarily in noncontent words, such as pronouns, conjunctions, articles, and prepositions. In this early stage, only a few of the stutterings are on content words, such as nouns, verbs, adjectives, and adverbs. Gradually, as the severity of stuttering progresses, content words begin to constitute a greater proportion of the stuttered words.

The covert, internal reactions of the speaker also go through an evolutionary process, beginning with little overt reaction to disfluency, through self-identification as a stutterer, to the eventual strong emotional reactions of fear and embarrassment. This gradually evolving pattern emphasizes the developmental nature of stuttering. Absence of an early developmental history should alert speech-language pathologists to the possibility that the disfluent speech produced by a client might not be stuttering. Bloodstein (1960) presents a four-phased transitional system that maps the developmental progress of stuttering from its inception to its possible full growth. The phases represent a typical, although not necessarily universal, pathway stutterers may gradually follow, each at their own rate. Table 2–2 is a summary of the developmental stages proposed by Bloodstein and widely accepted by speech-language pathologists as a guideline for tracking the development of stuttering.

Starkweather (1987) proposed that stuttering may be exacerbated when the demands of a child's environment exceed the child's capacity to produce fluent speech. These demands may be internal and linked, for example, to increasingly sophisticated language development, or they may be external from an environment that demands more fluency than the child can produce. In either event, this Capacitties and Demands Model further explains how stuttering can become more frequent and severe if left untreated. This conceptualization parallels the Bloodstein Developmental Phases, and it perhaps gives insight into why they occur.

Stuttering behaviors also vary in other significant ways from disfluent speech. Van Riper (1982) and Stromsta (1965) report that even the repetitions of stutterers are different from normal speakers. When stutterers repeat, they

Table 2–2.
Developmental Phases of Stuttering

Phase I

Age of onset: between the ages of 2–6 years.

Characteristics

1. Disfluencies are episodic in nature.
2. Disfluencies appear most under communicative stress, excitement, or presentation of lengthy information.
3. The dominant, although not exclusive, symptom is repetition.
4. Disfluencies are most present at the beginning of sentences or phrases.
5. Disfluencies occur on noncontent as well as content words.
6. Children show little evidence of concern about speech disfluencies.

Phase II

Age of onset: usually affects primary level school children; however, it may be found in 4-year-old children and as late as adulthood.

Characteristics

1. Disfluency has become chronic in nature.
2. The children identify themselves as stutterers.
3. Disfluencies occur predominantly on content words (nouns, verbs, adjectives, and adverbs).
4. Children continue to show little evidence of concern about speech.
5. Rapid speech or excitement increase disfluencies.

Phase III

Age of onset: most common in late childhood and early adolescence; it may occur at all ages between 8 and adulthood.

Characteristics

1. Disfluency becomes aligned with specific situations.
2. Specific words and sounds are identified as difficult to say.
3. Substitutions and circumlocutions are employed to avoid difficulties.
4. Little fear, embarrassment, or avoidance of speaking situations.

Phase IV

Age of onset: usually seen in later adolescence or adulthood; it may be evident in children as young as 10 years.

Characteristics

1. Vivid, fearful anticipation of disfluencies.
2. Identification of feared words, sounds, and specific situations.
3. Frequent use of word substitutions and circumlocutions.
4. Chronic avoidances of specific speaking situations.
5. Fear and embarrassment in speaking situations.

Adapted from Bloodstein O. (1960). The development of stuttering: part II. Developmental phases. *J Speech Hearing Disorders* 25: 366–376.

tend to insert the neutral schwa vowel /ʌ/ in place of the vowel that would ordinarily occur in a word. Thus, [bae-baesbaul] becomes [bʌ -bʌ -baesbaul]. Stuttering is also often characterized by an apparent struggle to produce sounds and words that have little to do with speech production. These often bizarre "secondary characteristics," such as jaw tremors, head shaking, eye closing, or total bodily gyrations, disappear during fluent communication productions.

True stuttering can be manipulated during the diagnostic session in several ways. These manipulations often help speech-language pathologists differentiate a stuttering pattern from other types of disfluency. For example, reduction in stuttering symptoms usually occurs with repeated readings of the same passage. This phenomenon, called the adaptation effect, was first mentioned in 1937 (Johnson and Knott, 1937). Although stuttering may decrease as much as 50% during the first five repetitions of a passage (Bloodstein, 1981), there is no transfer of this reduction in stuttering to other oral readings or to spontaneous speech. Although of no lasting therapeutic value, the adaptation effect is useful for differential diagnosis. Quite often, absence of the adaptation effect is a clue that the speech-language pathologist is dealing with a form of disfluency other than stuttering.

The distractibility of stutterers often sets them apart from other individuals who display unusual disfluency patterns. "White noise" or other masking sounds presented at high intensity (Cherry et al., 1955; Shane, 1955), speaking in time to a metronome (Barber, 1940), singing, group recitation, finger tapping, or arm swinging can all alter or eliminate stuttering for brief periods. In fact, any temporary distraction may produce transitory fluency. Most stutterers will be able to sing fluently or take part in choral reading exercises with little or no disfluency. An important fact to consider during the diagnostic session is how manipulable the disfluent symptoms are under varying conditions similar to those identified. These temporary shifts to fluent speech are a clue that the type of speech being diagnosed is stuttering.

People who are stutterers often have internalized a belief system about communication that differs from the perceptions of other speakers. Even as children, they often identify themselves as victims of some mysterious force that makes speaking a difficult task. It is not unusual for clients to report that "I can't say that word" or "my mouth is locked-up." Normal speech is a mystery to them, and as they grow, they develop lifestyles designed to avoid specific, anticipated speaking situations during which disfluency is expected. However, with the exception of their fears of communication, stutterers represent a wide variety of personality types and essentially the entire range of emotional adjustments (Bloodstein, 1981). They do not comprise an identifiable subgroup by their emotional make-up. Stuttering does not seem to be the result of specific emotional trauma. Most parents are at a loss to explain any specific conditions that might account for initiation of stuttering.

Stuttering does tend to run in families. Stutterers are much more likely to have relatives who stutter than fluent speakers (Kidd, 1980). However, the presence of a "stuttering gene" has not been isolated, and a widely held belief among speech-language pathologists supports the model that some environmental factors interact with an existing predisposition to cause stuttering behavior.

In summary, many of the following characteristics are necessary for a disfluent speaker to be labeled a stutterer.

1. The behavior must have a developmental history beginning in childhood.
2. There are no identifiable etiological or maintaining factors.
3. The repetition patterns differ from normal speakers.
4. The symptoms can be modified by any number of clinical manipulations.
5. Allied or "secondary characteristics" are not evident during fluent periods.
6. The speaker has internalized a belief system concerning communication that acknowledges stuttering and recognizes the difficulty of specific communication situations.

If a client does not present a case history consistent with this outline or seems at odds with the discussion presented thus far, the speech-language pathologist should be alerted to the idea that the speaker might be disfluent for reasons other than stuttering.

The following case history might help clarify the concepts discussed. This history and the others presented in this chapter demonstrate the differing types of disfluency clinicians encounter.

ILLUSTRATIVE CASE HISTORY
Stuttering
John, age 13

John reports a history of stuttering beginning at approximately 4 years of age with what his parents report was an abnormal number of repetitions of whole words as compared with both his older brother and younger sisters. His parents recall that they were told that John would "outgrow" his stuttering and that they should pretend it did not exist. John recalls that he knew, even at age 4, that there was something wrong, but he could sense that his parents did not wish to talk about it. His parents report that there were initial periods of time when John's speech was perfectly normal, followed by weeks when he could hardly talk. By age 6, there was a decrease in these swings between fluency and stuttering; John maintained a less severe but more consistent amount of stuttering. John reports that by the second grade he knew he was a stutterer, but that it did not bother him much. He reports that it got harder and harder to say words, but that he still answered in class. He was enrolled in speech therapy, but he cannot remember what was done in his school therapy group. Currently a freshman in high school, he reports that his speech is worse than ever. He avoids talking in class and especially on the telephone. Although his grades are good, John is not happy in school, and he fears he will have to face too many speaking situations in classroom presentations.

John tends to prolong the initial syllables of words, force his eyes closed, and have periods of 2 to 3 seconds when he is silent after beginning a word. He often repeats the sounds "umma umma umma" before initiating a sentence. He is active in his local church youth group and he sings in the choir with no difficulty. He reports no difficulty in unison response during prayer services.

NEUROGENIC DISFLUENCY

Neurogenic disfluency is the result of an identifiable neuropathology in a speaker with no history of fluency problems prior to occurrence of the pathology (Culatta and Leeper, 1987). Speech disfluencies often appear at the onset or soon after neurological trauma or progressive disease. Specific medications have also been reported to affect fluency (Helm-Estabrooks, 1987). It is critical to identify these speech breakdowns as the result of specific systemic dysfunction rather than the disfluencies of stuttering, which are unknown in origin. Calling neurogenic disfluency "neurogenic stuttering" or any similar term can be misleading as well as inaccurate. It is misleading because it implies that treatment might somehow parallel the treatment provided stutterers; it is inaccurate because it is confusing a neurologically based communication disorder with one of unknown origin (Culatta and Leeper, 1987). Kent (1983) suggests that the term *stuttering* in the case of developmental disfluency is a diagnostic label, whereas disfluency following neurological damage is only one symptom of a more pervasive problem. This is not simply an academic argument. The emotional trauma, frustration, guilt, and sense of failure that neurologically impaired speakers feel when attempting to modify their speech production with inappropriate stuttering therapy techniques can be devastating. The likely failure of these techniques may inadvertently add a sense of failure to an already traumatized client, and it is often an unwittingly cruel blow.

Neurogenic disfluencies are often different in form from those presented by stutterers. For example, Rosenbek (1984), describing the repetitions of incorrect sounds and words produced by aphasic or apraxic speakers, notes that these repetitions stop once the phonemically correct target or close approximation is achieved. By comparison, stutterers repeat sounds that are correctly articulated except for their frequency of occurrence. Aphasic patients who experience dysnomia or who exhibit dementia may display disfluencies in the form of interjections, pauses, and circumlocutions while attempting to search for the correct word. Once again, such behavior ceases once the target word is accessed. In contrast, stutterers are well aware of the word they are attempting to articulate prior to initiation of the disfluent behavior.

The different dysarthrias that result from lesions in the neuromotor speech system often include disfluencies such as prolongations, repetitions, and dysrhythmic phonation (Darley et al., 1975). These behaviors are usually accompanied by other communication deficits, such as imprecise articulation, dysphonias, and dysprosody, disorders that occur as infrequently in stutterers as in the general population.

Unfortunately, the disfluencies that appear after neurological disfunction often closely resemble stuttering behavior. Correct sounds and syllables may be prolonged, syllables may be changed to include the schwa vowel (Rosenbek, 1984), and secondary characteristics, such as facial grimaces, also may appear. Studies by Canter (1971), Caplan (1972), and Rosenbek and colleagues (1978) indicate that even when neurogenic disfluency behaviors parallel those of stuttering, some differences do exist. A grammatical influence on the location of disfluencies was reported in all three studies. Neurogenic disfluencies may frequently occur on function words, such as prepositions and conjunctions, as contrasted to stuttering in adults, with which the disfluencies are much more likely to be on nouns and verbs (Canter, 1971). Moreover, the "adaptation effect" discussed previously does not appear to decrease neurogenic disfluencies as a function of repeated practice.

It might also be expected that the rapid onset of neurogenic disfluency would affect client self-image differently than the developmental nature of stuttering. The person with a lifetime of experience as a fluent speaker might initially feel little concern about increased levels of disfluency after trauma, and may initially display little in the way of secondary coping or avoidance behaviors. Disfluency is a normal speech behavior, thus a short-term increase in disfluency level would not result in a client immediately sharing the same view of oral communication that a stutterer might have developed over a lifetime. The patient would feel little need to develop coping behaviors. However, if disfluency levels remained unusually high for a prolonged period, the patient with neurological dysfunction might develop attitudes similar to those of stutterers (Rosenbek, 1984).

The onset of neurogenic disfluency is usually abrupt. Stroke is a common condition under which neurogenic disfluency often occurs. Helm and associates (1980) point out that the necessary conditions for the appearance of disfluency following stroke were either bilateral brain damage or multiple, unilateral cerebrovascular accidents (CVAs). When the stroke occurs in the cortical, precentral motor programming area of the dominant hemisphere, such as in Broca's aphasia, a speech apraxia may also occur with associated disfluency symptoms, such as repetitions, blocks, perseverations, and circumlocutions (Johns and Darley, 1970).

A gradual onset of neurogenic disfluency is also possible when repeated disruption of neurological function occurs subsequent to the original insult. Helm and co-workers (1980) describe individuals in whom seizure disorders developed following closed head injury or tumors. In these patients, speech disfluencies were observed to appear simultaneously with seizure activity.

Unfortunately, unlike other neurogenic speech-language deficits, disfluency is not a symptom that by itself can be useful in the differential diagnosis of the site of lesion. Disfluency has been observed as a symptom in such diverse conditions as postencephalitic parkinsonism (Canter, 1971), ataxic dysarthria (Darley et al., 1969), apraxia (Rosenbek, 1980), and dialysis dementia (Rosenbek et al., 1975). Disfluency is a symptom associated with damage to virtually all areas of the central nervous system except, as Rosenbek (1984) points out, the occipital lobe.

Although it may be difficult, it is not impossible to distinguish between neurogenic disfluency and stuttering. As mentioned, stuttering is a developmental disorder of childhood. Children demonstrate the disfluencies characteristic of stuttering while they develop and refine their communication skills. In contrast, a neurogenic disfluency must be associated with an identified neuropathology in an individual who, prior to that identification, did not demonstrate abnormal disfluency in speech. The following summaries should help alert speech-language pathologists to the possibility of speech disfluencies resulting from three neurogenic bases: motor speech disorders, neurolinguistic disorders, and chemical reactions.

Motor Speech Disfluencies

The different dysarthrias that result from lesions to the neuromotor system often include disfluencies that superficially might be confused with stuttering symptoms. These behaviors, however, are usually accompanied by other communication deficits, such as imprecise articulation, dysphonias, and dysprosody disorders. Children with known disorders, such as cerebral palsy, present a special challenge because it is often difficult to determine if their disfluencies are solely attributable to the motor speech mechanism damage. Because it is possible that the neurological damage present prior to birth precluded the possibility of developing normally fluent speech, it becomes the task of speech-language pathologists to determine whether the disfluencies are the result of congenital, environmental, or a combination of factors that initiate or maintain disfluency (Culatta and Leeper, 1987).

Neurolinguistic Disfluencies

Aphasic patients who experience dysnomia or dementia may display highly disfluent speech while searching for words. Interjections, unusual pauses, and circumlocutions are all probable. However, these behaviors will usually cease once the target word is located. These speech manipulations by neurolinguistically impaired speakers maintain speech flow while searching for an elusive word. When stutterers employ similar tactics, they delay articulation of an already identified and feared word. Failure to distinguish between these processes can lead to frustration for clients and clinicians trying to remediate them.

Chemical Reaction Disfluencies

Helm-Estabrooks (1987) reported that drugs which affect the basal ganglia may affect speech fluency. She reports three studies that link disfluent behavior with concurrently administered medications in clients with no previous history of disfluency. Quader (1977) described two patients in whom administration of amitriptyline, a tricyclic antidepressant, resulted in "stuttered speech." In both patients, speech resumed its normal fluency when the drug was discontinued. Severe disfluencies developed in a 4-year-old child reported by McCarthy (1981) after administration of theophylline, a bronchodilator used to treat asthma. In a study reported by Nurnberg and Greenwald (1981), different dosages of phenothiazine with psychotic patients drastically affected fluent speech production.

Although most label warnings do not include information about the effects that medications have on fluency, speech-language pathologists should inquire concerning any recent introduction of medication in a patient's treatment plans, especially if the disfluency reported is of recent onset.

Neurogenically based disfluencies of these three types can usually be distinguished by alert clinicians. Many of the behavioral manipulations effective in changing stuttering behavior will have little or no effect on neurologically disfluent clients. Although these guidelines should sensitize readers, they are by no means absolute or totally definitive. The following illustrative case history of disfluency resulting from a motor speech disorder highlights how what seems a simple process in the safety of a text book can become a good deal less precise in the clinical world.

ILLUSTRATIVE CASE HISTORY
Motor Speech Disfluency
Kenny, age 9

The speech-language pathologist at Kenny's school began treating Kenny when he moved from another district. By age 9, he had been seen by two public school clinicians and two private practitioners. He was classified as a severe stutterer. His speech was characterized by prolongations, hesitations, and repetitions. Secondary characteristics included head nodding, hand and arm movements, facial grimaces, and eye aversion. Speech failure was often met with tearful frustration and negative self-evaluations.

An in-depth stuttering evaluation revealed that Kenny's speech did not noticeably change under shifting testing conditions. He was disfluent in choral speaking, in repeated readings of the same passage, and in monologues with a tape recorder. His repetitions tended to contain the appropriate vowels and not the intrusive schwa vowel. Delayed auditory feedback as well as high intensity white noise presentations had little effect on speech production. Kenny was adopted at age 3; therefore early speech development information was not available. However, his adoptive parents reported that his speech had not changed since he lived with them. All attempts at traditional speech therapy aimed at increasing fluency were ineffective. Kenny did not fit the expected profile for a young stutterer.

As part of an in-depth medical and educational evaluation requested by his parents, Kenny underwent a computed axial tomography scan. The results of this evaluation revealed cerebellar lesions that suggested a series of prenatal or early childhood CVAs, which caused a moderate ataxic dysarthria. As a result of this identification of site of lesion, speech therapy focused on decreasing rate, use of motor planning strategies to enhance fluency, and explaining to both Kenny and his parents the neurological basis for his disfluent speech.

PSYCHOGENIC DISFLUENCY

Speech disfluency can also appear in speakers for whom no evidence of neurological dysfunction is found and no history of developmental stuttering is reported. The most striking characteristics of this type of disfluency are its sudden onset and its relationship to an identifiable emotional crisis. Psychogenic disfluencies may be grouped into three categories: emotionally based, manipulative, and malingering. However, emotionally based disfluencies far outnumber manipulative disfluencies and malingering as documented phenomena.

Emotionally Based Disfluencies

An identifiable personal crisis and sudden onset of symptoms in otherwise fluent speakers are the most striking characteristics of this type of disfluency. Deal (1982) suggests eight comparison points that help differentiate emotionally based disfluencies from other classes of fluency failure.

1. The onset is sudden.
2. The onset is temporally related to a significant event . . . which seems to reflect extreme psychological pressures.
3. The pattern is primarily repetition of initial or stressed syllables.
4. The pattern is affected little by choral reading, white noise, . . . singing and different communicative situations.
5. (There are) . . . no islands of fluency: even automatic, over-learned social responses are (disfluent).
6. (The patient) . . . does not express any interest in . . . stuttering.
7. (The patient) . . . does not exhibit secondary symptoms, . . . does not avoid words, sounds or speaking situations; . . . (and there is) no attempt to inhibit.
8. (The patient) evidences the same pattern of repetition during mimed reading aloud, which is not characteristic with developmental stuttering or associated with disfluency secondary to brain damage (p. 304).

Once again, although the presenting symptoms may superficially resemble stuttering, speakers who display these signs should not be labeled as stutterers. In addition, speakers in this disfluency class have not suffered demonstrable neurological insults that might cause the disfluent speech pattern. It is not unusual for the frequency of repetitions in this category of disfluency to far exceed the frequency of disfluencies displayed by stutterers. Emotionally based disfluencies that affect 90% of all utterances are not unusual (Culatta and Leper, 1987).

The nature and the degree of the traumatizing event responsible for the disfluency is unique to each client. Deal (1982) reports a patient who suddenly became disfluent after each of two separate suicide attempts. Dempsey and Granich (1978) describe the sudden onset of disfluent speech after a patient's ship received a direct hit during a wartime experience. One of the authors was called to consult with a college quarterback who spontaneously became disfluent when faced with the possibility of starting an important game when the four players ahead of him on the team roster were injured or ineligible to play. As with previously described neurogenically disfluent clients, the disfluency patterns exhibited by emotionally traumatized patients are not usually as manipulable as those of stutterers.

Although treatment for these clients is usually best provided by counselors, psychologists, psychiatrists, social workers, or other appropriately trained professionals, speech-language pathologists are often contacted first due to the inappropriately labeled "stuttering problem."

Manipulative Disfluency

Disfluent speech used to control others has been anecdotally described in the literature (Shames and Sherrick, 1963; Van Riper, 1982). Van Riper reports that "one can sense the controlling, punishing, wheedling, exploitive urges behind the behavior. . . . These (disfluent speakers) . . . suffer less than their listeners." Manipulative disfluency is usually a childhood phenomenon.

Differentiating symptom patterns may include demand and insistent inflection and intonation, lengthy repetition of fluent words, and a variety of secondary characteristics that are not modified over time. These speakers are rarely emotional about their disfluency patterns, and they develop few avoidance behaviors or speaking fears (Van Riper, 1982).

Malingering

Disfluency used purposefully to avoid responsibility or assignments is a conceivable but undocumented possibility. Not only is a conscious volitional component of the disorder needed for diagnosis, but also a recognizable gain from the behavior needs to be obvious before the disfluency could be labeled malingering in nature. As Stevens (1986) points out: " . . . in malingering the symptom production is under the individual's voluntary control and is in pursuit of a goal that is obviously recognizable, given the individual environmental circumstance; this goal frequently involves the prospect of material reward or the avoidance of unpleasant work or duty" (p. 249).

For example, during the Vietnam War, the authors treated a client who was able to display fluent speech during therapy sessions and field trips outside the clinic. This 20-year-old man had been previously granted a deferment from military service due to his stuttering. The client decided it was in his best interests to maintain his stuttering for the foreseeable future. He attempted to swear his speech-language pathologist to secrecy regarding his fluency, and he terminated therapy until "after the war is over or until I am too old to go."

Sodium amytal hypnosis, which is believed to be a reliable test of many other types of behavioral malingering, does not distinguish between voluntary and involuntary disfluency. The test has been demonstrated to affect speech in patients with developmental stuttering as well as neurogenic disfluency. Nevertheless, evidence to support the existence of malingering disfluency might be found with careful examination. If speech-language pathologists document atypical disfluency characteristics (e.g., repetitions occurring consistently at the end of utterances), extremely high disfluency rates, and unusual responses to behavioral manipulations (e.g., maintained disfluency levels in the presence of masking noise), a diagnosis of malingering might be supported (Culatta and Leeper, 1989a). Such documentation would require a knowledgeable observer who could detail and weigh the subtle differences in quantity and quality of speech behaviors, such as those discussed in previous sections. Gorman (1982) suggested four steps in approaching such a problem.

1. Note the specific signs, symptoms, complaints, conditions or behaviors suspected of being malingered.
2. List the diagnoses that may account for these signs, symptoms, complaints, conditions, or behaviors, with proof that these diagnoses are not correct.
3. Mention the individual's circumstances that clearly account for the signs and symptoms.
4. State that these specific signs and symptoms are therefore consistent with malingering (pp. 401–407).

Fortunately, as the following illustrative case history and previous examples highlight, it is often not too difficult to isolate a psychogenic disfluency.

ILLUSTRATIVE CASE HISTORY
Emotionally-Based Disfluency
Jenna, age 10

The speech-language pathologist at Jenna's school was contacted several months into the school year by the fourth grade teacher who reported that Jenna was "suddenly stuttering her head off" in class. The child had been screened each year since the first grade, and she had no previous history of speech problems. During the ensuing clinical contact, the speech-language pathologist noted that Jenna was highly disfluent (approximately 80% of all utterances). Disfluencies took the form of easy repetitions on the initial sounds of words, and there were no noticeable secondary speech characteristics. The disfluencies did not change in frequency or form under conditions of rhythmic speech, white noise, or repeated readings of a speech passage well within the child's reading level. In addition, the speech-language pathologist noted that Jenna seemed both listless and distracted during tasks. During the course of the diagnostic interview, the child revealed that she had overheard her parents discussing the possibility of a divorce. Tearfully, Jenna expressed a fear that she and her sister would be placed in an "orphanage like in the movie *Annie*" and be separated from friends and family. During a subsequent conference with the school counselor and the child's parents, it was determined that divorce was indeed imminent and that it had not been discussed with the children. Jenna was informed by both parents that they would be separating and that she would remain with her mother most of the time and visit with her father on week-ends and spend longer periods with him during school vacations. She was assured that confinement to an "orphanage" was not in her future. Symptoms of disfluency soon disappeared, and there has been no recurrence in the following 36 months.

LANGUAGE DISORDERS

Language disorders in children, as well as the development of linguistic sophistication, can have an impact on the ability to speak fluently. Although the relationship between stuttering and language delay is not clearly understood, the effect of language disorders on fluent speech are beginning to be explored (Culatta and Leeper, 1988). Hall (1977) reported that after initiating language therapy with two severely language-impaired children, both became highly disfluent. However, he reported that as their linguistic skills improved as a result of a language-centered treatment program, their disfluencies decreased. D.E. Hall and associates (1986) also reported markedly increased disfluency with a severely language-delayed child during the initial stages of language therapy. These disfluencies accompanied increases in expressive language output. As was the case in Hall's study (1977), disfluencies decreased as the child's language skills increased. In both studies (involving a total of 3 children), the type of disfluencies reported were primarily part-word repetitions, prolongations, and dysrhythmic phonation.

The disfluencies exhibited by these language-delayed children appear to be different from those of both stuttering children and normal developmentally disfluent children. The available literature seems to support this conclusion. In their review of the literature, Wall and Myers (1984) report, "the two characteristics that would most likely be associated with stuttering, dysrhythmic phonation and tense pause, rarely occur in normal speaking children." Merits-Patterson and Reed (1981), in their study of the differences between language-disordered children who received therapy and those who did not, reported that the children who received therapy were more disfluent and that these disfluencies were characterized by part-word repetitions. Yairi and Clifton (1972) revealed that the disfluencies exhibited by normal language-learning children were characterized by revisions in the form of incomplete sentences, and word repetitions occurred frequently. The part-word repetitions of language-delayed children were not a significant portion of the disfluency sample presented by normal children.

Researchers are not in agreement as to why emerging language skills and increased disfluency seem to exist. Colburn and Mysak (1982a, 1982b) speculate that the disfluencies might serve a language-learning function by allowing practice of newly acquired structures. Disappearance of the disfluencies once newly learned linguistic structures are mastered has been reported in a literature review by Helmreich and Bloodstein (1973). Pearl and Berenthal (1980) hypothesized that functions such as semantic complexity may contribute to the disfluencies of nonstuttering preschoolers. Culatta and Leeper (1987) interpret the information presented thus far as an indication that complex language tasks increase the disfluent behaviors of all children, and that the demands of language treatment may have the side effect of increasing the disfluencies of language-delayed children. A critical point seems to be that the increase in disfluencies seems to occur with a child's attempts to use the new linguistic processes learned in language treatment.

How the disfluencies of language-impaired children are identified will have a major impact on treatment. If they are identified as "stuttering," then the treatment provided will utilize tactics to modify stuttering. If they are identified as "language-based," the treatment will focus on improving language skills, and it will not directly target disfluencies. Because these disfluencies do not meet the criteria that would enable them to be labeled stuttering, perhaps they may be viewed, as Sabin and colleagues (1979) suggest, as "vocal hesitations" that are a part of learning language. As "hesitations," these disfluencies may signal a temporary failure in the organizational aspects of verbal planning or the verbal execution phase of speaking (Butterworth and Goldman-Eisler, 1979), rather than within a stuttering-based framework. For example, reformulations of thoughts in a stuttering-based conceptualization are classified as "revisions," which correct an error in production, clarify, or change meaning (Adams, 1982). As "linguistic hesitations," they are identified as "false starts," which are interpreted as the "best indicators of high level verbal planning failure" (Butterworth and Goldman-Eisler 1979).

The implication derived from this limited review of the literature is that misdiagnosis of language-based disfluency as developmental stuttering could waste limited and valuable intervention time by providing therapy aimed at an inappropriate target. In addition, the probable ineffectiveness of stuttering-based therapy for a language problem will lead to failure and frustration for the child and the speech-language pathologist. Hall and associates (1986) suggested that clinicians should consider the primary nature of the communication disorder when planning treatment strategies. Clinical reports seem to indicate that the initial increase in disfluency in language-delayed children is not indicative of an emerging stuttering problem, but rather the result of the struggle by the child to meet newly introduced and more stringent language rules imposed by treatment.

Adams (Personal communication, 1987) suggested another possibility. He speculates that as language treatment progresses, a child gains more internal language. However, the child may not yet be facile in making appropriate selections of new language responses and in inhibiting older, less appropriate ones. Furthermore, the child may not yet be skilled in the translation of internal language into motor commands. Fluency failure may then result because of linguistic or motor immaturity. Adams believes that, "if that were indeed the case, the fluency failures could legitimately be viewed as disfluencies much (or exactly) like the ones evidenced by normal youngsters." For speech-language pathologists, these conflicting explanations of the disfluencies displayed by language-impaired children can be resolved. The somewhat limited data seem to indicate that maintaining language treatment and increasing communication skills in spite of the emerging disfluencies will eventually alleviate what appears to be a temporarily created fluency failure. The following case history illustrates a typical pattern of disfluency allied with language disorder.

ILLUSTRATIVE CASE HISTORY
Language Disorder Disfluency
Scott, age 3

Hall and colleagues (1986) described Scott (age, 3 yr, 6 mo), who was diagnosed as exhibiting severe receptive-expressive language delay. Both expression and comprehension were approximately 1 year behind his chronological age, and his verbal abilities lagged to the greatest degree. His conversational mean length of utterance did not exceed one word, with occasional inclusion of automatic phrases. Audiological testing revealed normal speech reception thresholds.

Speech and language therapy targeted the following goals:

1. on-task attending behavior,
2. recall and sequencing of verbal commands and critical story elements,
3. comprehension and production of prepositions,
4. expansion of linguistic constructs,
5. development of age-appropriate pragmatic skills, and
6. improvement of oral motor sequencing.

Five months into the therapy program, a severe disfluency pattern developed that consisted of whole-word repetitions, prolongations, repetitions of initial consonants, and interruption of air flow. The disfluencies were noted along with increases in expressive language. Speech and language therapy continued into the first grade; reports indicated substantial growth in expressive language and articulation skills, as well as other gains. At this point, disfluencies had decreased and were simply being monitored by the speech-language pathologist. By the second grade, according to Scott's mother, his disfluencies were confined to highly emotional situations, and his normal conversation was characterized by minimal occurrence of disfluencies.

MIXED DISFLUENCIES

We live in an imprecise world in which the model clients described in text books often do not exist. The preceding discussion outlined the major explanations for fluency failure. Speakers may be developmentally disfluent or stutterers; they may suffer from neurogenic or psychogenic disfluency; they may even be disfluent as the result of language disorders. However, falling into one category does not automatically exclude the speaker from all others. Circumstances arise in which the causative factors for disfluency may overlap. A precedence for this overlap exists in motor speech disorders. Darley and associates (1975), in attempting to classify the different types of dysarthria, suggest that in clinical practice, speech-language pathologists encounter multifocal or defuse disorders that display mixtures with differing degrees of complexity of the "pure" types initially described. Their argument, which is applicable to the current categorization system, is that examples of mixed dysarthrias "serve to document further the principle that motor speech disorders . . . are predictable and lawful."

Mixed types of disfluency, wherein the speech pattern observed is the result of a blend of two or more of the factors outlined in this chapter, are only documented anecdotally. Unlike the precise descriptions available of the mixed dysarthrias, precise descriptions of mixed disfluencies have yet to emerge. Thus, a person who is already a stutterer may suffer neurological dysfunction or emotional trauma, and their resulting unique disfluency characteristics will be independent of the prior existing stuttering problem. The possibility of emotionally based disfluency blending with neurogenic disfluency, or vice versa, is unexplored, as is the possibility of stuttering developing concomitantly with the failure to develop language appropriately. Clinical implications of these yet to be described fluency failure possibilities should give speech-language pathologists cause for concern with any patients in whom multicausality might be an issue. Clinical decisions must be made as to which aspect of the disfluency is most debilitating, which is most correctable, and which will lead to the most normal communication. The following case report illustrates the problems clinicians may face with disfluencies that are the result of multiple etiologies.

ILLUSTRATIVE CASE HISTORY
Mixed Disfluencies
Nicole, age 12

Nicole was referred to a university-based clinic by her school speech-language pathologist primarily as the result of a conflict with the child's mother, who was "argumentative, hypercritical, and unwilling to follow programs suggested" at school. The child presented a history of disfluency initially reported at age 4 and sporadically treated during the intervening years by a number of therapists. Nicole tended to repeat and prolong initial syllables in words, and to avert her gaze during silent pauses of 2 or more seconds while talking. Stuttering and fluency counts of the number of syllables stuttered versus the number of syllables uttered revealed a fluency rate of approximately 80%. She identified herself as a stutterer, and she was able to isolate specific words, sounds, and situations she anticipated as being difficult for fluent speech production. She did not avoid any speaking situations. Symptoms were manipulable under several fluency-enhancing conditions. Nicole was diagnosed as a stutterer, and she was enrolled in a program that emphasized rate reduction and continuous phonation. She rapidly improved, and she was fluent on 98% of all utterances at a normal rate of speech prior to a semester break.

After the semester break, Nicole appeared to have a dramatic setback. Her fluency rate dropped to 73%, and she was not able to replicate the gains she had previously made in her therapy program. However, conversations with her peers as observed through observation windows were normally fluent. This pattern continued for several sessions. In addition, the child appeared more subdued and emotionally labile than previously noted.

Conferences with the school speech-language pathologist and the school social worker revealed that during the semester break, Nicole's older sister (age, 14 yr) had contacted social service agencies to report that both she and her sister were the victims of sexual assault by their biological father. The case was in process with both children living at home. Nicole's mother refused to comment on the charges, but she did voice dissatisfaction with the lack of progress in "stuttering" therapy.

Given the intransigence of the disfluency pattern and the current familial unrest, speech therapy was suspended while individual counselling for the child was initiated. Periodic check-ups by the school speech-language pathologist revealed a picture of periods of disfluency interspersed with periods of "normal" speech when communicating with adults at school. The child continues to remain fluent when observed with her peers.

SUMMARY

Although the symptoms of speech disfluency may be easily identified by trained or untrained listeners, accurate interpretation of these symptoms requires awareness of the underlying causes of disfluent speech. It is arguable that the inconsistent results achieved with stuttering therapy programs can be in part the result of misapplication of stuttering therapy strategies to disfluent but nonstuttering clients. This chapter attempted to sensitize readers to the possibilities that exist along the parameter of disfluency. The remainder of this text is based on the assumption that the client being treated is, as best as can be determined, a stutterer. Treatment of any other types of disfluent speakers with stuttering-based strategies will obviously affect the success of the procedures employed.

STUDY QUESTIONS

1. What are the six types of disfluencies?
2. What distinguishes normal developmental disfluencies from other types of disfluencies?
3. How can you distinguish incipient stutterers from normally developmentally disfluent children?
4. Describe Bloodstein's four developmental phases of stuttering.
5. What are the six characteristics necessary for a disfluent speaker to be labeled a stutterer?
6. How can you distinguish neurogenic disfluencies from stuttering?
7. What are the eight characteristics of psychogenic disfluency that distinguish it from stuttering?
8. How can a language disorder result in the occurence of disfluencies that may be confused with stuttering?
9. Describe a set of behaviors that would result from a mixed disfluency.

Section

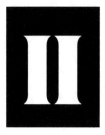

II

Diagnosis

A diagnostic assessment requires that clinicians understand the basic components of the assessment, how to assess behaviors and attitudes, and what behaviors to assess. In Chapter 3, the basic components of the diagnostic interview are discussed, followed in Chapter 4 with presentation of various protocols that have been developed for measuring overt and covert behaviors.

Chapter

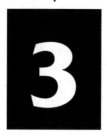

The Diagnostic Interview

The ability to describe and accurately measure a communication disorder facilitates successful treatment. The more imprecise the description and the less rigorous the available analysis techniques, the greater the likelihood of variable therapeutic results. In this chapter, the reasons for conducting a comprehensive assessment and the methods of achieving it are presented. Obtaining information requires that we understand and use not only the most widely accepted recording measures, but that we are skillful enough to go beyond mechanistic tabulations and to learn how to structure interviews to uncover critical information. With this information, clinicians can then develop treatment strategies. Detailed analyses of both overt and covert aspects of stuttering, along with specific tools to measure these characteristics, are presented in Chapter 4.

MEASUREMENT

Stuttering may be divided into overt and covert characteristics. Overt characteristics are the visible behaviors a stutterer displays; covert characteristics are the belief systems about communication a stutterer learns. For an assessment to be successful, both overt and covert aspects of the disorder must be measured and understood by clinicians. In addition, the role that significant others have in the client's life must be understood by speech-language pathologists.

Value of Measurement

We began by stating that the key to understanding and treating any disorder is directly tied to our ability to describe and measure the critical components of the disorder. To illustrate this, compare our skills in successfully treating clients with articulation disorders to our current skills in treating aphasic clients. Our current abilities enable us to describe articulation disorders on almost all possible parameters. We can describe them phonetically, motorically, phonologically, and developmentally. We have an excellent understanding of normal articulation. We know how to measure the behavior presented and, as a result, we can evaluate our intervention efforts. Our assessment techniques often provide clues to treatment.

We are significantly less adept in our ability to describe and measure the components of aphasia. Because we are still struggling to learn the parameters of neurolinguistics, we can only venture hypotheses on what causes dysfunction. We are still learning what occurs after trauma to motoric and sensory functioning. The consistency and the reliability of our measurement systems are far from perfect. As a direct result, our treatment strategies can best be classified as experimental.

We can provide much more effective treatment when we can measure and describe a disorder. Our current knowledge of the parameters of stuttering places us closer to our understanding of aphasia than our understanding of articulation disorders. However, there is a great deal we can learn about stuttering through careful measurement and description.

The real value of diagnosis and assessment is to provide information for therapeutic intervention and to facilitate generalization of new speech behaviors. Each question we ask and every measurement we take should help evolve a therapeutic strategy for stuttering clients. If we gather data for purposes we cannot explain, we do our clients a disservice. We should always be prepared to answer the questions, "why did you want the information you just requested?" and "why are you measuring my behavior?" All too often clinicians fall into the rut of following protocols that have little or no meaning to us or to our clients. For any given patient, a particular measurement may be appropriate; however, all measurements are not appropriate for all clients.

The Ideal Assessment Situation. For a moment let's construct the perfect assessment situation for a child. With some modifications, readers can use this example to construct the ideal assessment situation for an adult. We will superimpose realistic limitations later, but for now we describe the best assessment situation imagined. In this imagined setting, we could observe the client communicating freely in his or her natural environment, free of the contaminating presence of the speech-language pathologist. We could see and hear what the client "really sounds like" with little outsider interference. After observing our client for as long as we might wish, we would next conduct a masterful interview with his parents. Our mastery of interviewing techniques would enable us to search through the developmental stages and the social and familial factors important for our client. The parents would understand our goals and cooperate fully in sharing relevant information, which would help us discover or rule out specific active or precipitating factors that might differentiate chronic stuttering from temporary disfluency.

We would then interview the child using the same skills used with his parents to determine covert and overt factors that might be maintaining disfluency. Our interview questions and measurement techniques would yield a wealth of information that would directly impact on suggestions for future treatment. Our tabulation and coding procedures would yield information of value for treatment, and they would simultaneously describe the client's communication pattern. Finally, we would pull together all the information gathered through observations, interviews, and measurements and share them in a useful way with the client and his parents. This conference would help them not only to understand their current situation but also to understand the need for therapy and the methods necessary for change.

How close we can come to this ideal situation may often determine the success or the lack of progress our clients will experience. Now, let's realistically reconstruct the diagnostic session to see what is practical. Throughout this text, readers are encouraged to adopt, adapt, or dismiss the authors' suggestions as appropriate for their particular work setting. All suggestions are not possible for all settings; however, with a little imagination and persistence, most are feasible.

CLIENT OBSERVATIONS

Observations of client and parental behaviors can be one of the most important sources of diagnostic information. Observations of all types, if they can be accomplished efficiently, usually justify the time they consume. Observational data can be gathered outside and within the clinical setting.

Outside the Clinic

Although it can be very helpful to observe the client before any diagnostic intervention is started, observations of stuttering clients' behavior in a natural setting are not usually feasible. Time concerns and expenses involved usually preclude speech-language pathologists from observing the client at home. In addition, placement of a speech-language pathologist in the home setting changes the environment significantly and no longer ensures the validity of the sample obtained. However, this does not mean that outside clinic observations are impossible. Inexpensive technologies are available that enable parents and clients to audiotape and videotape scenes outside the clinic that might be helpful to speech-language pathologists. As video and tape recorders become more standard items in the average household, it is not too far-fetched to request that parents or clients send a tape prior to the interview, or to bring one to the diagnostic session. Obviously, it makes sense to provide instructions about the sample requested. If a sample is requested, it is usually better to get one that is spontaneous rather than one during which the client recites a rehearsed text or where a parent instructs the child to "say something into the recorder so that the speech teacher can hear how you stutter." Naturalistic recordings, when available, can often highlight different behaviors observed within a school or in a clinic.

Informal Clinic Observation

If observation suites are available, it is always of value to watch the client and his parents or other significant persons interact for a short time. These on-site observations can accomplish several functions. First, they allow the speech-language pathologist some time to watch the client and parents prior to any of the interactions of the interview setting. This "breathing time" is often of great value in last-minute interview strategy decisions. The speech-language pathologist can also observe the communication patterns that exist prior to any outside intervention. Because, in most cases, we cannot go into the home, we can observe the client and his family interacting without our interference.

During this period, we should observe the client's speech, the characteristics of the conversations, and the overall nature of the interactions. Is the child manipulative? Are the parents demanding? Is the tone harsh? Does all appear unremarkable? As mentioned earlier, the clinical intuition of the speech-language pathologist is always critical. The information obtained by simply watching parents and their children can be vital. At this point in the evaluation, it is usually more productive to be descriptive than judgmental. It is better to describe an interaction than classify it as "good" or "bad," especially because we are not sure if specific parental styles are automatically helpful or harmful toward achieving fluency. Shames and associates at the University of Pittsburgh ran an interesting series of studies on adult-child interaction styles. After observing a parent and a child interact, the parent's style of interacting was described. The clinician then assumed an opposite style of interaction with the child. Changing interaction styles had a positive effect in eliciting fluency (Egolf et al., 1972). It did not seem critical to propose a specific parenting style, but instead to suggest one different from the one currently being used. This information does not put clinicians on firm ground in making suggestions to parents about the "best way" to interact with their children. It usually is the most prudent course of action to describe and to analyze what we are observing before suggesting some preconceived solution that may cause unnecessary familial upheaval and be of limited value in changing speech behavior.

Preparing families to be observed is not terribly difficult. Usually, it is sufficient to inform the client and the parents that you would simply like them to talk to each other for a while to get used to the therapy room and that you will be watching from behind the observation mirror. After a few moments, most clients adapt to the situation, and the parental interactions obtained can be useful. On another level, this time alone in the therapy room without the speech-language pathologist often gives the fearful child some time to establish himself and to explore the setting. Parents also can be asked during the subsequent interview if the speech heard during the observation period is the type of speech they normally hear at home.

GUIDELINES FOR CONSTRUCTING INTERVIEWS WITH STUTTERERS AND THEIR FAMILIES

The traditional way of obtaining information is to interview clients and their parents when appropriate. These question and answer sessions can often provide insights that cannot be gleaned from prediagnostic intake forms or referral notes from other professionals. Diagnostic interviews, however, involve more than simply asking questions.

When we look at what we do as speech-language pathologists, the one common thread is interviewing. We talk to our clients and they talk to us. It goes on with children, adults, parents, husbands, and wives. Each aspect of speech-language pathology may emphasize a different aspect of interviewing, but several fundamental parts are always the same. Purposes and specifics may vary, but client focus does not change. As Shames and Florance report (1980), the focus of the clinical interview is the stutterer. The needs, the issues, and the problems of the stutterer dominate. The interview is not an even-handed situation; the goal is not sharing of mutual needs or concerns. Speech-language pathologists must see themselves as people with the goal of facilitating their clients' thoughts and feelings. During the brief interactions of the diagnostic interview, we try to establish a trusting relationship with our clients, which is neither a casual nor an unimportant aspect of what we do to eventually effect change. The special relationship we establish with our clients is initiated through the interviewing process.

There are two types of initial interviews: those that are initiated by the client, and those that are initiated by the therapist (Benjamin, 1974). Each calls for a different beginning strategy with stuttering clients and their families.

Client-initiated Interviews

It makes the most sense when someone wishes to speak with you to give them the opportunity to tell you why they wanted the meeting. It does not always work out that way. For example, before a client's mother can tell us the purpose of the requested meeting, we might say "I guess you want to find out about Susan's stuttering problem?" If you have guessed incorrectly, the mother is now in an awkward situation. She may feel that perhaps she should be concerned with the problem you suggested and, fearing to contradict you, discuss stuttering rather than her real concerns. Perhaps she will correct you and say "No, what I really came here to talk with you about is . . . " While setting the topic, she may be thinking, "Who are you to tell me why I'm here? If you give me a chance I'll tell you why I came to see you." Neither of the preceding examples can lead to smooth openings and effective communication. The least intrusive and possibly the most effective way to initiate the interview is to ask the person why they wished to see you. An example of this would be, "My name is Susan Smith. I'm the speech-language pathologist at Johnson Elementary School. Please tell me why you wanted to talk with me?" This direct approach often enables the client to immediately share the problem with minimal distraction from the interviewer.

Speech-Language Pathologist–initiated Interviews

Interviews begin differently in speech-language pathologist–initiated interviews. In this circumstance, it may be best to get to the point of the interview with as little delay as possible. An example might be: "My name is Rich Culatta. I'm the speech-language pathologist at Garth Elementary School. I want to talk with you about Bill's speech. Is the way that Bill talks of any concern to you or your husband?" Now the interviewer is in a position to listen. Although it is often necessary to provide more information in the interviewer-initiated conference than in the client-initiated conference, Benjamin (1974) warns that interviewers should be careful not to turn interviews into lectures or monologues. If interviewers become so involved in explaining why they think there is a problem, why the interview is necessary, and what the implications of an untreated disorder might be, the whole purpose of an interview could be defeated. Although it is both necessary and appropriate to explain the reason for the interview, it may not be necessary to justify it in great detail. Benjamin (1974) suggests the following opening statements:

> I suppose you know why I asked you to come in" or "We both know why you are here" or "Can you guess why I asked you to stop by" are openings . . . (that) can come across in a threatening light. Such pointless coyness has no place. The interviewee may not know and fear our disbelief. He may think he knows and wish not to tell. He may . . . become confused. He may consider this a challenge . . . and decide to fight rather than cooperate. (p.14)

The goal in interviewing is to establish a relationship based on understanding and mutual cooperation. Quite often, how we begin the session can set the tone for the entire interview.

THE DIAGNOSTIC INTERVIEW

Along with direct or indirect observations of the clients' behavior, the diagnostic interviews with parents or clients can help fill the informational gaps that lead to successful treatment planning. The interview process can be divided into several parts. There are specific types of information that only parents can provide, whereas an interview with the client can provide information about covert feelings and enable us to measure overt behaviors that parents can only describe.

Information from Parents

The information we need to get from parents is related to their reasons for seeking professional help, descriptions of their child's behavior, historical information, previous treatment experiences, their reactions to their child's speech, and their belief system regarding stuttering. This information can be obtained through asking specific questions based on the content outlined in Table 3–1. Obviously, speech-language pathologists will wish to rephrase these questions into a style with which they are comfortable.

Reasons for Seeking Professional Help. We need to obtain information before we can suggest strategies for improvement. There is no better way of

Table 3–1.
Question Outline for Parents

Questions	Answers
1. Why are you here today?	
2. Tell me about your child's problem	
3. Who referred you?	
4. Please describe the stuttering behavior	
a. Frequency	
b. Duration	
c. Overt behaviors	
d. Covert behaviors	
e. Variability	
5. Tell me about normal speaking times	
6. Please describe your child's daily activities	
7. How does your child speak with other people?	
8. What do teachers report?	
9. How do you help your child to speak better?	
10. Has anything changed during the last 6 months?	
11. Tell me about previous therapy	
12. Does anyone in your immediate or extended family stutter?	
13. Summarize your child's medical history	
14. Summarize your child's educational history	
15. What do you believe causes stuttering?	

getting information than to ask for it. "Why are you here?" and "tell me about your child's problem" are excellent beginning questions. The goal is to hear from the parents the current status of the problem as they are experiencing it. By discussing the reasons for the interview, including who referred the client to the speech-language pathologist, we can often uncover valuable information about parental concern. The parent who says that she came to see you only because the child's grandmother insisted on the visit is providing different information than the mother who tearfully reports that she was sure from the moment her child began speaking he was a stutterer, despite reassurances to the contrary from the family pediatrician, a nurse practitioner, and two previously consulted speech-language pathologists.

Description of the Behavior. Assuming that some type of observation of the client has previously occurred, it is usually efficient to ask the parents for a description of the stuttering behavior, which accomplishes at least two functions. First, the speech-language pathologist can compare the recently observed behavior to the behavior the parent describes. Obviously, any discrepancies become fertile ground for an in-depth discussion. Second, the parental description highlights their concerns. What may be of most concern to the speech-language pathologist or the child may not be of major concern to the parent. The clinician can be led far afield of the client and the parent's real concerns by assuming that what the clinician thinks is of concern to parents and clients is valid. Despite any observations, it is helpful to ask for a detailed description of the problem, including frequency of occurrence, duration of stuttering episodes, overt behaviors, and covert reactions.

It is appropriate to ask the parents during the session for a description of their child's daily activities, especially speaking times. Are there people with whom the child is more fluent than others? Are there friends or relatives with whom the child is particularly disfluent? What do the child's teachers report? Are there links between these performances that the parents suspect might be meaningful? The more specific and descriptive these questions are, the better the information they uncover will be.

Finally, we also need to learn what the parents are doing when the child stutters and when she is fluent. Many parents are told that they should "do nothing" when their child stutters. As a result, when the child stutters, the parent assumes a stiff trance-like state approaching total paralysis for the duration of the block. This, in all probability, is not a natural or effective response. However, many other parental responses and attempts to control stuttering are effective. We need to know which strategies are effective and which are ineffective. Encourage parents to be as descriptive as possible when they describe their approaches to modifying stuttering behavior. Speech-language pathologists should not feel uncomfortable asking which of the parental approaches seem most successful in eliminating stuttering or maintaining fluency.

Episodes of stuttering can be extremely variable (Bloodstein, 1981). This variability, especially in the young child, can be useful in determining appropriate intervention techniques. Thus, it is always appropriate to ask if there has been any change during the past 6 months in symptomatology, overall communication behavior, or attitudes. Information about the variability of the problem may be critical. Parents should be encouraged to talk about the good speaking times, as well as the bad. All too often the natural inclination is to focus on the presenting problem, which prevents both the parents and the speech-language pathologist from obtaining information about normal speaking times. Because most stutterers are fluent more than they stutter, this information is critical to treatment strategies.

Previous Treatment. Previous treatment details can help speech-language pathologists gain an understanding of what the family has experienced and their current beliefs about the etiology and the treatment of stuttering. A parental explanation as to why previous treatment was either unsuccessful or transitory will also be helpful in understanding the family's current views and expectations. It may be important to allow for a period of parental ventilation. Do they believe their child is a victim of some unknowable force? Do they feel that he might be reacting to some unsettling factors in his environment? Perhaps they see stuttering episodes as manipulative events the child is using to control family interactions. Because there are so many theories and therapies that attempt to explain the cause and continuation of stuttering, it is always a good idea to determine under which belief system a family is operating.

Case History Data. Case history questions 12 to 15 in Table 3–1 are easily justified. Information about stuttering relatives can often provide a warning that a young child may be an incipient stutterer. In addition to the behavioral data gathered, this historical data may prove very helpful in arriving at a diagnosis that points toward stuttering rather than normal developmental disfluency. Medical and educational history information may, as we have seen in Chapter 2, alert us to disfluency possibilities other than stuttering. For most stutterers, there will be no remarkable medical or educational history information that will point away from stuttering and toward some other type of disfluency. However, it is critical to determine whether complicating medical and educational factors coexist with the presenting disfluency. An analysis of social history can reveal if there are any compensations the child is making for disfluent speech. Not every shy, withdrawn, or lonely child is a stutterer; however, it is important to uncover if negative attitudes toward communication can be translated into deviant social behavior.

Belief System. As we obtain the case history, we should also construct a belief system under which we think the parents are functioning. The beliefs that parents hold about stuttering will influence how they interact with their children on all parameters. As the parents are encouraged to recount the history of the problem, clinicians can often begin to piece together parental views on etiology, maintenance, and treatment. These views form the parents' belief system regarding stuttering. Sometimes simply recounting these beliefs clarifies them for both the parents and the speech-language pathologist.

Parental Guilt and Defensiveness. Parental feelings of responsibility and guilt are a natural occurrence with many developmental problems, and stuttering is no exception. Most parents wish to know "did I cause this problem? Perhaps I caused it unwittingly through poor parenting or perhaps I failed to provide some needed positive experiences for my child." The bottom line with most parents is "is stuttering my fault?" Parents are often defensive, especially those parents who have been exposed to the diagnosogenic theory of stuttering (Johnson, 1955), which, in essence, places the responsibility for initiation and maintenance of stuttering on faulty perceptions of essentially normal speaking behavior. It may be appropriate to ask parents the larger questions "what do you believe causes stuttering" or "what have you been told causes stuttering?" It is not unusual to have an outpouring of feelings of guilt, defensiveness, and hostility in response to this line of questioning. We often hear comments such as, "we tried to ignore early stuttering and pretend that it just wasn't there, but we knew he sounded different," and "we never did any of the things that we have been told caused stuttering, yet she still stutters." Parents will report that "we didn't do anything differently with this child than our others. They don't stutter, why does he?" These attitudes often contribute to parents being less candid than they might otherwise be with speech-language pathologists.

Attacking the credibility of a parental informant, no matter how well meaning, is not productive. For treatment to be productive, parents must be on the "same side" as the clinician. It is truly unfortunate that several generations of parents have been counseled and continue to be told that it was their naive judgments that caused their children's fluency problems. It may be appropriate to share with parents early in the interview that most of the current information we have about stuttering reveals that there is no proof that parental reaction to normal speech causes stuttering. In fact, recent reports (Andrews et al., 1983) indicate that there were no significant differences in the reports of parenting behaviors in a matched sample of 50 stuttering families and 50 nonstuttering families. Furthermore, stutterers and their parents show no greater evidence of neurotic symptoms than nonstuttering children and their parents. Finally, Andrews and colleagues (1983) reported that very young children regarded as stutterers display three times as many part-word repetitions and prolongations as nonstutterers. It appears that the parents of stuttering children, rather than being the cause of stuttering by misperceiving normal speech, are often simply good listeners who react appropriately to the deviant speech productions of their children. It is quite possible that some children become stutterers due to their reactions to their world in the same way that other children become nail-biters or bed-wetters.

We may also wish to inform parents that stuttering tends to be more prevalent in some families than in others and that perhaps the eventual cause of stuttering, which is currently unknown, will be linked to some combination of internal factors and experiences in growing up. However, it is important to stress that children experiencing similar conditions do not all become stutterers. Normal speakers, as well as stutterers, experience stress, good and bad times, understanding or neglectful environments, quiet or noisy homes, or being only children or having brothers and sisters. It is important to share with parents that their child's experiences may be critical, and that the more information they can provide, the easier it might be to change things for the better.

Parental behavior is not necessarily good or bad with regard to its effect on a child's fluency. Some behaviors may have more of an effect on a child than others, and they should therefore be modified. It is usually appropriate to share with parents that most of the information gathered during the interview will not be linked to initiation of their child's stuttering. Our professional obsession with the cause of stuttering has led to generations of frustrated parents and clinicians wasting energy that could be more profitably spent on modification or elimination of the unwanted behavior.

Clinicians must never pass judgments in the absence of some verifiable behavior. If a particular parental practice is leading to disfluency on the part of a child, then, by all means, that behavior must be changed. However, we must protect ourselves and our clients from ambiguous prescriptions of a "healthy speaking environment" when we do not know what that environment might be for a given child.

Information from Clients

A successful client interview should provide the data that will enable the speech-language pathologist to (1) understand the stutterer's conceptualization of his pathology, (2) analyze the client's strengths, and (3) construct a preliminary intervention plan. Ideally, this information will be in the form of baseline data.

The client's belief system (covert factors) and observable behaviors (overt factors) should be measured and analyzed. In an ideal world, we would be able to ask our client a series of questions similar to those detailed in the previous section. Answers to these questions would guide us in understanding how the client functions as a disfluent speaker. Questionnaire outlines for children, adolescents, and adults appear, respectively, in Tables 3–2, 3–3, and 3–4. These questions parallel those presented to the parents during the initial interview. Any differences in the perceptions between clients and their parents will obviously be of importance in constructing a meaningful diagnosis. Tables 3–2, 3–3, and 3–4 do not represent every question a speech-language pathologist might wish to ask; however, they do provide a starting point for diagnosis.

Reasons for Coming. *Why are you here today?* Children often have no idea who speech-language pathologists are and why they are seeing them; others are well aware. Asking "why are you here today?" allows us to either clarify or explain the function of the diagnostic setting. It is critical to try to work with a motivated client rather than a confused, suspicious, or misinformed one. Age is not a factor for excusing client awareness. It is the task of speech-language

Table 3–2.
Question Outline for Children

Questions	Answers
1. Why are you here today?	
2. Tell me about your speech	
3. Tell me what you do when your speech is bumpy	
4. Tell me what you think about when your speech is bumpy	
5. Tell me how you feel when your speech is bumpy	
6. Is your speech sometimes smooth and sometimes bumpy?	
7. Why do you think your speech is bumpy?	
8. Tell me about the times when your speech is smooth	
9. What happens when you go from smooth to bumpy speech or from bumpy speech to smooth speech?	
10. Can you make your speech become smooth or bumpy?	
11. What do you do to make your speech smooth?	
12. Has anyone helped you before to speak smoothly?	
13. Tell me what they did to help you	

pathologists to be certain that the diagnostic process is as clear to the young child as it is to the parents. The question "why are you here?" helps the client understand the purposes of the diagnostic session. In addition, a knowledge-able client, regardless of age, can be a partner in the search for relevant information.

Although most adolescents are aware of why they are in the diagnostic session, they may wish to avoid announcing the reason from a sense of embarrassment. Also, the reason they give may not be complete. For example, the client who answers "because the counselor told me to," may have an intense desire to change his speech, but may be reluctant to be that honest with an adult.

Adults will almost always be aware of why they are attending the diagnostic session. Although their reasons may be informative, even more critical information can be derived from understanding their timing. For example, "you have been stuttering for 42 years, why have you decided to begin therapy **now**?"

Table 3–3.
Question Outline for Adolescents

Questions	Answers
1. Why are you here today?	
2. Tell me about your speech	
3. Who referred you?	
4. Please describe the stuttering behavior	
a. How often	
b. How long	
c. Things people can see	
d. Things no one else can see	
e. How does it change	
5. Tell me about the good speaking times	
6. Tell me about speech therapy you have had	
7. Why do you think you stutter?	
8. Has anything big changed recently?	
9. Tell me the kind of things you do each day	
10. Tell me about the times when your speech is good	
11. What changes when you go from easy speech to stuttering or from stuttering to easy speech?	
12. What do you do that allows you to go from one to the other?	
13. What do you do when you really try to speak fluently(smoothly)?	
14. Have you ever been in speech therapy before?	
15. Tell me what you did in speech therapy	

Description of the Behavior. *Tell me about your problem.* The speech-language pathologist has thus far observed the parent and child interaction, and she has spent time with the parents obtaining a description of how they perceive the problem. Now it is the client's time to talk about stuttering. How the client describes his problem can provide insight into appropriate therapeutic strategies and information for initial intervention planning. Although the words used to describe the problem will differ, children, adolescents, and adults are all equally capable of describing the actual speech behaviors.

Table 3–4.
Question Outline for Adults

Questions	Answers
1. Why are you here today?	
2. Tell me about your problem?	
3. Who referred you?	
4. Please describe the stuttering behavior	
a. Frequency	
b. Duration	
c. Overt behaviors	
d. Covert behaviors	
e. Variability	
5. Tell me about normal speaking times	
6. Please describe your daily activities	
7. Tell me about the times when your speech is good	
8. What changes when you go from normal speech to stuttering or from stuttering to normal speech?	
9. How much control do you have over these changes?	
10. What do you do if you wish to be fluent?	
11. Have you ever been in speech therapy before?	
12. Tell me what you did in speech therapy	
13. Has anything changed in the last 6 months?	
14. Does anyone in your immediate or extended family stutter?	
15. Summarize your medical history	
16. Summarize your educational history	
17. Summarize your social history	
18. What do you believe causes stuttering?	

Behaviors During Stuttering. *What do you do when you stutter?* Minimally, a description of overt features informs clinicians which aspects of stuttering are most important to the client. Descriptions also provide a measure of awareness or lack of awareness of the behaviors the client displays when stuttering.

Thoughts During Stuttering. *What do you think about when you stutter?* Answers to this question often provide insights into the client's belief system. Speech-language pathologists can also learn if the client uses any particular strategy to deal with episodes of stuttering.

Feelings During Stuttering. *How do you feel when you stutter?* An honest answer about feelings and thoughts can in the best of circumstances provide a basis for many subsequent sessions of clarification of perceptions about communication. Absolute refusal to deal with these questions also provides information about needs to suppress feelings and recognition of a potential problem.

Speech Changes During the Last 6 Months. *Has your speech changed during the last six months?* Stuttering is a developmental disorder. Changes in speech behavior during an extended period often provide clues regarding the direction in which the disorder is moving. Disfluencies may lessen or become more frequent and severe. The child's perception of the course of stuttering can be vital in establishing a program to achieve normal communication. If speech is reported as becoming more fluent, speech-language pathologists may wish to emphasize that communication is becoming less effortful. If the child reports worsening speech, speech-language pathologists may wish to use this information to confront the implications. It is also valuable to compare the child's view with those of parents and teachers.

By the time the child reaches 10 or 11 years of age, the variability associated with the development of stuttering has ceased. However, a variety of environmental and emotional factors are prevalent, as they are with adults. Information received from this question can provide clinicians with an understanding of a real or a perceived relationship that exists between the client's speech and his environment.

Cause of Stuttering. *What do you think is the cause of your problem?* As it did with parents, this question allows speech-language pathologists to gain insight into the belief system of the client. Very often, superstitious beliefs and unfounded bits of trivia can combine to maintain an unhealthy attitude toward talking. Simply allowing the child to tell why she thinks she stutters can lead to explanations of behavior that will provide a great deal of comfort to the child.

By the time the stutterer reaches adolescence, his belief system regarding the cause of stuttering is often an amalgamation of fears, false conceptions, and guilt. Although the adult may possess some factual knowledge regarding the etiology of stuttering, his increased age has also allowed him more time to acquire additional false conceptions. It is important for the clinician to determine not only what beliefs about stuttering the client has, but also how they may impact on the intervention program. For example, if a client says, "I know I can't be fluent unless I'm completely relaxed," the clinician will have to either train the client to be fluent under stressful situations or convince him that the relationship between relaxation and fluency is not necessarily causal.

Happenings During Fluent Speech. *Tell me about the times when your speech is good.* All too often we focus on the negative behavior without emphasizing to the client that he is fluent more often than he stutters. This question serves two purposes. First, it can provide speech-language pathologists with information about times, people, and situations that the client sees as successful talking times. This approach will lead to an analysis of the positive aspects of these times and hopefully some abstraction of the common elements that make talking positive. Second, this question shifts the focus of the diagnostic inter-action from stuttering toward normal speech experiences, which is the goal of therapy. The client is helped to recognize the fluency she already exhibits during at least some occasions. She is led not only to recognize these times, but also to report them in detail to the speech-language pathologist.

Occurrences When Speech Changes. *What changes when you go from good speech to stuttering or stuttering to good speech?* This question leads the client to begin to understand that articulatory postures, thinking postures, and other behaviors change as a function of fluency or stuttering. It also provides the speech-language pathologist with an indication of how sensitive the client is to these changes.

Control Over Changes. *How much control do you have over these changes?* This question helps the speech-language pathologist understand in greater detail if the client is consciously manipulating his speech. It also suggests to the client that control is possible. The speech-language pathologist may gain insight into the client's feelings of victimization as she responds to this question, as well as to the preceding 3 questions.

Efforts to Speak Fluently. *What do you do when you wish to be fluent?* Once again this question may also be more valuable in establishing the concept that a person has control over communication than it is in obtaining clinically useful information.

Previous Speech Therapy. *Tell me about previous speech therapy?* It is vital that speech-language pathologists understand the client's perception of both the content and the value of previous therapy. The fact that there was previous therapy means that the client may be appropriately skeptical about the thera-peutic process and its value. In addition, clinicians may wish to review or to take advantage of the gains of a previous experience.

RESISTIVE CLIENTS

In an ideal world, insightful answers to these questions would leave little left than to measure overt characteristics and the client's insightful abilities to manipulate his manner of speech. However, in a world populated by real clients instead of text book examples, achieving the goals of the diagnostic session are often significantly more difficult than simply rattling off the suggested questions and waiting for meaningful responses. Older clients come to us with a history of trying to hide their problems from strangers, or perhaps with a history of failures in therapy that make them unwilling to trust yet another speech-language pathologist. Younger clients may be frightened by what they experience, and they may try their best to hide stuttering from themselves and everyone else. Emotional reactions to both the disfluency and the reaction of loved ones may make logical analysis of the process of talking very difficult for these people. In addition, some may lack the skills needed for instant insight into their communication behaviors. Many children and young adults we see clearly do not wish to verbalize their inner feelings initially. They desire to escape the spotlight, and they wish that stuttering "would go away and leave them alone," which may make them unwilling to give more than monosyllabic answers to the important questions. In some instances, speech-language pathologists are seen as teachers or authority figures, and they may represent exactly the type of person with whom these children have a difficult time talking.

Finally, the larger portion of children and young adults we interview do not see us by choice. They have been led to us or screened by us because they are failing to communicate normally. Even though the questions listed contain an outline for the information we vitally need, we often cannot either ask them directly or rely on the content of the responses obtained. We must sometimes rely on other clues and obtain the information needed less directly. For example, we recently saw an 11-year-old boy who insisted that stuttering was " no big deal" in his life, but he turned away from the clinician and wept during the course of the diagnostic interview each time the speech-language pathologist focused the questioning on stuttering. It did not require the powers of Sherlock Holmes to determine that this child was deeply upset by the whole process.

Some clinicians succeed by changing the focus of the questions so that the child or the adolescent may feel as though he is reporting other people's behaviors. An example of how to modify questions to make them less threatening appears in Table 3–5. Questions similar to these, which will provide speech-language pathologists with the same information as previously discussed, are sometimes effective in allowing the child to talk about stuttering in a less threatening way. Sometimes they are no more effective than the original set of questions. With children, puppets, role-playing techniques, as well as use of drawing materials, clay, and finger paints can sometimes overcome initial reticence. A well-structured interview that simply adheres to some basic principles of effective interviewing often makes obtaining information possible.

Speech-language pathologists often find it is easier to deal with the overt aspects of stuttering first. Then, after they have measured and manipulated the clients' way of talking, it is often more comfortable to discuss reactions to the overt measures.

Table 3–5.
Less-threatening Questions for Children and Young Adolescents

Questions	Answers
1. Do you know why your Mom and Dad brought you here?	
2. Has anyone ever said anything to you about how you talk?	
3. Who?	
4. What did they say?	
5. Has anyone ever told you things you can try to make it easier to talk?	
6. What did they say to do?	
7. Did it work?	
8. Who do you like to talk to at school?	
9. Who do you like to talk to at home?	
10. Who don't you like to talk to at school/home?	
11. Why?	
12. Who are the best talkers at your school?	
13. Who are the worst talkers at your school?	
14. Where do you fit in?	

WRITTEN QUESTIONNAIRES

Pencil and paper questionnaires such as the Fluency Assessment Instrument (Goldberg, 1981), the Stuttering Attitudes Checklist (Cooper and Cooper, 1985), the Severity Scale and Adjective Checklist (Erickson, 1969), and the Perceptions of Stuttering Inventory (Woolf, 1967) can help speech-language pathologists understand the client's perceptions of how he talks. With young children unable to read, speech-language pathologists might even adapt the questionnaires and present them orally. Sometimes the fact that the questions delve into areas the child thought were a private problem can be helpful. These instruments and others are discussed in greater detail in Chapter 4.

SUMMARY

This chapter began by providing an explanation of why we should spend our time gathering information about stuttering prior to initiating treatment. We suggested that the real value of assessment is to obtain information that will be used in treatment. This information may be gained by observing the stutterer and through diagnostic interviews. Stutterers and their parents can usually help in our search for meaningful information. We outlined the specific information that might be valuable, and we listed what we need to know from parents and clients of different ages. Gathering information, however, is more than simply asking lists of questions. Structuring an environment that will enable the client to share experiences and beliefs is critical so that we may structure a meaningful intervention program. Speech-language pathologists should be well-versed in interviewing procedures and knowledgeable about effective interviewing techniques. Once these ancillary skills to diagnosis are mastered, the interviewing process will facilitate gathering the critical information we outlined. The next chapter presents some specific techniques and commonly used instruments that provide further help during the diagnostic process.

STUDY QUESTIONS

1. What clinical value is there in accurately measuring both overt and covert behaviors of stutterers?

2. Describe the procedures and techniques for observing clients and their families inside and outside the clinic.

3. What are the differences between client- and speech-language pathologist–initiated interviews?

4. Describe the types of information you would wish to get from the parents of children who stutter, and why each is important.

5. Describe the types of information you would wish to get from clients who stutter, and why each is important.

6. What techniques should be tried with resistive clients?

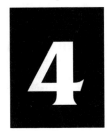

Assessment Techniques

Stuttering behaviors can be both overt and covert. If an assessment of stuttering is to be complete, both types of behaviors must be identified and measured. The purposes of this chapter are to first present established methods for identifying each type of behavior, and then to describe a comprehensive testing procedure that will allow clinicians to develop treatment strategies from the information obtained.

OVERT CHARACTERISTICS OF STUTTERING

We referred to the overt characteristics of stuttering as the visible and auditory components of the disorder. The overt aspects are what the stutterer does when talking that set him apart from the normally fluent speaker. Although each stutterer will develop a pattern that is unique, the components of that pattern are both predictable and fairly easy to measure. To identify the overt characteristics of stuttering, clinicians should be able to identify specific behaviors, be knowledgeable about measurement procedures, and have a basic understanding of the various published overt behavioral protocols currently available.

Overt Stuttering Behaviors

The behaviors listed in Table 4–1 were cited by Williams and colleagues (1978) more than 25 years ago, and they are a partial compilation of the professionally accepted code words still used to describe the overt verbal aspects of stuttering. All speech-language pathologists need to do is match any given clients'

Table 4–1.
Observable Characteristics of Stuttering

Behavior	Definition	Example
Hesitation	Any nontense break in the forward flow of speech	I __ am going home
Broken words	With unacceptable within-word hestitations	Partially uttered words: I am g__oing home
Repetition	Repeated utterances of parts of words (PWR), words (WR), and phrases (PR)	I am g going (PWR) I am am going (WR) I am I am going (PR)
Interjections	Use of sounds, syllables, and words that are independent of context of utterance	I er er am uh going
Prolonged sounds	Unacceptably prolonged sounds, usually at the start of a word	I am s-s-s-so late
Dysrthymic phonation	Distortion of the prosodic elements within a word, with improper stress, timing, or accenting	I am going (rising inflection) home
Tension	Audible manifestation of abnormal breathing or muscular tightening between words, parts of words, or interjections	I am (forced breathing) going home
Revisions, modifications	Grammatical or content	I am, I was going.
Incomplete phrases	Failure to complete an initiated unit of speech	I am— but not today.

Adapted from Williams, D.E., Darley, F. L. & Spriestersbach, D.C. (1978). *Diagnostic Methods in Speech Pathology.* New York: Harper & Row.

symptoms to this list to describe the overt stuttering being emitted. In addition, "secondary characteristics" (Bloodstein, 1981), or associated nonspeech activities such as eye blinks, facial grimaces, and unusual head, arm, or trunk movements that occur concurrently with the overt stuttering behaviors are usually described.

Although these descriptors help speech-language pathologists construct a pretreatment portrait of the client, they often provide little in the way of helping devise overall treatment strategies. Although they may serve as markers to help speech-language pathologists identify the occurrence of stuttering, these behaviors are usually absent when the client produces stutter-free speech. Clinicians often become fascinated with the variety, complexity, and combinations of overt behaviors that clients develop. However, there is little justification to dwell at length on these descriptors in the clinical setting. It is probably most efficient simply to describe and tabulate the occurrence of these behaviors and to move on to more clinically productive measures.

Tables 4–2 and 4–3 are illustrations of the type of forms designed to tabulate the frequency of occurrence of the observable characteristics of stuttering described.

Linguistic Revisions. These behaviors are often used by stutterers either to initiate the flow of stutter-free speech or to gain the time needed to deal with an anticipated moment of stuttering. For example, a stutterer might repeat a word or sound until he feels able to complete an utterance. The repetitions used might thus be considered postponement or avoidance behaviors used to gain the time necessary to communicate. The client may use whole phrases, spoken fluently, to "ease" into the speech flow. These often stilted and marginally appropriate phrases such as "let me see" or "as you know," when used as transitions to stutter-free speech, are labeled starter devices for the role they have in getting the stutterer into the meaningful part of his utterances.

Awkward phrases and distorted grammatical forms may be used to navigate around feared words. Identified as circumlocutions, they often stretch the stutterer to his creative limits. For example, a client may say "I live in a small town in the mountains" when anticipating difficulty with the specific name of his community. One client reported answering the telephone as follows: "this is the Smith residence, 1221 Harper Street, John speaking" to circumlocute around the feared word, "hello." Circumlocutions, starter devices, postponement tactics, and avoidance behaviors are often attempts to disguise stuttering behavior from listeners. Over time and with practice, many clients become adept at quickly substituting nonfeared words for those preidentified as likely to be stuttered. These word substitutions are often only marginally appropriate, and they can distort the meaning of the speaker's message. Examples of substitutions might be the use of "money changer" for the feared word "Philistines" by a stuttering minister, or the word "yes" in place of "hello" when answering the telephone.

The extent to which any given client uses these devices can only be determined partially by observation. Usually the client is the best source to identify which of these tactics he uses in conversational speech. Most clients will report that even if fluent utterances are the result of these manipulations, there is a lack of satisfaction with the process and a high degree of tension as a result of the vigilance necessary to use these techniques.

Measurements of Duration. Many of the behaviors detailed have a similar effect on a stutterer's speech. They distort the temporal expectations the listener brings to the communication moment. Stuttering is a disorder of the "time aspect" of speech. The broken words, repeated syllables, and sounds that characterize the speech of many stutterers do not meet our societies' expectations for speech production within a specific time frame. As a result, many of the descriptors we used are based on an underlying time judgement.

Table 4–2.
Measures of Disfluency of Speaking and Oral Reading

Name _____ Age _____ Sex _____
Examiner _____ Date _____
Reading passage used: No.1 _____ No. 2 _____ Other (specify) _____
Speaking procedure used: Job Task _____ TAT Task _____ Other (describe) _____

	Reading Passage			Speaking Task		
	No.1	No. 2	Other	Job	TAT	Other
A. Number of words	—	—	—	—	—	—
B. Number of disfluencies						
a. Interjections per 100 words = a/A × 100	—	—	—	—	—	—
b. Part-word repetitions per 100 words = b/A × 100	—	—	—	—	—	—
c. Word repetitions per 100 words = c/A × 100	—	—	—	—	—	—
d. Phrase repetitions per 100 words = d/A × 100	—	—	—	—	—	—
e. Revisions per 100 words = e/A × 100	—	—	—	—	—	—
f. Incomplete phrases per 100 words = f/A × 100	—	—	—	—	—	—
g. Broken words per 100 words = g/A × 100	—	—	—	—	—	—
h. Prolonged sounds per 100 words = h/A × 100	—	—	—	—	—	—
i. Dysrhythmic phonations in words per 100 words = i/A × 100	—	—	—	—	—	—
j. Tension pauses per 100 words = j/A × 100	—	—	—	—	—	—
k. Total repetitions (b+c+d) per 100 words = i/A × 100 = Repetition Index (RI)	—	—	—	—	—	—
l. Total disfluencies = (a+b+ . . . h) per 100 words = j/A × 100 = Total Disfluency Index (TDI)	—	—	—	—	—	—

Reprinted from Williams, D.E., Darley, F. L. & Spriestersbach, D.C. (1978). *Diagnostic Methods in Speech Pathology*. New York: Harper & Row.

Prolongations, for example, are sounds that exceed the standard time allowed for their utterance. Repetitions can be seen as a violation of the number of times within an utterance sounds are allowed to be spoken. Duration of stuttering episodes, as well as measures of speech rate, also place evaluation of stuttering into a temporal framework. On a more global level, the presence of stuttering will often reduce the speed with which a message is conveyed to a

Table 4–3.
Checklist of Stuttering Behavior

Name _____ Age _____ Sex _____

Observer _____ Date _____

Instruction to Observer

Observe the stutterer as he or she speaks or reads aloud. Focus your attention on such disfluencies and related reactions as you would classify as stuttering. Observe these reactions as they are associated with the speaking of specific words. Write each such word at the top of a column and make a check mark in the appropriate space to indicate each type of disfluency or other reaction observed. Note by the use of 1, 2, 3, et cetera, the sequencing of the behaviors. Under "Supplementary Observations" add descriptive details concerning any of the numbered items checked, and comment on apparent emotionality of the speaker, general degree of tension, relevant remarks made by the speaker, et cetera.

Types of Reaction	Word 1	Word 2	Word 3	Word 4	Word 5	Word 6
1. Repeating part of word	___	___	___	___	___	___
2. Repeating whole mono-syllabic word	___	___	___	___	___	___
3. Repeating this and other word(s)	___	___	___	___	___	___
4. Saying "uh—uh" or the like	___	___	___	___	___	___
5. Prolonging sound(s)	___	___	___	___	___	___
6. Pausing in middle of word	___	___	___	___	___	___
7. Failing to complete the word	___	___	___	___	___	___
8. Holding breath	___	___	___	___	___	___
9. Gasping	___	___	___	___	___	___
10. Inhaling irregularly	___	___	___	___	___	___
11. Exhaling irregularly	___	___	___	___	___	___
12. Speaking on exhausted breath	___	___	___	___	___	___
13. Delay in starting word	___	___	___	___	___	___
14. Pressing lips together	___	___	___	___	___	___
15. Pressing tongue against teeth or palate	___	___	___	___	___	___
16. Closing eyes	___	___	___	___	___	___
17. Protruding tongue	___	___	___	___	___	___
18. Enlarging eyes	___	___	___	___	___	___
19. Opening mouth irrelevantly	___	___	___	___	___	___
20. Dilating nostrils	___	___	___	___	___	___
21. Turning head sideways	___	___	___	___	___	___
22. Bending head downward	___	___	___	___	___	___
23. Moving head up or back	___	___	___	___	___	___
24. Moving hands or fingers	___	___	___	___	___	___
25. Moving legs or feet	___	___	___	___	___	___
26. Moving body	___	___	___	___	___	___
27. Other (specify)	___	___	___	___	___	___
28. _____	___	___	___	___	___	___
29. _____	___	___	___	___	___	___
30. _____	___	___	___	___	___	___

Supplementary Observations:

Reprinted from Williams, D.E., Darley, F. L. & Spriestersbach, D.C. (1978). *Diagnostic Methods in Speech Pathology.* New York: Harper & Row.

listener. Even "symptom-free" utterances that are produced too slowly or too quickly are unacceptable when judging the "normal" flow of speech.

Because timing is such a critical aspect of communication, and because it is an aspect most often violated by stutterers, the diagnosis of stuttering behavior must include detailed measures of timing in several forms. The duration of disruptions, as well as the duration of normal utterances, needs to be considered. In addition, the overall speaking rate of clients should be compared, if possible, to their peers. Analysis of a client's speech should include the temporal aspects of stuttering, the descriptors mentioned, some measures of frequency of occurrence, and a perception of the severity of the disorder.

The duration measurements of most interest to speech-language pathologists are measures of the longest periods of fluency and stuttering produced by clients during speech samples. The most commonly accepted way to measure the length of fluent or stuttered utterances is to simply time the three longest occurrences of the behavior and to average the time recorded to arrive at a measure of duration in seconds.

Measurements of Frequency. The frequency of the occurrence of stuttering, reported as the percentage of moments of stuttering, is the most familiar and often used measure. It has been routinely considered part of the diagnostic battery since the 1930s (Bloodstein, 1987). There are two measures of stuttering frequency that are valuable during the initial description of stuttering. The first is the number of words stuttered on during the sample, and the second is the number of syllables stuttered on. Each tabulation can provide different but equally important information.

To calculate the percentage of words stuttered during the sample, first count the number of words uttered (WU). Next, total the number of words stuttered (WS). By dividing the words stuttered by the words uttered and multiplying by 100, the percentage of words stuttered on is derived.

$$\frac{30 \text{ (WS)}}{300 \text{ (WU)}} \times 100 = 10\% \text{ stuttering}$$

Calculating the percentage of syllables stuttered is a bit more complex. Costello and Ingham (1984b) suggest that speech-language pathologists count "moments of stuttering." Moments of stuttering are "each speaker's attempt to produce a given syllable, irrespective of the duration of that attempt" (p. 311). Thus, production of the word "ba-ba-ba-ba-ba-ba-baseball" is considered one moment of stuttering, with one syllable stuttered in a two-syllable word. In multisyllabic words, more than one moment may be counted if the stutterer stutters on more than one syllable of that word.

Prior to calculating the percentage of stuttered syllables, the total number of syllables uttered needs to be determined. This figure can be obtained in one of two ways. The first is to count the number of syllables spoken during the sample. A suggested short cut is to select varied and representative segments from a sample tape on which the client is talking and to count the number of syllables spoken in each segment until 2 minutes have elapsed. Divide the number of syllables obtained during this segment by 2 to calculate the number of syllables spoken per minute (SPM). Then listen to the entire sample, clocking the client's talking time and discounting any pauses of more than 2 seconds. Multiply SPM by total talking time, and an estimate of the total number of syllables spoken is derived.

To calculate the percentage of syllables stuttered, divide the total number of moments of stuttering by the total number of syllables spoken and multiply the results by 100.

$$\frac{100 \text{ (moments of stuttering)}}{500 \text{ (syllables spoken)}} \times 100 = 20\% \text{ syllables stuttered}$$

Regardless of the method selected for counting syllables, it is more difficult to count syllables than words. Justification of this expenditure of time is that counting syllables is a more accurate measure of total communication than counting words. Clients using multisyllabic words would appear to produce less speech in the same time frame if only words were counted. Most of us can produce more small words than large words in 1 minute.

Measures of Speech Rate. Rate of speech and judgments of how normal speech sounds to the listener are directly related. Reduced rates of speech convey less information than the listener is expecting. Even when speech is stutter-free, if it is unusually slow, the speaker will be perceived by listeners as abnormal (Ingham and Packman 1978; Runyan and Adams, 1978). The evaluation process should include a measure of rate in addition to the descriptive measurements discussed. There are a variety of techniques for the measurement of rate (Costello and Ingham, 1984a; Perkins, 1975; Adams, 1976). These authors favor compiling at least a 2-minute segment of fluent speech and then counting the number of syllables uttered during this fluent segment. This method is preferable to measuring the rate of the stutterer's speech that includes both fluent and disfluent productions. The co-mingling of these two behaviors can result in an abnormally fast rate of speech appearing to be significantly slower than it actually is. This increase occurs when the stutterer has either frequent repetitions or extended blocks.

During and after treatment, new measures need to be compared with this initial measurement to determine whether the client's rate of speech was altered. Expected speaking rates for fluent speakers have been presented by several authors. Ingham (1984b) suggested that the normal rate of speech falls between 170 and 210 SPM for adults. In Table 4–4, Culatta and Leeper (1989b) provide a useful breakdown of syllable rates by age for adults. In Table 4–5, Culatta and associates (1987) present SPM rates for children between the ages of 3 and 8. Other studies that have analyzed speaking rates of adults and children have been presented by Meyers and Freeman (1985), Purcell and Runyan (1980), Pindzola and colleagues (1989), and Andrews and Ingham (1971).

Table 4–4.
Adult Syllable Rates

Age (yr)	Mean Syllables/min (SPM)	Range	SD
25–34.11	187.83	121–180	44.23
55–64.11	209.56	125–309	54.97
65–74.11	190.25	83–286	55.60
75–84.11	204.75	57–303	70.23
85+	211.85	63–319	62.79

From Culatta, R. & Leeper, L. (1989). Speech rates of elderly speakers. American Speech-Language and Hearing Association Annual Convention, St. Louis, MO.

Perceived Severity of Stuttering. The descriptions and measurements considered contribute to listeners' and clients' judgment of the severity of stuttering. However, all the components do not have equal weight in affecting judgments. A person who produces only one instance of stuttering during an analyzed segment is markedly different than one who produces 50 instances of the behavior during a similar period. Similarly, a moment of stuttering that lasts 3 seconds will be perceived as more severe than one that lasts a fraction of a second. Severity judgments are based on the total visual and auditory performance package the client presents. Statements of severity range from judgments of how deviant a speaker sounds to estimates of how "natural or unnatural" the speech evaluated might be (Martin et al., 1984). The Scale for Rating the Severity of Stuttering (Williams, 1978) (Table 4–6) is a traditional attempt at blending the components of stuttering into an analyzable form. It assumes that each component will become more deviant as judgments of severity increase.

Martin and co-workers (1984) took a symptom-free approach. They found that listeners could produce reliable ratings of stutterers' speech when asked to evaluate samples using a 9-point scale. On this scale, a rating of 1 signified

Table 4–5.
Child Syllable Rates

Age (yr)	Mean Syllables/min (SPM)	Range	SD
3.0–3.11	157.21	96.84–198.36	26.28
4.0–4.11	168.72	141.70–215.66	19.71
5.0–5.11	158.84	98.33–206.85	27.21
6.0–6.11	169.38	114.16–217.58	27.78
7.0–7.11	172.57	117.02–213.15	24.83

From Culatta, R., Page, J.L. & Wilson, L. (1987). Speech rates of normally communicative children. American Speech-Language and Hearing Association's Annual Convention, New Orleans, LA.

Table 4–6.
Scale for Rating Severity of Stuttering

Speaker _____ Age _____ Sex _____ Date _____
Rater _____ Identification _____

Instructions:

Indicate your identification by some such term as "speaker's clinician," "clinical observer," "clinical student," or "friend," "mother," "classmate," et cetera. Rate the severity of the speaker's stuttering on a scale from 0 to 7, as follows:

0   No stuttering
1   Very mild—stuttering on less than 1 percent of words; very little relevant tension; disfluencies generally less than one second in duration; patterns of disfluency simple; no apparent associated movements of body, arms, legs, or head.
2   Mild—stuttering on 1 to 2 percent of words; tension scarcely perceptible; very few, if any, disfluencies last as long as a full second; patterns of disfluency simple; no conspicuous associated movements of body, arms, legs, or head.
3   Mild to moderate—stuttering on about 2 to 5 percent of words; tension noticeable but not very distracting; most disfluencies do not last longer than a full second; patterns of disfluency mostly simple; no distracting associated movements.
4   Moderate—stuttering on about 5 to 8 percent of words; tension occasionally distracting; disfluencies average about one second in duration; disfluency patterns characterized by an occasional complicating sound or facial grimace; an occasional distracting associated movement.
5   Moderate to severe—stuttering on about 8 to 12 percent of words; consistently noticeable tension; disfluencies average about 2 seconds in duration; a few distracting sounds and facial grimaces; a few distracting associated movements.
6   Severe—stuttering on about 12 to 25 percent of words; conspicuous tension; disfluencies average 3 to 4 seconds in duration; conspicuous distracting sounds and facial grimaces; conspicuous distracting associated movements.
7   Very severe—stuttering on more than 25 percent of words; very conspicuous tension; disfluencies average more than 4 seconds in duration; very conspicuous distracting sounds and facial gestures; very conspicuous distracting associated movements.

Reprinted from Williams, D.E., Darley, F. L. & Spriestersbach, D.C. (1978). *Diagnostic Methods in Speech Pathology*. New York: Harper & Row.

highly natural speech, and a rating of 9 signified highly unnatural speech. The value of this system is that it does not rely on an intimate knowledge of the components of stuttering, and it probably comes closer to evaluations the speaker will encounter outside the clinical world.

Measurement Procedures

Instrumentation and Setting.   An audio or videotape recorder, a stop watch, and an event recorder (digital counter) are the primary tools needed to clinically analyze a client's speech. More sophisticated and expensive equipment may be helpful with a particular client, but it is not critical to obtain a thorough and meaningful initial analysis. One of the most critical aspects of the assessment process is recording a representative speech sample. Speech in the diagnostic room may be different from speech at home. Talking to the unfamiliar speech-language pathologist for the first time may differ from talking with a familiar friend or a brother or sister. Periods of remission in developing stutterers provide information about fluency potential, whereas periods of stuttering highlight the disorder. In fact, speech samples during which clients do most of the talking are probably foreign to most stutterers who may never be the primary communicators in conversations. Obtaining an unbiased sample for analysis is extremely difficult. However, the practicing speech-language pathologist does not always have the luxury of the clinical researcher to obtain "pure samples."

Guidelines for Recording Speech Samples. Common sense and an awareness of a particular client's presenting problems can help clinicians obtain a valid sample for analysis. Andrews and Harvey (1981) suggest that initial measurements might show a client at his worst, and that as stuttering returns to its usual form, faulty initial measures might not provide accurate baseline or pretreatment data. A logical conclusion seems to be that repeated measurements may be needed and that initial assessments should be made, when possible, in a variety of settings. Costello and Ingham (1984a) suggest the following conditions be considered for recording speech samples:

1. Speech with the speech-language pathologist in the clinical setting
2. Speech with a parent in the clinical setting
3. Speech at home with the other parent, caretaker, spouse, or close friend, as appropriate
4. Speech with a brother or sister
5. Telephone conversation speaking
6. Speech in a familiar activity at school or with someone at work
7. Speech with the speech-language pathologist outside of the therapy room (p. 306).

This list of situations is not totally inclusive. There are other situations and conditions that merit sampling for any given client. Goldberg (1981) suggests recording samples in four different situations: (1) reading, (2) describing, (3) monologue, and (4) dialogue. This type of sampling has been referred to as "molecular analysis." The more varied and meaningful the measurements, the more complete the evaluation. It should be possible to obtain at least the sample with the client and the speech-language pathologist and, when necessary, the client and a parent. Costello and Ingham (1984a) recommend that these samples be at least 10 minutes in length. Sharing the purpose of the request for the sample often helps parents understand what is needed and usually leads to better results. Once parents understand that the clinician wishes to hear the child's speech in a fairly typical conversation, they are usually better able to create the appropriate atmosphere that will allow the speech-language pathologist to hear an adequate sample. Although clinicians may wish to experiment with the effects of various speech demands (i.e., interruptions, disagreements, questions), it is probably wisest to obtain as much of an uninterrupted sample as possible during the initial recording. Once the initial samples have been collected, descriptive analysis may begin.

Overt Assessment Protocols

In this section of the chapter, several available assessment protocols that can help speech-language pathologists describe and measure the overt aspects of stuttering are briefly summarized. Each protocol can be used to measure several of the overt behaviors previously discussed. However, none of the protocols will measure all of the categories presented. Table 4–7 lists the parameters that comprise overt stuttering. Each instrument included in the following review is represented, and the parameters it measures are listed in the table.

Measures of Disfluency of Speaking and Oral Reading.   This form, presented by Williams (1978), provides a measure of the percentage of occurrence of each type of disfluency the stutterer emits. Both reading and speaking tasks are used to derive the sample to be analyzed. The total frequency of repetitions and disfluency may also be calculated.

Checklist of Stuttering Behavior.   This checklist, provided by Williams (1978), is a word-by-word analysis of the types of reactions the stutterer displays while speaking or reading. The "Supplementary Observations" section allows speech-language pathologists to add descriptive details not listed on the checklist form.

Scale for Rating Severity of Stuttering.   This form (Williams, 1978) is a global rating of the perceived severity of stuttering. The scale is segmented from 0 to 7; 0 indicates no stuttering, and 7 indicates very severe stuttering. Criteria for the selection of each rating point are included on the form.

Concomitant Stuttering Behavior Checklist/Stuttering Frequency and Duration Estimate Record.   Both these forms appear in the Cooper Personalized Fluency Control Therapy, Revised program (Cooper and Cooper, 1985). The first form allows speech-language pathologists to record as many as 32 behaviors that may occur in the five general categories of posturing, respiratory, facial, syntactic/semantic, and vocal behaviors. The second form allows judgment of severity of stuttering based on frequency and duration measures.

Fluency Baseline Record.   The Fluency Baseline Record, as described by Culp (1984), is designed for preschool children. It assesses speaking under five conditions: monologue, dialogue, retelling a story, play, and a pressure situation. An analysis of overt stuttering behaviors is tabulated during each condition, and percentages of disfluencies are calculated.

Table 4 7.
Overt Measurements

Instrument	Child/ Adolescent or Adult	Speech Characteristics	Nonspeech Characteristics	Duration	Frequency	Rate	Perceived Severity	Locl. Linguistic Unit	Consistency	Adaptation
1. Meas. of Disfl. of Speech or Reading	C/A	X			X					
2. Checklist of Stuttering Behavior	C/A	X	X		X					
3. Scale for Severity of Stuttering	C/A		X	X	X		X			
4. Concom. Stutt. Behavior Checklist	C/A	X	X		X					
5. Stuttering Frequency & Duration Est. Rec.	C			X	X					
6. Fluency Baseline Record	C/A				X					
7. Child Fluency Assess. Inst.	C	X	X	X	X	X				
8. Adolescent Fluency Assess. Inst.	A				X	X				
9. Adult Fluency Assess. Inst.	C				X	X	X			
10. Stuttering Diagnosis and Evaluation Checklist	C/A	X	X						X	X
11. Stuttering Severity Instrument	C		X	X	X					
12. System. Fluency Train. Assessment	C/A	X	X		X	X				
13. Stuttering Assessment Protocol	C/A			X	X	X	X			

1. Measures of Disfluency of Speaking and Oral Reading. Williams, D.E., Darley, F.L & Spriestersbach, D.C. (1978). In F.L Darley & D.C. Spriestersbach, (Eds.). *Diagnostic Methods in Speech Pathology.* New York: Harper & Row.

2. Checklist of Stuttering Behavior. Williams, D.E., Darley, F.L & Spriestersbach, D.C. (1978). In F.L Darley & D.C. Spriestersbach, (Eds.). *Diagnostic Methods in Speech Pathology.* New York: Harper & Row.

3. Scale for Rating Severity of Stuttering. Williams, D.E., Darley, F.L & Spriestersbach, D.C. (1978). In F.L Darley & D.C. Spriestersbach, (Eds.). *Diagnostic Methods in Speech Pathology.* New York: Harper & Row.

4. Concomitant Stuttering Behavior Checklist. Cooper, E.B. & Cooper, C.S. (1985). *Cooper Personalized Fluency Control Therapy, Revised.* Allen, IX: DLM Teaching Resources.

5. Stuttering Frequency and Duration Estimate Record. Cooper, E.B. & Cooper, C.S. (1985). *Cooper Personalized Fluency Control Therapy, Revised.* Allen, IX: DLM Teaching Resources.

6. Frequency Baseline Record. Culp, D.M. (1984). The preschool fluency development program: Assessment and treatment. In M. Peins (Ed.), *Contemporary Approaches to Stuttering Therapy.* Boston: Little Brown & Company, 39–71.

7. Child Fluency Assessment Instrument. Goldberg, S.A. (1981). *Behavioral Cognitive Stuttering Therapy (BCST): The Rapid Development of Fluent Speech.* Tigard, Oregon: C.C. Publications.

8. Adolescent Fluency Assessment Instrument. Goldberg, S.A. (1981). *Behavioral Cognitive Stuttering Therapy (BCST): The Rapid Development of Fluent Speech.* Tigard, Oregon: C.C. Publications.

9. Adult Fluency Assessment Instrument. Goldberg, S.A. (1981). *Behavioral Cognitive Stuttering Therapy (BCST): The Rapid Development of Fluent Speech.* Tigard, Oregon: C.C. Publications.

10. Stuttering Diagnostic and Evaluative Checklist. Luper, H.I. & Mulder, R.I. (1966). *Stuttering Therapy for Children.* Englewood Cliffs, NJ: Prentice-Hall.

11. Stuttering Severity Instrument. Riley, G. (1972). A stuttering severity instrument for children and adults. *Speech Hearing Disorders, 37,* 314–322.

12. Systematic Fluency Training Assessment Form. Shine, R.E. (1980a). *Systematic Fluency Training for Children.* Tigard, OR: C.C. Publications.

13. Stuttering Assessment Protocol. Culatta, R. & Goldberg, S.A. (1995). *Stuttering Therapy: An Integrated Approach to Theory and Practice.* MA: Allyn and Bacon.

Behavioral Cognitive Stuttering Therapy. As a part of the Behavioral Cognitive Stuttering Therapy system, Goldberg (1981) devised three assessment instruments—one for children, one for adolescents, and one for adults—that objectify many aspects of stuttering behavior. The overt measures are primarily frequency counts of stuttering and fluent behaviors.

Stuttering Diagnostic and Evaluative Checklist. A form similar to that of Williams (see Table 4–1) was presented by Luper and Mulder (1966). Their Stuttering Diagnostic and Evaluative Checklist helps clinicians tabulate the occurrence of repetitions, prolongations, hard contacts, and interjections. It also provides for scoring of processes such as consistency and adaptation.

Stuttering Severity Instrument. A widely used format for assessing stuttering severity is the Stuttering Severity Instrument for Children and Adults (SSI), developed by Riley (1972) (Table 4–8). The SSI tabulates the frequency of stuttering, the duration of moments of stuttering, and any concomitant physical movement that might accompany stuttered speech. Points are allotted in each of the three areas. The total of these points translates into a five-point severity scale ranging from very mild to very severe.

Systematic Fluency Training. The Systematic Fluency Training For Young Children program was developed by Shine (1980a). The diagnostic portion of the program includes assessments of rate, the SSI severity instrument, a stuttering analysis, and a checklist highlighting any affected physiological processes during speech.

Stuttering Assessment Protocol. The SAP, which was developed by the authors, provides descriptive baseline data and a series of probes of changeability that enables clinicians to develop treatment strategies. This instrument is discussed in greater detail later in this chapter.

This section of the chapter on assessment techniques detailed the overt characteristic of stuttering, including suggestions for recognizing and charting observable behaviors, techniques for measuring these behaviors, and suggested protocols that might be of interest. Pindzola (1986) provides a comprehensive listing of selected instruments that are currently used to measure stuttering. Interested readers are encouraged to read this review article.

COVERT CHARACTERISTICS OF STUTTERING

The covert aspect of stuttering is comprised of the belief system stutterers develop about talking. Belief systems develop over time, and they are different for each stutterer. However, despite the unique specific views about communication a given client may develop, overall views can be categorized, defined, and understood. Stutterers develop beliefs about their individual abilities to talk, the effect of situations on their speech, and the effects of listeners on their fluency.

Table 4–8.
Stuttering Severity Instrument

NAME _____ SEX M F GRADE _____

SCHOOL _____ DATE OF BIRTH _____

EXAMINER _____ DATE _____ AGE _____

READER _____ NON-READER _____

FREQUENCY Use *Readers Table* 1 and 2 or *Non-Readers Table,* not both.

READERS TABLE

1. Job Task		2. Reading Task	
Percentage	Task Score	Percentage	Task Score
1	2	1	2
2-3	3	2-3	4
4	4	4-5	5
5-6	5	6-9	6
7-9	6	10-16	7
10-14	7	17-26	8
15-28	8	27 and up	9
29 and up	9		

NON-READERS TABLE

3. Picture Task	
Percentage	Task Score
1	4
2-3	6
4	8
5-6	10
7-9	12
10-14	14
15-28	16
29 and up	18

Frequency Task Score 1 and 2 or 3 ☐

DURATION

Estimated Length of Three Longest Blocks	Score
Fleeting...	1
One half second	2
One full second	3
2 to 9 seconds	4
10 to 30 seconds (by second hand)	5
30 to 60 seconds.......................................	6
More than 60 seconds...................................	7

Duration Score ☐

PHYSICAL CONCOMITANTS

Evaluating Scale: 0 = none; 1 = not noticeable unless looking for it; 2 = barely noticeable to casual observer; 3 = distracting; 4 = very distracting; 5 = severe and painful looking.

Distracting Sounds: Noisy breathing, whistling, sniffing, blowing, clicking sounds   0 1 2 3 4 5

Facial Grimaces: Jaw jerking, tongue protruding, lip pressing, jaw muscles tense 0 1 2 3 4 5

Head Movements: Back, forward, turning away, poor eye contact, constant looking around...................................0 1 2 3 4 5

Movements of the Extremities: Arm and hand movement, hands about face, torso movement, leg movements, foot tapping or swinging........0 1 2 3 4 5

Total Physical Concomitant Score ☐

Total Overall Score ☐

CHILDREN'S SEVERITY CONVERSION TABLE (I)

Instructions: To convert the total overall score to a percentage, circle the appropriate number below.

Total Overall Score (circle one)	Percentile	Severity
0-5	0-4	Very Mild
6-8	5-11	
9-13	12-23	Mild
14-15	24-40	
16-19	41-60	Moderate
20-23	61-77	
24-27	78-89	Severe
28-30	90-96	
31-45	97-100	Very Severe

ADULT'S SEVERITY CONVERSION TABLE (II)

Instructions: To convert the total overall score to a percentage, circle the appropriate number below.

Total Overall Score (circle one)	Percentile	Severity
0-16	0-4	Very Mild
17-19	5-11	
20-21	12-23	Mild
22-24	24-40	
25-27	41-60	Moderate
28-30	61-77	
31-33	78-89	Severe
34-36	90-96	
37-45	97-100	Very Severe

Reprinted from Riley, G. (1972), A stuttering severity instrument for children and adults. *Journal of Speech and Hearing Disorders, 37,* 314–322.

Covert Stuttering Behaviors

There are six measurable major types of covert stuttering behaviors: (1) emotional reactions, (2) avoidance, (3) expectation of stuttering, (4) expectation of fluency, (5) motivation, and (6) self-perception. All types are related to the stutterer's belief system, and none are observable. To quantify them, diagnosticians must rely on the stutterer's self-assessment. This lack of verifiable data is viewed by some as introducing an unnecessary amount of subjectivity into the study of stuttering (Ingham, 1990). Others believe, however, that even though measuring covert behaviors is not as easily accomplished or objective as overt behaviors, understanding the stutterer's belief system is essential for understanding how to proceed in therapy (Perkins, 1990a; Cooper and Cooper, 1985).

Emotional Reaction. Each stutterer's reaction to both fluent and disfluent speech is unpredictable. The fear of fluency may be as great as the fear of stuttering. Clients may become withdrawn, aggressive, passive, hostile, or depressed by their manner of speech. Speech-language pathologists need a window into these feelings to help construct an effective therapy plan.

Avoidance. Stutterers may tend to avoid production of not only feared sounds or words, but also situations and encounters with specific people. Regardless of the type of therapy the stutterer is involved with, clinicians will almost always ask the stutterer to engage in feared situations. By having an understanding of what is currently being avoided, clinicians can design therapy that can eventually confront these avoidances.

Expectation of Stuttering. To a large extent, we are a product of our past experiences. Stutterers who expect to stutter may be engaging in a self-defeating exercise, regardless of the therapeutic techniques taught to them by their clinicians. By understanding the extent to which a stutterer believes that control and normal communication are impossible, clinicians can begin addressing the problem in therapy.

Expectation of Fluency. It is important to determine if the stutter believes that some form of control over speech is possible. The expectation that one can be fluent is an indication that the use of fluent speech is a possibility for that person.

Motivation. Changes in long-term behaviors can be difficult to accomplish, whether they involve behaviors such as smoking, procrastination, or stuttering. Assessments of motivation are less likely to involve general questions of whether the individual would like to develop fluency, and more likely to examine the extent of commitment and effort an individual is willing to make to effect behavioral change.

Self-Perception. How an individual sees him- or herself is important in the structuring of intervention protocols. For example, different treatment protocols may be developed for two individuals who have similar covert behaviors but who differ dramatically on the degree of severity each perceives.

Measurement Procedures

The two most common ways of getting information about how a stutterer's beliefs can affect speech are through the interview and use of questionnaires. Questionnaires may require either forced-choice answers or rating scale evaluations. Examples of forced-choice questions are ones that can be answered with "yes" or "no" answers, or those that require the stutterer to choose between self-descriptive statements, such as "a mild stutterer" or "severe stutterer." A rating question asks the stutterer to describe his or her perceptions through the use of a scale with end points such as "calm" and "anxious," "mild" and "severe," or "strongly agree" and "strongly disagree." It is important to realize that the answers derived from these test instruments do not necessarily provide a picture of reality, but rather they describe how stutterers view themselves within their world.

Covert Assessment Protocols

Following are brief reviews of some of the more commonly available instruments used to measure attitudes and beliefs about stuttering. Most of the protocols go directly to the source of the behavior: the stutterer. Some ask for pertinent information from significant others in the speaker's environment, usually parents. Each instrument included in the following review is summarized in Table 4–9, which indicates the instrument's appropriateness for children and adults, individuals who will be supplying the requested information, and categories measuring emotional reactions, avoidances, expectation for stuttering, expectation for fluency, motivation, and self-perceptions.

Stutterer's Self-Ratings of Reactions to Speech Situations. This instrument (Table 4–10), which has been in use since 1955, is described in detail by Williams (1978). The stutterer is asked to list his reactions to 40 common speaking situations on four parameters: avoidance, reaction, stuttering, and frequency. Each reaction is scaled on a 1 to 5 continuum. Shumak (1955) found that these self-ratings and categories tended to interact in terms of the severity of the stuttering problem and the client's perceptions of difficulty.

Perceptions of Stuttering Inventory (PSI). Woolf (1967) devised this 60-item paper and pencil test battery that seeks to measure a client's awareness of struggle, avoidance, and expectancy behaviors that comprise his stuttering. As the client checks whether statements are "characteristic of me," a pattern will emerge as to how the client perceives his stuttering. Questions such as "I avoid talking to people in authority" or "I rearrange what I plan to say to avoid a hard word" reveal avoidance tendencies in daily communication, whereas

Table 4 9.
Covert Measurements

Instrument	Child/ Adolescent or Adult	Client/ Other	Emotional Reaction	Avoidance	Expectation of Stuttering	Expectation of Fluency	Motivation	Self-perception
1. Stut. Self-Rat. Reaction to Sp. Situations	A	C	X	X	X			
2. Perception of Stutt. Inven.	A/C	C		X	X			
3. Stuttering Severity Scale	A/C	C	X	X	X	X		
4. Stuttering Problem Profile	A/C	C	X	X	X	X	X	
5. Child Fluency Assessment Inst.	C	C/O				X	X	X
6. Adolescent Fluency Assessment Inst.	A	C/O			X		X	X
7. Adult Fluency Assessment Inst.	A	C			X	X	X	X
8. Stutt. Attitudes Checklist	A/C	C			X		X	X
9. Sit. Avoid. Behav. Checklist	A/C	C	X	X		X	X	
10. Par. Attitudes Toward Stut. Checklist	A	O	X	X	X	X	X	

1. Stutterers Self-Ratings of Reactions to Speech Situations. Williams, D.E., Darley, F.L. & Spriestersbach, D.C. (1978). In F.L Darley & D.C. Spriestersbach, (Eds.). *Diagnostic Methods in Speech Pathology.* New York: Harper & Row.

2. Perceptions of Stuttering Inventory. Woolf, G. (1967). Perceptions of stuttering inventory. *Brit J Disorders Commun, 2,* 158–177.

3. Stuttering Severity Scale. Lanyon, R.I. (1967). The measurement of stuttering severity. *J Speech Hearing Res, 10,* 836–843.

4. Stuttering Problem Profile. Silverman, F. (1980). The stuttering problem profile: A task that assists both client and clinician in defining therapy goals. *J Speech Hearing Disorders, 45,* 119–123.

5. Child Fluency Assessment Instrument. Goldberg, S.A. (1981). *Behavioral Cognitive Stuttering Therapy (BCST): The Rapid Development of Fluent Speech.* Tigard, Oregon: C.C. Publications.

6. Adolescent Fluency Assessment Instrument. Goldberg, S.A. (1981). *Behavioral Cognitive Stuttering Therapy (BCST): The Rapid Development of Fluent Speech.* Tigard, Oregon: C.C. Publications.

7. Adult Fluency Assessment Instrument. Goldberg, S.A. (1981). *Behavioral Cognitive Stuttering Therapy (BCST): The Rapid Development of Fluent Speech.* Tigard, Oregon: C.C. Publications.

8. Stuttering Attitudes Checklist. Cooper, E.B. & Cooper, C.S. (1985). *Cooper Personalized Fluency Control Therapy, Revised.* Allen, IX: DLM Teaching Resources.

9. Situation Avoidance Behavior Checklist. Cooper, E.B. & Cooper, C.S. (1985). *Cooper Personalized Fluency Control Therapy, Revised.* Allen, IX: DLM Teaching Resources.

10. Parent Attitudes Toward Stuttering Checklist. Cooper, E.B. & Cooper, C.S. (1985). *Cooper Personalized Fluency Control Therapy, Revised.* Allen, IX: DLM Teaching Resources.

Table 4–10.
Stutterer's Self-Ratings of Reactions to Speech Situations

Name _____ Age _____ Sex _____
Examiner _____ Date _____

After each item put a number from 1 to 5 in each of the four columns.

Start with right-hand column headed Frequency. Study the five possible answers to be made in responding to each item, and write the number of the answer that best fits the situation for you in each case. Thus, if you habitually take your meals at home and seldom eat in a restaurant, certainly not as often as once a week, write the number 5 in the Frequency column opposite item No. 1, "Ordering in a restaurant." In like manner respond to each of the other 39 items by writing the most appropriate number in the Frequency column. When you have finished with this column fold it under so you cannot see the numbers you have written. This is done to keep you from being influenced unduly by the numbers you have written in the Frequency column when you write your responses to the 40 situations in the Stuttering column.

Now, write the number of the response that best indicates how much you stutter in each situation. For example, if in ordering meals in a restaurant you stutter mildly (for you), write the number 2 in the Stuttering column after item No. 1. In like manner respond to the other 39 items. Then fold under the Stuttering column so you will not be able to see the numbers you have written in it when you make your responses in the Reaction column.

Following the same procedure, write your responses in the Reaction column, fold it under, and, finally, write your responses in the Avoidance column.

Numbers, for each of the columns, are to be interpreted as follows:

A. Avoidance:
   1. I never try to avoid this situation and have no desire to avoid it.
   2. I don't try to avoid this situation, but sometimes I would like to.
   3. More often than not I do not try to avoid this situation, but sometimes I do try to avoid it.
   4. More often than not I do try to avoid this situation.
   5. I avoid this situation every time I possibly can.
B. Reaction:
   1. I definitely enjoy speaking in this situation.
   2. I would rather speak in this situation than not.
   3. It's hard to say whether I'd rather speak in this situation or not.
   4. I would rather not speak in this situation.
   5. I very much dislike speaking in this situation.
C. Stuttering:
   1. I don't stutter at all (or only very rarely) in this situation.
   2. I stutter mildly (for me) in this situation.
   3. I stutter with average severity (for me) in this situation.
   4. I stutter more than average (for me) in this situation.
   5. I stutter severely (for me) in this situation.
D. Frequency:
   1. This is a situation I meet very often, two or three times a day, or even more, on the average.
   2. I meet this situation at least once a day with rare exceptions (except Sunday, perhaps).
   3. I meet this situation from three to five times a week on the average.
   4. I meet this situation once a week, with few exceptions, and occasionally I meet it twice a week.
   5. I rarely meet this situation—certainly not as often as once a week.

(Continued)

Table 4–10.
Continued

	Avoidance	Reaction	Stuttering	Frequency
1. Ordering in a restaurant	____	____	____	____
2. Introducing myself (face to face)	____	____	____	____
3. Telephoning to ask price, train fare, etc.	____	____	____	____
4. Buying plane, train, or bus ticket	____	____	____	____
5. Short class recitation (ten words or less)	____	____	____	____
6. Telephoning for taxi	____	____	____	____
7. Introducing one person to another	____	____	____	____
8. Buying something from store clerk	____	____	____	____
9. Conversation with good friend	____	____	____	____
10. Talking with an instructor after class or in his office	____	____	____	____
11. Long distance telephone call to someone I know	____	____	____	____
12. Conversation with father	____	____	____	____
13. Asking girl for date (or talking to man who asks me for a date)	____	____	____	____
14. Making short speech (one or two minutes) in familiar class	____	____	____	____
15. Giving my name over telephone	____	____	____	____
16. Conversation with my mother	____	____	____	____
17. Asking a secretary if I can see her employer	____	____	____	____
18. Going to house and asking for someone	____	____	____	____
19. Making a speech to unfamiliar audience	____	____	____	____
20. Participating in committee meeting	____	____	____	____
21. Asking instructor question in class	____	____	____	____
22. Saying hello to a friend going by	____	____	____	____
23. Asking for a job	____	____	____	____
24. Telling a person a message from someone else	____	____	____	____
25. Telling a funny story with one stranger in a crowd	____	____	____	____
26. Parlor games requiring speech	____	____	____	____
27. Reading aloud to friends	____	____	____	____
28. Participating in a bull session	____	____	____	____
29. Dinner conversation with strangers	____	____	____	____
30. Talking with my barber (or beauty operator)	____	____	____	____
31. Telephoning to make appointment, or arrange meeting place with someone	____	____	____	____
32. Answering roll call in class	____	____	____	____
33. Asking at a desk for book, or card to be filled out, etc.	____	____	____	____
34. Talking with someone I don't know well while waiting for bus or class, etc.	____	____	____	____
35. Talking with other players during a playground game	____	____	____	____

(Continued)

Table 4–10.
Continued

	Avoidance	Reaction	Stuttering	Frequency
36. Taking leave of a hostess	___	___	___	___
37. Conversation with friend while walking along the street	___	___	___	___
38. Buying stamps at post office	___	___	___	___
39. Giving directions or information to strangers	___	___	___	___
40. Taking leave of a girl (boy) after a date	___	___	___	___
Total	___	___	___	___
Average				
No. of 1s	_____			
No. of 2s	_____			
No. of 3s	_____			
No. of 4s	_____			
No. of 5s	_____			

Reprinted from Williams, D.E., Darley, F. L. & Spriestersbach, D.C. (1978). *Diagnostic Methods in Speech Pathology.* New York: Harper & Row.

selection of items such as "I make my voice softer or louder before stuttering" reveals expectancy levels.

Selection of responses such as "I make sudden jerky or forceful movements with my head, arms or, body during speech . . ." reveals an awareness or perception of struggling behaviors. These perceptions may exist throughout treatment. Table 4–11 contains the PSI. A profile will emerge by simply totaling the number of responses to the 20 questions in each area.

Stuttering Severity Scale. This protocol, developed by Lanyon (1967), consists of a 64-item inventory of behaviors and attitudes that differentiate stutterers from nonstutterers and that also points to three levels of stuttering severity. It requires that the client respond "true" or "false" to the items presented.

Stuttering Problem Profile. Designed by Silverman (1980), the Stuttering Problem Profile in Table 4–12 is designed to help the speech-language pathologist define therapy goals important to the client. Eighty-six statements are evaluated by the client to help determine in which areas the stutterer is most motivated to improve. The author suggests that the value of this instrument is in designing intervention programs.

Fluency Assessment Instruments. Goldberg's (1981) three separate assessment instruments are comprehensive systems for assessing many aspects of stuttering, including covert reactions. Each instrument is designed for a specific age range: children, adolescents, and adults. Although the wording differs

Table 4–11.
Perceptions of Stuttering Inventory (PSI)

Name _____   Age _____   <u>S</u> <u>A</u> <u>E</u>
Examiner _____   Date _____

Directions

Here are sixty statements about stuttering. Some of these may be characteristic of <u>your</u> stuttering. Read each item carefully and respond as in the example below.

<u>Characteristic</u> <u>of</u> <u>me</u>
_____ Repeating sounds.

Put a check mark ( ) under <u>characteristic</u> <u>of</u> <u>me</u> if "repeated sounds" is part of <u>your</u> stuttering; if it is <u>not</u> characteristic, leave the space blank.

<u>Characteristic</u> <u>of</u> <u>me</u> refers only to what you do now, not to what was true of your stuttering in the past and which you longer do; and not what you think you should or should not be doing. Even if the behavior described occurs only occasionally or only in some speaking situations, if you regard it as characteristic of your stuttering, check the space under <u>characteristic</u> <u>of</u> <u>me</u>.

<u>Characteristic</u>
<u>of</u> <u>me</u>

_____ 1. Avoiding talking to people in authority (e.g., a teacher, employer, or clergyman). (A)
_____ 2. Feeling that interruptions in your speech (e.g., pauses, hesitations, or repetitions) will lead to stuttering. (E)
_____ 3. Making the pitch of your voice higher or lower when you expect to get "stuck" on words. (E)
_____ 4. Having extra and unnecessary facial movements (e.g. flaring your nostrils during speech attempts). (S)
_____ 5. Using gestures as a substitute for speaking (e.g., nodding your head instead of saying "yes" or smiling to acknowledge a greeting). (A)
_____ 6. Avoiding asking for information (e.g., asking for directions or inquiring about a train schedule). (A)
_____ 7. Whispering words to yourself before saying them or practicing what you are planning to say long before you speak. (E)
_____ 8. Choosing a job or a hobby because little speaking would be required. (A)
_____ 9. Adding an extra and unnecessary sound, word, or phrase to your speech (e.g., "uh," "well," or "let me see") to help yourself get started. (E)
_____ 10. Replying briefly using the fewest words possible. (A)
_____ 11. Making sudden jerky or forceful movements with your head, arms, or body during speech attempts (e.g., clenching your fist, jerking your head to one side). (S)
_____ 12. Repeating a sound or word with effort. (S)
_____ 13. Acting in a manner intended to keep you out of a conversation or discussion (e.g., being a good listener, pretending not to hear what was said, acting bored, or pretending to be in deep thought). (A)

(Continued)

Table 4–11.
Continued

_____	14. Avoiding making a purchase (e.g., going into a store or buying stamps in the post office). (A)
_____	15. Breathing noisily or with great effort while trying to speak. (S)
_____	16. Making your voice louder or softer when stuttering is expected. (E)
_____	17. Prolonging a sound or word (e.g. m-m-m-m-my) while trying to push it out. (S)
_____	18. Helping yourself to get started talking by laughing, coughing, clearing your throat, gesturing, or some other body activity or movement. (E)
_____	19. Having general body tension during speech attempts (e.g., shaking, trembling, or feeling "knotted up" inside). (S)
_____	20. Paying particular attention to **what** you are going to say (e.g., the length of a word, or the position of a word in a sentence). (E)
_____	21. Feeling your face getting warm and red (as if you are blushing) as you are struggling to speak. (S)
_____	22. Saying words or phrases with force or effort. (S)
_____	23. Repeating a word or phrase preceding the word on which stuttering is expected. (E)
_____	24. Speaking so that no word or sound stands out (e.g., speaking in a singsong voice or in a monotone). (E)
_____	25. Avoiding making new acquaintances (e.g., not visiting with friends, not dating, or not joining social, civic, or church groups). (A)
_____	26. Making unusual noises with your teeth during speech attempts (e.g., grinding or clicking your teeth). (3)
_____	27. Avoiding introducing yourself, giving your name, or making introductions. (A)
_____	28. Expecting that certain sounds, letters, or words are going to be particularly "hard" to say (e.g., words beginning with the letter "p"). (E)
_____	29. Giving excuses to avoid talking (e.g., pretending to be tired or pretending lack of interest in a topic). (A)
_____	30. "Running out of breath" while speaking. (S)
_____	31. Forcing out sounds. (S)
_____	32. Feeling that your fluent periods are unusual, that they cannot last, and that sooner or later you will stutter. (E)
_____	33. Concentrating on relaxing or not being tense before speaking. (E)
_____	34. Substituting a different word or phrase for the one you had intended to say. (A)
_____	35. Prolonging or emphasizing the sound preceding the one on which stuttering is expected. (E)
_____	36. Avoiding speaking before an audience. (A)
_____	37. Straining to talk without being able to make a sound. (S)
_____	38. Coordinating or timing your speech with a rhythmic movement (e.g., tapping your feet or swinging your arm). (E)
_____	39. Rearranging what you had planned to say to avoid a "hard" sound or word. (A)
_____	40. "Putting on an act" when speaking (e.g., adopting an attitude of confidence or pretending to be angry). (E)
_____	41. Avoiding the use of the telephone. (A)
_____	42. Making forceful and strained movements with your lips, tongue, jaw, or throat (e.g., moving your jaw in an uncoordinated manner). (S)

(Continued)

Table 4–11.
Continued

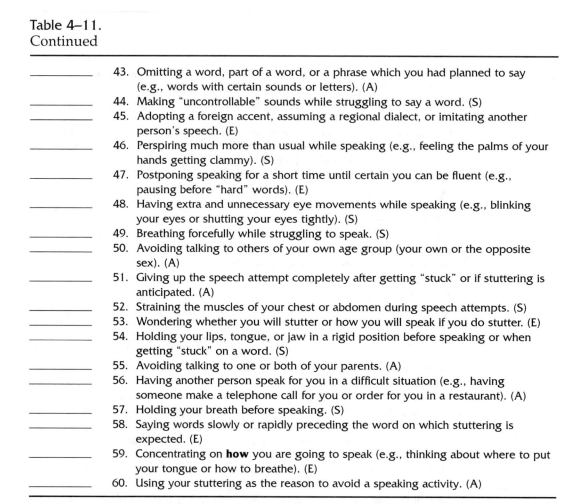

_____	43. Omitting a word, part of a word, or a phrase which you had planned to say (e.g., words with certain sounds or letters). (A)
_____	44. Making "uncontrollable" sounds while struggling to say a word. (S)
_____	45. Adopting a foreign accent, assuming a regional dialect, or imitating another person's speech. (E)
_____	46. Perspiring much more than usual while speaking (e.g., feeling the palms of your hands getting clammy). (S)
_____	47. Postponing speaking for a short time until certain you can be fluent (e.g., pausing before "hard" words). (E)
_____	48. Having extra and unnecessary eye movements while speaking (e.g., blinking your eyes or shutting your eyes tightly). (S)
_____	49. Breathing forcefully while struggling to speak. (S)
_____	50. Avoiding talking to others of your own age group (your own or the opposite sex). (A)
_____	51. Giving up the speech attempt completely after getting "stuck" or if stuttering is anticipated. (A)
_____	52. Straining the muscles of your chest or abdomen during speech attempts. (S)
_____	53. Wondering whether you will stutter or how you will speak if you do stutter. (E)
_____	54. Holding your lips, tongue, or jaw in a rigid position before speaking or when getting "stuck" on a word. (S)
_____	55. Avoiding talking to one or both of your parents. (A)
_____	56. Having another person speak for you in a difficult situation (e.g., having someone make a telephone call for you or order for you in a restaurant). (A)
_____	57. Holding your breath before speaking. (S)
_____	58. Saying words slowly or rapidly preceding the word on which stuttering is expected. (E)
_____	59. Concentrating on **how** you are going to speak (e.g., thinking about where to put your tongue or how to breathe). (E)
_____	60. Using your stuttering as the reason to avoid a speaking activity. (A)

From Woolf, G. (1967). Perceptions of stuttering inventory. *Br J Disorders Commun, 2,* 158–177.

in each instrument, all measure the same covert aspects of stuttering. Included in each instrument are appropriate case history questions, suggestions for frequency counts, situational rating scales, self-perception questionnaires, and, in the child and adolescent instruments, parental attitude questionnaires.

Personalized Fluency Control Therapy Program. There are three checklists in the Personalized Fluency Control Therapy program (Cooper and Cooper, 1985) that delve into the covert aspects of stuttering for the client and the client's parents. The Stuttering Attitudes Checklist consists of 25 statements used to gauge an adolescent or an adult client's attitudes toward stuttering. It is suggested that analysis of individual statements will point toward specific topics that will be a concern during intervention. The Situation Avoidance Behavior Checklist is used to help the client identify which of 50 common speech situations the client is likely to avoid. The authors suggest that this

Table 4–12.
Stuttering Problem Profile (June 1973 Revision)

NAME: _____ AGE:_____ DATE: _____
ADDRESS: _____

INSTRUCTIONS

On the following pages are a list of statements made by stutterers about their stuttering problem following a period of therapy. In order to help you and your clinician to define goals for therapy, please circle the numbers of those statements that YOU WOULD LIKE TO BE ABLE TO MAKE AT THE TERMINATION OF THERAPY **THAT YOU DON'T FEEL YOU COULD MAKE NOW.** If there are statements you would like to be able to make that aren't included in the list, write them on the last page.

1. I am usually willing to stutter openly.
2. I have learned to speak on exhalation rather than on inhalation.
3. I don't usually have trouble with the first sounds of words.
4. I no longer have a great deal of difficulty speaking in school.
5. I am able to give myself assignments and carry them out to my own satisfaction.
6. I am usually willing to use the telephone.
7. I am as cheerful as most people.
8. I don't usually experience a great mounting of tension and feeling of panic before speaking engagements.
9. I repeat sounds, syllables, and words infrequently.
10. I have a strong desire to do something about my stuttering problem.
11. I used to be quiet and shy. Now I tend to be outgoing.
12. My attitude toward my stuttering is no longer one of embarrassment.
13. I am not in a rush to respond when talking with people.
14. I don't usually experience emotional depression after stuttering in front of other people.
15. I can usually control the level of tensing when involved in speaking situations.
16. I can read relatively fluently.
17. I have learned to live with my problem.
18. I have learned not to be afraid of people.
19. I no longer have the feeling that stuttering is a miserable abnormality.
20. I am putting more emphasis on communication than on words.
21. I have learned how to stutter in a way that is more acceptable to the listener.
22. I have gained a better overall understanding of the problem.
23. I am confident that if I work at it, I can do something about my stuttering.
24. I understand how fluent speakers react to stutterers and why.
25. I usually don't hold myself back from talking when with a group of people.
26. I am not as ashamed as I used to be because of my stuttering.
27. I usually don't stutter much when giving a formal report to a group of people.
28. I have gained increased courage to participate in conversations, answer phone calls, and talk to strangers.
29. I am reasonably tolerant of nonfluency in general.
30. I usually don't avoid feared words and situations.
31. I no longer have a feeling of hopelessness about my stuttering.

(Continued)

Table 4–12.
Continued

32. My mental attitude toward my stuttering has changed. The gist of my present attitude is "true acceptance of the fact that I **am** a stutterer."
33. I talk as much as most people.
34. When around other people, I don't usually hold back my feelings because of fear of stuttering.
35. I usually am not preoccupied with myself.
36. I am usually willing to discuss my problem with other people.
37. I no longer object to my therapy program.
38. I have expanded my activities, both social and business.
39. I usually don't have strong feelings of shame and embarrassment when I block.
40. I now feel I could change what I do when I stutter if I would wake up and do it.
41. I no longer anticipate stuttering on certain sounds.
42. I am convinced that I can talk without having to struggle.
43. I don't usually become very anxious when I have to initiate a phone call.
44. My breathing while speaking usually isn't irregular.
45. When I stutter, related movements such as hand jerks and eye blinkings rarely occur.
46. I no longer speak at an excessive rate.
47. I usually am not afraid of public reading.
48. I find it relatively easy to ask a clerk for something in a store.
49. I can purposely speak the way I want in the majority of situations.
50. I would be willing to become an officer in a club where I would have to give speeches.
51. I have learned that speaking can be an enjoyable experience.
52. I don't usually worry about entering speaking situations.
53. I don't usually become extremely depressed when in a period of "regression" in my speech.
54. I no longer consider myself an oddity because I stutter.
55. I usually am willing to say what I feel like saying.
56. I usually am not afraid to stutter in front of people.
57. My self-confidence has increased considerably.
58. It doesn't bother me to hear other stutters speak.
59. I try to avoid changing words I think I will stutter on.
60. Words that I used to use as "starters" have all but completely disappeared.
61. I am getting involved in many speaking situations.
62. I believe I can overcome my problem to the extent I can live comfortably with it.
63. I look upon my stuttering as something that can be changed or modified.
64. I have as many friends as most people.
65. I have learned to modify some of the overt behavior, e.g., facial grimaces.
66. I am relatively relaxed in speaking situations.
67. I am sure I can completely conquer the problem.
68. I recognize the worth of experimenting and playing around with my stuttering.
69. I don't usually experience feelings of failure when in a period of "regression" in my speech.
70. I no longer try to avoid looking at the person with whom I am talking while I am stuttering.

(Continued)

Table 4–12.
Continued

71. I now rarely anticipate stuttering.
72. I feel that I have learned to accept the fact I stutter.
73. I have quit being a lone wolf.
74. I do not react violently to my nonfluencies.
75. I feel fairly confident I can do something about my stuttering.
76. I have finally accepted the fact I am a stutterer. Before I never felt like I was one and always tried to "hide" it.
77. I push myself to enter situations in which I know I will stutter instead of avoiding them.
78. I probably talk to as many people as most persons.
79. I am usually willing to modify my stuttering blocks outside the therapy situation in the manner recommended by my therapist.
80. I usually don't worry very much about the reactions of others when I have a speech block.
81. I am paying more attention to my strengths than my weaknesses.
82. I tend to be relatively relaxed when giving a formal report to a group of people.
83. I usually am not afraid to approach people and talk to them.
84. I realize that improving my speech must be a day-to-day affair with specific goals and assignments set up.
85. I have accepted a certain amount of nonfluency as normal speech behavior.
86. I recite in the classroom as much as most students.

Additional Statements

From Silverman, F. (1980). The stuttering problem profile: A task that assists both client and clinician in defining therapy goals. *J Speech Hearing Disorders, 45,* 119–123.

form may be helpful to establish a hierarchy of tasks for direct intervention. The Parent Attitudes Toward Stuttering Checklist is a 25-item questionnaire designed to identify parental attitudes and feelings. Counselling sessions may be designed around any misperceptions or specific concerns uncovered by this questionnaire.

Our review of the instruments should present readers with a cross-sectional overview of the types of tools available to measure attitudes and beliefs that stutterers and their families hold about stuttering. Each tool has its own focus, and each may be more applicable to some clients than others.

A COMPREHENSIVE TESTING PROCEDURE

In the previous sections of this chapter, we reviewed a number of assessment procedures that can be used for the diagnosis of stuttering; many are both effective and valuable. However, none address all of the requirements of a comprehensive diagnostic assessment. Missing is an initial screening device to determine if clients are exhibiting a form of disfluency that is really stuttering. In addition, existing protocols rarely provide guidelines for developing individualized intervention protocols based on presenting symptoms. To accomplish these goals, the Comprehensive Testing Procedure was developed.

The first step in the procedure is to determine if the client is a stutterer or an individual with another type of disfluency problem. The Differential Screening For Stuttering (DSS) is designed to perform this function. If the screening results indicate the client is a stutterer, then assessments of both overt and covert behaviors are performed. The instrument used to assess overt behaviors is the Stuttering Assessment Protocol (SAP). The SAP not only provides a descriptive analysis of the stutterer's speech behaviors, but also provides valuable information for the development of intervention protocols. Covert behaviors are assessed through the use of already existing instruments that we have found adequate for our purposes.

Differential Screening for Stuttering

The DSS requires clinicians to: (1) obtain a case history, (2) obtain behavioral information, and (3) perform a speech analysis. A checklist taken from the DSS appears in Table 4–13.

Case History Information (Indicators 1–4). A client's case history can provide clinicians with a vast amount of information important for the differential diagnosis. Of particular importance is information relating to onset, development, family history of stuttering, and etiology. No one factor should be used to diagnosis stuttering. Rather, clinicians should look for the presence of multiple factors that would lead to a diagnosis of stuttering or another type of disfluency. As previously discussed, stuttering is a disorder of childhood. Reports of *onset* past the age of 7 should alert speech-language pathologists that the disfluent client may not be a stutterer. Stutterers pass through a series of well-defined *stages of development* prior to stabilization as chronic stutterers (Bloodstein, 1960). A developmental history, as compared with sudden onset of the disorder, will provide further clues toward confirmation of the diagnosis of stuttering. Stutterers are more likely to have a *family history* of stuttering than fluent speakers or speakers with different types of disfluencies. The incidence of stuttering within families of stutterers ranges from 25 to 52% (Yairi and Ambrose, 1992). Thus, reports of familial incidence also provide data that can confirm a diagnosis of stuttering. As discussed in Chapter 1, the *etiology* of stuttering is unknown. The ability of a client to point to a specific, verifiable cause for disfluency will usually negate the diagnosis of stuttering.

Behavioral Information (Indicators 5–10). Certain speaking conditions often bring about increased fluency with stutterers, and they can help speech-language pathologists differentiate stutterers from other disfluent speakers. These activities include adaptation, automatic speech, choral reading, and singing. For stutterers, repeated readings of the same passage will often result

Table 4–13.
Differential Screening Test for Stuttering Checklist[a]

Number	Indicator	Associated with Stuttering	Associated with Other Forms of Disfluency
1	Onset	Before 7 years of age	After 7 years of age
2	Stages of development	Progressive	Abrupt
3	Family history	History of stuttering in family	No history of stuttering in family
4	Etiology	Unknown	Appears immediately following a specific event
5	Adaptation	Number of disfluencies reduces through fifth reading	Little or no reduction of disfluencies through fifth reading
6	Automatic speech - 1 (days of the week)	Relatively fluent	Little or no change
7	Automatic speech - 2 (months of the year)	Relatively fluent	Little or no change
8	Automatic speech - 3 (count to 20)	Relatively fluent	Little or no change
9	Choral reading (reads for 1 minute, 30 seconds; disregard first 30 seconds)	Fluency level improves	No effect on fluency
10	Singing	Fluency level improves	No effect on fluency
	Total checks		

[a]*Instructions:* Check the appropriate box for each indicator. Although there is no specific number of checked indicators that unequivocally differentiates a stutterer from a person with another form of disfluency, a preponderance of checked items in one column can provide substantial evidence.

in a significant decrease in stuttering (Johnson and Innis, 1939). Called *adaptation*, this phenomena, although of limited usefulness in therapy, can be highly significant for differential diagnosis. As the meaningfulness or propositionality of a response decreases, quite often so does the stuttering that accompanies it (Sheehan 1958; Eisenson and Horowitz, 1945). Ask the client to recite the days of the week, the months of the year, or to count or perform other similar speaking tasks. This *automatic speech* will often bring a degree of fluency to stutterers that will not occur with other types of disfluency. Reading with another person or participating in any *choral reading* activity will often increase the fluency level of stutterers (Barber, 1939; Johnson and Rosen, 1937; Ingham and Carroll, 1977; Ingham and Packman, 1979; Adams and Ramig, 1980). *Singing* will often result in a fluent performance from a stutterer. Asking for a well-known and emotionally neutral song such as "Happy Birthday To You" will provide some differential diagnosis data.

Speech Sample Analysis. If this analysis indicates that the client may be a stutterer, then a speech sample analysis should be performed. This previously described speech analysis will provide additional information that can confirm the diagnosis. A specific item of importance is the loci of disfluency. The vast majority of disfluencies that occur in the speech of stutterers are located in the beginning of linguistic units, such as words, phrases, and sentences (Bloodstein, 1987). A large percentage of disfluencies that appear in the middle or end of words and phrases would be a counterindication of stuttering.

Stuttering Assessment Protocol (SAP)

The second component of the comprehensive testing procedure is the SAP, which was derived from the work of Costello and Ingham (1984a). The SAP provides descriptive baseline data and a series of probes of changeability that ultimately enable clinicians to develop treatment strategies. Table 4–14 is the data sheet for the SAP.

The SAP is divided into two sections. The first section is a compilation of measurements and judgments about the client's current communication status. It provides both a way to quantify the speech behavior speech-language pathologists encounter initially, and a fairly comprehensive series of baseline measures. Part two of the protocol probes the changeability of the client's speech. By allowing speech-language pathologists to briefly manipulate the conditions under which a client communicates during the diagnostic session, this protocol may provide a rationale for selecting a particular therapeutic regimen. Although the SAP primarily assesses overt behaviors, some significant covert behaviors are also examined. For more in-depth analysis of covert behaviors, several of the instruments previously described are used. Two suggested instruments are the Perceptions of Stuttering Inventory (Woolf, 1967) and the Behavioral Cognitive Stuttering Therapy instrument (Goldberg, 1981).

Baseline Data Collection. Baseline measures are those taken prior to any therapeutic intervention. In an ideal setting, several baseline measures should be attempted. Usually these speaking performances prior to intervention are either audio- or videotaped. The minimal samples required with children are a tape of the child speaking with his parents, either at home or in the clinical setting, and a similar tape of the child talking with the speech-language pathologist. For an adult, a conversation with a familiar listener can substitute for the parental tape. A 10-minute sample the speech-language pathologist and the client or his parents feel is representative will usually suffice. It is important that the speech-language pathologist obtain this sample with the client doing most of the talking and the other participants refraining from dominating the conversation. Time is calculated in minutes and seconds of client talking time.

Table 4–14.
Stuttering Assessment Protocol

NAME _____ DATE OF BIRTH _____ AGE _____
DATE _____ TEACHER _____ GRADE_____

BASELINE DATA

		With Parent	**With Speech-Language Pathologist**
BASELINE TIME TO BE ANALYZED		_____ minutes	_____ minutes
PERCENT OF SYLLABLES STUTTERED	$= \dfrac{\text{syllables stuttered}}{\text{total syllables}}$	_____ = [ ]	_____ = [ ]
PERCENT OF WORDS STUTTERED	$= \dfrac{\text{stuttered words}}{\text{total words}}$	_____ = [ ]	_____ = [ ]
DURATION OF MOMENT OF STUTTERING (average of 3 longest moments)	$= \dfrac{a + b + c}{3}$	$\dfrac{+ \; + \; +}{3} = [\quad]$	$\dfrac{+ \; + \; +}{3} = [\quad]$
FLUENT SPEECH RATE	$= \dfrac{\text{syllables spoken}}{\text{minutes of sample}}$	_____ = [ ]	_____ = [ ]
LENGTH OF STUTTER FREE UTTERANCES (average time of 3 longest utterances)	$= \dfrac{a + b + c}{3}$	$\dfrac{+ \; + \; +}{3} = [\quad]$	$\dfrac{+ \; + \; +}{3} = [\quad]$
(average number of syllables uttered for a, b and c)	$= \dfrac{a + b + c}{\text{time}}$	$\dfrac{+ \; + \; +}{\text{time}} = [\quad]$	$\dfrac{+ \; + \; +}{\text{time}} = [\quad]$
PERCEPTION OF SPEECH QUALITY: 1–9 (1=highly natural 9=highly unnatural)	Stutterer's Self = Perception [ ]	Parent's Perception [ ]	Speech-Language Pathologist Perception [ ]

PROBES OF CHANGEABILITY OF STUTTERING

CONDITIONS
  A = Client's usual speech
    Clinician says "Now speak the way you ususally do."

  B = Probe condition
    Clinician states instructions as written under each probe

TIME FOR EACH SAMPLE
  A = 1 minute
  B = 1 minute

DATA
  For all conditions use the following formula:

  $\dfrac{\text{syllables stuttered}}{\text{total syllables}} = \text{Data}$

(Continued)

Table 4–14.
Continued

STRATEGY	TACTIC	A	B	A
PHYSIOLOGICAL ADJUSTMENT	**1. Light Contact** " . . . keep the contacts between lips, lips and tongue, and tongue and teeth as gentle as possible."	— =	— =	— =
	2. Whispering " . . . whisper like this."	— =	— =	— =
RATE MANIPULATION	**3. Reduce Rate** " . . . talk slowly like this."	— =	— =	— =
	4. Prolonged Speech " . . . talk slowly like this. Stretch out your words and keep your voice working the whole time."	— =	— =	— =
OPERANT CONTROLS	**5. Verbal Punishment** " . . . no (or wrong)" said contingent on stuttering	— =	— =	— =
	6. Reinforcement of Fluency " . . . as you talk I will drop a coin for you to keep for each 10 seconds of fluent speech."	— =	— =	— =
LENGTH AND COMPLEXITY OF UTTERANCE	**7. Single Word Response** " . . . tell me what these pictures are."	— =	— =	— =
	9. Abstract Response " . . . tell me a story about this picture."	— =	— =	— =
ATTITUDE	**10. Control of Speech** " . . . do you believe that stuttering is curable or only modifiable."	— =	— =	— =
	11. Role " . . . what will be your role in therapy?"	— =	— =	— =
MONITORING	**12. Cognitive Control** " . . . use your very best speech and try not to stutter."	— =	— =	— =
	13. Self-Recording " . . . keep talking, but every time you stutter make a mark on this paper."	— =	— =	— =

Using the guidelines previously discussed in this chapter, the speech-language pathologist would next analyze a representative 2-minute segment and determine the *percent of syllables stuttered* by the client. This measurement is made for samples with both the familiar listener and the speech-language pathologist. These percentages and the syllable counts from which they were derived should be entered on the appropriate lines on the form. Similarly, the data for *percentage of words stuttered* are entered on the next line on the SAP. To calculate the *duration of moments of stuttering*, the speech-language pathologist should select and time the three longest moments of stuttering that occur in the segments analyzed. The *fluent speech rate* on each tape should be entered on the form. The importance of this measurement was previously discussed in this chapter. The *length of stutter-free utterances* may be determined in two ways. The first is to time the three longest segments of stutter-free speech emitted by the client and to enter the average time of these utterances on the SAP. The second is to count the total number of syllables uttered during these stutter-free times and to enter the average number of syllables produced on the form. The final baseline judgment is a measure of *perception of speech quality*. The parent, the speech-language pathologist, and the client should listen to the segments analyzed and make judgments as to their perception of how normal or natural the speech analyzed sounded. A scale of 1 to 9 is used, with 1 being a judgment of highly natural speech, and 9 being a judgment of highly unnatural speech.

After completing the first part of the SAP, clinicians will have recorded 15 data points on six behaviors. This fairly comprehensive analysis can be referred to repeatedly during treatment to help determine whether progress occurs. These measures may and should be repeated as often as the judgment of the speech-language pathologist dictates.

Probes of Changeability.   The second section of the SAP consists of 13 probes of behavioral changeability. These probes are derived from clinical reports suggesting their effectiveness in changing stuttering behavior. We limited the probes in the SAP to those related to the six major therapy approaches we will discuss in chapter 7 to allow clinicians to move directly from probe findings to intervention strategies. These strategies are: (1) physiological adjustments of the mechanisms used for speech, (2) rate control, (3) operant controls, (4) length and complexity of utterance strategies, (5) attitude manipulations, and (6) monitoring of speech. The presentation methodology follows a standard ABA research format. The "A" conditions involve no treatment. The "B" condition involves treatment. By using an ABA design, clinicians can compare the client's normal speech with use of a specific technique and the effects of removing the technique on the client's speech. Costello and Ingham (1984a) suggest that by combining therapy techniques with a single subject research design format, an indication of their effectiveness for a particular client may be forthcoming. The ABA format we suggest is an instruction for the alternation of treatment and nontreatment conditions. The initial A is a 1-minute segment during which no treatment is applied. The B segment is a 1-minute segment during which treatment (probe) is applied. The second A is a 1-minute segment of no treatment. Thus, each probe is 3 minutes long, and it is divided into sequential segments of no treatment and treatment conditions. A more powerful measure would be an ABAB design, wherein the second B is a 1-minute segment during which the treatment is reintroduced. Because this procedure might add 15 minutes to an already lengthy assessment, it is not suggested.

There is evidence to suggest that the ABA design is sufficiently powerful to provide clinicians with prognostic information (McReynolds and Kearns, 1983). However, clinicians are encouraged to use an ABAB format whenever it is warranted or appropriate. The data collected for each probe consist of the number of syllables stuttered during each separate segment and the number of syllables uttered during each segment. The number of syllables stuttered is divided by the total number of syllables to derive a percentage of syllables stuttered for each segment.

$$\frac{\text{Syllables stuttered}}{\text{Total number of syllables}} = \text{Percentage of stuttered syllables}$$

Analysis consists of comparative results. For each probe, the effects of the treatment technique are compared with no treatment conditions. The analysis can be as simple as merely rank ordering the effects of the probes, or as complex as performing an analysis of variance to determine if differences are significant. Clinician preferences can determine the level of sophistication used to analyze the results of the probes. The usefulness of the results will be dependant on the level of analysis. If, for example, a rank ordering procedure was used, the clinician will be able to determine a priority of intervention techniques, some of which may not be significantly different. If an analysis of variance was performed, then a variety of options becomes available to the clinician, which range from determining what techniques are most appropriate to deciding what approaches may have the possibility of generating generalization effects.

Physiological adjustment probes entail consciously manipulating the speech mechanism by changing phonation or the articulatory postures used for speech. The two probes based on this approach are the use of light articulatory contacts and whispering. One of the earliest methods suggested for changing the speech of stutterers was use of "loose contacts" (Van Riper, 1973). The method consisted of using reduced tension in the lips, tongue, and vocal cords while speaking (Daly, 1984). Luper and Mulder (1966) reported that some children treated with this technique improved greatly and required no further treatment. "Loose contacts," "light contacts," and "easy speech" (Williams, 1971, 1979) all refer to the easing of tension in the upper articulators. After recording 1 minute of the clients' usual speech for condition A, the B or treatment phase of this Probe begins when the speech-language pathologist tells the stutterer, "when I ask you to, speak trying to keep the contacts between your lips, lips and tongue, and tongue and teeth as gentle as possible." At the end of the 1-minute segment of attempted "light contact," the clinician requests that the client, "please return to your regular way of talking now." The final minute of spontaneous speech is then collected for subsequent analysis.

Unless otherwise indicated, all samples for probes should be of spontaneous speech. Pictures, discussion topics, themes, and other speech-enhancing activities should be employed to help the client generate the volume of spontaneous speech needed during the probes. Ingham (1984b) reports that stuttering may be reduced when stutterers whisper. Johnson and Rosen (1937), Perkins and colleagues (1976), Commodore and Cooper (1978), Commodore (1980), and Bruce and Adams (1978) report that whispering is effective in reducing stuttering. For the treatment segment of this probe, the stutterer is instructed to "when I ask you to, please whisper like this [clinician demonstrates] until I ask you to stop." The speech-language pathologist then collects a 1-minute sample of speech produced while whispering and compares it to the nontreatment (A) segments.

Rate manipulation probes of two types are suggested. The first involves an instruction to the client to slow the rate of speech. The slower rate is still one that is perceived to be within normal rate limits. The second probe involves a drastic reduction of rate, resulting in an extensive prolongation of speech. Simply reducing the rate of speech is sometimes an effective initial manipulation of stuttered speech (Ingham et al., 1974; Perkins et al., 1979; Johnson and Rosen, 1937). Prior to this probe, the speech-language pathologist provides a model of slowed speech for the client. The client may practice this slowed form of speech briefly before the probe begins. The same format as previously described is used. After the first A minute the speech-language pathologist instructs the client to "when I ask you to, please talk slowly like this." During the probe, data are collected for later analysis. The clinician may remind the client to maintain a slow rate during the B segment.

Prolonged speech, the result of delayed auditory feedback, was reported by Goldiamond (1965) to produce speech that was stutter-free. Shames and Florance (1980) and Goldberg (1981) reported that prolonged speech can be obtained and shaped without the use of delayed auditory feedback via modeling of the prolonged speech desired by the clinician for the client. As with the previous probe, a brief practice session is appropriate prior to instigating the probe. The B condition instructions are "please talk very slowly like this. Stretch out your words and keep your voice working the whole time." Costello and Ingham suggest that a rate of 70 SPM or the speech that results from 250 msec of continuous delayed auditory feedback be modeled for the client.

Operant control probes of two different types can be used. The first involves a form of verbal punishment contingent on each stuttered syllable or word. The second uses positive reinforcement for the production of fluent speech. Negative comments contingent on the production of stuttering have been shown by several researchers to depress the frequency of occurrence of stuttering (Cooper et al., 1970; Martin and Siegel, 1966a, 1966b; Quist and Martin, 1967; Reed and Godden, 1977; Martin and Haroldson, 1979; Christensen and Lingwall, 1982). During this probe, the client is told that, "I want you to keep talking. However, each time you stutter I will make a comment." During the B phase, the clinician says "no!" or "wrong!" immediately contingent on each moment of stuttering.

The results of studies that positively reinforce speakers for production of fluent stutter-free speech are consistently positive (Shaw and Shrum, 1972; Peters, 1977; Johnson, 1980; Hegde and Brutten, 1977). Reinforcement techniques have ranged from tangible presentation of money contingent on fluent speech to social praise. During the reinforcement phase of the probe, clinicians present either a chip or a coin contingent on 10 seconds of stutter-free speech. The instructions for the experimental (B) condition are: "As you talk, I will drop a coin for you to keep, for each 10 seconds of fluent speech you produce."

Length and complexity of the utterance modifications have been shown to effect the rate of stuttering in significant ways. The Length and Complexity of Utterance Probes test three variables: single word responses, concrete utterances, and abstract utterances. Costello-Ingham (1993), Costello (1983a), and Ryan (1974b, 1986) present programs based on evidence that manipulation of speech along the parameters of simplicity of utterance can affect fluency of production. The three probes suggested in this section of the SAP manipulate the variables of length, complexity, and abstract conceptualization. For the single-word response probe, the client is instructed during the B segment to "tell me what these pictures are as soon as you see them." Any set of easily identifiable flash cards may be used. The authors have been most successful using the flip card pictures that are a part of the McDonald Deep Test of Articulation (McDonald, 1964) as stimulus material.

The Concrete Speech Probe requires longer utterances with a low level of abstractness. The client is shown a picture and instructed to "please, describe what you see in this picture." Several thematic pictures fairly common in diagnostic language tests may be used. During the A segments of this probe, the client simply returns to conversational speech for the required minute. The Abstract Speech Probe mandates another layer of complexity by requiring the stutterer to increase the abstractness, complexity, and informational level of her speech. The instructions during the B segment of this probe are "please tell me a story about this picture, or tell me what happened just before this scene."

The data from these three related Probes may be analyzed several ways. First, the levels of fluent speech at each level may be determined. Second, the effects of the different conditions may be compared (i.e., probes 8 and 9 to probe 7; probe 9 to probe 8; probe 9 to probe 7; probe 8 to probe 7). Resultant analysis may reveal if the particular client's speech is manipulable by controlling the length or the complexity of speech.

Attitude probes examine the attitudes and the self-concepts that may influence treatment outcome. Some researchers believe that the clients' pre-therapeutic attitudes may affect therapy success (Guitar, 1976; Andrews and Craig, 1988). Others believe that specific attitudes about speaking and the role that the client has in the therapeutic process are critical factors (Shames and Florance, 1980). Long-term maintenance of therapeutic gains may be less likely with clients who begin with highly negative attitudes (Guitar, 1976; Guitar and

Bass 1978). In addition, clients who do not assume "ownership" or feelings of control over the problem may also be at risk (Craig et al., 1981). As Costello (1984b) states, "negative attitudes may not cause stuttering, but in some individuals at least, the attitudinal consequences of stuttering may interfere with treatment" (p. 441).

The goal of these two attitude probes is to attempt to identify attitudes that might put a potential client at risk. They are the only probes in the SAP that rely on speech-language pathologist's interpretation of the client's responses to determine therapeutic needs. As such, they do not use an ABA format, but instead they challenge clinicians to identify client needs from brief responses. The Control of Speech Probe requires the client to elaborate on the possibilities offered by speech therapy. The client is asked "do you believe that stuttering is curable or only modifiable?" Follow-up or clarifying questions are encouraged. The Role in Therapy Probe is an attempt to uncover the client's view of the involvement needed in future treatment, and it may provide information in structuring subsequent sessions. The client is asked "what will be your role in therapy?" Once again, logical follow-up questions that will uncover attitudes are encouraged.

Monitoring probes involve cognitive control and self-recording. Eventually, a client's ability to monitor his or her speech may determine the difference between successful therapy or relapse to previous stuttering. Whether the skill is called monitoring (Culatta and Rubin, 1973), self-instruction (Shames and Florance, 1980), or instructional control (Martin and Siegel, 1966b), the awareness stutterers have about their speech is a vital skill to measure. The Cognitive Control Probe tests the ability of a specific client to manipulate speech when instructed to do so by the examiner. Studies have shown that stutterers might be able to modify their speech pattern when asked to do so by a listener (Martin and Siegel, 1966b; Culatta and Rubin, 1973; Martin and Haroldson, 1979). The instructions for the 1-minute B segment is "please use your very best speech and try not to stutter at all." At the end of the segment, the speech-language pathologist requests the client to "please return to your usual way of talking now."

The Self-Recording Probe is based on the work of La Croix (1973). He described an unusual way to both affect the frequency of stuttering and measure clients' awareness of the behaviors' frequency of occurrence. During the B condition, the client is instructed to "keep talking, but every time you stutter, make a mark on this piece of paper." If the probe responses have been visually- or auditory-recorded, speech-language pathologists can compare this record of stuttered moments with that of the client. Thus, this probe provides a measure of the perceived frequency of occurrence by the client as compared with the clinician. Although not a part of this probe, a similar task can be used if identification of frequency by parents differs from those of the clinician or the child.

Once the client has completed this part of the SAP, the speech-language pathologist will have as many as 11 conditions that have enabled the client to demonstrate the ability to manipulate speech. The speech-language pathologist will also have been able to measure any changes that occurred during these procedures, and they will be better able to plan intervention strategies. Often clients, especially children, are unaware of the communication options available to them. The probes of changeability provide a relatively rapid, yet effective way to demonstrate to the client their communication skills already present.

Other Probes. In addition to the probes suggested, speech-language pathologists might wish to try some other manipulations. These probes are less general in their application, but they may still provide valuable information for given clients. Rhythmic speech is a commonly accepted device for the temporary reduction of stuttered speech (Brady, 1969; Barber, 1940; Hutchinson and Norris, 1977; Brayton and Conture, 1978; Martin and Haroldson, 1979; Martin et al., 1985). A metronome set at 90 beats per minute can be used to apply this probe. Many clients are able to produce the rhythmic model by speaking in time to tapping provided for them by a speech-language pathologist. The instructions provided for the B condition is "please say each syllable in time to my tapping." Shadowing is the technique whereby the client repeats words that clinicians say as soon as they are said. This overlapping form of imitation, where the repetition is a fraction of a second behind the model, has been shown to affect stuttering behavior (Cherry and Sayers, 1956; Kondras, 1967; Andrews, et al. 1982). This probe requires practice. At first it is best for speech-language pathologists to shadow the client to demonstrate the skill. When the switch is made to client production, the speech-language pathologist should use words and short sentences. Although children may find this task difficult at first, it is usually an enjoyable activity, with no shortage of laughter on the part of the client or the clinician. The same format used with the other probes is employed during shadowing. Instructions are "you say what I say as soon as you can."

Time-out probes measure the effect of punishment contingent on stuttered speech. This technique has been shown experimentally to reduce the frequency of stuttering (Haroldson et al., 1968; Martin and Berndt, 1970; Adams and Popelka, 1971; Egolf et al., 1971; Martin and Haroldson, 1971; James and Ingham, 1974; Martin and Haroldson, 1979). This "time-out" from talking should last approximately 5 seconds after each moment of stuttering. Instructions for the B segment are, "please keep talking until I say STOP. Don't begin talking again until I say Go Ahead." The client is to stop immediately, even midword, when possible. The time-out period is approximately 5 seconds.

Choral reading is a long-standing practice used to demonstrate the stutter-free potential of stutterers (Barber, 1939; Johnson and Rosen, 1937; Ingham and Carroll, 1977; Ingham and Packman, 1979; Adams and Ramig, 1980). Appropriately selected reading material is necessary for this probe. During the A segments, the client is asked to read aloud. During the B segment, the client is asked to read in unison with the speech-language pathologist. As with all other probes, percent of stuttering is tabulated for each 1-minute cell.

SUMMARY

In this chapter, we presented a variety of tools, protocols, and techniques to measure the overt and covert aspects of stuttering. The wisest strategy would be for speech-language pathologists to familiarize themselves with the goals and purposes for which each of these instruments was designed and to then pick and choose among them as they deem necessary for any given client. Most of the insights clinicians will obtain will be derived from the probing that takes place during the diagnostic interview. There is really no substitute for face-to-face interaction between clients and clinicians. A well-structured interview and subsequent in-depth data collection will enable speech-language pathologists to bring their training, knowledge, and clinical intuition into sharp focus. The resulting understanding of clients and their families will facilitate the structuring of the intervention program.

STUDY QUESTIONS

1. Describe and provide examples of each type of overt stuttering behavior.
2. Describe and explain the procedures you would use for audiotaping or videotaping a client's (child, adolescent, adult) overt stuttering behaviors.
3. Thirteen overt measurement protocols are summarized in this chapter. Briefly indicate the strengths of each.
4. Describe and provide examples of each type of covert stuttering behavior.
5. Ten covert measurement protocols are summarized in this chapter. Briefly indicate the strengths of each.
6. Describe each component of the Differential Screening for Stuttering Checklist (DSS).
7. Presented with a client (child, adolescent, adult), describe how you would administer each component of the Stuttering Assessment Protocol (SAP).
8. How would you use the results from the SAP to contruct an intervention protocol?

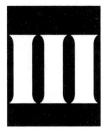

Treatment

To construct effective treatment plans, speech-language pathologists must be knowledgeable in many areas. Each of these areas will eventually contribute to successful treatment. In Chapter 5, the role of culture in diagnosis and therapeutic processes is discussed. Basic differences in relevant clinical behaviors of various cultures are presented, with emphasis on how to make acceptable clinical activities culturally sensitive. Chapter 6 highlights eight of the most critical variables that can affect both the process and the outcome of therapy. Chapter 7 presents a model that is helpful in understanding the various strategies and techniques available to speech-language pathologists. In Chapter 8, this model is applied to 32 approaches to the treatment of stuttering. Chapter 9 is a tutorial for constructing treatment programs.

Chapter

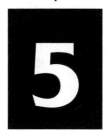

5

Culture and Stuttering

We live in a multicultural and ethnically diverse society in which individuals develop and often act in accordance with culturally related values. The importance of acknowledging the effects of culture on all clinical interactions has been emphasized by various authors (Cole, 1989; Shames, 1989).

Most appeals for cultural sensitivity in the area of communicative disorders result from the ethnic diversity of clients. Although critically important, ethnicity is only one of many cultural categories. "Culture," according to Goodenough (1987), is a shared way of perceiving, believing, evaluating, and behaving. When culture is viewed in this manner, it becomes apparent that culture is not only limited to ethnicity, but also to different sources of shared values and methods of communication. Gollnick and Chinn's (1990) approach to understanding cultures can serve as an important foundation for developing clinical sensitivity. They maintain that within the United States, there exists a macroculture and many microcultures. The macroculture of the United States, and all other countries, consists of values on which most political and social institutions are based. The 10 values they believe are inherent in the macroculture of the United States are:

1. status based on occupation, education, and financial worth;
2. achievement valued above inheritance;
3. work ethic;
4. comforts and rights to such amenities;
5. cleanliness as an absolute value;
6. achievement and success measured by the quantity of material goods purchased;

7. egalitarianism as shown in the demand for political, economic, and social equality;
8. inalienable and God-given rights for every individual that include an equal right to self-governance or choice of representatives;
9. humanitarianism that is usually highly organized and often impersonal; and
10. new and modern perceived as better than old and traditional (p. 13).

Although macrocultural values bind the population together as a whole, they are not sufficient for understanding individual value systems. Each individual not only is a member of a macroculture, but also shares values with members of subcultures. These cultures are known as "microcultures," and each is differentiated from others by specific values, speech and linguistic patterns, learning styles, and behavioral patterns. Gollnick and Chinn list eight types of microcultures that individuals can identify with.

1. Ethnic or national origin
2. Religion
3. Gender/sex
4. Age
5. Exceptionality
6. Urban-suburban-rural
7. Geographic region
8. Class

From these microcultures, values emerge, and from values, styles of communication and interactions develop. Cultural identification for most Americans involves a blending of various microcultures. To illustrate the concept of blending, imagine the components of the value system of a 24-year-old Mexican American woman, with a PhD from Stanford, who is a vice-president of a large bank in Los Angeles. She grew up in Dallas and was the only daughter of parents who were corporate executives. Although she might share many of the same ethnic values as a 50-year-old religious Mexican American woman with a 5th grade education who works as a migrant farm worker in the midwest, vast differences in values would also exist.

Values, styles of interaction, and methods of communication develop from various experiences. The complexity clients bring into speech and language clinics is no less than our examples of the vice president and the migrant farm worker. Clients come to the clinic with an amalgam of values, beliefs, and behaviors from the macroculture and their various microcultures. Although cultural identification with one microculture may be dominant in the values and behavioral patterns of an individual, it rarely is sufficient for understanding that person. It is imperative that clinicians be sensitive to how various cultural components effect the communicative disorder, the client, and the clinical interaction. In the following sections, crosscultural information on incidence and occurrence, principles of interaction, specific speech behaviors, and diagnostic instruments are presented.

Sensitivity to both macrocultural and microcultural values in the study of communication in general, and stuttering in particular, is a relatively recent development. As a result, much of the information presented in this chapter is in its formative stages. It is the task of readers to synthesize and apply the concepts presented to individual situations. The day when we are able to fill in the blanks left in this chapter and answer all the questions posed is hopefully not too far in the distant future. However, the need to be aware of the issues is current, immediate, and often vital to successful treatment. We do not have the luxury of waiting for all the answers before attempting diagnosis and providing treatment for multicultural and linguistically diverse populations. Our macroculture places an emphasis on fluent, precise communication, and all its members suffer the consequences of their communication failures.

INCIDENCE AND OCCURRENCE

Incidence and occurrence of stuttering is an area of investigation that has been examined for many years, although rarely within a crosscultural framework. Much of the early research was done to confirm or dispute assertions that stuttering was environmentally based. If the etiology of stuttering was environmentally based, then its occurrence should be found to vary with different cultures. To test their premise, many early investigators pursued macrocultural studies of societies that were isolated and preindustrial. Although some of the early research was flawed, a wealth of crosscultural information is available.

Macroculture

Researchers examining differences in stuttering related to ethnic or national origin were driven to find definitive evidence that stuttering did or did not have a genetic base. By the mid-1950s, anthropological studies had convinced Kluckhohn (1954) to conclude that stuttering was found in all ethnic and national cultures. Continuing evidence of the existence of stuttering in all examined cultures led Lemert (1979) to conclude that:

> If cultures can be found in which there is neither current incidence of stuttering nor historical evidence of stuttering, then the notion of a genetic basis for stuttering can be summarily set aside. The alternative would be to conclude that whole populations or races differ in their biological potentialities for stuttering, which, within the scope of present knowledge concerning race, does not seem tenable (p. 173).

Most of these early studies focused on preindustrial or aboriginal societies that had minimal contact with other ethnic cultures. By examining relatively isolated groups, it was thought that a better understanding of the relationship that existed between stuttering and child-rearing practices could be determined.

Preindustrial/Aboriginal Cultures.   As early as 1915, Satir reported the existence of stuttering among the Nootka Indians of the east coast of Vancouver Island (Lemert, 1979). Later, the often-quoted studies by Johnson (1944) and Snidecor (1947) asserted that stuttering did not exist among the Bannock and Shoshone Indians of Idaho. The absence of a word for stuttering led Johnson and Snidecor to conclude that the diagnosogenic theory of stuttering was valid. That is, stuttering is a disorder created by labeling and treating normal disfluencies as deviant. The view that stuttering did not exist among North American Indians was dispelled by Lemert (1953). He reported finding numerous stutterers among the Kwakiutl, the Nootka, and the Salish tribes of Canada. The findings of Johnson and Snidecor continued to be widely accepted despite Lemert's work, because they functioned as evidence for an environmental basis of stuttering. They lost their persuasive power when Van Riper (1971) reported the existence of two unpublished articles that refuted Johnson and Snidecor's findings. Van Riper maintained that not only did stuttering exist in the Bannock and the Shoshone tribes, but also that the Indians had a name for it.

These early studies of isolated cultures were not confined to North America. Anthropological studies in South America and Africa revealed the presence of stuttering in other preindustrial societies. A study of the Fulnio tribe on the Pernambuco River of Brazil indicated the presence of stutterers (Lemert, 1979). In Africa as early as 1953, Morgenstern (1953) found the occurrence of stuttering among Ibo and Idoma children of West Africa to be 2.67%. Later, Aron (1962) found the existence of stuttering and a word to describe it among school children of the African Bantu Tribes. Lemert (1962) found stuttering in a number of Polynesian societies.

Although most of the studies of preindustrial or aboriginal cultures resulted in finding stuttering and a word to describe it, the absence of both have been noted. Bullen (1945) found stuttering to be rare or nonexistent in certain tribes of New Guinea, the South Pacific, among the Australian Aborigines and the Polar Eskimos. Although there are many questions regarding these studies, no attempts have been made to replicate or refute them. Currently, it would pose a methodological problem, because the isolation of these ethnic cultures that was present in 1945 no longer exists.

Many of the early studies attempting to relate the presence or absence of stuttering to macrocultural values and linguistic concepts were fraught with methodological problems. Investigators often spent a minimal amount of time with the people they were investigating, or they gathered data prior to being accepted by their subjects. Where anthropologists often spent years of daily interaction prior to making any conclusions, many of the researchers on stuttering spent only weeks, or worse, based conclusions on second- or third-hand reports. In one article presented in 1969 at the Annual American Speech-Language-Hearing Association in New York, a researcher, after spending a considerable amount of time with the Bancock, was told that when the investigators came asking if anyone stuttered, they said no only because they were ashamed of their stutterers. Not only did they have a word for stuttering, but active stutterers had always been a part of their society.

With increased globalization of cultures, it is difficult to find a macroculture that has not been influenced by western, industrialized values. Acculturation results in a blending of values that presents very difficult methodical problems for individuals attempting to find a pure environmental etiology for stuttering. Stuttering has been reported to exist in virtually every society in which anthropological data have been gathered. Reports of it not existing in isolated aboriginal societies have been tainted by inadequate or inappropriate information gathering techniques.

Some individuals (Lemert, 1979; Bloodstein, 1981) argued that even if stuttering was absent in a society, it would not constitute definitive evidence that the etiology of the disorder was cultural, because cultural values may act as precipitating agents for what may be a physiological or a neurological anomaly. The rareness or absence of stuttering in an ethnic culture would indicate only that the values of that society are not causative factors in the development of stuttering. It would not be evidence that stuttering does not have a genetic basis.

Microcultures

Although knowledge of the macroculture does provide clinicians with a basic framework for understanding the client's core cultural traits, it may not prevent insensitivity toward the client's microcultural values. Each person is the product of both macrocultures and microcultures. In many situations, lack of sensitivity to an individual's microcultural values may result in little more than some annoyance on the part of the offended person. An orthodox Jew who is asked to attend a dinner and then is served pork may be offended by his host's ignorance or insensitivity, but the event will probably be shortly forgotten or even become the centerpiece of a humorous story he will relate to his friends. The clinical situation, however, is very different.

Stutterers enter the clinic as vulnerable individuals. They not only have a communication problem, but they have also failed to find its solution. They also give permission to the clinician to probe feelings they may not have previously shared with anyone. Even more threatening, they may allow clinicians to place them in embarrassing situations, or to guide them into changing the way they perceive themselves and others. Because of the very intrusive nature of the clinical interaction, insensitivity to the client's microculture will have more serious consequences than a host's ignorance about Jewish kosher laws. At the very least, clients may become defensive and refuse to allow themselves to be vulnerable with an individual who does not respect or understand their values. At worst, clients may begin to evaluate their values as inappropriate, unacceptable, or, worse, deviant.

Speech-language pathologists cannot be expected to be experts in anthropology. Nor can we be expected to be intimately aware of all the microcultural variables of each cultural subgroup in our country. Sensitivity toward the existence of differences within a pluralistic society, however, is critical. The field of speech pathology has been late in understanding the importance of microcultural values in clinical settings. The available information on stuttering and microculture, circa 1994, follows. Information on some microcultures has been available for many years and is well documented, such as sex and age. In other areas, such as religion, geographic region, and urban-suburban-rural settings, there currently exists little or no reported information about stuttering or stutterers.

Class. Class studies of stuttering are often related to child-rearing practices. For example, an argument has been presented that stuttering is the result of perfectionistic parents demanding or expecting children to be perfectly fluent during the period of language learning when disfluencies are normal and developmental. Glasner's (1949) study of child-rearing practices identified harsh discipline, humiliation, and indulgence as directly affecting the occurrence of stuttering. The relationship posited by Glasner was persuasive to many, and it added credence to the environmentalist's belief that stuttering was a learned behavior.

Glasner's etiological viewpoint was incorporated within a more general theory of child-rearing practices known as the diagnosogenic theory of stuttering (Johnson, 1955). Johnson maintained that misidentification of normal developmental disfluencies as deviant led children to associate normal disfluencies with negative emotions and negative listener reactions. These disfluencies then become stuttering. Some of the early researchers of stuttering believed that child-rearing practices conducive to the development of stuttering could be related to specific social classes. Schnidler (1955) identified parental attitudes of the middle and upper social classes as being most conducive to causing stuttering.

Probably the best known and most quoted study on the relationship of class to the occurrence of stuttering was conducted by Morgenstern (1956). He studied the occurrence of stuttering in Scotland in nine socioeconomic classes determined by the occupation of the father. His findings indicated that occurrence of stuttering for some classes differed significantly from the general population. The lowest classes had a lower occurrence of stuttering, and the semiskilled classes had more. His explanation for the differences was that social mobility, with its corresponding pressures, affected the occurrence of stuttering. The lowest classes had little expectation of bettering the status of their children, and they therefore placed little pressure on them to improve. The semiskilled classes had the greatest potential for improving the status of their children, and they therefore placed extensive pressure on them to rise above their origins. According to Morgenstern, the pressure to improve and to perfect speaking skills was directly related to the occurrence of stuttering.

There is very little current research on the occurrence of stuttering within socioeconomic classes. It may in part be due to methodological problems associated with class identification. We need to identify not only the specific class of the parents, but also the class they identify with. The difficulty of gathering socioeconomic ethnographic data was presented by Lemert (1979), who maintained that if socioeconomic variables affect the occurrence of stuttering, then the relationship should be between the child who stutters and the reference group to which the parents identify.

Although examination of social classes may not yield convincing data regarding the etiology of stuttering, it may provide relevant information for treatment. Undoubtedly, parent's reactions toward stuttering and fluent speech will impact on treatment. Clinicians should be aware of the extent that these reactions reflect class values.

Ethnic or National Origin. In our examination of macrocultures, it is evident that the phenomenon of stuttering exists in every industrialized society, and probably in most, if not all, aboriginal societies. If stuttering is somehow related to ethnic values, we would expect to see differences in percent of occurrence in different countries or ethnic identities. Table 5–1 is a compendium of reported percentages of stuttering in various ethnic groups. With the limited data available, it does appear that the percentage of occurrence is lower for aboriginal cultures than industrialized societies, which may be the result of a less stressful or demanding life style or other microcultural values that have not been identified.

Most of the available data comparing the occurrence of stuttering in ethnic populations within the United States cannot be used to make inferences about the general population. Studies that have reported significant differences have been limited to small samples, such as a city's schools (Cooper and Cooper, 1991; Gillespie and Cooper, 1973); they are fraught with methodological problems (Waddle, 1934); or they cite unpublished data (Cooper and Cooper, 1993). This is not to imply that differences in the occurrence of stuttering do not exist between ethnic populations within the United States. Rather, until more carefully controlled, larger studies can be undertaken, comparative statements may be premature. Our concern is both methodological and ethical. Methodologically, we believe that an individual does not have a single microcultural set of values. As noted earlier, individuals have values derived from the macroculture and various microcultures. Can the sex ratio differences between the African American and white communities reported in the literature (Goldman, 1967) be attributed to ethnic values or are they related to socioeconomic val-

Table 5–1.
Occurrence of Stuttering in Various Ethnic Cultures

Ethnic Culture	Source	Percent of Occurrence
Bantu	Aron (1962)	1.26
South Dakota Indians	Clifford (1965)	3.00
England	Andrews and Harris (1964)	4.80
United States	Bloodstein (1981)	4.50–10.00

ues? Comparative studies not only need the rigor associated with scientific methodology, but also the sensitivity to cultural variables required of anthropological studies.

The finding of population differences can have ethical implications as well. For example, can differences be related to genetic predispositions to stutter, or do they imply that the values associated with the cultures studied are less healthy than the values of other cultures? A more fundamental question is, are any differences related to referral patterns, rather than either the stutterer's cultural values or genetic predisposition? In an interesting study by Lambert and colleagues (1989), it was found that the referral for services for children with special needs was influenced by the ethnicity of the person making the referral. Until more conclusive, rigorously designed studies have been reported, speech-language pathologists should be cautious regarding conclusions that may be unsubstantiated, incorrect, or culturally insensitive. If generalizable data exist showing significant differences in the occurrence of stuttering in the ethnic cultures of the United States, we are unaware of them.

Religion. There are no published studies on the occurrence of stuttering within various religions. We could hypothesize that the occurrence would not differ in religions that shared similar values, and we might expect to find differences in the percent of occurrence in religions with vastly different values and world views. A personal experience of one of the authors may shed light on how religion may affect the occurrence of stuttering. On a trip to Egypt, the author had numerous conversations with devout Muslims regarding stuttering and its treatment. When asked how stutterers are treated, he was told that they were not. Stuttering, according to these Muslims, was an affliction from Allah that tested the individual and his family's faith. Many western fundamentalist religions view physical illness and disorders in a similar way. It is viewed as a sign that they have offended a deity or that their faith is being tested (Briggs, 1977). Because it is unlikely that traditional speech therapy would be an available or an acceptable avenue of treatment for these individuals, an increased prevalence of stuttering within these populations may be more related to absence of treatment, rather than to values that may be related to the etiology of stuttering.

Gender/Sex. There is unequivocal evidence that more males than females stutter in every society in which stuttering has been studied (Table 5–2). Early explanations for this occurrence involved reference to child-rearing practices. Schuell (1946) maintained that because parents' expectations for boys were greater than for girls, the resulting increased pressure on boys was a precipitating factor for the development of stuttering. Although child-rearing practices have changed since Schuell presented her hypothesis, there is no evidence that the gender ratio has changed. This constancy of sex ratio despite more equitable child-rearing practices has led many researchers to believe that the ratio is genetically determined (Kidd, 1980). The available crosscultural data also support this view.

Table 5–2.
Occurrence of Stuttering by Gender

Ethnic Culture	Source	Males	Females
Bantu children	Aron (1962)	3.28	1
Egypt	Okasha et al. (1974)	3.00	1
Poland	Glogowski (1976)	3.00	1
African Americans	Goldman (1967)	2.40	1
White Americans	Goldman (1967)	4.90	1
Americans	Brady and Hall (1976)	3.90	1

Language. The occurrence of stuttering does not appear to be dependent on native language, regardless of the language's phonemic structure. At best, the phonemic loci of stuttering may differ between each language, but the grammatical loci is constant (Bloodstein, 1987). Stuttering tends to occur at the beginning of words, phrases, and sentences. There is no evidence to suggest that the occurrence of stuttering is related to the native language of the speaker.

Age. Age is definitely a factor in the occurrence of stuttering. Prior to the age of 2 years, few cases of stuttering are reported. Disfluencies until the age of 3 years are usually identified as a normal part of speech. Bloodstein's (1981) comparison of the various onset studies indicates that a considerable amount of variability exists. Explanations for the inconsistency may be related to problems of parents remembering when the behavior began. A more reliable but less precise method of identifying the age of onset was used by Goldberg and Culatta (1991) when they asked stutterers about the onset of stuttering and grouped the data into two categories: (1) prior to 7 years, and (2) beyond 7 years.

Some general conclusions regarding age are possible. First, most stuttering occurs prior to the age of 7 (Goldberg and Culatta, 1991). Disfluency that occurs after the age of 7 is more likely to be psychogenic disfluency caused by an emotional trauma rather than developmental stuttering (Culatta and Leeper, 1987). The incidence increases from the beginning of speech to the beginning of elementary school (Bloodstein, 1981), when it remains fairly constant until middle or junior high grades, at which point a gradual decline through high school begins (Brady and Hall, 1976), continuing through old age (Andrews and Harris, 1964).

SPEECH BEHAVIORS

Crosscultural studies of speech behaviors have generally been limited to their occurrence within age ranges or various ethnic/linguistic groups. There is no published comparative data for the other six cultural groups.

Age

The literature presents extensive data differentiating stutterers from nonstutterers at various ages (Johnson et al., 1959). Data of this type become reference points for outlining the developmental stages of stuttering (Bloodstein, 1981). During its early stages, stuttering is less effortful and numerous than later stuttering (Van Riper, 1982). The form stuttering takes within various age ranges may have little relationship to maturation and more relationship with compensatory behaviors. As stutterers experience increasing negative speaking situations, new behaviors may be developed that the stutterer hopes will terminate the block or shorten a repetition. As one compensatory behavior fails, others are substituted or merely added on to the repertoire (Brutten and Shoemaker, 1967).

Ethnic and Language Groups

There have been some efforts to identify certain speech characteristics that occur more often in one ethnic or language group than in others. Leith and Mims (1975) found that interjections and modifiers may be more common in the speech of African Americans using black dialect than speakers of the standard white English reference group. By inference, this finding would imply that speech-language pathologists should take greater care not to mistakenly identify normal linguistic components of African American dialects as stuttering. Leith and Mims also maintained that fewer hesitations and prolongations are present because these speech characteristics were socially less acceptable within the African American culture. Montes and Erickson (1990) did not find any significant differences in the occurrence of stuttered speech behaviors in English and Spanish bilingual children. However, they did note that the type of disfluencies associated with second language learning were often misidentified as stuttering.

The difficulties associated with identifying culturally or linguistically related disfluencies was noted by Goldberg and Culatta (1991). In a nationwide study, they found that no particular stuttering pattern predominated among white Americans. It is quite likely that large-scale studies of various ethnic cultures will yield similar results. There is not sufficient data to make any generalization regarding the types of disfluencies most commonly associated with any ethnic culture.

HOW CULTURAL DIFFERENCES MAY AFFECT THERAPY

Cultural clashes or insensitivity on the part of speech-language pathologists can change or subvert both assessment and therapy. For example, one important determinant in the success of the diagnostic interview is clients' perceptions of clinicians. Not only is the professional competence of clinicians evaluated by clients, but also their worth as caring, protective, and supportive individuals. Many of these judgments are made on the basis of the clinicians' nonverbal and verbal behaviors, some of which are very obvious and direct, and others are extremely subtle. These behaviors derive their meaning from their own referent culture, and they often have a different meaning in other cultures. Eye contact avoidance, for example, which is a sign of respect for authority within the Japanese culture, could be interpreted as disrespectful within a white American culture and could result in the clinician misperceiving the client's intentions. The integral relationship between values and behaviors is one that is often unseen by the individual exhibiting them (Hall, 1959). Culturally sensitive clinicians not only must have a general awareness of their clients' cultural values, but also must understand how verbal and nonverbal behaviors will be interpreted.

Ethnic or National Origin

Ethnic identity for many individuals constitutes their dominant culture. It ties them to other individuals with common history, values, attitudes, and behaviors (Yetman, 1985). The commonality may involve physical characteristics, behaviors, language, values, or where they reside. It would be difficult for speech-language pathologists to become knowledgeable of all ethnic cultures. They should, however, familiarize themselves with the basic behavioral patterns of the ethnic cultures from which their clients are most likely to come. The east, west, and southern coastal areas, and large cities throughout the country have the most diverse ethnic cultures. On the west coast, for example, it is very likely that clients will come from various Asian, South Pacific, Central American, South American, Far Eastern, European, and African American ethnic cultures. In San Francisco, for example, the New Comer High School has students from more than 27 ethnic cultures.

Clients do not necessarily expect clinicians to be familiar with all aspects of their culture. They do expect and should receive the clinician's acceptance of their value system, and a basic understanding of the intent of verbal and nonverbal behaviors. There are many types of ethnic differences that can have an impact on clinical interactions. A review of the literature reveals five significant areas: (1) child-rearing practices, (2) learning styles, (3) emotions, (4) interaction rules and behaviors, and (5) referral patterns.

Child Rearing. Child-rearing practices are not only an expression of an ethnic culture's values, but also the primary method for its perpetuation. The father who instructs his son on how to treat his elders may be conveying both ancient beliefs and his own personal needs. The interplay of culture and parental needs has led some researchers of cultural diversity to re-examine theories of child rearing (Hoffman, 1988). Of primary interest to these researchers is to what extent the personal needs of the parents modify the teaching of a culture's traditional values. For clinicians, the issue is more than academic. There is much evidence to suggest that specific parental behaviors are conducive to the development of fluency, whereas others reinforce the continuation of stuttering (Egolf et al., 1972; Cooper, 1979; Costello and Ingham, 1984b). Culturally sensitive clinicians need to determine which behaviors are expressions of traditional values and which are reflections of individual parental needs and beliefs. Counselling parents to change individual child-rearing styles is easier and far less-threatening than asking them to change a behavior that is an integral part of their heritage. If counselling is to be beneficial, it must be compatible with the parents' culture (Saleh, 1986).

A similar sensitivity is necessary when treating young stutterers. Children, to a large extent, are products of their parent's behaviors and values. Critical comments directed toward their behaviors may unintentionally convey a negative assessment not just of them, but more cruelly, of their parents. By understanding that the cultural components of parents' child-rearing practices are expressed through their childrens' behaviors and values, the focus of counselling and suggestions for change can be more effective.

Even early identification of disfluencies that require professional intervention may have cultural concomitants. Studies of parental reactions to children's behaviors indicate that parents from various cultures will react differently to the same behavior (Zeskind, 1983). Whereas the stuttering behavior of a child in one culture may be viewed merely as a different form of speaking that requires little attention, the same speech pattern in another culture may result in shame to the family and an intensive effort by the parents to find help.

Learning Styles. Development of a more fluent speaking pattern usually requires learning new strategies and specific behaviors. It may necessitate decisions to engage in activities, monitoring of feeling states, or initiation of specific behaviors. The assumption has always been that these strategies and behaviors could be uniformly taught to clients. Whether one chose an operant approach (Shames and Egolf, 1976), a cognitive approach (Rubin and Culatta, 1971), a symptomatic approach (Van Riper, 1971), or any of the more eclectic approaches found throughout the history of stuttering therapy, an equality of client learning styles was assumed. Reinforcement paradigms were thought to be equally effective for all clients. The assumption was made that clients had the same ability to cognitively make a decision to be fluent, or that methods of bouncing, cancellation, and pull-out could be learned and implemented by all clients.

Recent experiments on children's learning styles reveal a very different picture. Research in crosscultural learning styles should not be confused with ill-conceived attempts to support arguments of genetic inferiority or superiority. On the contrary, the research offers explanations for why children with similar cognitive abilities from different cultures can have widely disparate scores on standardized tests, even when they are culturally balanced. For many years, two explanations for the differences were offered. One was based on genetics, and the other addressed the inappropriate referents used in some of the tests. It became disturbing for those who supported the inappropriate referent model to find that even when test referents were normed for different ethnic cultures, significant differences existed. What became apparent to researchers in the area of instructional technology (Cronbach and Snow, 1977) was that many of the ethnically normed tests did not account for different learning styles. Large scale crosscultural studies revealed that children have preferred, culturally dependent learning styles (Dunn et al., 1990). If children are asked to respond to a standardized test or to engage in a learning situation that is not compatible with their learning style, the outcome results will be negatively affected.

When teaching elements of fluency to clients, clinicians need to be cognizant of the most appropriate method of instruction. For example, whereas learning through repetition may be effective with Japanese children, it could prove to be less useful with Mexican children (Resendiz and Fox, 1985).

Emotions. Stuttering can have an immense psychological impact on the speaker. It is a disorder that the person can rarely escape, because speech is so central to our lives. An individual who maintains that his stuttered speech has no effect on his life is either deceitful, unaware, defensive, or lives in a fantasized world. There is no question that stutterers experience strong feelings about their speech. However, the feelings individuals have about their problem may to a large extent be related to their culture and to the reactions of those individuals within that society. One would expect, for example, that an individual from a society that places great importance on fluent speech, such as the Japanese, would feel differently about the problem than someone from a Central American culture in which basic survival is not as dependant on communication skills.

Understanding how the members of each culture express various emotions can be an enormous benefit when interpreting a client's statements or responses. For many Asian cultures, outward display of certain emotions with nonfamily members would be unthinkable (Cheng, 1987), whereas the same emotions might be freely displayed by African Americans (Taylor, in press) or Hispanics (Ramirez and Castaneda, 1974). Although the feelings may be identical for each client, their culture dictates how their feelings will be displayed.

Interaction Rules and Behaviors. Individuals bring into the clinic their own cultural rules of interaction. Although specific differences can be found between various microcultures, the greatest differences exist between Eastern and Western cultures (Farver and Howes, 1988). Compare, for example, the Indian and American methods of introduction. In India, the hands are clasped together and the head is bowed, signifying a reference for the divine in the person who is being met (Campbell, 1988). Contrast this with the Western custom of extending an open hand and looking directly at the person, which is thought to be symbolic of showing the person being greeted that the greeter has no weapons. The hand clasping of India and the extended open hand of the Western cultures both signify a greeting. Yet, each contains within it a vastly different history and communicative intent.

Interaction rules are analogous to the syntax of a language: It gives form and structure to the interaction. The specific behaviors of the interaction are analogous to the words of a language. Understanding the interaction rules and the behaviors of a culture can reduce an enormous amount of communication problems.

Referral Patterns. Patterns of referral for children needing services are more complicated than merely objective identification of a problem. Some studies have found that an important determinant of whether a child is referred for special services is the cultural values of the individual responsible for making referrals (Lambert et al., 1989). Sometimes, children who are learning a second language have normal disfluencies that are often identified as stuttering (Montes and Erickson, 1990). Conversely, the cultural values of the person making the referral may place little importance on the presence of stuttered speech and may therefore allow the child in need of help to struggle alone.

Religion

During an average week in the United States, approximately 42% of all adults attend a church or a synagogue, and nearly 143 million individuals claim affiliation with a religious group (Gollnick and Chinn, 1990). Although religion for many people is a formal institution that has little influence on the development of their values and behaviors, for others it can have the greatest impact on their lives. Awareness of a client's religious values can be important in avoiding embarrassing situations that might have a negative impact on the therapeutic relationship. Knowing that a client has strong Mormon values would prevent clinicians from offering a cup of coffee, because this beverage is forbidden by Mormon doctrine. Even having a Halloween party during the time designated for therapy might prove offensive to some fundamentalist religions who view the holiday as a form of Satanic worship. Similarly, scheduling an important clinical event on the last day of Ramadan would be viewed as insensitive by most Moslems.

Gender/Sex

Behavioral Expectations. The gender history of the United States has been one of clearly defined behavioral expectations (Frazier and Sadker, 1973). Little boys were expected to be dominating, strong, good at the sciences, and to love baseball. Little girls were expected to be sweet and nice, loveable, great spellers, and collectors of cute dolls. The behaviors taught to children were considered to be the method of indoctrinating values that would carryover to adulthood (Stockard and Johnson, 1980). As the social values of America changed, the expectations of children's behavior also changed. The values that were once considered to be "male" and "female" now have less rigidly defined boundaries for both children and adults. The implication for clinicians is that what is appropriate for young male and female clients is not a foregone conclusion, but it is dependent on individual differences and not sexual stereotypes.

Male-Female Interactions and Culture. A potential disruptor of the diagnostic and clinical processes can be role expectations for men and women. In white, middle-class culture, it is usually of no consequence for females in authority roles to ask direct questions of men who either individually or with their families seek assistance. Also, within the same culture, it is appropriate for male therapists in the privacy of the clinic room to inquire about very private family relationships. Neither of these interactions are appropriate in certain other cultures. For example, a female therapist questioning a male about his beliefs and practices may be seen as insulting and disrespectful without the proper explanation of why the questions are being asked. Or it might be unthinkable for a woman to share a clinic room with a male therapist and to discuss the intimacies of family relationships without her husband or another family member present. What might appear to be the intrusive meddling of a mother-in-law in one culture might be seen as fulfilling a matriarchal responsibility in another.

As is usually the case, sensitivity to the situation and tactful requests for guidance can often prevent clashes. For example, rather than asking a father, "how do you punish your son when he misbehaves," clinicians might say, "I need to understand how your household deals with discipline problems. I don't wish to criticize, just to understand. Could you explain to me how you express your displeasure toward your son?" Instead of ignoring the presence of a mother's adult female relative, clinicians may ask the mother if she would like her relative to come with her into the clinic room. Even within the session, clinicians must be alert to inadvertent offenses. In gathering data, we often focus on the most knowledgeable member of a family. For case history information, this is usually the mother or the female guardian of a child. In this situation, ignoring an accompanying adult male may prove to be insulting and detrimental to the entire clinical process. Sensitivity, common sense, and the ability to quickly confess and to apologize for inappropriate acts can often save a perilous situation.

Homosexuality. Gradual acceptance of homosexuality has allowed many men and women to openly express cultural values that in the past would have remained hidden. There is no available evidence that the occurrence of stuttering within the lesbian and gay population differs from that of the heterosexual population. It is imperative that clinicians be sensitive to the gender-specific values of their gay and lesbian clients. Conversely, clinicians should realize that one microcultural variable is not sufficient for understanding clients. Sexual orientation is only one of many cultural values clients bring into the clinical situation, and it is usually one that has limited importance in treating stuttering.

EVALUATION AND INTERVENTION

Culture can impact on the diagnostic evaluation in four ways: basic principles of interaction, construction and selection of test instruments and intervention protocols, procedures for gathering data, and procedures for presenting data.

Instruments and Protocols

Test instruments are usually based on normative data gathered from a target population. In the past, the reference group of speech and language clients tended to be white, middle-class Americans of various ages. With increased sensitivity to ethnic differences, standardized, age-related tests for language and articulation became available for African Americans, Hispanics, and Asians (Cheng, 1987; Cole and Deal, in press). However, in the area of stuttering, instruments have been differentiated only according to one culture, age. The acceptability of directly questioning members of various cultural groups may also affect evaluations and assessment outcome.

Age. Some test instruments are designed only for a particular age range, such as children (Shine, 1980a), adolescents, and adults (Woolf, 1967). A few modify the instrument to be appropriate for more than one age range. One example of sensitivity to age factors is found in the Behavioral Cognitive Stuttering Therapy program (Goldberg, 1981). Goldberg designed three different sets of interview questions for children, adolescents, and adults. Although the information desired by the interviewer is identical for all ages, each set of questions uses age-appropriate terminology, phrasing, and concepts.

Direct Questioning. In various stuttering assessment instruments, the task of clinicians is not only to determine the specific behavioral components of the disorder, but also to gain an understanding of how clients view the problem, the impact it has on their lives, and their feelings about it. One of the most important distinctive features that differentiates various cultures is how directly an individual is willing to discuss and confront openly an issue that is both embarrassing and debilitating. Stuttering is often both. In examining various assessment protocols, clinicians should be aware that although the directness of some instruments will result in obtaining unambiguous information with certain clients, it can also result in deliberate attempts to distort information with others.

Although some of these client differences may be attributable to personality differences, cultural values may also be the cause. For example, during an assessment, one of the authors was attempting to determine if a Filipino client believed his stuttering was seriously affecting the ability to find a satisfying job. In response to the direct question "is your stuttering preventing you from satisfying your employment goals?" the client responded with "no, not really." Yet when asked a very similar question through the use of a five-point rating scale, the client circled "5," indicating that stuttering was a problem significantly impacting on his employment. After being in therapy for many weeks, the clinician asked the client to explain the discrepancy. The client responded that in his culture it was not appropriate to openly state that one's own behavior was preventing success. The use of the rating scale, however, was more acceptable. There are no hard and fast rules for when to be direct and when to be indirect. The more familiar clinicians are with the cultures of their clients, the more likely appropriate decisions will be made.

Procedures for Gathering Data

Assessment procedures presented in Chapter 4 should be viewed as models amenable to change based on individual and cultural variability of clients. Modifications may be necessary in the areas of (1) obtaining a case history, (2) requiring the client to engage in activities that elicit stuttering, and (3) use of a translator.

Obtaining a Case History.   Obtaining a case history may be viewed by clinicians as critical, but by some clients, it is viewed as embarrassing or traumatic. For example, when asked to describe her child's developmental history, the Laotian mother through a translator responded with limited information. According to the translator, she said that everything developed normally. Following the session, the translator told the clinician that for the mother to provide the information requested, she would have had to describe the horrific events her son was required to endure before they escaped their country. Not only would the description be traumatic for the mother, but also it would have caused her to experience a terrible shame in the presence of a professional individual.

Not all cultures view traumatic or embarrassing occurrences as private events never to be shared with individuals outside of the family. One individual who began stuttering when he was placed in the Auschwitz concentration camp in Germany unabashedly related to the clinician the details of his parents' death and his own grim survival. For this individual, there was a historical and a cultural reason for never allowing the trauma of genocide to recede from his memory, regardless of how painful it became.

Engaging in Activities to Elicit Stuttering.   In the Stuttering Assessment Protocol (SAP), probes were used to determine if the introduction of specific techniques would alter the production of stuttering. Although use of these probes would be acceptable to most stuttering clients, they may prove to be embarrassing or threatening to some. A West Virginia coal worker who has a limited education may feel that being asked to read a passage is an attempt by someone in a higher socioeconomic class to reinforce the class differences that exist between them. An African-American woman who endured years of humiliation in the South and who now feels liberated might feel enraged when a verbal punishment resulted when she stuttered during the probe portion of the SAP. A Korean bureaucrat may find it unbearable to be asked to speak in the presence of four unknown individuals to determine how audience size affects fluency.

Many such problems involving cultural differences can be avoided by disclosure and explanation. Clinicians should explain that the purpose of the activities is to determine under what circumstances the client can produce the greatest amount of fluent speech and that they are not intended to humiliate or to embarrass them. Furthermore, if there is anything that the client would care not to perform, it would be acceptable and respected.

Use of a Translator. When using a translator to gather information, the individual is in a unique position to transform questions and requests into more culturally acceptable linguistic forms. This transformation can have both positive and negative consequences. Clinicians who insensitively ask an Iranian father if anyone in his family punished the client when she stuttered might have the question transformed by the translator into one that asks how people reacted to his daughter's stuttering. Although this change may prevent the father from walking out of the session, it may also distort the type of information the clinician will get. Translators should be instructed prior to the session as to its purposes, and they should also receive a list of questions that will be asked. Translators should be informed that although it is appropriate and desirable for them to transform questions into acceptable cultural forms, the intent of the question should not be distorted. In a movie a number of years ago, an American adventurer comes into a village in the South Pacific to find only one person who speaks English. After the chief requires the American to do something disagreeable, the American tells the translator to tell the chief that "he is the off-spring of a pig." As the translator talks to the chief, the chief smiles and indicates approval of what is being said. The American grabbed the translator and asked what he said. "I said that you would be honored if the chief would allow you to buy a pig for his esteemed mother." When asked why he did not relay the correct message, the translator responded that although he did not care what the chief did with the American, he too would be killed for even conveying such an insult. Translators need to understand that some of the questions they may be asked to convey can be embarrassing to the client or family. Although they should try to convert the question into the most appropriate form, the conversion should not distort the intention of the question.

Methods of Recording Information. Not all methods of recording information are equal in all cultures. In some South American countries, when an individual in authority begins writing down information on a pad, it may be the signal for adverse consequences. Use of cameras and videotape recorders is forbidden in cultures that believe these methods of recording result in a "freezing" of the person's soul. Use of video tapes to record the behaviors of children are viewed by some parents receiving financial assistance as ways of documenting inadequate parenting. What the speech-language pathologist might view as the best objective methods of recording data may conjure up images of more sinister objectives for the parent of a different culture. Many of these misunderstandings can be avoided by merely explaining why a certain method is being used and by asking if the client or parent approves.

Procedures for Conveying Information

In various cultures, there may be certain socially accepted rules as to when and how information is provided. For example, after asking a question about her child, an African American woman would probably not be satisfied with the clinician saying she will answer that question later. However, a Vietnamese woman who asked the same question might find the answer to be more appropriate.

If an interpreter is used, it is hoped that the information will be accurately conveyed in the client or the family's native language. If the client or the family is using limited English and the services of an interpreter are not used, clinicians should use a form of English that is simplified and nontechnical, and they should often ask the individual if he understands what is being said. The rate of speech should also be slowed to allow time for the individual to translate. Because some clients and their families may be embarrassed to indicate that they do not understand something, written information should also be provided. This approach allows limited English-speaking individuals to follow graphically what is being conveyed or asked auditorily.

SUMMARY

This chapter emphasized the importance of avoiding cultural clashes; it has been anecdotal in nature and sparsely factual. Readers might be tempted to ask why we do not wait until there is more data prior to discussing the impact cultural differences may have on service delivery. The answer is as simple as the demographics of speech-language pathologists. As of 1993, 91% of those providing services are female, and 94% are caucasian (ASHA, 1993). Although training programs, federal agencies, and ASHA are sponsoring recruitment programs, the trend for the past 10 years does not indicate that any significant changes have occurred or are about to occur (ASHA, 1993) in minority demographics. Yet the population we serve is multicultural and becoming more so every year. For example, in San Francisco, more than 40% of all school children are of nonwhite parents (California Department of Education, 1993). In Los Angeles, the percentage is even higher. It has been predicted that by the year 2000, the demographics of the entire state will begin to reflect that of Los Angeles and San Francisco.

This is not an isolated phenomena. Throughout the country, populations are changing, more rapidly in large cities than in small ones. But all are changing. Members of our professions clearly do not match the cultural and linguistic diversity of our country, and it is unlikely that the demographics of our profession will ever match that of the populations we serve. Fortunately, the provision of culturally sensitive, quality service is not dependent on matching the cultures of clients and clinicians. It is dependent on a willingness to appreciate and to accept the values of our clients' cultures.

Just as ignorance of the law is not a valid excuse in the jurisprudence system, ignorance of cultural differences cannot be a justification for providing ineffective or offensive therapy. We are a nation of minorities, with a multitude of dialects, primary languages, and cultural values. According to Orlando Taylor (1989), "clearly, communication disorders specialists will increasingly work with culturally and linguistically diverse populations who will bring to the clinical situation a variety of cultural and linguistical behaviors that differ from the Eurocentric and English-speaking norms that predominate in our field" (p. 73).

Culture, therefore, is the starting point at which any model of communication and therapeutic intervention must begin. It is the context in which all communication takes place. Its importance in understanding a client's language and behaviors and as a guideline for designing effective therapeutic programs cannot be overemphasized.

STUDY QUESTIONS

1. How do macroculture and microcultures differ?
2. Past studies attempting to relate cultural values to the occurrence of stuttering have been fraught with methodological problems. Describe them.
3. Gollnick and Chinn identify 8 types of microcultures. Describe how each can affect the process and outcome of therapy.
4. What information is known about the occurrence of specific stuttering behaviors in various microcultures?
5. What information is not known about the occurrence of specific stuttering behaviors in various microcultures?
6. Why is it important to differentiate between a parent's individual child-rearing needs and culturally determined child-rearing practices?
7. How may cultural learning styles affect the construction on intervention protocols?
8. Given the large number of diverse cultures that our clients bring to the clinical interac tion, what can you do to minimize misunderstandings and increase cultural awareness?

Variables Affecting Stuttering Therapy

Effective stuttering therapy involves more than just rote application of prescribed intervention protocols. Therapy is an intensive process that is often guided by variables external to clients and clinicians. In this chapter, we identify nine of the variables that impact significantly on what is done in therapy. These variables should not be viewed as all-inclusive. Rather, they are the ones that in our clinical experience can have the most dramatic effect on both the process and outcome of therapy. For organizational purposes, we ordered them chronologically in terms of the sequence of decisions that speech-language pathologists encounter.

THE INFORMED CLIENT

Although there is still much we need to learn about stuttering, there is a wealth of knowledge about the disorder. Stutterers and families often enter a therapeutic relationship with important gaps in their understanding of the disorder. Their view of stuttering may be based on information that is inaccurate. Self-evaluations may be inappropriately based on feelings of guilt related to how stuttering began or why it continues. A knowledgeable client becomes a clinical partner in the therapeutic process; a misinformed client may be a liability to therapy.

It is the responsibility of clinicians not only to answer the direct questions of the client, but also to provide information that may be beneficial in developing attitudes that enhance therapeutic progress. In the last 20 years, more than 1,400 research articles have been published on stuttering. Although some of the findings have been repeatedly validated, others have not. Some studies are of little immediate value to clients, whereas others may be of critical importance. The more controlled the study, the more likely the results will be unequivocal. These studies include voice onset, electromyographic studies (EMG), electroencephalographic (EEG) studies, and demographic data. The more environmentally or personality-based, the more likely the results will be equivocal. These studies include the effects of certain types of behaviors on the variability of stuttering or use of specific clinical techniques to increase fluency or to decrease stuttering. Both types of information can be shared with clients. It is a clinician's responsibility to determine what information will be beneficial. Some of the information that is known and may be beneficial to adult and some adolescent clients appears in Table 6–1. This information should be made available to parents and guardians of children and adolescents, along with the additional known facts that appear in Table 6–2.

Although we have learned much about stuttering, there are still many facts that need to be uncovered. Just as it is important to share our knowledge with our clients, it is also important to share our ignorance. When the available data or your clinical experience cannot be relied on to answer a client's question, it is important for legal, ethical, and therapeutic reasons to say "I don't know." Some critical topics about which we lack definitive knowledge are:

1. What are the causes of stuttering?
2. How or do environment and genetics interact?
3. What is the best treatment practices for a given individual?
4. What are the prognostic indicators for success or failure?
5. What are the effects of various parental practices on stuttering?
6. How is stuttering genetically passed on to subsequent generations?

Answers to these questions cannot come from unsubstantiated theories or clinical impressions alone. They require careful and deliberate research. Scholars in the area of speech-language pathology have labored over these topics for many years. Each topic has slowly given up bits of new information following careful study. Only by continuing research will our knowledge of stuttering increase and eventually benefit our clients.

WORK SETTINGS

Stuttering therapy is not conducted in a vacuum. There are five settings in which it usually occurs. Each of these settings may shape the quality of the interaction between the speech-language pathologist and the stutterer. Every

Table 6–1.
Information About Stuttering to Share with Clients and Parents

Stress and stuttering are not always related.	Reed and Lingwall (1976)
There is a greater likelihood of stuttering to occur in families of stutterers than families of nonstutterers.	Kidd (1980); Andrews et al. (1991)
Reinforcing the occurrence of fluent speech results in its further occurrence.	Halvorson (1971)
The frequency of stuttering is highly variable.	Bloodstein (1944)
Bilingual stutterers stutter more in one language than the other.	Nwokah (1988)
Elimination of stuttering will not result in the substitution of another "symptom-like" behavior.	Nurnberger and Hingtgen (1973)
For stuttering therapy to be effective, new behaviors and attitudes must be generalized.	Ingham (1980); Goldberg (1981); Craig et al. (1987)
If there is a physiological component associated with stuttering, it most likely is neurological, not motor or laryngeal.	Perkins (1981); Webster (1990)
Stuttering is found in almost all cultures.	Bloodstein (1987)
Stutterers have more syllable repetitions than word repetitions and more word repetitions than sound prolongations.	Yairi (1983)
Fluency is greater in situations where attitudes are positive.	Ulliana and Ingham (1984)
The larger the audience size, the more likely stuttering will occur.	Siegel and Haugen (1964)
More males stutter than females.	Morgenstern (1956)
Short-term intensive therapy appears to be equivalent to traditional forms of therapy in producing positive long-term results.	James et al. (1989)
Not all disfluency is stuttering.	Culatta and Leeper (1988); Kent (1983)
Disfluency that is not stuttering may not respond positively to traditional stuttering therapy.	Culatta and Leeper (1988); Kent (1983)
The length of time necessary to achieve maximal success is variable, although it appears that the more severe the stuttering behavior, the longer it tends to take to achieve fluency.	Goldberg (1981)
The use of drugs to treat stuttering is still not warranted.	Brady (1991)
Although cultural attitudes toward stuttering differ, there is no indication that the attitudes cause stuttering. Nor is it clear what relationship exists between cultural attitudes and the maintenance of either stuttering or fluency.	Bebout and Arthur (1992); Shames (1989); Stewart (1971)
There is no one best treatment program for all stutterers.	Chapter 9, this text; Andrews et al. (1982)
Neither children nor adults who stutter appear to be more anxious than children or adults who do not stutter.	Fink and Niebergall (1975); Kraaimaat et al. (1991); Miller and Watson (1992)

Table 6–2.
Information About Children and Stuttering to Share with Parents

Approximately 68% of children who stutter have other speech, language, or learning problems.	Blood and Seider (1981); Cantwell and Baker (1985); Homzie et al. (1988); Ryan (1992); St. Louis and Hinzman (1988)
Children who stutter rate their parents lower on control and hostility and higher on love and autonomy than nonstutterers.	Yairi and Williams (1971)
Girls begin to stutter sooner than boys.	Yairi (1983)
Approximately 1% of school-age children stutter.	Brady and Hall (1976)
There is no evidence to suggest that personalities of young stutterers are different than nonstutterers.	Baker and Cantwell (1985)
Stuttering children do not differ from nonstuttering children in terms of prenatal care, development, medical conditions, or general anxiety levels.	Cox et al. (1984)
Distinctions in speech between recovering and chronic stutterers become apparent by 20 months after onset.	Yairi and Ambrose (1992)
Stutterers are randomly distributed among the birth ranks.	Gladstein et al. (1981)
The frequency of stutterers in birth ranks before the proband and the frequency of stutterers in birth ranks after the proband are not significantly different.	Gladstein et al. (1981)
Stuttering children do not differ scholastically from nonstuttering children. Positive attitudes toward school develop with long-term stuttering therapy.	Bubenickova (1977)
Early intervention is important in the amelioration of stuttering.	Costello (1984b)
There is no clear indication that the motor speech abilities of stuttering children are different from those of nonstuttering children.	Healey and Adams (1981); Riley and Riley (1980, 1986)
The relationship that exists between stuttering and the linguistic interaction patterns of parent and child are complex and unclear.	Weiss and Zebrowski (1991); Meyers and Freeman (1985)
The more teachers know about stuttering, the more positive or realistic will be their attitudes toward stuttering children.	Crowe and Walton (1981); Nekrasova (1985); Yeakle and Cooper (1986)

work setting has its own unique features. There is no efficient way to completely describe each and every setting; however, there are enough features the various service provision facilities share that it is possible to evaluate their strengths and weaknesses and to suggest appropriate overall therapy approaches. Stuttering therapy is offered in five major settings: (1) public schools,

(2) hospital clinics, (3) university clinics, (4) private practice clinics, and (5) special intensive programs. Special intensive programs are available in almost every setting; however, we have set them apart because they usually share several traits, regardless of setting, that make them more like each other than the setting in which they are provided. Each setting has its own strengths and weaknesses. All too often the frustrations of a system can lead speech-language pathologists to focus on the restraints faced and to ignore the positive aspects of the job setting. This is analogous to concentrating on a client's stuttering and ignoring demonstrations of fluency.

Quite often the only way in which a speech-language pathologist can keep from being overwhelmed by the constraints of the job setting is to doggedly accentuate the positive. An old story seems very appropriate. Two little boys wandered into a pen that was four inches deep with manure. The first thought that he was in a terrible place to play and that there was no way to have any fun in such a horrible setting. His thoughts were of escaping this terrible place. The second surveyed the scene and thought "There must be a pony around here somewhere" and began an excited search for adventure. Somehow this tale seems very appropriate when describing some of the conditions we face as speech-language pathologists and the skills we need to be successful. This does not imply that we should blindly ignore the limits of our work setting and pretend we may implement any therapy program we wish. Indeed, ignoring the restraints of the work place will lead to improper selection of a therapeutic strategy and ensure failure. What is mandated is a clear appraisal and understanding of what can and cannot be attempted and how to structure a program that will be most likely to succeed. The goal of this section is to present examples of the challenges and strengths of various job settings.

Public Schools

By far, most of the service provided for children and young adults who stutter is school-based. In many ways, school-based speech-language clinicians face the greatest number of restraints in providing meaningful service to stuttering clients. Because the requirements of schools vary greatly, the challenges and strengths explained will not identically match every setting.

Challenges. We often visualize typical public school clinicians as being at the bottom of an upside-down triangle; not only the point of the triangle but its entire weight rests on them. As you go up the triangle, in our field, you have increased deniability. For example, speech-language clinicians in private practice may choose to see only those clients with whom they feel knowledgeable. Those working in hospital settings may be able to establish specializations that they rarely have to abandon. University clinicians and researchers can sometimes not only determine the exact type of client they wish to see but they can also refuse to see clients with whom they do not feel particularly comfortable. Not so for public school speech-language pathologists. By law (Public Law 94-142), they must provide service to all the communicatively handicapped in their school or schools. By definition, administrators expect them to be able to deal competently with any and every type of communication disorder that exists. Quite often they are encouraged to work prior to obtaining the minimal competencies required by the American-Speech-Language-Hearing Association (ASHA) by states that can hire them at a more economical wage than an ASHA-certified speech-language pathologist. Thus, in many instances, we have a bright capable person with little experience who has not yet finished her training who must face responsibilities that her more highly trained and experienced colleagues would never consider.

In addition, regardless of experience and training, many school-based speech-language pathologists face a professional isolation that can be numbing. In all but the largest urban school districts, it is not uncommon to have one or two speech-language clinicians per district responsible for all those with communication disorders in that district. Rarely, if ever, is there more than one speech pathologist in any given school. Immediate supervisors are quite often special educators with little understanding of the needs of the speech-language pathologist. Principals may be unaware of how speech-language pathologists differ from classroom teachers, and classroom teachers can be resentful and unconcerned about scheduling needs. Both the individual school principal and the nonspeech-language pathologist supervisor may apply unfair pressure for larger than manageable caseloads. The speech-language pathologist may also work in a physically isolated area in the school building, making it difficult to interact with the teaching and administrative faculties of the school. Factor in traveling and the mixed loyalties that being assigned to multiple schools imposes on speech-language pathologists, and we have a picture of a lonely, isolated, misunderstood professional who is not a classroom teacher but who works in the schools.

Clients may also come with their share of problems. Speech-language therapy in schools is one of the few settings in which clients are assigned or recruited for clinical intervention. Thus, school-based clinicians are often in the position of being the first to inform parents, administrators, and children that there is a communication problem. Parents often receive garbled, legally correct, but unintelligible forms with a "Special Education" heading informing them of their legal due process rights before they have an opportunity to fully understand that their child has a communication disorder and not necessarily an overall learning disability. It is quite common for parents to respond to administrative inquiries about the quality of special education services their children are receiving by reporting that their children are not receiving "special education service" only "speech therapy." In addition, quite often parents are simply not available for conferences, team meetings, or therapy planning sessions. Often the clinician's schedule is such that home visits are impractical on a regular basis. These situations can obviously lead to initially low motivation on the part of the client, especially if he or she is taken from art classes, physical education classes, or study halls for speech therapy.

Additional challenges may include a seemingly unending stream of scheduled and unscheduled breaks, such as snow days, school carnivals, assemblies, spring and fall breaks, fire drills, and summer vacations. Procedurally, school-based speech-language pathologists more than any other professional in our field face a bewildering array of forms and legal processing requirements. Unfortunately, if they are not ASHA-certified, they suffer further isolation. Culatta (1990) compared uncertified speech-language pathologists to mainland China before diplomatic recognition by the United Nations. Even though the field recognizes that there are thousands of service providers in the schools, some in desperate need of help, there is no formal mechanism to reach them. They do not formally exist because they are ineligible for membership in the most powerful and appropriate professional organization. Thus, many of their needs cannot be addressed by the almost 80,000 members of an organization that is dedicated to improving the lot of speech-language pathologists. Finally, they may have been trained at a university where instructors often have little experience in the school setting and evidence even less concern or understanding for the restraints under which school speech-language clinicians function.

That's a whole lot of lemons out of which to make lemonade!

Disguising or ignoring what is a reality for many speech-language pathologists does not alter the facts. Given this litany of possible problems, we must now look at the positive aspects of the school setting and derive an overall strategy that recognizes the limits of the setting.

Strengths. First, the bleak scene pictured does not describe all the speech-language pathologists or their work settings in every school. Many work with sensitive, understanding supervisors and caring administrators well aware of their needs and value to the educational process. Some school facilities are appropriate and conducive to optimal service delivery. In addition, approximately 46%, or 35,000, speech-language pathologists certified by ASHA (ASHA, 1993) provide services in the school setting. These professionals have access to special educational opportunities and a political structure provided by ASHA to continue to improve their professional lives.

A major advantage of working in the school setting is access to stuttering clients. Unlike other settings, distance and financial constraints are not as imposing on school-based speech-language pathologists. Busses bring stutterers and take them home. Within the restraints of a given case load, families can afford as much service as the speech-language pathologist chooses to provide. Peer-group interaction, if a part of therapy, does not have to be as forced as it is in other settings. It is also possible to observe stuttering clients interacting with peers, teachers, and other adults.

Ancillary services are obtainable for appropriate clients in the school setting. Social service referrals can be made and followed, as well as opportunities to select from a host of educational services ranging from special reading groups to informal conferences with homeroom teachers. Mandating of interdisciplinary and transdisciplinary teams encourages a team approach. Professional educators with special and regular educational skills are on the scene for consultation and feedback. Within reason, sessions may be client-driven and restricted to a few minutes in length when appropriate or allowed to go longer when needed, which can be of great value in transitional stages of carryover or generalization. Follow-up or generalization is most easily accomplished in the school setting, where assignment and monitoring of generalization tasks can be highly efficient.

Given this partial description of strengths and weaknesses of the school setting, let us attempt to outline general therapy strategies that might be effective. Remember, in this setting, as with all other settings, it is the responsibility of the speech-language pathologist to modify the methods she chooses to fit her work setting. Very few of the approaches available are custom-made for a specific job setting. To be successful, they must be meaningfully modified.

Guidelines. In most cases, the therapy should be child-based. Because families are often not available for in-depth participation, the structure of the therapy should heavily involve the child and his or her ability to modify stuttering behavior. Thus, programs that require a high degree of family involvement might not be best applied in the school context. Strategies must be considered which bring about early behavioral change that is meaningful to a client who might not be highly motivated during initial sessions. Techniques that suggest and initiate behavioral change help the client experience control and are more highly motivating than passively being the recipient of well-meaning lectures on the value of "good speech" in one's future life. Thus, the skills or beliefs obtained at each session should be able to stand by themselves so that the "danger" of leaving the child "stranded" in the middle of a therapy program is minimal. These guidelines can be used to devise therapeutic intervention strategies that can facilitate success and decrease both clinician and client frustration.

Hospital Clinics and Private Practice Clinics

Because hospital clinics, private practice clinics, and private practice share many of the same strengths and weaknesses, they are considered together in this section.

Challenges. Time, money, and distance are three of the major constraints of hospital and private practice settings. All three interact in the selection of appropriate intervention strategies. Because clients must either travel or be brought to sessions, usually after a busy school day, work day, or on a Saturday, sessions must usually be of uniform length and on a fixed schedule. In addition, the stutterer's ability to pay for services often dictates the intensity of the contact. A speech-language pathologist cannot often justify the time and expense involved in bringing a family 100 miles to conduct a short session, nor can she afford to travel that far to see a client for the same reasons. Similarly, few families can afford the economic strain of four $75.00 sessions per week. Peer-group observation and interaction can sometimes be difficult, and attempts to "bring in a friend" or go "out on assignments" are often clumsy, time-consuming, and unnatural. As a result, most of the information gathered by the speech-language pathologist is anecdotal in nature and suffers from the bias of being presented by the client.

There are other challenges that may not be shared by hospitals and private practitioners. The first is that some private practitioners may not have the access to social service personnel available in many hospitals. The second is that private practitioners may face the same type of professional isolation experienced by some school-based speech-language pathologists.

Strengths. There are many positive aspects of the hospital- and private practice–based setting on which speech-language pathologists can rely. Not the least of which is client motivation. Families are not often "assigned" to hospital clinics or private practice. Although a given child may resist the notion that he or she has a problem, there almost necessarily has to have been some family discussion prior to the initial appointment. Clinicians are rarely the first person to uncover the problem. Unencumbered by federal or state mandates to provide service, speech-language pathologists are free to set preconditions for treatment. Whether it be a commitment for family involvement, client purchase of a tape recorder, or simply mandated attendance requirements, clinicians have the right to terminate service for noncompliance.

Many hospital clinics have more than one person on staff, which facilitates the discussion of problems with colleagues and often provides insights into therapy strategies. The status of the speech-language pathologist is often enhanced by affiliation with a hospital or a recommendation by a respected referral source. This often provides both the clinician and the strategy she chooses some credibility with the stutterer. Although this initial credence cannot be relied on for very long, it often provides initial cooperation on which the speech-language pathologist can capitalize.

Guidelines. Speech-language pathologists in a hospital or a private practice often have the option to work with families as a unit or parents by themselves. It is conceivable that this option can be a very valuable tool in some circumstances. Programs may require an "orientation" period or some initial start-up time, because the clinician can be reasonably sure of client contact on a regular basis. Particular attention should be paid to carryover or generalization phases of programs because hospital-based speech-language pathologists or private practitioners may have limited opportunities to observe performance outside the therapy room. Programs and strategies that stress objective rather than anecdotal reporting of out-of-therapy session activities should be strongly considered. In addition, speech-language pathologists must take extra care to follow-up on dismissed clients because, unlike school-based clinicians, they will not "run into" former clients in the halls.

Although important in formulating a strategy, these guidelines do not appear to impose unbearable restrictions on the service provider in these settings. Obviously, there are other restrictions and benefits in these settings in addition to those mentioned. However, clinicians can identify and work around the restrictions of a specific setting.

University Training Clinics

Most university-based clinics are primarily training clinics in which beginning students, under the direct supervision of experienced supervisors, provide service to stutterers while they learn to be speech-language pathologists.

Challenges. The obvious weakness in this setting is the level of skill attained by the students prior to their contact with the stutterer. A related secondary problem is the quality and the quantity of the supervision provided by the clinical supervisor. The client must also survive the frequent change of clinicians as students progress through a variety of clinical experiences. The university academic calendar is often used in establishing clinic schedules, which means that many university-based clinics are not in operation for the full year. In addition, time is required to shuffle clients and clinicians to provide the experiences needed by student-clinicians, and, as a result, it is rare that clinics are in session for even the full academic term. University clinics may also be less facile in their abilities to make appropriate social service referrals. The status of the clinician-in-training, as well as the understanding that service is being provided at a "training clinic," can lead to a lack of respect for the service provided. This lack of respect is often mirrored in poor attendance and lack of commitment on the part of the client and his family.

Strengths. In a more positive light, university clinic settings offer some benefits to stutterers that cannot be matched by other services. In most instances, the financial abilities of the client are of little concern because many clinics are essentially public service operations supported by the university and student tuition. This means that intensive service can be offered, and many different types of schedule variations are possible. Student clinicians have a small number of clients for whom they are responsible and a relatively unlimited amount of time to plan for therapy sessions. They also have access to both supervisors and other faculty members interested in the particular client's communication problem. Parents and other family members are usually available and cooperative. It is not unusual for parallel programs or family support groups to be available at the university setting. The opportunity for parents to observe sessions and to participate is a major strength of the university setting. Many university clinics also run special summer programs that enable school-aged stutterers to maintain their therapy programs during the public school summer vacation period.

General Therapy Guidelines for University-based Clinics. There are two questions that university-based student clinicians must ask as they select an intervention strategy. The first is, "do I fully understand what I am attempting to do with this client?" The second is, "will I be assigned to this client long enough to accomplish my goals or does it appear likely that I will be removed from the case with no assurance that my plans will be continued by the next clinician?" The answers or attempted solutions and the ultimate ethical responsibility lies with the supervisor. In formulating the long-term goals for a client who stutters, it is the supervisor's task to make certain that the student clinician has a firm understanding of the principles involved in a specific therapy regimen. It is also the supervisor's responsibility to judge whether the student clinician is capable of providing the strategy as it was intended to be implemented. The second responsibility of the supervisor is to be as certain as possible that the academic term goals are realistic. The supervisor and the student-clinician should keep in mind that a program which emphasizes a steady progression of positive performance-based experiences is more likely to be successful than one based on a long-term relationship with the speech-language pathologist. Clients, especially young children, must be aware of the idea that a number of people are going to help them and that this is not because they are not "good clients." In fact, generalization and maintenance may be more easily enhanced through interactions with a number of clinicians. Regardless of the approach selected, it is also important that someone, preferably the supervisor, be available for consultation during breaks in the university schedule.

Special Intensive Programs

Special intensive programs usually involve training periods that span a limited number of days, but require daily prolonged contact between the stutterer and the clinic staff. Therapy usually takes several hours each day, requiring the client to engage in behavioral modifications or training activities in a variety of settings. Live-away speech camps for children and residential training programs for adults are typically special intensive programs.

Challenges. The major problems with these programs can be summarized very easily. Cost can be a problem; they are often self-supporting programs that must generate adequate funds to provide the level of service essential. Service must also be provided by speech-language pathologists trained in the specific therapeutic philosophy that structures the experience. Stutterers may also have to travel great distances to participate in these programs. In addition to the expenses for lodging and meals that clients must incur, these programs often must change normal family routines, at least for their duration. Special intensive programs are limited in their availability to the public, and they often have waiting periods and scheduling delays that may be of concern for parents and children in early or critical stages of stuttering problems. Although most reputable intensive programs attempt to provide for the carryover and maintenance aspects of therapy, their distance from the stutterer can present problems. In addition, referral to local speech-language pathologists cannot always ensure that the same or similar philosophy and therapeutic rational will be maintained, which may be of concern if clients suffer a relapse after completing the intensive program.

Strengths. On the positive side, many believe that the intensive nature of the therapeutic contact is critical to success (Shames and Florence, 1980; Ingham et al., 1972). The constant experience of control and positive behavioral activities under the guidance of an available speech-language pathologist can bring about rapid change. This change can often be highly meaningful to the client and his family. There is a short wait between sessions during these programs for either the client or the clinician. The client can easily monitor daily performance and get direct feedback about concerns. The speech-language pathologist can confer with other clinicians on site and ask for insights from others who share the same belief system. Scheduling, once the client is on site, poses no problems, because clients are available for all experiences scheduled. Specific interactions may be as lengthy or as brief as are needed. During intensive programs, the usual constrains of the "50-minute hour" are forgotten, and the stutterer and the speech-language pathologist are free to work on the problem. Because these programs require restructuring of family life and finances, parents and significant others are usually available and cooperative. The status of any given program, the length of time a client has waited to come to the program, and the commitment to attend usually lead to a high degree of client motivation.

Guidelines. Special intensive programs have a number of restrictions that must be met before they may be considered as viable alternatives to traditional treatment. The biggest concern of speech-language pathologists considering intensive scheduling is whether they can provide the intensive schedule necessary. Not only the clinician but also the client must be available. The clinician must also decide if an intensive program will allow the client time to adjust to the behavior change accomplished during the intensive work. Shames and Florence (1980) believe that an initially intensive schedule is valuable due to its ability to bring about rapid behavioral change, and that after the initial intensive period, a more traditional schedule can help maintain the change. The carryover and maintenance phases of intensive programs cannot be ignored. Clients cannot maintain the intensive level of contact or the possible dependence on the initial programs. Clinicians must plan for some form of prolonged contact past the initial intensive program itself. The danger to the client becomes one of rapid success followed by uncertainty and relapse. The client, remembering his initial success, often totally blames himself for subsequent failure and is hesitant to recontact the speech-language pathologist for needed follow-up help. Thus, the initial success becomes a burden that emphasizes current failure.

THERAPEUTIC APPROACHES

One of the first decisions that speech-language pathologists must make prior to treating a client is the manner in which therapy is to be structured. Therapy can be either directive, nondirective, or some combination of the two. These approaches differ in basic philosophy, methodology, and participant responsibility. They are more easily described than compared. Because most of the speech therapy provided is directive, this section of the chapter begins by discussing the underpinnings of a directive approach to stuttering therapy.

Directive Therapy

The underlying principle of directive therapy is that the speech-language pathologist's training, experiences, and insight make it possible to guide clients toward resolution of their problems. Directive therapy includes diagnosis, prognosis, baseline data collection, treatment plans, goals, objectives, contracts, exercises, and client evaluation. Problems are labeled and measured. Goals for the client are discussed and agreed on. A logical plan is conceived by the speech-language pathologist that leads in an organized way to a specific conclusion. Finally, success is evaluated in terms of achieving the stated goals.

Diagnosis. During the diagnostic session, speech-language pathologists gather and share information with clients. They share their insights and knowledge about approaches that might be used to change the stutterer's speech. Both immediate and long-range goals for therapeutic management are discussed. After acknowledging the client's input and analyzing the data, clinicians develop an individualized treatment plan.

Treatment Plans. Exercises and trial experiences are agreed on and performed under the guidance of the speech-language pathologist. Behavior during these and other speaking experiences is measured and compared with those measures taken during diagnostic baseline sessions to gauge improvement. When the stutterer masters the techniques suggested by the clinician and reaches some agreed on predetermined level of proficiency, he is dismissed from therapy. Periodic follow-up measurements are made to see if the agreed on behavior is being maintained. Although the ultimate responsibility for behavioral change is placed on the person who stutters, clinicians are responsible for showing the client the way to achieve goals. Speech-language pathologists judge adequacy of progress, need for new or different strategies, how and when activities begin, and when they end. In essence, clinicians take the responsibility to tell the client what to do to get better. The understanding is that if the client does what he is told, he will attain the behavior promised during the diagnostic interview. Although speech-language pathologists are sensitive to the needs and wishes of stutterers, they are in charge and they share their authority with clients as they see fit. The clinician is the director and has a master plan for the client. The plan is certainly amenable to client input, and although very little happens without client agreement, the pace of the sessions is usually dictated by the clinician.

Advantages. On the positive side are the definite, measurable goals that clients and clinicians can aspire to achieve. Their attainment can be documented and referred to in case of future relapse. The activities necessary to attain the goals are specific, and both clients and clinicians can be held accountable for attempting to carry them to a conclusion.

Disadvantages. On the negative side, this model of therapy can foster dependance on the part of the stutterer by shifting responsibility for at least initial modification away from the client and toward the clinician. "I'm doing what you told me to do, why am I not getting better quicker?" is a possible client question that places the therapist under pressure to continually provide strategies for client improvement. Client motivation and dedication to the process of therapy can be difficult to monitor when the clinician takes responsibility for leading the client through therapy. It is also an intimidating responsibility to take control of another person's behavior and become prescriptive in dictating behavior change. Finally, the directive clinicians can never be sure that the direction in which they guide clients is the one clients would have chosen if they were able to decide the plan of action most suited to their needs.

Most therapy provided for stutterers is directive in nature and is based on some set of underlying principles that will lead to various degrees of improved speech. The therapies outlined in Chapter 8 are examples of directive therapies. They each share a predetermined ideal of what both stutterers and speech-language pathologists need to do to help the stutterer improve speech.

Directive speech-language pathologists must also consider the role that the symptoms of stuttering will have in therapeutic strategies. How important are the unacceptable speech behaviors the client emits? Are they to be the main focus of therapy, a part of therapy, or possibly of no consequence to the treatment process? The diagnostic chapters of this book presented sample forms that could be used to describe and measure the overt symptoms of stuttering. A portion of the discussion dealt with recognizing both the existence of symptoms and differentiating between their differing forms. Some theorists and clinicians believe that we may control the disorder by reducing the severity of overt stuttering behaviors (Van Riper, 1973; Ham, 1986). Others believe that emphasis on the overt stuttering behaviors may be less important in a therapy process that focuses on the development of fluency. They argue that because clients can easily and rapidly produce various controlled forms of fluency without exhibiting stuttering behaviors, modifying these behaviors is of little value (Culatta and Rubin, 1971; Costello and Ingham, 1984b; Goldberg, 1983). A third group of directive therapists fall somewhere between the first two groups. These speech-language pathologists attempt to help the stutterer use as many of the behaviors he can to achieve fluency while attempting to simplify the stuttering (Cooper and Cooper, 1985; Peters and Guitar, 1991; Conture, 1990).

In general, those who believe that working to simplify the overt characteristic of stuttering is a productive way to control stuttering provide a symptom modification approach to their directive therapy. Those who believe that encouraging the stutterer to utilize more of the behaviors he performs when producing normal-sounding speech use a fluency enhancement model to treat stutterers.

The directive model is not the only model available to speech-language pathologists. Nondirective or client-centered approaches based on a significantly different perception of the goals of the therapeutic encounter are also available for consideration.

Nondirective or Client-Centered Therapy

Nondirective or client-centered therapy was developed by Carl Rogers (1942, 1951). Much of what we do as speech-language pathologists can be traced in whole or in part to the conceptualizations of Rogers. The manner in which we often talk to stutterers and their families has been filtered through the belief system of Rogerian nondirective therapy. A basic tenet of client-centered therapy is that the client brings to the encounter the ability to heal himself. It is the clinician's job to structure the therapy session in a manner that will facilitate client growth. The stutterer can realize his potential in the presence of a permissive therapist who understands, accepts and reflects the feelings the client expresses. The individual, not the problem, is the focus. The goal of therapy is neither to identify nor solve a client's problem, but rather to help the person gain insight into his behaviors so that he may better cope with them in an integrated manner.

What follows is a highlighting of some basic nondirective principles and the therapeutic techniques that have evolved from them. Although some of the philosophical underpinnings of nondirective therapy may not be instantly recognizable to speech-language pathologists, the techniques they produced should be recognized.

Clarification of Perceptions. Client-centered clinicians believe that client perceptions influence their behavior. Because only clients can fully understand these perceptions, it would be both inappropriate and futile for clinicians to attempt to label or explain to clients their own ways of perceiving their world. For behavior to change, perceptions must change. Intellectualization is no substitute for self-discovery. Telling a stutterer that his preconceived views of the difficultly of specific situations affects his speech is nowhere near as powerful as having the client realize this concept on his own. Clients cannot be expected to be told what to do and to mature as a result of the telling. Nondirective counselors have a bedrock belief that the client has the ability to direct himself and to find solutions to his problems. Rogers maintained that if a counselor believes that a client does not have the ability to reorganize himself, and as a result shifts to a therapy in which the counselor takes responsibility for client reorganization, the counselor confuses the client and subverts therapy (Rogers, 1951). Stutterers therefore are seen as people who have the innate capacity to improve and change their behaviors, including speech behaviors, in the appropriate therapeutic environment.

> One of the most revolutionary concepts to grow out of our clinical experience is the growing recognition that the innermost core of man's nature, the deepest layers of his personality, the base of his 'animal nature,' is positive in character— is basically socialized, forward-moving, rational and realistic (Rogers, 1951; p. 56).

In the nondirective or client-centered therapy situation, stutterers have the responsibility for their own growth, and sessions proceed at the clients' pace. The clinician totally accepts, without judgments and without qualifications, what the stutterer chooses to reveal. The clinician's role is to recognize and to reflect attitudes and feelings the client expresses. Speech-language pathologists hope to identify the feelings the client is relating. They then try not only to restate these feelings but also to clarify the theme the client is expressing. The goal is to help the stutterer perceive more clearly what he is expressing. For example,

Stutterer: I'm smart enough to understand that I'm making a big deal out of answering the phone, but I'm still scared when it rings.

SLP: You feel that your awareness of the situation should help you.

Stutterer: Yes it should, but I need to do more than be aware.

SLP: So you feel that simply being aware of a feeling doesn't change your behavior.

These probes help clarify without making the client defensive, and they will enable him to evolve his own coping strategies. These "insights" enable the client to attain desired goals of therapy. The stutterer will pass through several stages while gaining the "insight" needed to deal with his problems. Initially, the stutterer must be willing to accept the idea that help is needed. If he accepts the responsibility of seeking therapy, he will need to accept the responsibility for working on his problem. Speech-language pathologists can help define the situation by confirming the fact that they do not have the answers, but can provide a place where the client can work out his own problems. Speech-language pathologists should encourage expressions of feeling and keep from responding in any way that might block these feelings. For example,

Stutterer: Are you just going to sit there and repeat every thing I tell you? I'm paying you a hell of a lot of money to be my echo.

SLP: You sound angry.

Stutterer: You're damn right I'm angry. All we ever do in here is repeat what I say. How does that help me?

SLP: It sounds like you'd like me to come up with solutions to your problems. You know I'm not able to do that, but I'd sure like to help you find the answers you're looking for.

Speech-language pathologists accept, recognize, and clarify negative feelings by responding to the feelings rather than the content of the message. This acceptance results in the stutterer beginning to express more positive feelings. Positive expressions are accepted in the same nonjudgmental way as were the negative expressions. Clients and not clinicians will pick and choose the concepts that are most relevant.

Intermingled with this process is clarification of possible decisions and courses of action. The goal is to help the stutterer recognize his fears and clarify possible decisions, not to urge any specific actions. If successful, this process will be followed by positive actions by the client, which will lead to further insights. The stutterer will be more and more in control of his own behavior, and the need for the relationship will weaken and end.

Diagnosis. Nondirective clinicians have no need for diagnosis, prognosis, or baseline data. Symptoms are neither recognized nor measured. Actual speech behavior is discussed only as the stutterer sees fit. The client must be free to talk. Speech-language pathologists do not attempt in any way to explicitly guide the stutterer. Specific questions may uncover beliefs that the client is not yet willing to face and are therefore counterproductive to the process. Evaluation responses of either a positive or negative nature have no place in nondirective therapy. Judging a client, even in a positive way, can suggest that other material is not as valid and can potentially silence the client. Nondirective therapy removes the stutterer from judgments of all kinds. Stutterers may say anything they wish to their clinician, who accepts all statements without evaluating them.

Treatment. Examination of the process of client-centered therapy reveals the following sequence of events when therapy is successful (Hejna, 1960). At first, the sessions revolve around the reasons why the stutterer came to therapy. The clinician encourages free expression of feelings while the client tests to see if the clinician is really as accepting as she appears. In this way, the therapeutic situation is defined.

During subsequent sessions, significant material, often emotional in nature, is revealed while the clinician serves as a clarifier and a reflector for the stutterer. The client will then enter a period of self-evaluation and understanding. This self-actualization often leads to decisions regarding the original problem. Lastly, the stutterer will report the results of his positive actions and deal with their consequences.

Advantages. When successful, a client-centered approach places the responsibility for change on the most appropriate person in the encounter, the client. Therapy is not "done to him," but rather "with him" in the lead. Feelings of accomplishment necessary to combat the feelings of victimization stutterers often bring to therapy are a natural by-product of the process. Similarly, the issues selected and the order in which they are considered are in the control of the client. The speech-language pathologist has no agenda for the client to meet. The trust that the clinician places in the client is rewarded by the client's selection of an agenda that is most meaningful to that client.

Disadvantages. Obviously, nondirective therapy is not always as smooth a process as described here. Sometimes stutterers are unwilling or unable to accept the clinician's belief that stutterers have within them the seeds for their own solutions. The frustration encountered in the search can lead to client termination of the process. Nondirective therapy, by relying on client self-discovery, may be time-consuming as compared with other approaches. It is also difficult to use in situations demanding diagnostic reports and progress statements as prerequisites to continued services or fee payment. However, the concepts of client freedom of expression and speech-language pathologist acceptance must be considered when establishing a therapy protocol. As a field that endeavors to increase effective communication, we may not totally ignore the principle of nondirective therapy when constructing a strategy to work with stuttering clients.

AGE-RELATED CHARACTERISTICS

In this section, we attempt to delineate some of the special features that clients of different age groups bring to the therapy process. These generalizations may help speech-language pathologists select the most appropriate therapeutic regimen. Describing clients by age characteristics can be risky. Our intent is not to construct stereotypes of our clients; however, certain generalizations are appropriate, as any parent who has ever experienced the "terrible 2s" can verify. Like all generalizations, exceptions can always be found. Most speech-language pathologists have treated 40-year-old "children" and 4-year-old "adults." The four age groups described are:

1. preschool-aged children,
2. primary school-aged children,
3. teenagers, and
4. mature adults.

Preschool-aged Children

Generalizations. The joy of working with preschoolers is that most come to us without a history of failure in speech therapy. As a group, they are open to suggestions and they are willing to demonstrate the control that they have over the ways in which they can communicate. Even those with the most severe of presenting symptoms can quite readily manipulate their speech and take great delight in the results. The parents of these children are usually both available and concerned. The task becomes one of channeling parental energy into constructive intervention. We experience the best prognosis and the most options in dealing with preschool-aged children. Approaches ranging from increased contact with other children, fluency modeling, to creative dramatic and materials-oriented strategies can be useful. It is not often necessary to present these clients with long-winded explanations of the purpose for each activity presented. In addition, the restricted environment in which most of these children function make data collection and evaluation of progress a reasonable task.

Challenges. The most obvious drawback in planning a program for young children is the burden on speech-language pathologists to clearly explain the function of the therapeutic contacts to the young child in a jargon-free manner. This is sometimes hard to accomplish. It is our responsibility, regardless of the approach selected, to be certain that our preschoolers know exactly what we are asking of them and perhaps why we are asking it. Costello (1984b) differs with this opinion. She states that in her experience, it has been neither necessary nor particularly helpful to explain treatment strategies to very young clients. Explanations may actually confuse rather than help young children. Often simply directing their behavior with appropriate evaluative comments is sufficient.

In most circumstances, it is not only appropriate, but also more efficient to work directly with preschool-aged children. Costello (1984b) reports that if a child is old enough to use connected speech and to be diagnosed as a stutterer, that child is old enough to receive direct treatment to enhance fluent speech and to discourage stuttering. She reports that, for the most part, very young stutterers are not particularly difficult to treat.

Primary School-aged Children

Generalizations. The speech of primary school-aged children is often more difficult to change simply because they have had more time to experience fluency failure. Stuttering may not be a novelty but rather a companion of several years. These children may also come to thespeech-language pathologist with a history of previous therapy failure, and they may be more suspicious of attempts to help than preschoolers. They may also be carrying a heavier burden of guilt and helplessness than younger children. In addition, these children function in a larger environment with less parental influence than as a preschooler.

Challenges. It is more critical with these children than with younger children to honestly present therapeutic goals and a clear plan of obtaining them. These children are physically available, especially to school-based clinicians. Parents may or may not be available, which will help determine the focus of therapy. As a group, these children are still open enough and in many cases trusting enough of adults that significant inroads are attainable. They may not be initially motivated, but success in early therapeutic encounters can light the therapeutic fires quite easily. These children, more than those previously described, can begin to see the consequences of their communication problem. Although this insight may be uncomfortable for the child, it can provide the clinician with a motivational edge. The child's increased understanding of the problem may also make it a little easier for the speech-language pathologist to relate therapeutic strategies to real life changes. Although their environment has expanded, it is still controllable enough to simplify the tasks of carryover and maintenance for clinicians.

Teenagers

Generalizations.   A positive quality of these clients is that they understand the implications of behavior change. Once they experience positive changes, their youthful exuberance will often carry the therapeutic process forward. Even though they are fairly independent by this stage of their lives, the school environment can be used for many carryover and maintenance activities. It is more important to obtain early behavioral change with these clients than any described thus far. This change is critical both to motivate the client and to demonstrate that, regardless of past failure, behavior change and success are still a possibility.

Challenges.   The greatest drawback in working with clients in this group is the predictable negativism of adolescence. Speech-language pathologists will, initially at least, fall into "the not to be trusted" adult category composed of parents and teachers. They may represent to the teenager the very group with which they are least comfortable communicating. Stuttering may also make it impossible to achieve conformity in peer-group relationships. Rather than embracing the prospect of therapy, more often these stutterers would like to "wish away" their problems so that they might be like everyone else. They are also likely to have had several experiences with unsuccessful intervention attempts. Although these clients may still be under the nominal control of their parents, quite often, in reality, they function independently. The degree of independence from parents will obviously have an effect on the therapy strategy selected.

Adults

Generalizations.   The positive generalization we can make about these clients is that they are usually in control of their lives and the decisions that will affect their behavior. In many cases, they either voluntarily come to therapy or at least have a great deal to say about attending sessions. They are not, as the previous three groups often are, assigned to therapy by a concerned parent or teacher. In addition, these adult clients are quite often in pain. They have suffered with their disorder for years and are now motivated to do what it takes to gain control over their speaking lives. These clients are speech-language pathologists's allies and partners. Adult clients can often be counted on to "help" the speech-language pathologist to the best of their abilities. Even when resisting or subverting suggestions, adults can often understand the implications of their unwillingness to cooperate. However, the adult population is the most difficult to treat simply due to the chronicity of their problem. Along with the genuine desire that often comes for change, the chains of previous experiences often bind adult stutterers to attitudes about the difficulty of speaking and fears resulting from previous failures and humiliations.

Challenges. In many ways, adult stutterers are the opposite of preschool stutterers. Preschoolers need very little information and only the positive experiences of successful communication. Adult stutterers, however, need to experience successful communication in the context of a lifetime of stuttering and the philosophical and emotional changes they have made to accommodate their disorder. They have to integrate any new information with past experiences and somehow balance it with their current lifestyles. Sheehan (1970) wrote about the "iceberg of stuttering." He conceptualized the visible and measurable aspects of adult stuttering as only the tip of an iceberg, with the greatest portion hidden below the surface. The challenge with adult stutterers is to make the therapeutic experience whole enough to enable the client to make and understand the changes needed to modify not only a communication pattern, but also a lifetime structured by a disorder.

Clients in this group have had the longest amount of time to stutter. As a group, they have been able to devote the most time and energy toward making negative lifestyle changes to accommodate stuttering. They, more than the others, come to speech-language pathologists with the most tricks, avoidances, and the longest histories of fear, shame, and helplessness. They are also the most likely to have had several experiences with unsuccessful intervention. In addition, the complexity of adult living sometimes makes both scheduling of sessions and devotion to therapy difficult.

This section of the chapter attempts to share some generalizations about the four age groups speech-language pathologists are likely to encounter in their practices. As we stressed at the outset of this section, these generalizations, like all generalizations, break down when confronted by specific clients. There are children who need a great deal of information before they are willing to change, and there are adults who require little information. Some teenagers trust adults and have little trouble relating to speech-language pathologists; some primary school level children have had experiences that make them highly distrustful. The goal of this section was not to lock speech-language pathologists into a rigid categorization system, but rather to share the most likely characteristics they will find among and between the groups of stutterers encountered in practice.

PARENTS AND PARENTAL COUNSELLING

Donahue-Kilburg (1992) views the family as a "medium" for communication growth. It is the context within which communicative disorders can be diminished or strengthened. Although most therapists have asserted the primacy of the family in the treatment of children and adolescent stutterers, there is disagreement as to what should be the functions of parent counselling and how it should be done. Van Riper (1973) counselled parents to create a less stressful environment in which the child's stuttering was ignored, whereas Goldberg (1981) had parents directly reinforce fluency and indirectly punish stuttering. Both differ from Riley and Riley's (1984) approach that structures counselling to facilitate remediation of any of the nine components they believe are related to the development of stuttering. There are as many approaches to parent counselling as there are approaches to the treatment of stuttering. To compare them, it may be helpful to understand their relationship to counselling in general and to stuttering in particular.

General Counselling Principles

Counselling parents of stutterers should not be viewed as a special treatment area isolated from more general counselling procedures. It is a part of the therapeutic relationship that allows clinicians to establish an environment in which clients and family can change both attitudes and behaviors (Scheuerle, 1992) As shown in Figure 6–1, it is merely a subcomponent of general counselling procedures with all of its concomitant principles. General counselling approaches are based on a set of convictions about how people become dysfunctional, how they can best become functional, and the role the counselor has in the process. Some of these beliefs are based on facts, others rely on unconfirmed theoretical notions. Although few authors in the area of stuttering specifically identify the particular principles on which their approach is

Figure 6–1.
Hierarchies of Counselling

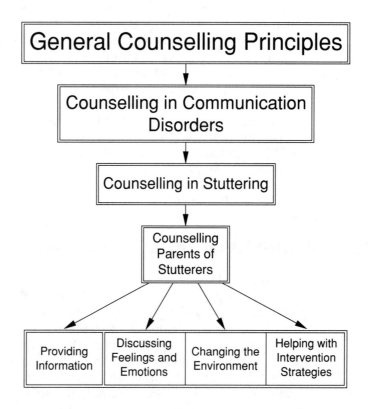

based, they are there, embedded in suggestions for how to interact with parents. Approaches may be as direct as rational-emotive therapy (Ellis, 1962), as introspective as Jungian therapy (Jung, 1968), or as nondirective as client-centered therapy (Rogers, 1951).

Although parent counselling is an important component of stuttering therapy, clinicians need to keep in mind that focus of all counselling activities is remediation of the communicative disorder. When counselling parents, there is always the danger that clinicians will be lured into providing suggestions for areas of parental concern that have little to do with stuttering (Rollin, 1987). Speech-language pathologists are not psychotherapists. They have neither the training nor the responsibility to provide general counselling for parents of stutterers. Discussions of parent-generated issues need to be within the boundaries of appropriate topics. These boundaries, according to Shipley (1992), should encompass issues that in some way impact on the communicative disorder. This does not mean that some feelings and emotions brought into the session can be cavalierly ignored. Rather, clinicians can either acknowledge their importance and indicate that they are not appropriate for the session, or they can be examined in relation to how they impact on the child's speech.

Counselling Parents of Stutterers

When counselling parents of stutterers, there are basically four things that clinicians can do: (1) provide information about the communication process and stuttering, (2) help parents understand their feelings and emotions, (3) ask parents to change the environment in which they are rearing their children, and (4) ask parents to help carry out specific aspects of intervention protocols. Not all counselling approaches give equal emphasis to these four activities.

Providing Information. Providing information about speaking and stuttering is the area in which there is most agreement among stuttering therapists. Quite often, accurate information is the best therapy. Parental guilt, hostility, defensiveness, and intransigence can be transformed into cooperativeness through education. There are many things we know about stuttering and many things we do not; both should be shared with parents. Some of the more common facts that should be shared with parents appear in Tables 6–1 and 6–2.

Discussing Feelings and Emotions. Many parents entering the clinical relationship bring to it emotional baggage that may be debilitating for them and their child. They may feel responsibility and guilt for the onset and continuation of stuttering. They may also feel inept as parents because they were unable to resolve the problem without professional help. Some parents also harbor resentment toward their child for being less than "normal." Regardless of what negative feelings a parent brings into the therapy process, the feelings should be confronted. Unresolved negative feelings can only hinder therapeutic progress. The methods chosen for dealing with parental feelings and emotions are usually determined by general counselling principles. These principles range from using an operant paradigm where positive attitudes are reinforced and negative attitudes are punished (Krumboltz and Thorensen, 1969; Shames and Egolf, 1976), to the use of role playing during which parents are encouraged to act out the feelings of others (Perls et al., 1951).

Changing the Environment. Parents are often asked to change the environment in which their child functions so that fluency may be enhanced or stuttering decreased. This is done as a form of indirect therapy for both developmentally disfluent children and chronic stutterers (Riley and Riley, 1984). There are many suggestions made to parents regarding how they should react to their child's speech. To parents, clinicians can say "don't interrupt your child," "allow your child to finish the utterance regardless of how long it takes," "give your child your full attention when stuttering occurs," "reduce your perfectionistic standards," "act calm," "don't call attention to the stuttering," "don't say the word stuttering," and "accept your child as a stutterer." Most of these suggestions and similar ones are based either on general counselling principles or theoretical concepts regarding the etiology and maintenance of stuttering. Few are based either on direct experimentation or extrapolations from experiments testing the effect of similar behaviors. In Table 6–3, a list of some suggestions is provided that have either an experimental or extrapolated basis.

Helping with Intervention Strategies. Most therapists would maintain that stuttering therapy is not just something that occurs during the clinical sessions. Rather, they believe that the success of stuttering therapy with children is very much dependent on parent involvement (Peters and Guitar, 1991; Conture, 1990; Cooper and Cooper, 1985). Parental involvement can be limited to carrying out suggestions of the type listed in Table 6–3, or they can be rather complex, including specific activities designed by the clinician (Ryan and Van Kirk, 1971; Goldberg, 1981; Riley and Riley, 1984). Regardless of the level of parent involvement sought, it is important that instructions are conveyed to parents in as unambiguous a manner as possible. Goldberg (1993) suggests that the following parent training strategy be used when asking parents to be involved in intervention.

1. Provide the parent with a description of one specific activity on a single typed sheet, in language devoid of jargon and adapted to the educational level of the parent.
2. With paper in hand, and after the parent has had an opportunity to read it, demonstrate for the parent the behaviors you wish them to perform.
3. With the parent, jointly perform the behavior.
4. Have the parent perform the behavior with the child and provide feedback; continue this step until the parent can perform the behavior without prompting or corrections.

Table 6–3.
Suggestions Provided to Parents for Environmental Manipulations

Suggestion	Illustrative Reference	Verification
Be consistent	Zebrowski and Schum (1993)	Numerous general articles on operant conditioning and the importance of applying appropriate consequences for specific behaviors.
Model slow speech when talking to children	Kelly and Conture (1991); Guitar et al. (1992)	Numerous general articles on the use of modeling as a method for emulation or self-monitoring.
Do not interrupt the child when speaking, especially if stuttering is occurring	Meyers and Freeman (1985)	On the basis of studies espousing the relationship between stuttering and anxiety.
Reduce nonspeech pressures	Sheehan (1975); Guitar et al. (1992)	See above.
Reduce speech pressures	Guitar et al. (1992)	See above.
Identify and increase fluency-enhancing situations	Van Riper (1973); Goldberg (1981); Peters and Guitar (1991)	On the basis of general and specific studies showing that fluent speech can be increased by increasing the factors associated with the occurrence of fluency.
Identify and decrease disfluency-causing situations	Van Riper (1973); Goldberg (1981); Peters and Guitar (1991)	On the basis of general and specific studies that show the occurrence of stuttering is reduced by reducing the factors associated with stuttering.
Remind the child to use an easier form of stuttering when a more severe form is occurring	Dell (1979)	Clinical impressions.
Reinforce the presence of fluent speech	Goldberg (1981); Ingham (1984)	On the basis of general and specific studies showing that reinforcement of fluent speech will increase its occurrence.

GENETIC COUNSELLING AND STUTTERING

The information currently available about genetic factors and the role of heredity in stuttering is beginning to impact on treatment. In Chapter 1, the overwhelming evidence regarding the role of heredity in more than 50% of developmental stuttering cases was presented. These findings should not be viewed as esoteric research data that have no relevance to clinic practice. A fundamental ethical issue is whether this information should be shared with clients and their families.

Information to be Conveyed

The first issue involves whether preliminary, but very solid evidence regarding the role of heredity in stuttering should be conveyed to parents. As discussed in Chapter 1, the data suggest that stuttering is a polygenic inheritance of a common dominant gene, with a multifactorial background and a sex-limitation mechanism (Goldberg, 1992). In other words, stuttering is caused by multiple factors that affect males and females differently and may skip generations. Admittedly, hard evidence for the causal relationship between genetics and stuttering is still unavailable; however, given the statistical occurrence of stutterers in families of stutterers and the occurrence of stuttering in identical twins, the relationship cannot be ignored. Offspring in families of stutterers are at greater risk for becoming stutterers than offspring in families without a history of stuttering. For clinicians, a decision to convey or to not convey this information can raise both ethical and possibly legal issues, and it can affect how parents view the disorder.

Ethical Issues. Given the knowledge currently at hand, is it ethical to withhold information about the role of heredity? Hard evidence may still be forthcoming, but incontrovertible statistical evidence is already available. Is the proper course of action to inform clients and their parents of this relationship? Specifically, because it appears that stuttering has a genetic component, should individuals who stutter and have a history of stuttering in their family be informed about the probability of their children becoming stutterers? Should a stutterer's parents who are thinking of conceiving another child be informed about the probabilities associated with their next child becoming a stutterer? The easy answer to this question for most people is that "it is not part of speech-language pathologist's responsibility to provide genetic counselling." Although this answer is technically correct, it is ethically misleading. It may not be the responsibility of speech-language pathologists to provide genetic counselling, but it is their responsibility to refer clients for appropriate services. If stuttering has a genetic component and speech-language pathologists do not do genetic counselling, then ethics requires speech-language pathologists to refer stuttering clients and their families to genetic counselors.

Legal Issues. Discussions of professional ethics are often transformed into the realm of law. Legal issues in the area of speech-language pathology have been primarily limited to contractual obligations, adherence to state and certifying bodies' codes of ethics, malpractice, and appropriate record-keeping (Silverman, 1983). If the cost of malpractice insurance is an indication of a profession's legal exposure to lawsuits, the practice of speech-language pathology has been mercifully spared extensive interactions with the legal profession. However, this respite may be disrupted as the information generated by genetic studies becomes more widely disseminated. Legal contentions could involve the concept of "disclosure," a new guiding principle in the practice of contractual relationships. According to disclosure laws, when sellers of property or services offer something for sale, they are obligated to reveal any and all conditions they have knowledge about that may negatively impact on the individual purchasing the property or service. In one highly publicized case, a buyer of a house successfully sued the seller for damages because he did not reveal that his neighbors were involved in the sale of illegal drugs. Establishments that serve alcohol now routinely post a sign indicating that alcohol consumption can lead to birth defects. Drug companies have for many years listed contraindications of their products. Gas stations post signs that inhalation of gasoline fumes has been shown to cause cancer in laboratory animals. Clearly, disclosure laws are fast becoming woven into the fabric of our society.

When the principle of disclosure is applied to stuttering therapy, various issues of legal exposure can develop. Take for example a case where a young adult woman is being treated for stuttering. During therapy the clinician did not suggest genetic counselling or inform her about the chances of conceiving a child who might develop into a stutterer. While having therapy, she conceives and eventually gives birth to a healthy baby boy. By the age of 4 years, the boy has developed all the classic signs of stuttering. The legal question would be, if the clinician knew of the probabilities associated with stutterers giving birth to children who would become stutterers and chose not to suggest genetic counselling or to disclose the information available on genetics and stuttering, can that clinician be sued for malpractice? Fortunately, at this point, this example is hypothetical; however, it is conceivable that in the near future legal issues relating to disclosure could become a major focus in clinical malpractice suits.

Parental Issues.   Many parents enter a clinical situation with guilt caused by believing that they were in some way responsible for the development of stuttering in their child. This belief may have been engendered by a variety of individuals, ranging from antagonistic relatives to well-meaning but uninformed professionals. To understand that their child's problem may be related to genetic factors rather than poor parenting can be immensely relieving and change a guilt-ridden parent into a valuable cotherapist. However, it does raise the concern of the parents that their child has a genetic defect, rendering the speech problem incurable and irreversible. It is the role of speech-language pathologists to bring balance to these seemingly opposing attitudes. Parents need to understand that a genetic predisposition toward stuttering is only a predisposition. Through active involvement by the family, the behavior can be greatly diminished and usually eliminated.

PREVENTION THROUGH EARLY INTERVENTION

Discussions of the prevention of stuttering need to begin with an understanding of basic terminology. In an official position paper of ASHA, it was suggested that speech-language pathologists adopt the health sciences distinction between primary, secondary, and tertiary prevention (ASHA, 1988). Primary prevention refers to preventing initial occurrence of a behavior; secondary prevention refers to treatment of a behavior during its very early identifiable stages; and tertiary prevention involves treatment of a communi-cative disorder to prevent other resulting behavioral disorders.

Although secondary and tertiary prevention have been addressed by many authors, primary prevention has received scant attention. In the last 15 years, little research has been done specifically on the topic (Gerber, 1990; Stark-weather et al., 1990). We believe that based on the information currently at hand regarding the relationship between stuttering and heredity, and given the mixed results of intervention at the secondary and tertiary levels, primary intervention should be an area of concern to speech-language pathologists. This concern can be expressed in the form of two questions: (1) is primary prevention a legitimate responsibility of speech-language pathologists? and, if so, (2) what techniques should be employed?

Primary Prevention as a Legitimate Treatment Practice

At issue is the concept of treating a child for a disorder that has not yet occurred and only has a statistical chance of occurring without any interven-tion. Specifically, if the available statistics indicate that a young child from a family with a history of stuttering has at least a 40% chance of developing into a stutterer, is it appropriate and ethical for speech-language pathologists to recommend preventative therapy for this child, who currently shows no signs of stuttering? Some perspective on the issue may be gained by examining how the medical profession deals with primary prevention. In the medical profes-sion, the concept of primary prevention is not only an accepted professional practice, but it is also willingly paid for by insurance carriers and government agencies. For example, providing prenatal care for expectant mothers is deemed important for preventing birth defects. Treatment of a mother with a venereal disease is proper medical practice to prevent the infection from being transmitted to the neonate during birth. It is expected that a physician would prescribe medicine to reduce the blood pressure of an individual with high blood pressure to prevent a stroke. If preventive practices in the medical profession can be seen as analogous to those in stuttering therapy, then it appears that primary prevention, even when the condition that is being pre-vented has only a statistical probability of occurring, is not only a legitimate professional activity, but also an ethical requirement.

Prevention Techniques

If speech-language pathologists are to be involved in primary prevention, then what types of activities should be recommended to the parents and what strategies used with the child? Unfortunately, there has been little written on the primary prevention of stuttering that can be used as guidelines (Stark-weather et al., 1990; Gerber, 1990). Suggestions for how to modify an early stutterer's environment tend to be based on ideology more than on research data (Gregory, 1984). Some have even suggested that most, if not all, popular suggestions given to parents have little empirical evidence to support them (Costello, 1984c). Possibly, the pragmatic clinical trial and error approach of

Starkweather (1992) is all that clinicians are currently left with when deciding what can be done with parents to forestall the development of stuttering.

Obviously, more factual information regarding the consequences of parental behaviors is needed. However, this area of research is woefully lacking in data. The following is a list of some research questions that need to be answered if primary prevention is to be a viable area of clinical practice in the treatment of stuttering.

1. What data-based advice should be given the parents of a child who is at risk?

2. Are there any specific speech modification techniques that should be used with fluent speakers who are at risk of becoming stutterers?

3. How should the environment be modified to reduce the probability that the child will develop a stuttering pattern?

4. When does a child who is at risk become an incipient stutterer? Can transition be determined by objective measurement?

If it is possible to prevent the occurrence of stuttering, then it appears speech-language pathologists have an ethical responsibility to engage in this form of professional practice, using appropriate factual information when available and engaging in research when it is not.

CLINICAL EFFICACY

Efficacy refers to the value and the effects of intervention protocols. It involves an examination of what we do for and to stutterers. It can be measured in terms of cost, physical effort, and psychological toll. In the simplest of terms, is the therapy worth the cost? Difficulties in answering this question are related to how outcomes are evaluated and measured. Baer (1990) suggests that those who are treated should determine what outcomes will become the measures of efficacy. In other words, let the stuttering client indicate to the therapist what should be accomplished in therapy. According to Baer, if the techniques selected can accomplish the task, they are efficacious; if they did not accomplish the task, then they are not efficacious. Although this approach is consumer-oriented, it assumes that the client has knowledge of the full range of outcome possibilities. Is it reasonable to expect clients to select a goal of fluency if they are unaware that it is a possibility? Even if Baer's unique approach was adopted, there are vast disagreements as to how outcomes can be measured (Ingham, 1990). For example, if the frequency of stuttering is to be a method of determining the efficacy of an approach, then it is necessary that moments of stuttering can be reliably identified. However, various studies have indicated that the task is not as easy as one would think (Young, 1984; Ingham, 1984; Kully and Boberg, 1988). Or, if "naturalness of speech" is to be the outcome measure, there would need to be general agreement about how the subjectivity of "naturalness" can be objectified.

Assuming that all these issues can be rationally addressed, then two questions regarding clinical efficacy can be examined: (1) is therapy better than no therapy? and (2) are some forms of intervention more valuable than others?

General Efficacy of Stuttering Therapy

Do we make a difference in the speech and lives of our stuttering clients? The answer received would depend on whom you asked and what you mean by a "difference." Some would maintain that when asked in this format, the question is unanswerable. However, if the question is transformed into the following two questions, then a meaningful discussion can follow: (1) is any therapy better than no therapy; and (2) is the level of success, regardless how one defines it, satisfactory?

Therapy Versus No Therapy. A number of years ago, there was a controversy between neurologists and speech-language pathologists regarding the efficacy of therapy for aphasic patients. Neurologists maintained that patients got better whether or not they received therapy during the first 6 months following the stroke. Through a careful study conducted at various Veterans Administration Hospitals across the United States, it was documented that even though most aphasics did improve during the first 6 months without therapy, those that did receive therapy improved significantly more (Wertz et al., 1981; Wertz et al., 1986). Efficacy in the area of stuttering therapy has not been as well examined as in the area of aphasia. One study, however, did look at the general efficacy of stuttering therapy. Andrews and colleagues (1983) believed the question of general efficacy could be addressed by employing a technique called "meta-analysis." They believed that the technique, often used to compare outcomes of different psychological approaches, could just as easily be implemented for comparing the outcomes of different stuttering programs. Andrews and colleagues examined more than 100 studies. They included a study in their analysis only if it met certain criteria. One of the most controversial aspects of the analysis was that the speech goals of improved fluency, reduced stuttering, and normal fluency were lumped together for the purposes of analysis. Their study revealed that there were significant differences in recovery between treated and untreated stutterers, and that there was great value in all of the approaches, although some were significantly better than others. They concluded that there could not be any question about the efficacy of stuttering therapy; it unquestionably produced significant positive results when compared with pretherapy conditions. Andrews and colleagues' study made it clear that almost any form of stuttering therapy is better than no therapy.

Outcome Satisfaction. Although few would disagree with Andrews and colleagues' conclusions that stuttering therapy in general is better than no therapy, there is concern if the results of therapy are adequate enough to justify its financial and emotional expense (Goldberg et al., 1992). Whereas a 50% success rate in articulation therapy for phonological disorders would be considered intolerable, a 50% success rate with stutterers using Andrews and colleagues' criteria would be considered laudable. The lack of critical self-examination becomes evident when looking at self-help groups. There are no self-help groups for individuals with lateral lisps, vocal nodules, or pragmatic linguistic difficulties. The formation of such groups would be viewed as ludicrous by our profession. However, self-help groups for stutterers are not only respected, but also receive the support of speech-language pathologists. The message is that for whatever reasons, professionals are failing more than a "comfortable" amount of time in the treatment of stutterers. These failures have resulted in many clinicians astutely avoiding doing stuttering therapy to minimize the clinical failures and frustration associated with not being able to help clients. This reaction may result in clinicians feeling better about themselves professionally, but it leaves many stutterers at a loss as to where to receive treatment.

Efficacy of Specific Intervention Programs

Are some intervention programs better than others or no therapy at all? Questions of this type tend to be more productive than asking if stuttering therapy in general makes a difference. As we have shown, therapy programs differ in a vast number of ways. To lump them together as Andrews and colleagues did offers little in the way of guidance to clinicians committed to treating stutterers. For these clinicians, the two most important questions raised are: (1) does this specific approach make a difference compared with no therapy? and (2) which of several approaches is most appropriate for a client?

Specific Approach Versus No Therapy. Studies comparing given approaches to no therapy usually involve references to spontaneous recovery, where stuttering disappears without any intervention having occurred. Sheehan and Martyn (1966) examined the value of stuttering therapy as practiced within public school settings. On the basis of their findings, they concluded that the type of therapy received in public school settings was no more effective than no treatment at all. Serious methodological issues posed many years after they completed the study raised questions regarding their findings. It does not seem fruitful to ask if the use of one approach is better than no therapy at all. Rather, questions comparing the value of programs and techniques have more clinical significance.

Comparing Programs and Approaches. The value of a program or an approach should be determined in relationship to specific clients. Some programs are written better than others. However, no program can be judged better than another with all clients. Comparing programs is not an abstract process; it should be based on experimentation and the needs of specific clients.

EXPLANATIONS FOR CLINICAL FAILURES

Although therapy is beneficial on a global level, for some clients, therapy does not work. Inevitably, the question is asked "who's at fault?" When fingers are pointed, they usually go in four different directions. Therapy failed because: (1) of the intractable nature of the disorder, (2) the client lacked motivation, (3) the clinician was not competent, or (4) the intervention program was inappropriate. How the clinician assigns blame for failures will have a fundamental impact on future clinical relationships.

Nature of the Disorder

Stuttering is viewed by many as a disorder distinctively different than other communicative disorders in terms of a clinician's ability to affect a meaningful change in its occurrence. Therefore, when clients are unable to achieve significant changes, it is argued that "that's what happens with stuttering." Some have argued that this belief has led to the demise of stuttering therapy, because many clinicians have little interest in treating clients who they believe cannot improve. By assigning the blame for clinical failure on the disorder, a sense of hopelessness and acceptance of a debilitating condition is conveyed to the client. This "let's do the best we can" attitude not only is limiting for the client, but it also allows the clinician and client to avoid examining other factors that may be contributing to failure.

Lack of Motivation

Blaming a client's lack of motivation for clinical failures is a classic reason used by some clinicians to explain why clients do not progress. Although the reason has been cited throughout the history of stuttering therapy, it gained added adherents when some learning theorists began to view stuttering as a purely learned behavior that continued only because it was reinforced. Although citing a lack of motivation may be appropriate for some clients, for others, it may obscure very different reasons for failure. Unfortunately for these clients, they may be convinced by their clinician to willingly accept the blame for failure. With repeated failures, the client's self-image as an incompetent communicator is reinforced. It is little wonder that stutterers who experience minimal clinical success and who are chastised for lack of progress drop out of therapy, especially if it is implied that their stuttering problems remain because of limited motivation. An excellent example of this problem appears in a study conducted by Goldberg and Culatta (1991). A questionnaire was sent to members of a national self-help group. More than 80% of those who completed the questionnaire felt they were currently moderate or severe stutterers. Of these individuals, more than 90% had been involved in stuttering therapy. Of these individuals, more than 70% no longer continued with therapy, even though they acknowledged they still had a communicative disorder that was extremely disruptive to their lives. For these individuals, the pain associated with clinical failures far outweighed its benefits. It is an important clinical maxim that we should initially assume clients are motivated to change their behaviors if provided the means to accomplish it.

Clinician Incompetence

The concept of clinician incompetence is one that is alluded to but rarely addressed in the literature. It was first confronted most directly in Sheehan and Martyn's classic article (1966) that maintained school-age stutterers who did not receive therapy fared no better or worse than school-age stutterers who received therapy in public schools. Although many people have raised methodological issues with the study, it did bring to the forefront a feeling openly expressed by many dissatisfied clients and quietly discussed by some clinical educators. Many clinicians have been and are currently inadequately trained to treat stutterers. With the recent elimination of ASHA's requirement for accumulating clinical contact hours with stutterers during graduate education, the problem will become more severe (Goldberg et al., 1992). Clinicians who question their own competence will most likely be tentative and possibly defensive, especially when the client's questioning or resistance relates to an area in which their knowledge is inadequate. When the competence of the clinician is questioned by the client, it is unlikely that the trust necessary for the development of a positive clinical relationship can ever be developed.

Use of Inappropriate Treatment Protocols

One of the more positive legacies of operant-based therapies is the philosophy that success and failure are meaningless terms for treatment provision. In their place is the concept that application of treatment techniques is either appropriate or inappropriate. Clients do not fail; clinicians must simply chose a more appropriate set of contingencies to modify (Shames and Egolf, 1976). Thus, the pressure is not one of finding a therapy that "will work," but rather modifying conditions so that stutterers can successfully modify their behavior. By assuming that the appropriate treatment paradigm has not been found, the negative feelings associated with the assignment of blame can be avoided. It is in evaluating the selection of treatment protocols that the assignment of failure should be initially placed, not only because it avoids making subjective judgments, but given the complexities associated with stuttering, it is the most likely reason why therapy fails.

SUMMARY

In this chapter, we described how eight variables can dramatically affect the course and outcome of therapy. Our intention was not to exhaust the subjects, nor imply that other factors could not impact on therapy. Rather, it was to call attention to how the dynamic relationships that exist between clients and clinicians can be affected by everything from work setting to genetic information. Therapy involves both process and content. In this chapter, some of the processes of stuttering therapy were examined; in the next three chapters, content issues are addressed.

STUDY QUESTIONS

1. There are many things that we know about stuttering and should be explained to clients and their parents. What are they?

2. What are the advantages and disadvantages of each type of work setting? How would these impact on the delivery of services?

3. How do directive and nondirective therapy differ? For what purposes should each be used?

4. There are certain general characteristics that are associated with age groups. What are these and how would they impact both assessment and intervention?

5. Describe the appropriate areas of counselling for parents of stutterers.

6. What are the ethical issues involved in the area of genetics and stuttering?

7. What is currently available for the primary prevention of stuttering?

8. In determining the efficacy of any given intervention protocol, what needs to be considered?

9. Clinical failures can be attributed to many factors. Describe each and explain how each assignment of blame could affect therapy.

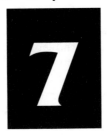

Intervention and Transfer Strategies: PROLAM-GM

Over the years, we have often heard well-intentioned but naive family members, usually grandmothers, tell their stuttering grandchildren some variation of the following: "Honey, don't work so hard to talk. If you believe in yourself, you can do it. Just remember to slow down, think before you talk, and keep it simple. But most of all, remember, no matter what, I love you." Is this charming folk-wisdom of no consequence or perhaps even harmful advice from meddling nonprofessionals? How does it compare with the techniques that have been presented in more than 50 intervention protocols published in the past 15 years? An examination of these treatment programs reveals six intervention strategies.

1. physiological adjustments (don't work so hard)
2. rate manipulation (slow down)
3. operant controls (I love you)
4. length and complexity of utterance (keep it simple)
5. attitude changes (if you believe in yourself)
6. monitoring (think before you talk)

Perhaps our professional sophistication is only a systematic and careful adaptation of information we all know on an intuitive level. And perhaps when all is said and done, the six major strategies outlined comprise the best treatment package available to stutterers. The acronym PROLAM-GM is useful as a way of organizing the various intervention and transfer strategies. PROLAM refers to the the intervention strategies, and GM stands for generalization and maintenance.

The first purpose of this chapter is to present each component of PROLAM, to provide a rationale for its use, and to describe general procedures for its application. We refrain from making judgments as to which of the PROLAM techniques are most effective. Each is appropriate for some clients. On the basis of our clinical experiences, we have concluded that many of the failures experienced by our clients result from inappropriate selection of intervention techniques rather than inherent properties of the techniques. For example, use of a technique with one client may result in complete unmonitored fluency, yet identical application with another client may result in dismal failure. Most of the current therapy protocols are comprised of some combination of tactics that rely on the six major categories named.

The second purpose of the chapter is to describe the GM components of PROLAM-GM, generalization and maintenance. Regardless of which strategy or combination of strategies we choose to treat a stutterer, the ultimate goal of therapy is to have the stutterer exhibit improved speech not only in the clinic, but also in nonclinical situations. A significant number of out-of-clinic failures are attributable to either absence of generalization and maintenance techniques, or poorly constructed ones. We believe that attention paid to generalization and maintenance in most intervention protocols is inadequate. At the end of this chapter, we provide both strategies and tactics that have been shown by various research studies to be effective in the establishment and maintenance of fluent speech.

Chapters 7, 8, and 9 are interconnected. In Chapter 8, summaries of 32 intervention and transfer programs are presented in terms of PROLAM-GM applications discussed in this chapter. In Chapter 9, a method for constructing individualized PROLAM-GM protocols along with an accompanying tutorial are presented.

PHYSIOLOGICAL ADJUSTMENTS

Physiological adjustment strategies are comprised of tactics that manipulate bodily components that are known or thought to be involved in the production of stuttered speech. An example would be the attempt to use gentle contact between the articulators when talking. The assumption underlying all intervention programs using this strategy is that the physiological components necessary for production of normal fluent speech are in some way used inappropriately when stuttering occurs. The therapy tactics used are therefore those that will result in a "readjustment" of the disordered component, or in use of compensatory behaviors and strategies. There are five types of physiological strategies: (1) phonatory adjustment, (2) stress reduction, (3) auditory feedback, (4) drug therapy, and (5) secondary characteristics elimination.

Phonatory Adjustment Strategies

Programs featuring phonatory adjustments are based on the premise that stuttering is the result of inappropriate phonatory behaviors, usually related to the onset of phonation (Borden et al., 1985). Purported differences in phonatory processes between fluent and disfluent speakers are based on research suggesting delayed voicing onset times for stutterers (Metz et al., 1976; Janssen et al., 1983). Although these delays may be related to various factors, ranging from laryngeal musculature anomalies to neurological processing problems, the intervention technique most often used to deal with laryngeal concerns involves reducing the abruptness of voice onset. The two techniques used most often in phonatory adjustment protocols are either initiating phonation in a very gentle manner (Webster, 1980), or beginning speech after exhalation has begun (Azrin and Nunn, 1974; Schwartz, 1977). A generic program for phonatory adjustments appears in Table 7–1. Table 7–2 represents a generic program for developing fluency by beginning speech after exhalation has begun.

Table 7–1.
Physiological Adjustments (Gentle Onset)

Step	Activity	Description
1	Initiation of effortless phonation	Instruct clients to phonate in a way that minimizes the possibility of completely adducting the vocal folds.
2	Incorporating effortless phonation within syllables	After clients have mastered the technique of effortless phonating, they incorporate the technique within the production of single syllables.
3	Increasing the length of responses	Following the mastery of fluent speech production of single syllables, the target response is increased, usually to single words.
4	Systematic approximation of normal fluency	Once clients are producing fluent productions of single words fluently and consistently using an effortless form of phonation, their fluent productions are shaped. With each subsequent step, normal fluent speech is more closely approximated.
5	Increasing the length of fluent utterances	The length of fluent responses is gradually increased from words, to sentences, to monologues and dialogues.

Table 7–2.
Physiological Adjustments (Speaking After Exhalation Begins)

Step	Activity	Description
1	Initiation of phonation	Instruct clients to inhale and exhale. Hand signals can be used when inhalation ends and exhalation begins.
2	Uttering syllables following phonation	Clients are asked to repeat step 1, but to utter a syllable shortly after exhalation begins.
3	Increasing the length of responses	Following the fluent production of single syllables, the target response is increased, usually to single words.
4	Systematic approximation of normal fluency	Once clients are producing fluent productions of single words fluently and consistently using an effortless form of phonation, their fluent productions are lengthened. With each subsequent step, normal fluent speech is more closely approximated.

Stress

Use of stress-reducing techniques is a common tactic in physiological adjustment protocols. They are based on the assumption that a specific component of speech production or groups of components experience a breakdown of normal functioning during psychological stress. This stress results in physiological changes, resulting in the occurrence of disfluencies (Wingate, 1962). Theoretically, the stress levels at which the stutterer's speech components "break down" are lower than those of normal speakers. Therapy that is based on this premise involves reducing stress levels of clients through a variety of techniques. The most frequently used techniques include: progressive relaxation (Jacobson, 1938), systematic desensitization (Wolpe, 1958), and visualization (Daly, 1988b).

Progressive Relaxation.   Progressive relaxation involves physical relaxation of the client followed by introduction of various speech situations. Clients are asked to tense one portion of their body and to then release the tension. The progression is generally from the head to the feet. As each new area of the body becomes relaxed, the client experiences deeper levels of relaxation. The rationale for using progressive relaxation is that by producing both a physical and a psychological state of relaxation, the threshold at which the physiological processes break down is increased. Various audiotapes are available that allow clinicians to use a standardized format, or to learn the sequence and to present instructions to the client in the clinician's voice. A generic program appears in Table 7–3.

Systematic Desensitization. Systematic desensitization involves use of hierarchies of stress-inducing experiences. Stutterers experience real or imagined situations divided into segments that run from least to most anxiety-producing. A stutterer with telephone fears, for example, may experience a hierarchy that begins with observing photographs of a telephone and then becomes more

Table 7–3.
Progressive Relaxation

Step	Activity	Description
1	Assuming a relaxing position	Clients either sit in a comfortable chair or lay in a prone position.
2	Easy comfortable breathing	Clients are asked to breathe easily and deeply, completely filling both lungs and then exhaling gently.
3	Facial muscles are relaxed	Clients are asked to visualize the tension in their face, increase it, then release it, visualizing all the tension dissipating.
4	Shoulders, neck/chest areas are relaxed	Same technique as in step 3.
5	Legs, feet areas are relaxed	Same technique as in step 3.
6	Whole body relaxation	Clients are asked to systematically go through each muscle group and identify any tension. When an area is identified, the procedures outlined in step 3 are applied.
7	Initiation of speech in relaxed position	Clients are now asked to begin speaking, still with their eyes closed, in a relaxed position.
8	Initiation of speech in a sitting position with eyes open	Clients are asked to speak with their eyes open in a more normal position.
9	Initiation of speech in a standing position	While standing, clients are asked to speak with the clinician.
10	Initiation of speech while walking	Clients are asked to remain as relaxed as possible and begin walking. As they walk, they begin talking.
11	Generalization instruction	Clients are taught how to initiate relaxation methods during their daily activities.

anxiety-producing through stages of seeing a toy phone, then a real phone, followed by a ringing phone, which is eventually held and finally answered. A sequence of hierarchial activities is arranged for each situation in which the stutterer reports a difficulty in maintaining fluent speech. The rationale for the approach is that by reducing or eliminating the stress-inducing features of various stimuli, such as large audience, the reflexive conditioning involved in initiation of stuttering will be deconditioned (Brutten and Shoemaker, 1967). The generic sequence appears in Table 7–4.

Visualization.   Visualization is a relatively new technique applied to stuttering that asks clients to visualize anticipated speaking situations in which they are

Table 7–4.
Systematic Desensitization

Step	Activity	Description
1	Assuming relaxing position	Client is asked to visualize a situation in which he or she is completely relaxed. This may involve progressive relaxation or visualization techniques. This step may be repeated in the beginning of each new session.
2	Presentation of a nonthreatening stimulus	A nonthreatening form of a feared stimulus is presented to the client and its effect on the client's level of anxiety is discussed. For example, the client who fears speaking to large groups of people is asked to speak only to the compassionate clinician. When the client feels no anxiety, the next activity begins.
3[a]	Systematic presentation of stimuli with increasing levels of threat	The stimulus presented in step 2 is slightly modified, possibly resulting in a slight increase in anxiety. For example, instead of having only the clinician in the room with the stutterer, a nonthreatening individual may join them. The anxiety-producing level of the stimulus is slowly increased through the use of various steps. Each new step is begun only when the client indicates that no anxiety remains.
4	Presentation of feared stimulus	The final presentation is of the feared stimulus. In this example, the client may be asked to make a presentation to a group of people.

[a]Can be more than one step.

in control and capable of speaking fluently or with reduced stuttering. The technique is similar to what athletes experience when they envision a likely event in a game, such as shooting a foul shot in a noisy arena. They not only place themselves into the situation, but they also "see" themselves performing successfully. Although visualization is relatively new in the area of speech-language pathology, its use has been reported for a number of years in other health professions (Korn and Johnson, 1983), in self-help literature (Sommer, 1978), sports psychology (Fetz and Landers, 1983; Hird et al., 1991; Vealey, 1986), and in general psychology texts (Samuels and Samuels, 1975; Paivio, 1971; Richardson, 1969). The generic sequence appears in Table 7–5.

Auditory Feedback

A number of years ago, there was an interest in determining if stuttering was somehow related to delays in auditory feedback. Specifically, if stutterers heard themselves speak a few milliseconds after they produced speech, was this sufficient to produce stuttering? Although many studies were done to determine if the auditory processes of stutterers differed from that of nonstutterers, findings appeared contradictory. Some researchers maintained that an unequivocal difference existed between stutterers and nonstutterers in terms of the amount of time required to receive auditory feedback (Toscher and Rupp, 1978; Hall and Jerger, 1978); however, other equally-qualified researchers found no significant differences (Hannley and Dorman, 1982; Karr, 1977).

Even though the findings were not conclusive, various intervention protocols were developed that attempted to provide the stutterer with a compensatory strategy for reducing the effects of impaired auditory feedback. Various devices were constructed that provided the stutterer with white noise or a

Table 7–5.
Visualization

Step	Activity	Description
1	Identification of problem	The client is asked to imagine and describe a likely speaking situation in detail.
2	Active visualization of the sequence	The client is asked to think of or verbalize the sequence of events leading up to the speaking situation. The client is to visualize his participation in the event.
3	Visualization of the successful completion of the event	As the client just begins to visualize his participation in the event, he is instructed to modify the scene so that it results in the successful use of fluent speech or fluency-inducing techniques.

rasping sound administered through an instrument that resembled a hearing aid (Dew et al., 1967). A typical device is the Edenborough Masker, which delivers noise to the stutterer's ears as he speaks (Dewar et al., 1979). The device has two components. The first is an ear piece designed to deliver the auditory signal, and the second is a signal-generating device in the form of a pendant worn around the neck and placed in the vicinity of the larynx. As the person speaks, a microphone picks up the vibration and generates either a rasping or a white noise sound to the ear piece. This noise somehow enables the user to produce fluent speech. A generic description of the techniques appears in Table 7–6.

Drug Therapies

As far back as the 1940s, therapists who used a medical treatment model had a long-standing interest in identifying biochemical differences between stutterers and nonstutterers (Hill, 1944). The belief was that if biochemical differences could be found, appropriate drug therapy could be instituted that would correct the problem. Most of the studies that found differences in the biochemistry of stutterers and nonstutterers found that those differences occurred

Table 7–6.
Auditory Feedback

Step	Activity	Description
1	Auditory feedback delivered at high volume levels	A noise is generated at a high level to the stutterer's ear immediately on initiation of phonation.
2[a]	Reduction of feedback volume	After the stutterer has been producing more fluent speech at desired levels, the volume of feedback can be reduced. This may involve a number of steps.
3[a]	Reduced wearing of the device	After the stutterer has been producing more fluent speech at desired levels, the amount of time the device is worn is gradually reduced. This may involve a number of steps.
4	Selective wearing of device	After the feedback volume and amount of time the device is worn is reduced, the stutterer is expected to be able to identify the specific situations in which the device is necessary. Only during those situations is the device used.

[a]Can be more than one step.

following an episode of stuttering (Moore, 1959; Edgren et al., 1970). Studies showing general differences not related to the actual stuttering response were either negative or disputed due to poor methodology (Hill, 1944).

There has been new interest in exploring the possibility that stuttering can be diminished or eliminated through the use of antidepressants that affect brain chemistry. Stager and colleagues (1994) compared the use of clomipramine and desipramine in the treatment of stuttering. They found that clomipramine was more effective than desipramine with some patients, whereas neither drug resulted in any significant changes in level of fluency under controlled situations in other clients. Stuttering was eliminated in none of the subjects. It is still premature to judge the long-term effectiveness of the various drugs being studied. Currently, use of medications to treat stuttering either has not produced notable success or has reduced the levels of stuttering temporarily. A generic sequence model is not presented in this chapter because use of various chemical therapies involves only drug administration.

Secondary Characteristic Elimination Strategies

Simplification of stuttering often requires that physiological modifications be made in the secondary characteristics that may accompany the verbal aspects of stuttering. These behaviors, such as eye blinks, head tremors, and bizarre limb or trunk movements, are the targets for those who believe that stuttering can be simplified. An example of an approach that calls for physiological adjustments of secondary characteristics is the Symptom Modification Approach (Van Riper, 1973). One of the tactics of this protocol is to have the client perform a "symptom analysis" of any and all secondary behaviors that might accompany his stuttering and then begin to eliminate or simplify them one at a time. A generic sequence of events is listed in Table 7–7.

RATE OF SPEECH MANIPULATIONS

Use of a reduced speech rate to modify stuttering has been recommended by many clinical researchers. Although there is agreement regarding its positive effects on reducing the occurrence of stuttered speech, there is disagreement regarding why slowing a stutterer's speech is an effective control (Ingham, 1990). Some researchers believe that reduction of rate results in simplification of the physiological speech processes, thus allowing easier synchronization (Perkins et al., 1976). Others maintain that reduction in rate of speech prevents the stutterer from anticipating feared stimuli that result in production of the stuttering response (Bloodstein, 1958; Goldberg, 1981).

Regardless of the rationale for its use, the methodology remains the same. The rate of a stutterer's speech may be reduced by (1) prolongation, (2) combining prolongation with continuous phonation, and (3) using an instructional rate control method.

Table 7–7.
Secondary Characteristics Elimination

Step	Activity	Description
1	Identification of secondary behaviors	Those behaviors that have nothing to do with the actual production of stuttering are identified. An individual program may be written for each behavior, or a program may include more than one behavior.
2	Monitoring of secondary behaviors	The client is instructed to carefully monitor the occurrence of each behavior and become intimately familiar with them.
3[a]	Elimination of the behavior	Various techniques are used to eliminate or reduce the severity of the behavior. These may include modifying the behavior into one that is less severe, or the use of positive and negative contingencies. More than one step may be involved.

[a]May involve more than one step.

Prolongation

Prolongation involves stretching out words by lengthening the amount of time required to produce each syllable. It may be at a very slow rate, such as 30 syllables per minute, or one that is significantly faster. A typical application of a prolongation strategy might use the following tactics. The client begins with a reduced rate, either modeled by the speech-language pathologist (Goldberg, 1981) or instilled via delayed auditory feedback (DAF) training (Golddiamond, 1965; Shames and Florence, 1980). Once the client is proficient, the delay is shortened and the rate of speech is gradually increased until it approximates a normal speech rate. The generic sequence appears in Table 7–8.

Combining Rate Reduction with Continuous Phonation

This technique is really a combination of rate reduction and phonological simplification. The sequence of combining the two techniques may differ with various approaches. Shames and Florence (1980), for example, ask clients to use both techniques simultaneously, thus prolonging a word and then using a form of continuous phonation with the final syllable of a word until phonation of the first syllable of the next word begins. By combining the two techniques, a continuous slow phonation occurs, resulting in a smooth nonstop transition between one phoneme and another. The generic sequence appears in Table 7–9.

Instructional Rate Control

It may not be necessary to require clients to prolong their speech to reduce their rate. Although Culatta and Rubin (1973) believed that rate reduction may

Table 7–8.
Prolongation

Step	Activity	Description
1	Extensive prolongation	The stutterer is asked to engage in a number of activities using an extensive amount of prolongation. It may approximate 60 syllables per minute.
2[a]	Reduced prolongation	As the stutterer successfully masters extensive prolongation, either producing fluent speech or reduced stuttering, the rate of speech is gradually increased. This may involve a number of steps.
3	Slow fluent speech	Eventually the client's speech is brought up to a speed that is slower than the original rate, but not slow enough to call attention to it.

[a]May involve more than one step.

be effective for increasing fluency, they did not believe that prolongation was necessary to achieve it. The rationale was that because stutterers were fluent for most of their speaking time, they already knew how to speak fluently. If they knew how to speak fluently, there was no need to shape fluent speech through the use of any successive approximation techniques, including prolongation. Therefore, if rate reduction was necessary, it could be accomplished by instruction. The generic sequence for reducing speech rate without using prolongation appears in Table 7–10.

Rate reduction techniques have been used by clinicians for many years. Although the rationale for its use and specific forms may vary, the technique has been proven to be effective with a significant number of stutterers. Clinicians who choose to use this technique have available the three variations of rate reduction. Through careful experimentation, scientific clinicians will rapidly discover which of these techniques is best suited to their clients.

OPERANT CONTROLS

Operant behaviors are those behaviors whose frequency or probability of occurrence are influenced by the consequences they generate. Simply put, if a behavior is an operant, then what happens immediately after it occurs will affect the probability of its future occurrence. For example, if stuttering is an operant behavior, then its frequency of occurrence will increase if it is reinforced, and its frequency of occurrence will decrease if it is punished. The terminology and concepts associated with operant intervention techniques are precise, and they require a prescribed administration of specific objects and

Table 7–9.
Prolongation and Continuous Phonation

Step	Activity	Description
1	Extensive prolongation with continuous phonation	The stutterer is asked to engage in a number of activities using an extensive amount of prolongation. It may approximate 60 syllables per minute. The client is further instructed to have the end of one syllable flow into the beginning of the next.
2[a]	Reduced prolongation with continuous phonation	As the stutterer successfully masters extensive prolongation, either producing fluent speech or reduced stuttering, the rate of speech is gradually increased. This may involve a number of steps. Continuous phonation continues.
3	Slow fluent speech with continuous phonation	Eventually the client's speech is brought up to a speed that is slower than the original rate, but not slow enough to call attention to it. It is at this step that the client is taught to modify continuous phonation into a more normal pattern of breaks between words.

[a]May involve more than one step.

events. Therefore, we chose to provide readers with a brief description of the basic foundation on which operant stuttering therapy is based and then to describe the various generic intervention programs available. Students familiar with operant conditioning may wish to go directly to the generic program section.

Basic Terminology

The language of operant conditioning is critical because it defines how therapeutic strategy is administered. This review of basic operant terminology is presented to ensure that the reader and authors share the same vocabulary. The

Table 7–10.
Instructional Rate Control

Step	Activity	Description
1	Instruction to reduce rate	The client is asked to consciously reduce the rate of his speech below that which he routinely uses.

critical terms necessary for understanding the operant programs reviewed are (1) discriminative stimuli, (2) positive reinforcement, (3) negative reinforcement, (4) punishment, and (5) extinction.

Discriminative Stimulus.   A discriminative stimulus (S^D) is a behavior, object, or event, in whose presence an observable response occurs. An example of S^D would be a hand signal given by the clinician indicating to clients that they should begin using certain behaviors that will produce fluent speech. The fluent speech is the response (R). Within an operant paradigm, there are consequences attached to responses. Consequences can involve positive reinforcement, negative reinforcement, and punishment.

Positive Reinforcement.   Positive reinforcement (RF+) involves administration of a positive reinforcer contingent on a desired response. In the example, when the client used the behaviors and produced fluent speech, the clinician could have responded with "that's wonderful." Just because an event is an RF+ in one situation, does not necessarily mean it will be an RF+ in another. Something is an RF+ only if it increases the likelihood that the response will occur in the future or that when it appears it will be stronger. In the example, if in future speech the client's fluency increased as a result of providing praise, then praise would be the positive reinforcer, and the entire sequence of providing it would be the RF+.

In the example, the client is dependent on the clinician for reinforcement. Some protocols do not rely solely on external reinforcers, because reinforcement is dependent on another person. Although this approach may be feasible in the controlled therapy situation, it is hardly possible in real life. Thus, many programs attempt to have clients, when they are capable, provide their own reinforcement for desirable behavior. This approach is obviously more efficient and will more likely lead to longer-lasting behavior change because the client can be reinforced when the clinician is not present. This step in therapy will usually involve extensive discussions of the client's attitudes and feelings when they produce the desired form of speech outside the clinic.

The second move from tangible to intangible reinforcers is equally vital. Giving a child an M&M for each fluent word will satiate the child as soon as he or she is full and thus decrease the reinforcing power of the candy. Intangible reinforcers, such as verbal praise or self-satisfaction, can be provided as contingent reinforcers, with less risk of satiation. The critical issue with all positive reinforcers is that they be experimentally verified as being truly reinforcing. One cannot assume without measuring the consequences of their application that any contingent responses are automatically positive reinforcers.

Negative Reinforcement.   Negative reinforcement is termination of an aversive stimuli contingent on a desired response. It is a technique that is not used often in stuttering therapy, because it is more complicated to construct than other consequences. To illustrate it, the example used in the preceding paragraph needs to be modified. The desired response that the clinician wants from the client is still production of fluent speech through the use of specific behaviors. The clinician might design an aversive situation by refusing to acknowledge the client, by looking way, until the desired response was emitted. At this point, the clinician might initiate eye contact, thus terminating the aversive situation of ignoring the client.

Punishment. Punishment may be administered in several ways. One way involves direct application of an aversive stimuli. An aversive stimuli is anything that reduces the strength of a behavior or the likelihood that it will occur in the future. In our original example, the behavior the clinician may wish to suppress is the client's use of a faster-than-allowable rate of speech. Whenever the client exceeds a specific syllable rate, clinicians says "no, slow down, you're going too fast." The utterance is an aversive stimuli if it reduces the occurrence or strength of the rapid rate in the future. If it has no effect, then technically it is not an aversive stimuli, no matter how angrily it is spoken.

Another way to administer punishment is called a response cost. A response cost involves removal of a previously received positive reinforcer when an undesirable behavior occurs. Again, we slightly modify the original example. The client this time is a child. Every time the child produces fluent speech by using the specific behaviors that were taught, he is given a token. The child understands that at the end of the session, every five tokens can be cashed in for a small toy. Whenever the child fails to use the desired behaviors, a token is removed from those already earned.

Extinction. Extinction occurs when the reinforcing conditions that once followed a desired behavior are removed. Thus, if the only satisfaction our young client received from producing fluent speech was the token, then removal of the reinforcer would lead to eventual cessation of task performance, which in this case is fluency.

Basic Concepts

Appropriate Consequences for Behaviors. The two basic controls most frequently developed into intervention protocols are use of positive reinforcers (Shames and Sherrick, 1963; Halvorson, 1971) and use of punishment (Flanagan et al., 1958; Siegel, 1970; Costello, 1975). There is controversy as to whether use of punishment is an appropriate procedure to reduce stuttering. Some researchers maintain that punishment is effective in reducing stuttering (Costello, 1975), whereas others assert that when punishment used in isolation is removed, increased stuttering occurs (Janssen and Brutten, 1973). Flanagan (1986) maintains that the differences reported in various research studies may have been related to the strength of the aversive stimuli.

Systematic Application of Consequences. The effectiveness of operant controls depends on their systematic application. This application involves a specific definition of the behaviors to be manipulated and a schedule for presentation of the consequent behavior. Haphazard application to undefined behaviors can lead to strengthening of competing responses and ultimate failure of any program designed to change behavior.

Reinforcement Schedules. Reinforcement schedules can involve reinforcement for a specific number of responses or for a behavior that is occurring after an amount of time transpires. The first schedule type is referred to as a *ratio schedule of reinforcement,* and the second is known as an *interval schedule.* Ratio reinforcement schedules can be fixed or variable. It is fixed if the number of correct responses required to receive a reinforcer remains the same. An example would be a 4:1 fixed ratio schedule of reinforcement, where one token would be received for every 4 minutes of fluent speech. With a variable ratio schedule of reinforcement, a token could be received after 2 minutes, 1 minute, then 10 minutes of fluent speech.

Interval schedules of reinforcement involve providing a reinforcer for a desired behavior following a given amount of time. The interval can be fixed or variable. An example of a 5:1 fixed-interval schedule of reinforcement would be providing a token to a child if the first word spoken would be fluent after 5 minutes of elapsed time. If the interval schedule was variable, then the amount of elapsed time would be continually changing. Reinforcement schedules can be manipulated to accomplish various tasks. For example, continuous reinforcement may be valuable in instilling a new behavior. This approach may be modified later to a fixed or a variable ratio schedule of reinforcement once a behavior is in place. The advantage of ratio schedules is that they prevent satiation from occurring, and they make the behavior resistant to immediate extinction once the contingent reinforcer is removed.

Reinforcement Protocols

Most intervention protocols utilize positive reinforcement. Positive reinforcers can take the form of tangible goods, such as chips that are redeemable for prizes, money, or, most often, verbal praise. The reinforcement schedules can be fixed, variable, ratio, or interval. The mechanics of reinforcement described in the previous section apply to all intervention protocols utilizing reinforcement as a method of establishing a specific behavior. Where programs differ is in what is selected as a target behavior. Basically, four categories of target behaviors can be selected: (1) fluency, (2) fluency-enhancing behaviors, (3) speech devoid of secondary characteristics, and (4) desired statements regarding speech.

Fluency. Shames and Sherrick (1963) and Halvorson (1971) conducted some of the pioneering experiments in which fluent speech was directly reinforced. From these early experiments and their replications, various intervention protocols were developed. The assumption underlying these approaches is that both fluent speech and stuttering are operant behaviors; therefore, by directly reinforcing production of fluent speech, fluency can be increased. The generic sequence of these protocols appears in Table 7–11.

Table 7–11.
Reinforcing Fluency

Step	Activity	Description
1	Identifying initial and final behaviors	A determination is made regarding the level of fluency that client currently has and the level of fluency that would be considered the final goal of therapy. The level can be either in terms of the number of fluent words, expressed as a percentage, or a number of minutes.
2	Construction of a successive approximation program	With the beginning behavior and the final target behavior specified, a program involving small successively increasing steps toward the target behavior is constructed.
3[a]	Implementation of the program	The program is implemented, with specific success criteria specified for each step. The number of steps in programs varies.
4	Specification of reinforcing contingencies	Clinician- and parent-administered contingencies are specified.
5	Generalization of program	The program is generalized to nonclinical settings, with particular attention given to the transfer of clinician- and parent-generated contingencies to client self-generated contingencies.

[a]May be more than one step.

Fluency-enhancing Behaviors. Some protocols do not reinforce fluency directly, but rather reinforce behaviors that facilitate fluency. These protocols may include continuous phonation (Cooper and Cooper, 1985), rate reduction (Shames and Florence, 1980), monitoring (Goldberg, 1981), easy onset (Webster, 1980), or speaking after phonation begins (Azrin and Nunn, 1974). Some approaches use combinations of various fluency-enhancing behaviors. The rationale offered for reinforcing fluency-enhancing behaviors rather than directly reinforcing fluency is that the former provides a strategy for utilizing compensatory behaviors. Compensatory behaviors are behaviors the stutterer can use to produce fluent speech. Most protocols that incorporate fluency-enhancing behaviors are based on the belief that stuttering is not just an operant behavior, but that it also involves an organic or a neurological component. Because stuttering is not just an operant behavior, application of reinforcing contingencies to fluent speech will not be completely effective. The generic sequence for reinforcing fluency-enhancing behaviors appears in Table 7–12.

Table 7–12.
Reinforcing Fluency-enhancing Behaviors

Step	Activity	Description
1	Identifying each fluency-enhancing behavior	Fluency-enhancing behaviors are identified. If more than one behavior is used in the protocol, the sequence of teaching each behavior is determined.
2	Construction of successive approximation programs	A successive approximation approach may be developed for each fluency-enhancing behavior, or all behaviors may be worked on simultaneously.
3[a]	Implementation of the program	The program is implemented, with specific success criteria specified for each step. The number of steps in programs varies. Criteria may be specified either in terms of percentage of fluent words spoken or number of fluent minutes.
4	Specification of reinforcing contingencies	Clinician- and parent-administered contingencies are specified.
5	Generalization of program	The program is generalized to nonclinical settings, with particular attention given to the transfer of clinician- and parent-generated contingencies to client self-generated contingencies.

[a]May be more than one step.

Speech Devoid of Secondary Characteristics. Those who view stuttering as a combination of both operant and reflexive behaviors (Brutten and Shoemaker, 1967) believe that only the operant aspects of stuttering are amenable to operant conditioning. Reflexive behaviors differ from operant behaviors in that they do not involve volition, nor must they be learned. An example of a reflexive behavior would be the elevated pulse rate associated with anxiety. Brutten and Shoemaker (1967) stress that only the secondary characteristics that stutterers develop to prevent, terminate, or minimize a stuttering episode are learned. Thus, they are amenable to operant procedures. The remaining "core of stuttering" is conditioned reflexive behavior to be treated using techniques other than operant conditioning.

When positive reinforcement is chosen to eliminate secondary characteristics, the stutterer is reinforced for producing speech devoid of secondary characteristics. Reinforcement is not related to the level of fluency achieved by the client, but rather to elimination of secondary characteristics. In protocols that attempt to eliminate these behaviors, they are treated before any attempts are made at increasing fluency or decreasing stuttering. Protocols that involve elimination of secondary characteristics as a separate step usually view the actual stuttering behaviors as a combination of operant and reflexive behaviors. The generic protocol for elimination of secondary characteristics appears in Table 7–13.

Types of Statements. What one chooses to speak about is an operant behavior and is therefore amenable to operant procedures. In many approaches, what one talks about can be an important component of therapy (Egolf et al., 1972). Within some approaches, it is important that the client speak in terms of responsibility (Rubin and Culatta, 1971); in others, statements involving feelings of control are sought (Perkins, 1990a). Still others find it desirous that clients relate how they felt when they were fluent (Rollin, 1987). Reinforcement for the type of statements desired is usually overt; the clinician reinforces the client's responses through either verbal or nonverbal responses. Examples of nonverbal behaviors would be smiles and positive head shakes. Verbal behaviors would be in the form of statements such as "that was a very insightful

Table 7–13.
Eliminating Secondary Characteristics Through Positive Reinforcement

Step	Activity	Description
1	Associated behaviors are identified	The stutterer may have one or more associated behaviors. Each are identified.
2	Familiarization with the behaviors	The stutterer learns to identify the occurrence of each of the associated behaviors.
3	Reinforcement for speech devoid of associated behaviors	The stutterer is reinforced for speech that lacks the target associated behavior. When more than one associated behavior exists, a reinforcement program may be developed for each, or a single program may involve all.
4	Successive approximations	The program is constructed so that the length of time or the amount of speech produced is reinforced for successively greater amounts of speech or time.
5	Specification of reinforcing contingencies	Clinician- and parent-administered contingencies are specified.
6	Generalization of program	The program is generalized to nonclinical settings, with particular attention given to the transfer of clinician- and parent-generated contingencies to client self-generated contingencies.

comment," or "I think it's great that you realize that." The generic sequence for reinforcing specific comments appears in Table 7–14.

Punishment Paradigms

Use of punishment in stuttering therapy is controversial. Some have ethical concerns regarding the use of aversive techniques, whereas others question the basic premises on which punishment is based. If both issues and concerns can be adequately addressed, then punishment may be applied to reduce or to eliminate (1) the frequency of stuttering, (2) secondary characteristics, and (3) undesirable statements.

Basic Issues and Ethical Concerns. Although certain forms of punishment undoubtedly reduce stuttering within experimental and clinical settings (Costello, 1975), their effects tend to be short-lived and difficult to generalize (Siegel, 1970). On a theoretical basis, punishment is appropriate to use if three conditions are met: (1) the behavior to be eliminated is viewed as a purely operant behavior; (2) the clinician is comfortable in increasing the strength of the aversive stimuli until the behavior is eliminated; and (3) the use of punishment is viewed as the elimination of a behavior and not the development of a new behavior (Goldberg, 1993).

As previously mentioned, some clinical researchers view stuttering as comprising both operant and reflexive behaviors (Brutten and Shoemaker, 1967).

Table 7–14
Reinforcing Types of Statements

Step	Activity	Description
1	Identifying types of statements	One or more categories of statements are identified as being desirable of reinforcement. These may include categories such as control, responsibility, or positive feelings.
2	Determining if reinforcement should be covert or overt	The clinician needs, if appropriate, to inform the client that only certain types of statements will be reinforced. The choice usually made is that reinforcement is covert.
3	Determining appropriate reinforcers	The clinician needs to determine what would constitute appropriate nonverbal and verbal reinforcers
4	Application of reinforcers	With the occurrence of the desired type of statements, the clinician administers the appropriate nonverbal and verbal reinforcers.

The operant portion of the behavior are the secondary characteristics. The reflexive components comprise the actual speech behaviors, such as repetitions and blocks. For these researchers, punishment paradigms would only be appropriate to use for secondary characteristics, and not for the speech behaviors they believe involve an organic or a neurological component.

Ethical concerns involve not only issues of usage, but also the strength of the aversive stimuli. The notion of being committed to increasing the strength of the aversive stimuli until the behavior is eliminated is one that causes great discomfort to many people in the helping professions. If a frown does not work, is the clinician willing to increase the strength of the aversive stimuli to a disapproving comment, then onto a more negative statement, or even the use of physically aversive behaviors?

Finally, although one could argue that use of punishment is appropriate for elimination of stuttering because it is not teaching a new behavior, others would argue that if the components of fluent speech are more than merely the absence of stuttering, then punishment would not be sufficient to establish fluency (Goldberg, 1981). Also, the stutterer who is establishing clinical fluency through the use of punishment is left neither with an understanding of the components of fluency nor the ability to maintain fluency when the aversive contingencies are removed.

When punishment is used for elimination of specific components of the stutterer's behavior, it can take two forms; either direct presentation of aversive stimuli or implementation of response cost procedures. Presentation of aversive stimuli may be as mild as a disapproving facial expression, or as controversial as use of mild electric shock. Response costs are generally used with children who, after accumulating tokens or similar tangible items for fluent speech, have a portion of them removed after each stuttering episode.

Reduce or Eliminate Stuttering. Initial experiments involving use of punishment to reduce stuttering were quite controversial. Aside from the ethical issues involved with the use of aversive stimuli, many believed that because the primary stuttering response was thought to be a conditioned reflexive behavior, use of punishment would result in increase of the stuttering response, not its diminution. However, the experiments of Flanagan and colleagues (1958), Siegel (1970), Costello (1975), and others showed that stuttering could be diminished through use of aversive stimuli. A generic sequence for using aversive control appears in Table 7–15.

Reduce or Eliminate Secondary Characteristics. Behaviors developed by the stutterer in an attempt to reduce, prevent, or eliminate a stuttering episode are operants. Regardless of one's beliefs about the organic components associated with stuttering, all agree that these behaviors are learned and can be reduced or eliminated through aversive control. The generic sequence for use of aversive stimuli to reduce or eliminate secondary characteristics appears in Table 7–16.

Table 7–15.
Reduction or Elimination of Stuttering Through Aversive Control

Step	Activity	Description
1	Selection of aversive controls	Before beginning any activity that relies on aversive control to eliminate a behavior, the clinician should determine the mildest and strongest form of aversive stimuli to be used. Each step between the mildest and the strongest aversive stimuli should be specified.
2	Selection of target behaviors to be eliminated	The clinician needs to determine the extent of stuttering behaviors that will be eliminated. The decision may involve administering aversive stimuli after every stuttering episode or following a specific number of episodes.
3[a]	Successive approximations of target behaviors	If a decision is made to administer aversive stimuli following a specific number of stuttering episodes, then a program involving successive approximations needs to be developed.
4	Administration of the aversive stimuli	The program is implemented.

[a]May involve more than one step.

Reduce or Eliminate Undesirable Statements. Procedures that can be used for reinforcement of desirable statements were described in the section on reinforcement. The other side of the coin would be use of punishment for reduction or elimination of undesirable statements. A generic sequence of events for this paradigm appears in Table 7–17.

Summary

Every intervention protocol utilizes some form of reinforcement or punishment. In some approaches, there is a casual and nonsystematic application. In others, a rigorous protocol with specific reinforcement schedules is provided. Positive reinforcement of fluency and punishment of stuttering are the two most frequently used operant procedures for treating stuttering. Although they may be used in isolation, they appear to be most effective when paired in a given protocol. Thus, it is rare when punishment for stuttering is used without pairing it with positive reinforcement for fluency, especially with response cost programs that allow the client to "bank" numerous positive, tangible reinforcers for fluent behavior prior to subtracting them for stuttering

Table 7–16.
Reduction or Elimination of Associated Behaviors Through
Aversive Control

Step	Activity	Description
1	Selection of aversive controls	Before beginning any activity that relies on aversive control to eliminate a behavior, the clinician should determine the mildest and the strongest form of aversive stimuli to be used. Each step between the mildest and strongest aversive stimuli should be specified.
2	Selection of target behaviors to be eliminated	The clinician needs to determine if all associated behaviors are to be punished simultaneously or if a program involving the addition of each behavior will be used. The second decision involves deciding if aversive stimuli will be administered following each associated behavior or after a specified number of associated behaviors.
3[a]	Successive approximations of target behaviors	If a decision is made to systematically add associated behaviors to a punishment paradigm, then a successive approximation program will need to be constructed. If a decision is made to administer aversive stimuli following a specific number of stuttering episodes, then a program involving successive approximations needs to be developed.
4	Administration of the aversive stimuli	The program is implemented.

[a]May involve more than one step.

responses. In addition, research has suggested that punishment by itself does not seem to have lasting effects in reducing stuttering (Siegel, 1970). The matrix that appears in Table 7–18 offers readers a graphic way of identifying what occurs with each type of intervention protocol.

LENGTH AND COMPLEXITY OF UTTERANCE

Controlling the length and the complexity of a stutterer's language reduces stuttering and increases fluency. Experimental programs (Rickard and Munday, 1965) and clinical programs (Ryan, 1974, 1981; Mowrer, 1975; Johnson et

Table 7–17.
Punishing Undesirable Statements

Step	Activity	Description
1	Identifying types of statements	One or more categories of statements are identified as being undesirable. These may include categories such as lack of control, lack of responsibility, or negative feelings.
2	Determining if punishment should be covert or overt	The clinician determines if it is appropriate to inform the client that only certain types of statements will be punished. The choice usually made is that punishment is covert.
3	Determining appropriate aversive stimuli	The clinician needs to determine what would constitute appropriate nonverbal and verbal aversive stimuli.
4	Application of aversive stimuli	With the occurrence of the undesirable type of statement, the clinician administers the appropriate nonverbal and verbal aversive stimuli.

al., 1978; Costello, 1980) have utilized this technique to increase fluent speech. Most of the approaches combine manipulation of the length and the complexity of the clients' language with punishment of stuttering and reinforcement of fluency.

Length

Programs may begin by requiring fluent production of isolated vowels, consonants (Johnson et al., 1978), multisyllabic words (Ryan, 1974b), or two-syllable words (Costello, 1980) and then proceed in a logical step-by-step manner to longer and more complicated utterances. Most programs end with some type of timed fluent monologue. Usually the client is reinforced at each step for fluent utterances and remains at that step until criteria for advancement are met, at which point the length of allowable utterances is escalated. These approaches appear to be particularly powerful with children and adolescents. The generic sequence for this approach appears in Table 7–19.

Complexity

Manipulation of length of utterance is a simpler task for clinicians than manipulation of complexity, because linguistic complexity is a multifaceted concept that can be measured in terms of syntax, semantics, morphology, pragmatics, and metalinguistics. Programs that simplify the linguistic complexity of utterances rarely differentiate between these areas of language

Table 7–18.
Operant Paradigms for the Treatment of Stuttering

Activity	Positive Reinforcement	Punishment	
	Administering Reinforcers (Reinforcement)	Administering Aversive Stimuli (Punishment)	Withdrawal of Positive Reinforcers
Establishment of fluent speech	X		X
Establishment of fluency-enhancing behaviors	X		X
Speech devoid of secondary characteristics	X	X	
Increase in use of desirable statements	X		
Reduction of undesirable statements		X	
Reduction of Stutterings		X	X

(Stocker and Gerstman, 1983; Ryan and Van Kirk, 1971). The steps in the simplification usually involve at least two components, most often syntax and metalinguistics. Most programs provide suggestions and guidelines to help establish a logical progression. A generic sequence of steps for this approach appears in Table 7–20.

Table 7–19.
Generic Sequence for Length of Utterance

Step	Activity	Description
1	Deciding on initial and final length of utterance	The clinician needs to specify the initial and final step of therapy. The initial step will usually involve the production of a single sound or word and end with the production of sentences of a specified number of words.
2	Decision of sequential steps	After deciding on initial and final steps of the program, the intermediate steps are designed.
3	Implementation of the program	The length of the utterance is increased in small steps; movement from one step to another is dependent on the client meeting a specific criteria level.

Table 7–20
Generic Sequence for Complexity of Utterance

Step	Activity	Description
1	Decision on target behavior	The clinician needs to specify the initial and final step of therapy. The initial step will usually involve the production of a simple response, such as a single word response or a simple description of an object. The final step will involve more complex utterances, such as asking questions or providing responses to open-ended questions.
2	Decision of sequential steps	After deciding on initial and final steps of the program, the intermediate steps are designed.
3	Implementation of the program	The complexity of the utterance is increased in small steps; movement from one step to another is dependent on the client meeting a specific criteria level.

ATTITUDE

Stuttering has two major components: the feelings that accompany stuttering and the speaking behaviors that are the result of stuttering. According to some clinical researchers, treating one aspect and ignoring the other dooms any therapeutic approach to failure (Starkweather, 1980). Most of the programs currently available have some form of attitude manipulation either as a mandated component or as an optional branch to be used if needed. A clinician's decision of whether to attempt to modify clients' attitudes is often based on how the clinician answers the five questions posed by Shames (1986).

1. Is attitude change necessary or desirable?
2. Do all stutterers evidence the same negative attitudes prior to their involvement in stuttering therapy?
3. Should attitudes be worked on directly in therapy?
4. What comes first, attitude change or behavioral change?
5. Do all therapeutic protocols focus on the same attitudes?

Is Attitude Change Necessary or Desirable?

When attempting to answer this question, one finds very little in the way of data, but much logical opinion emanates from specific theoretical constructs. More psychologically oriented clinicians (Wolpe, 1958; Sheehan, 1970; Luper and Mulder, 1966) believe that appropriate attitudes are critical to behavior change. Van Riper (1973) states categorically that exploration of attitude change is the exploration of behavior change. Most other clinicians (Guitar and Peters, 1980; Starkweather, 1980; Shames and Florance, 1980) fall somewhere between emphasizing the need for both attitudinal and behavioral change for lasting success. Those adhering to a strictly operant view of stuttering (Webster, 1980; Ryan, 1986; Costello, 1984a) tend to focus on observable behavior and demand clear evidence for the need to adjust attitudes before attempting to treat them. Conversely, if a child has specific word fears, repeated production of those words in an acceptable manner may remove the fear and change the attitude indirectly. Thus, although attitudes must be taken into account, they do not always have to be faced directly (Shames and Rubin, 1986).

Do All Stutterers Evidence the Same Negative Attitudes?

Do stutterers share the same attitudes toward communication prior to therapy? Although there are a wide variety of positive and negative attitudes toward speech and stuttering, there is no indication that the beliefs of stutterers are homogenous or that speech-language pathologists can assume that clients hold specific beliefs simply because they are stutterers. However, there are many negative attitudes that, when present, can impact on the progress of therapy. Silverman and Zimmer (1982) document how speech attitudes can effect stutterers' lives in pervasive ways. In their study, stuttering students took little part in classroom activities, and they avoided speaking privately with teachers. As adults, they reported that they took jobs for which they were overqualified and experienced little success because of their inappropriate attitudes toward communication. Bloodstein (1960) believes that negative attitudes toward speaking develop over time. They are, in fact, criteria points that help differentiate stutterers developmentally. A reoccurring theme addressed in some protocols is the relationship the stutterer believes exists between stuttering, success, and failure (Goldberg, 1981). Confused attitudes about the general effects of stuttering might make therapy more difficult, even if they do not cause or maintain stuttering (Howie and Andrews, 1984).

Should Attitudes Be Worked on Directly in Therapy?

Can attitudes be treated directly? Clinicians must decide if a relationship exists between specific negative attitudes and clinical progress. Many clinical researchers believe that the relationship exists in terms of both what the stutterer brings into the therapy session and how it affects progress. Attitudes, according to Gregory (1968), result in predispositions that affect the way stutterers respond to intervention efforts. They are feelings that become part, due to emotional conditioning, of a personal belief system (Peters and Guitar, 1991). It is hypothesized that positive attitudes toward speaking can facilitate successful therapy. Conversely, negative attitudes about speaking may prevent adequate generalization of fluency (Guitar, 1976). Negative attitudes may take the form of experiencing stuttering with anger, fear, frustration, helplessness, feelings of victimization, or the belief that one's speech can be controlled by external factors. Cooper (1979) suggests that any program that does not at some point in its application assist the stutterer in assessing and clarifying feelings and attitudes about stuttering and fluency control is not only inadequate but also may be detrimental to the client. Howie and Andrews (1984) believe that if we can develop measures of attitude that predict outcome, perhaps we can identify those attitudes that place clients at risk.

In contrast, Costello (1984b) articulates the viewpoint of many clinical researchers by questioning the role of attitudes in precipitating and maintaining stuttering. She believes that it has not been clearly shown that adults entering therapy with negative attitudes are less successful in therapy. Nor does she think that stuttering children as a group evidence attitudinal problems that set them apart from their fluent peers. The resulting recommendation of these clinicians is to treat the overt behavior unless or until there is a compelling reason to deal with attitudes.

Perkins (1979) perhaps summed up the mixed feelings best when he reported that speech-language pathologists believe that maintaining appropriate attitudes is essential to the lasting use of normal speech and that this conviction is held by clinicians with little hard evidence.

What Comes First, Attitude or Behavioral Change?

Although behaviorists believe that attitude change is the result of behavioral change, their attitudinally oriented counterparts believe that attitude change can be brought about on a cognitive level, which makes behavioral change possible. There is no substantial proof that either view is inaccurate. Shames and Rubin (1986) suggest that there is nothing that prevents clinicians from simultaneously working on attitudes and behavior.

Do All Therapeutic Protocols Focus on the Same Attitudes?

No. The belief systems of speech-language pathologists often shape the attitudes of their clients. Currently, approaches that attempt to shape attitudes are based on three major belief systems. Some clinicians believe that the end goal of therapy is for clients to control their stuttering. Clients treated with this approach must maintain their identity as stutterers and prepare to spend their lives adapting to their problem. Other clinicians believe that the end goal of therapy is monitored fluency. Stutterers can now see themselves as fluent speakers, but only at the price of constant or periodic monitoring of their speech. The third school of thought hopes to instill normal fluency with no remaining concern about speech once therapy is successfully concluded.

Attitudes to Be Changed

If clinicians decide it is important to directly work on a client's attitude to facilitate successful accomplishment of the desired goals, then it is necessary to determine what goals should be selected. A review of the literature reveals there are essentially five types of attitudes, not all compatible, that clinicians attempt to develop in their clients: (1) acceptance of responsibility for behavioral change, (2) realistic understanding of both negative and positive effects of stuttering on the client's life, (3) acceptance of stuttering as a life-long condition, (4) acceptance of monitored fluency as a life-long condition, and (5) acceptance of nonmonitored normal fluency as a life-long condition.

Responsibility for Change. Williams (1979) writes that belief in external control leads stutterers to believe that other people can be the cause of their stuttering. For example, if a stutterer believes that the ability to control speech on any level rests in the hands of the listener, then exercising stressing self-initiated behavioral change may be difficult. Although the specific behavioral changes and goals vary among programs, all assert the importance of having the client accept the responsibility for change, regardless how change is defined. The form this counseling takes may rely on logical argumentation, discussion of client history, and practical demonstration. A generic sequence appears in Table 7–21.

Control of Stuttering. Some clinicians believe that an end goal of therapy is for the client to control his stuttering (Peters and Guitar, 1991). The client treated with this philosophy must maintain his identity as a stutterer and

Table 7–21.
Acceptance of Responsibility for Change

Step	Activity	Description
1	Obtaining client's acceptance of responsibility of behavioral change	Through discussion, the clinician determines to what degree the client is depending on him/her to affect behavioral change. If the client accepts responsibility and views the clinician as a facilitator of behavioral change, no further counselling in this area is warranted. If the client does not accept responsibility, counselling continues.
2	Historical evidence that all client changes are the result of client decisions to act	Events in the client's past are discussed, with emphasis on showing the client that all changes resulted from the client deciding to do specific behaviors.
3	Current evidence demonstrating client responsibility for changes	The clinician can ask the client to engage in certain activities with an understanding that regardless of what the client was asked to do, the client had to make a decision to proceed and therefore is responsible for the change.
4	Client commitment of roles	The clinician requires the client to acknowledge that the clinician is the facilitator and the client is the responsible individual.

prepare to spend his life adapting to stuttering in various prescribed ways. Approaches selecting this attitude usually couple it with stuttering modifications that allow the client to substitute in place of a severe form of stuttering one that is less obvious and traumatic to the stutterer (Van Riper, 1982). The generic sequence for this approach appears in Table 7–22.

Monitored Fluency. Other clinicians believe that the end goal of therapy is monitored fluency. Stutterers can now see themselves as fluent speakers, but only at the price of constant or periodic awareness of their manner of speaking.

Normal Nonmonitored Fluency. The third school of thought hopes to instill normal fluency with no remaining concern about speech once therapy is successfully concluded. Williams once said that "stuttering therapy is training your client to see his problem the same way that you do"; the wisdom of this remark is easily applied to attitude manipulation as a component of stuttering therapy.

MONITORING

Monitoring is described differently by different researchers. It may be as simple a process as "becoming aware of what you are doing at the time you are doing it" (Sheehan, 1984). It can be the "real-time monitoring by the client of speech to regulate the extent to which fluent pervasive patterns are being emitted" (Hillis, 1993). For some, monitoring means guaranteeing fluency word by word (Rubin, 1986), whereas for others it is more difficult to define other than a "feel of fluency" used to enhance awareness and strengthen feedback (Peins et al., 1984). Its distinguishing characteristics may be suprasegemental indications of deliberateness and reduced rate (Rubin, 1986),

Table 7–22.
Generic Program for the Acceptance and Control of Stuttering

Step	Activity	Description
1	Acceptance of stuttering	Clients are brought to understand the intractable nature of the problem.
2	Confronting the role of stuttering in one's life	Clients begin to examine how stuttering is impacting on their lives.
3	Developing strategies for control	Clients, with the help of the clinician, begin developing strategies for exercising control.
4	Implementing strategies for control	Activities are designed during which clients can practice the control strategies.

the need to "really listen" to self-speech to increase auditory awareness (Peins, 1984), or the need to expend mental effort to the manner as well as to the content of any given message. The key concepts appear to be self-awareness, deliberate control, and self-feedback. As Rubin (1986) eloquently suggests, "monitoring is not a gimmick. It is a very specific form of consciousness raising, of raising the act of speaking from an automatic level to a very purposeful one."

How does one monitor? The task appears to be a formless one. It requires increased concentration, awareness, and commitment. Although the process is difficult to describe, clients seem well able to learn it, as well as to signal its presence to themselves and others (Culatta and Rubin, 1971; Goldberg, 1981; Shames and Florance, 1980). Often clinicians do not suggest specific techniques. Instead they instruct their clients to attend to the words that they are about to utter and to make certain they are "doing whatever it takes" to say the words fluently. Rubin states that the "task is an imageless one. All I am aware of is the determination that the word I am uttering and the next one are fluent" (Rubin, 1986). Monitoring behavior is not unlike what normal speakers do during moments when a high degree of fluency is critical. It can be the cautious, deliberate speech manner that can signal the difference between helplessness and control. Monitoring is a decision about manner of speech made prior to any specific utterance. Monitoring does not enable the client to deal with stuttering; rather, clients deal with marshalling the skills needed for purposeful fluency. As one might expect, measurement of such a hazy concept is difficult. Like love, truth, and beauty, the difficulty of definition and measuring may not weaken the importance of the concept. Therapies that propose fluency as a goal tend to use monitoring as an intermediate step toward that goal. In fact, the vigilance required by monitoring becomes one of the final steps toward normal unmonitored fluent speech (Culatta and Rubin, 1973; Shames and Florance, 1980; Goldberg, 1981).

The programs summarized in this text use many different monitoring techniques. However, they all share the need for the client to at some point take control over production of his or her speech in a way that will bring about the desired goals of therapy. Unless and until the client assumes this responsibility, therapy, regardless of its philosophy, is unfinished.

Up to this point, we introduced and discussed the types of intervention strategies available to speech-language pathologists and stuttering clients. These six options are:

1. (P) physiological adjustments,
2. (R) rate manipulation,
3. (O) operant control,
4. (L) length and complexity of utterance manipulations,
5. (A) attitude change,
6. (M) monitoring,

used in whatever combination and order the clinician finds needed will provide the strategies for instillation of behavioral change. The last two components of the model, generalization and maintenance, consider those strategies employed to infuse the gains of therapy into nonclinical, real-world speech.

GENERALIZATION

Development of stutter-free speech within a controlled clinic environment can be accomplished through a variety of strategies. Real problems often occur when the client attempts to use a new speaking pattern in a nonclinical setting. The ability of the client to generalize clinically mastered behaviors outside the clinical setting has been and continues to be an area of major concern. Perhaps this transfer of skills is the most critical issue in the treatment of stutterers (Costello, 1989). The technical definition of generalization was developed by Stokes and Baer (1977): "the occurrence of a relevant behavior under different, nontraining conditions (i.e., across subjects, settings, people, behaviors, and/or time) without the scheduling of the same events in those conditions as had been scheduled in the training condition." Simply put, generalization of fluent speech or reduced stuttering occurs when clients can use their new speaking pattern outside the clinic, in a variety of situations and with a variety of people.

Often in the literature the terms *transfer, carryover,* and *generalization* are used interchangeably. Usually, they refer to the display of a behavior in a new setting. In this chapter, "generalization" will be used instead of either "transfer" or "carryover," because it has a standard definition. "Maintenance," which is discussed in the next segment, refers to procedures that facilitate continuation of the new speech behaviors in nonclinical settings.

Uses of Generalization

The study of generalization of behavior serves two different purposes. As a research tool, generalization may be a measure used to compare the effectiveness of various intervention programs. As a stage of therapy, it becomes the method to establish new behaviors in nonclinical settings.

Comparing Effectiveness. The effectiveness of various intervention techniques is often determined by examining the degree to which each results in the generalization of new behaviors. Ryan and Van Kirk (1983), for example, examined the efficacy of four different fluency development techniques for children by comparing the degree of fluency maintained after therapy ended. Other studies that demonstrate the effectiveness of a technique include those offering support for a portable DAF unit (Craven and Ryan, 1984), incorporation of psychological counselling (Evesham and Fransella, 1985), and the equality of intensive versus traditional therapy sessions (James et al., 1989). A more difficult comparison approach involves assessing entire therapeutic protocols. This assessment is done when for various reasons it is not possible or practical to assess specific components of each approach. An excellent example of the use of this research approach is Andrews and colleagues'(1983) comparison of more than 100 stuttering therapy studies. One of the ways that the approaches were compared was the degree to which generalization of new behaviors occurred. For practicing speech-language pathologists, however, the role of generalization as a process within therapy has the most immediate impact.

A Stage in Therapy. Stuttering therapy programs incorporate generalization either as the final stage of therapy or while establishing new behaviors. As the final stage of therapy, the established target behaviors are practiced in a variety of nonclinical settings. These behaviors, which can either be fluent speech or reduced stuttering, are practiced in a variety of nonclinical settings utilizing self-monitoring techniques, specific activities, or even electronic feedback devices. Regardless of the approach, the basic generalization procedure is to teach a behavior within a protective environment (the clinic), to establish it, then to replicate it in a nonclinical setting. For example, in the GILCU (Ryan, 1974b), lengthy fluent productions are gradually taught to the client. The client is then asked to produce constructions of a similar length in nonclinical settings. In the Stutter-Free Speech program (Shames and Florence, 1980), a client's speech is shaped through DAF and prolongation until it approaches a normal rate. The client then practices this rate outside the clinic through the use of behavioral contracts. Ingham's (1984) program of teaching fluent speech also involves establishment of normal fluency within a clinical setting before generalization occurs.

An Integrated Part of Therapy. Generalization is also used as an ongoing process in therapy. Van Riper's (1973) early forms of stuttering therapy incorporated generalization within, rather than at the end of, therapy. He emphasized the importance for the stutterer to continually practice new reduced stuttering patterns in social situations. In Webster's Precision Fluency Shaping Program (1974), clients begin generalizing each new step of their fluency development from the beginning of therapy. In Goldberg's Behavioral Cognitive Stuttering Therapy program (1981), clients are required to generalize exaggerated forms of fluency from the first day of therapy.

Sheehan (1980), a strong advocate of immediate generalization application, maintained that if a separate generalization stage was required, then inadequate therapy procedures were probably applied. According to him, if the procedures were appropriate, generalization would be a logical consequence of their mastery rather than something that required an additional stage. This position finds support in the results of generalization experiments in other areas. In the area of psychotherapy for example, Ager (1987) found that the degree to which his clients were able to generalize new behaviors were related more to the components of the establishment procedures than to any other variable. This important relationship that exists between establishment procedures and generalization is also found in other areas, such as teaching social communicative behavior to retarded adolescents (Hunt et al., 1986), generalizing speech skills in hearing-impaired children (Perigoe and Ling, 1986), and generalizing production of new phonemes in misarticulating children (Gierut et al., 1987). In each of these studies, it was clearly shown that the procedures used during establishment of new behaviors can have a significant effect on the length of time required and the extent to which generalization can take place.

Generalization of a new behavior is more complex than it may appear. Clinicians often have difficulty understanding why it is so difficult for clients to continue to display a behavior taught in the clinic. For example, explanations as to why a client cannot remain fluent outside of the clinic might include distractions not present in the clinic, speech anxieties that do not exist in the safety of the clinic, or even a lack of motivation to implement gains. Regardless of the explanation, the fault is usually seen as unrelated to the establishment procedures. However, generalization studies clearly indicate that the success or failure of generalizing behaviors is most often a function of the establishment procedures.

Structure of Generalization

The first step in understanding generalization is to understand its structure. When we talk about the structure of generalization, we look at the logical relationships that exist between stimuli and responses. Two types of structures exist: stimulus generalization and response generalization.

Stimulus Generalization. Stimulus generalization occurs when a specific response can be elicited by the presence of two or more stimulus configurations that are similar in some aspects but different in others. A stimulus configuration is a set of stimuli that is present when a specific response is elicited. The configuration may involve only a few critical variables, or it may encompass a much greater number. Table 7–23 illustrates a training sequence for generalizing fluent responses to questions that begins with only a few critical variables and ends with a large number of variables. In this illustration, four stimulus configurations result in the same response. The first two are in training situations, and the last two are in untrained situations. A training situation involves teaching a behavior during which as many aspects of stimulus configuration, response, and consequences are controlled. During the untrained situation, some aspects of the sequence are not controlled. In this illustration, the two training stimulus configurations differ only in terms of one element, the linguistic requirements of the interaction.

In stimulus configuration one, the clinician attempts to facilitate the development of fluent speech in a relatively calm situation. The client has already been taught a form of controlled fluency. The clinician is now attempting to begin the process of stimulus generalization. Both the client and the clinician sit in a quiet clinic room, facing each other across a table, and the clinician allows the client to complete a response to a question before the clinician asks another question. In this situation, the desired response is the fluent response

Table 7–23.
Stimulus Generalization

Situation	Stimulus Configuration	Response
1. Trained	**People:** clinician and client. **Physical situation:** client and clinician sitting at table in clinic. **Linguistic requirements:** clinician asks question, waits for response to be completed before continuing.	Fluent speech while responding to a question.
2. Trained	**People:** clinician and client. **Physical situation:** client and clinician sitting at table in clinic. **Linguistic requirements:** clinician asks question, but does not wait for response to be completed before continuing.	Fluent speech while responding to a question.
3. Untrained	**People:** specific individuals agreed on by the clinician and the client. **Physical situation:** specific daily activities agreed on by the clinician and client. **Linguistic requirements:** individual will ask question.	Fluent speech while responding to a question.
4. Untrained	**People:** anyone. **Physical situation:** all daily activities. **Linguistic requirements:** individuals will ask question.	Fluent speech while responding to a question.

to questions. The activity may continue over a number of sessions until the client is able to respond fluently to questions at a specific criterion level. With success, the clinician attempts to generalize the stimulus.

In stimulus configuration two, the desired response remains the same, but one stimulus variable changes: the linguistic requirements of the situation. This time, the clinician purposely interrupts the client's response. If the client can successfully produce fluent responses when interrupted, the process of stimulus generalization begins to occur. Between sessions, the client may be instructed to use the controlled form of fluency in specific situations, with specific people, when asked to respond to a question. This is stimulus configuration 3 in Table 7–23. If the clinician is satisfied with the client's success, further generalization activities can be tried. An example would be stimulus configuration 4.

The rationale for designing activities that incorporate stimulus generalization is that it prepares clients to produce a specific desired response in a variety of situations.

Response Generalization

Response generalization occurs when a specific stimulus configuration can elicit two or more responses that are similar in some aspects but different in others. During stimulus generalization, the response stayed the same throughout the procedures. During response generalization, the reverse is true: The stimulus remains the same, but the response changes. In our stimulus generalization example, the clinician desired the stutterer to produce fluent responses to questions. Obviously, the stutterer's speech consists of more than responses to questions. The clinician may have made an intervention strategy decision to initially choose one form of speech, to generalize it, then to proceed to another form of speech. The clinician could have chosen to use another intervention strategy that focused on response generalization rather than stimulus generalization.

An example of response generalization appears in Table 7–24. In this example, the stimulus configuration remains the same throughout the intervention. The clinician and the client engage in a conversation in the therapy room in each step of the intervention, but the form of client response changes. In this example, the clinician attempts to shape fluent speech. To do this, three variables associated with the form of fluent speech being taught are modified: (1) signaling, (2) rate, and (3) phonation. In each of the first three training situations, one new variable is modified. In the final situation, which is untrained, the client is instructed to "just talk" and to not consciously monitor any of the three variables associated with production of the controlled fluency.

Combinations of Stimulus and Response Generalizations

There is obvious merit in using both stimulus and response generalization techniques. Each contributes to the ability of the client to generalize new behaviors in untrained situations because the client often encounters new stimulus configurations that require complex response patterns. For example, although the client was taught to be fluent with the clinician during arguments, substitution of the clinic director may result in disfluent speech. In this case, the "authority" the client associated with the director may have created a stimulus configuration that was so different from the trained stimulus configuration that the failure is understandable. It is not possible to anticipate all the situations in which clients will be required to produce target behaviors. However, the greater the emphasis in therapy on stimulus and response generalization, the more likely it will be that the critical variables found in nonclinical situations will have been incorporated within the training sequence during therapy.

Methods for Enhancing Generalization

Generalization depends on many things. In the preceding section, the importance of structure in developing generalization activities was emphasized. Although an intervention protocol may be logically structured, its components may not add anything to the process of generalization. The literature suggests

Table 7–24.
Response Generalization

Situation	Stimulus Configuration	Response
1. Trained	**People:** Clinician and client. **Physical situation:** sitting at table in clinic. **Linguistic requirement:** conversation about topic of interest to the client.	1. Signal: hand is raised as signal to use controlled fluency. 2. Rate: 60 syllables per minute. 3. Phonation: effortless initiation of initial sounds.
2. Trained	**People:** clinician and client. **Physical situation:** sitting at table in clinic. **Linguistic requirement:** Conversation about topic of interest to the client.	1. Signal: fingers are squeezed together as signal to use controlled fluency. 2. Rate: 60 syllables per minute. 3. Phonation: effortless initiation of initial sounds.
3. Trained	**People:** clinician and client. **Physical situation:** sitting at table in clinic. **Linguistic requirement:** conversation about topic of interest to the client.	1. Signal: fingers are squeezed together as signal to use controlled fluency. 2. Rate: 120 syllables per minute. 3. Phonation: effortless initiation of initial sounds.
4. Untrained	**People:** clinician and client. **Physical situation:** sitting at table in clinic. **Linguistic requirement:** conversation about topic of interest to the client.	1. Signal: none. 2. Rate: unmonitored. 3. Phonation: unmonitored.

that the effect of generalization activities can be substantially increased if three things are done: (1) enhance sensory awareness, (2) emphasize critical features, and (3) develop associations.

Enhance Sensory Awareness. The stimulus configuration will result in a greater likelihood of acquisition if it can stand out from other things that occur at the same time, which can be accomplished by enhancing sensory awareness. For example, when teaching the technique of easy phonation on the initial sound of each word, the clinician may wish to emphasize the importance of easy initial phonation by barely phonating on the first sound and then loudly producing the second one.

Emphasize Critical Features. Within any stimulus configuration, there may be some features that are more important than others. If the clinician can highlight these critical features for the client, their importance is emphasized. In signaling to be fluent in the Stutter-Free Speech program (Shames and Florence, 1980), for example, the client's use of an upheld hand emphasizes the importance of focusing on monitoring fluent speech. The upraised hand provides a stronger monitoring signal than a slight finger tap on a table top.

Associations. The memory of how to perform a specific behavior can be enhanced by associating it with some other, more familiar concept. For example, when explaining reduced rate to a young child, it can be presented as speech similar to someone slowly crawling on the floor. The visual image may make it easier for the child to remember how to produce speech at a slow rate.

Generalization Activities

Selection of activities during which new speech behaviors are taught should, as much as possible, be approximations of the activities that occur naturally outside the clinic. Naturalistic activities within a clinic setting are more likely to result in generalization of behaviors than activities that are more contrived (Woods, 1987). The design of the learning activities in the establishment phase of therapy may be critical for later generalization. The activities should focus on those elements that may have a direct effect on the client's ability to produce fluent speech. Some of the most common aspects of communication that clients report affect their fluency are the (1) status of the listener, (2) content of the message, (3) sex of the listener, (4) age of the listener, (5) emotional state of the stutterer, (6) past speech history with a specific listener, and (7) number of listeners.

Status. Clients will often indicate that their speech varies with the type of person to whom they are speaking to (Sheehan et al., 1967). If this is a factor with any given client, speech-language pathologists may construct status hierarchies mirroring the types of people the client encounters. Role playing each of the types may be effective in establishing stimulus generalizations.

Content. The content of what is being said can have an effect on fluency. Some view the stutterer's difficulty with fluency that is related to content to be an indication of problems with communicative intent (Sheehan, 1958); others view it as an indication of difficulty with emotionality (Rollin, 1987). Although there is disagreement on why stutterers have difficulty with some forms of utterances and not others, many programs incorporate content within their fluency training. When teaching a new speaking pattern, clinicians should have the client practice the pattern during various types of utterances. Examples of types of utterances that might be appropriate are: descriptions, questions, aggressive speech, providing specific directions, answering direct questions, or defending a specific belief.

Sex. Some stutterers report that the sex of their listener is a factor in their ability to speak fluently (Bloodstein, 1987). It is important that stutterers practice their new speaking patterns with members of both sexes throughout therapy.

Age. For some stutterers, the age of their listener is perceived to be a factor influencing their fluency. Usually, individuals who are younger than the stutterer have no negative effect on production of fluent speech. As the listener approaches the age of the stutterer, it becomes more of a factor (Ramig et al., 1982). Throughout therapy, the client should practice the new speaking pattern with individuals of varying ages, but especially individuals who are of a similar age or older.

Emotional State. Stutterers report that their ability to speak fluently is affected by their emotional state (Allen and Daly, 1978). The relationship of emotional states to speech differ widely between stutterers. Some can be fluent only when they are angry, whereas others are extremely disfluent when angry. However, it may be difficult to artificially create various emotional states in which the stutterer can practice the new speech pattern. It may be possible to use the emotional state the client brings to the clinic. Communication attempts might be attempted while approximating the following emotional states: anger, anxiety, happiness, relaxation, fear, concern, and helplessness. Obviously, the genuineness of the feelings attempted may be questioned. For some, visualization exercises might be effective.

Past Speech History. The past history of success or failure a client has had with an individual or a situation will be a determinant on future success. Therefore, clinicians should be sure that the new speaking pattern is practiced in each situation the client has identified as having resulted in failure in the past.

Number of Listeners. Perhaps the easiest variable to manipulate is the size of a given audience for a client. The advantages of increasing or decreasing the size of an audience in a systematic manner are obvious.

MAINTENANCE

Unfortunately, once clients attain fluency, they do not automatically maintain it. Andrews and colleagues (1980) found that a planned maintenance program is needed for stuttering therapy to be successful. Maintenance refers to a variety of after-treatment activities that are applied to help clients keep intact the gains of a treatment program. It is the long term continuation of fluency in a wide variety of settings. Maintenance is seen as an integral part of therapy. The client experiencing the maintenance aspects of a therapy is still in therapy (Ryan, 1979). Maintenance programs should not be confused with follow-up activities. Follow-up is simply a post-therapy evaluation of a client's long-term performance after a period of no clinical intervention (Boberg et al., 1979). Maintenance strategies are fairly straightforward, and most programs of therapy share some or all of the following procedures to maintain their gains.

Enhancing Activities

Daily Self-monitoring Activities. Dismissal from intensive therapy does not excuse a client from the need to purposefully engage in self-monitoring activities of all types, ranging from monitored fluency to visualization. Many programs provide activities the client should review independently as home practice once intensive therapy is terminated (Ryan and Van Kirk, 1974; Daly, 1984).

Regular Clinic Contacts. Scheduling of periodic contacts on a diminishing frequency ranging from monthly to semiannually to yearly serve as maintenance markers for many clients (Ryan and Van Kirk, 1971). Each visit allows clients to review immediately past behavior and to analyze their fluency status.

Refresher Programs. If a client begins to backslide or evidence loss of gains made in therapy, it may be appropriate to "recycle" appropriate segments of the previously completed therapy program (Boberg, 1981; Ryan and Van Kirk, 1974; Webster, 1980). Clinical judgment usually determines how much of a given program must be repeated or if aspects originally deleted or modified should be introduced the second time around.

Self-help Groups. From time to time it is possible for a client to either form a self-help group or to join an existing one. Often these groups are valuable for ventilation, practicing therapy techniques, or even socialization (Howie et al., 1981). Appendix B lists and describes some self-help groups.

Ingham (1993) summed up the goals of generalization and maintenance programs with four major objectives.

1. To have the client use therapy practices that reduce or eliminate stuttering in the absence of formal therapy.
2. To have the client demonstrate that the factors associated with therapy (e.g., situations and/or people) are not necessary for the client to continue to evidence therapy benefits.
3. To have others regard the client as a normally fluent speaker.
4. To have the client no longer "do things with his or her speech" to sound fluent (p. 167).

Relapse

Any discussion of maintenance naturally leads to an examination of relapse. Stuttering differs from most other communication disorders in terms of relapse. For some still unknown reasons, short-term mastery of program goals by stutterers does not always lead to long-term application. Relapse seems especially problematic in older, postadolescent clients. The term *relapse* is ill-defined because it covers all forms of client regression, from occasionally stuttered words to the resumption of a speaking pattern similar to pretherapy patterns. However, whatever the decline in clinically achieved gains, current facts indicate that stutterers do not maintain clinical gains, especially normal-sounding fluency. Silverman (1992) reports that fewer than 50% of older children and adults who acquire normal-sounding fluency during treatment are able to maintain fluency permanently. Others (Bloodstein, 1987; Kamhi and McOsker, 1982; Perkins, 1981; Martin, 1981; Starkweather, 1990) report similar negative percentages. The good news is that relapse rate, however measured, appears to be much lower for preschool-aged children (Starkweather, 1990; Starkweather et al, 1990). Perkins (1983) concluded from his study of both published and unpublished reports of fluency-shaping programs that the single most predictable outcome is relapse in some form or another. Although all progress is not always lost, the goal of permanent, natural-sounding unmonitored speech is not regularly achieved. Why does relapse plague stutterers more than clients with voice problems or articulation disorders? The answer still lies beyond the knowledge of researchers; however, we can speculate on a few possible explanations summarized below by Boberg et al. (1979).

Slow Decay Due to Similar Stimuli.   We can hypothesize that over time, fluent clients will begin to experience the old tensions they felt prior to achieving fluency. Boberg calls these "microstutterings." These tensions and the stutterer's response to them are, at first, unnoticed by either listeners or by the speaker, and as a result, they are not controlled. Over time, these "microstutterings" increase in both magnitude and frequency and become overt stuttering. This chipping away process leaves a behavior that may be even more resistive to change than the original stuttering.

Failure to Practice.   Practice for fluency and the inherent monitoring it entails comes to be viewed over time as both unnecessary and punishing. Clients may view it as unnecessary because they can produce the behavior they wish most of the time accidentally, with no conscious attention, and they simply hope this fluency will continue. Monitoring may be seen as punishing because it may compromise the spontaneity of any given speaking moment. As Boberg implies, the control techniques become identified as abnormal, and they contradict the reason for seeking change in the first place, which was to get rid of abnormal communication processes.

Genetic Implications.   The risk of relapse may depend on the severity of the presenting problem (Guitar, 1976), which may be related to familial history of stuttering (Kidd, 1980; Goldberg, 1992). The implication of this yet unproven hypothesis is that if such individuals do exist, these clients must accept maintenance as a life-long process (Boberg et al., 1979).

The reality of relapse does not mean that speech-language pathologists and their clients must be helpless victims to this success-dissolving process. Several strategies have been suggested to pre-empt the occurrence of relapse.

Client Assumption of Responsibility. Many clinical researchers have come to the same conclusion despite different initial philosophies. Clients must assume responsibility for their ongoing success. Stutterers must become self-therapists. Once clients achieve the goals of an approach, they must adopt those goals as their own and apply them independently (Culatta and Rubin, 1971; Ryan and Van Kirk, 1974; Costello, 1975; Guitar, 1976; Hanna and Owen, 1977; Peters and Guitar, 1991). Peters and Guitar (1991) provide their clients with a written handout explaining the need for stutterers to become their own clinicians by analyzing behavior, establishing therapy goals, and systematically achieving those goals in an independent manner.

Attitude Change. Although some may find "attitude therapy" of little value (Ingham et al., 1972), most programs have components that deal either directly or indirectly with attitudes that encourage stutterers to be more positive about their speaking abilities. We described the role of attitude change in the overall PROLAM-GM model as a factor in attaining speech change. In this context, we suggest that appropriate attitudes toward fluency and fluency failure may have an effect on potential relapse.

Normalization of Speech Fluency Prior to Termination. Just as it is inappropriate to dismiss a client with a chronic voice problem simply because that client displays an appropriate voice in therapy, it is becoming increasing clear that achieving fluency in the therapy room is not a sign that therapy is over. This initial "egg-shell fluency," described by Ryan and Van Kirk (1971), is neither durable nor the end product of therapy. Adams and Runyan (1981) report that stutterers most likely to escape relapse are those whose speech is objectively and perceptively indistinguishable from normal speech. Clients who are free of stuttering but still show signs of incomplete fluency are much more likely to relapse.

Prepare for Relapse. The occurrence of relapse is no surprise to speech-language pathologists and it should be no surprise to clients. Forewarned is definitely forearmed. Perkins (1984) prepares "clients to recover from relapse as a predictable eventuality" (p. 180). Clients discuss their weakness in anticipation of relapse, and they practice the steps needed to recover should the need arise. In practice, they violate the principles that brought them fluency so that they might practice recovery without fear. This practice recovery is a vital part of treatment, and it prepares clients to not only face but also plan contingencies for recovery.

The unpredictability of generalization and maintenance, coupled with the reality of relapse, must lead beginning clinicians to question the value of stuttering therapy. Is it all a horrible, depressing waste of time? Apparently not. Studies are beginning to show that some stutterers' lives are better for the experience. Andrews and colleagues (1980) examined 42 studies that met their criteria for analysis and found reassuringly upbeat information. Stutterers receiving treatment were more normal in their speech than 92% of their stuttering peers not in treatment. However, success did not come easily or in a haphazard manner. Approximately 100 client contact hours were needed, in addition to systematic generalization plans, possible attitude change, cooperation of significant others, and a planned maintenance program. There may be a lot of ifs, ands, and buts in the therapy picture, but the message seems to be that good therapy gets good results.

SUMMARY

We presented a model for therapy that encompasses the components of effective therapy. We tried to explain the purpose that each component of the PROLAM-GM acronym might have in provision of treatment to any given client, as well as to highlight both theoretical and practical factors of each component of the model. Obviously, each segment could not be exhaustively reviewed. However, the bibliographic references as well as the suggested readings should help speech-language pathologists understand the components of the model. Finally, we discussed the need for systematic generalization and maintenance components regardless of the implementation strategies selected. The next chapter illustrates how specific therapy protocols can help speech-language pathologists implement the techniques for each of the PRO-LAM-GM components.

STUDY QUESTIONS

1. There are 5 physiological strategies that can be used to affect the speech of stutterers. Describe how each would be used with a child, an adolescent, and an adult.

2. There are 3 rate modification strategies that can be used to affect the speech of stutterers. Describe how each would be used with a child, an adolescent, and an adult.

3. Describe in detail the structural components of an intervention program that use both postitive reinforcement and aversive control.

4. How would you use modifications in the length and complexity of utterances to affect the speech of child, adolescent, and adult stutterers?

5. Most clinicians believe that the attitude of a client can be a significant predictor in the success of therapy. In what ways would you facilitate the development of positive attitudes in child, adolescent, and adult stutterers?

6. What strategies would be appropriate for facilitating the development of monitoring behaviors in child, adolescent, and adult stutterers?

7. Describe the process for developing stimulus generalization in child, adolescent, and adult stutterers.

8. Describe the process for developing response generalization in child, adolescent, and adult stutterers.

9. Describe the three strategies for structuring therapy that will enhance generalization of fluent speech in child, adolescent, and adult stutterers.

10. Construct comprehensive maintenance programs for child, adolescent, and adult stutterers who successfully complete a therapy program.

11. Relapse is a problem experienced by most clients. Describe what can be done to minimize the problem.

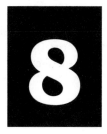

Synopsis of Approaches to the Treatment of Stuttering

This chapter summarizes 32 strategies for treating stutterers. It should serve as a first step in the understanding of the various treatment approaches. When possible and appropriate, copies of the summaries were shared with those most responsible for an approach. The various authors were asked to suggest readings they believed would be most helpful to readers of the summaries. Approaches marked with an asterisk have been read by their authors, and the readings that appear in the Suggested Readings category for these approaches are those they suggested. We would like to thank the authors for their graciousness and cooperation. They have all contributed much to our field and to the lives of our clients. We hope readers will learn as much as we did in preparing and reviewing these approaches.

In listing 32 separate approaches, an attempt was made to be reasonably comprehensive. However, it is not possible to list and summarize all available approaches in one chapter. Nor was it possible to use the format when an approach contained combinations of general suggestions, philosophies, and various approaches. This does not mean that these approaches are any less valuable than the ones reviewed. They were usually contained within comprehensive texts on stuttering that emphasized understanding the theories involved in stuttering therapy more than the specific techniques (Conture, 1990). The format used for each protocol contains the following 10 components.

Program:

the name or most common descriptor of the program summarized.

Person:

person or persons most responsible for the approach.

Age Range:

suggested client ages the authors believe are appropriate for their strategies.

Objectives:

end results of the program.

Summary:

a brief narrative description of the therapy.

PROLAM-GM Components:

only those PROLAM-GM components used by the authors are listed.

Research Findings:

when available, a partial listing of research findings are included.

Special Features:

any unusual or special features that may make an approach particularly useful for a specific client are highlighted.

Suggested Readings:

a listing of readings is presented that will enable readers to gain in-depth knowledge of a particular strategy.

The absence of a component in our analysis does not mean the author does not use it in his or her intervention protocol. Rather, its omission may mean that it was not sufficiently detailed enough to aide clinicians in utilizing the technique without significant improvisation. The use of "generalization" is a good example. Although virtually all authors believe generalization is important, not all provide readers with a methodology for implementing it. It is hoped that this format, or its modification, can be used by readers, to analyze those approaches not reviewed. In Chapter 9, a strategy is presented that allows clinicians to selectively choose those techniques from the various approaches that are appropriate for specific clients.

Comprehensive Alberta Stuttering Program

Person: Einer Boberg and D. Kully.

Age Range: Adults and adolescents.

Objectives: An intensive residential program involving structured activities designed to increase fluency skills. Transfer and maintenance activities are an integral component of the program (Boberg & Kully, 1984).

Summary

This is an intensive, residential 6 hours/day, 3-week program consisting of 11 steps: (1) pre-clinic testing, (2) measures in group setting, (3) identification, (4) introduction to prolongation and fluency skills, (5) slow prolongation, (6) medium prolongation, (7) slight prolongation, (8) controlled-normal rate, (8) preparation for transfer, (9) transfer, (10) post-testing, and (11) maintenance program. Groups consist of between 4 and 12 clients, with 2 to 6 clinicians. The program integrates strategies to systematically modify speech with techniques to promote attitude change, avoidance reduction, and interpersonal skill development. The collection of data is through use of audio and videotape recording, with an emphasis on recording the number of stuttered and fluent syllables within a unit of time.

Following the collection of data, clients are taught to identify and describe their stuttering behavior. Then the skills of easy breathing, gentle starts, smooth blending, and light touches are taught, beginning with single syllables, and progressing gradually to longer and more complex utterances. Fluency skills are taught in the framework of prolongation, beginning with a rate of approximately 40 syllables/minute, and progressing systematically to near-normal rates of speech. To progress from one rate to the next, clients must complete a specified number of sessions with accurate skills and 1% or less stuttering and pass a self-evaluation test. In addition to fluency skills, clients are taught to recover from stuttering using a self-correction strategy. Throughout the program, activities are incorporated to promote development of self-management skills, including self-evaluation, self-monitoring, and problem-solving.

In parallel with the fluency-shaping procedures, cognitive-behavioral strategies are used to promote open, accepting attitudes about stuttering and controlled speech and to encourage identification and elimination of avoidances. These changes are achieved through discussions and readings, as well as through training in effective self-talk and specific speech exercises.

Transfer activities begin once clients achieve consistent and accurate skill use at near-normal rates in conversation within the clinic. There are 50 assignments progressing from easy to more challenging in each of five categories;

(1) conversations, (2) phone calls, (3) shopping, (4) self-correction, and (5) special challenges. Assignments are recorded for later analysis by the client and the clinician. Maintenance activities consist of individualized home programs and a variety of scheduled clinic visits, including 5-day booster sessions and refresher weekends.

PROLAM-GM Components:

Physiological Adjustments	Use of breath control, easy onset of speech, gentle articulatory contacts.
Rate	Use of prolongation, with increase in rate to approximate normal speech.
Attitude	Group discussion, readings, and exercises to foster effective self-talk and attitudes that facilitate the development and transfer of controlled fluent speech.
Monitoring	Client is responsible for monitoring performance throughout the establishment and transfer phases.
Generalization	Structured program with criteria for advancement.
Maintenance	Scheduled clinic visits, home program, booster sessions.

Research Findings:

Boberg, E. & Kully, D., Long-term results of an intensive therapy program for adult and adolescent stutterers. *JSHR*, in press.

Langevin, M. & Boberg, E. Results of an intensive therapy program. *JSLPA*, in press.

Special Features: None.

Suggested Readings:

Boberg, E. (1980). Intensive clinical program. In W.H. Perkins (Ed.) *Strategies in stuttering therapy: Seminars in speech, language and hearing.* New York : Brian C. Decker.

Boberg, E. (1984). Intensive adult-teen therapy program. In W. Perkins (Ed.) *Current therapy of communication disorders.* New York: Thieme-Straton.

Boberg, E. & Kully, D. (1985). *Comprehensive stuttering program.* College Hill Press.

Boberg, E. & Kully, D. (1984). Techniques for transferring fluency. In W.H. Perkins (Ed.). *Current therapy of communication disorders.* New York: Thieme-Stratton.

Two-factor Behavior Therapy

Person: Gene J. Brutten and D.J. Shoemaker.

Age Range: All.

Objectives: To reduce the frequency and occurrence of stuttering through both classic conditioning and instrumental conditioning procedures.

Summary

Two-factor behavior therapy is based on the assumption that stuttering results from the interaction of genetic and environmental factors. Genetic predisposition is based on the sex-limited polygenic model of inheritance. Although an individual may be genetically predisposed to stuttering, the behavior will not occur unless certain environmental factors are present. These factors tend to result in a level of stress that can cause emotionally induced disorganization, leading to the motor discoordination of speech. These factors differ among stutterers. To individualize therapy, a molecular analysis of the stutterer's behavior is performed. Molecular behaviors are derived by analyzing an individual's fluency failures in terms of respiration, laryngeal movements, oral motor control, and speech timing. Stuttering is therefore the involuntary result of organismic conditions and environmental circumstances that affect motor performance.

Two-factor behavior therapy is not a set, predetermined approach that should be used for all stutterers without modification. It is not, however, an eclectic approach, but rather one that is internally consistent with the basic two-factor learning theory, and it is modifiable depending on the client's specific molecular behaviors. There are two types of behaviors associated with stuttering, those that develop through emotional learning (factor I behaviors) and those that result from operant conditioning (factor II behaviors). Because each behavior resulted from a specific learning paradigm, each requires a different form of intervention.

Factor I behaviors, which are classically conditioned, can be modified either through deconditioning or counterconditioning. Deconditioning involves returning a conditioned stimulus to its originally neutral status (e.g., teaching a stutterer that the approach of a sales person does not necessarily result in negative consequences). Procedures for deconditioning involve repeated presentation of the conditioned stimulus without negative consequences. Counterconditioning involves learning a new response to a conditioned stimulus. For stutterers, this approach results in the replacement of a negative emotional response with a positive emotional response to the same stimulus (e.g., being able to say one's name fluently when asked, where in the past, an embarrassing fluency failure usually resulted). The procedure involves repeated presentation of the conditioned stimulus in various negative emotion–producing situations, beginning from the least negative to the most negative (e.g., initially saying one's name in a room with no listeners to eventually saying one's name in front of an audience consisting of strangers).

Factor II behaviors are instrumental responses that have been operantly conditioned over a number of years. The stutterer developed these behaviors in an attempt to prevent, reduce the severity of, or terminate a fluency failure. These behaviors may remain even after factor I behaviors have been eliminated. They can be eliminated through reinforcement, nonreinforcement, or punishment. Of the three procedures, reinforcement of fluency-enhancing skills, such as breath control, easy voice onset, continuous voicing, slow transition from one articulatory gesture to another, and rate reduction, is the most desirable because it affects both respondant and operant behaviors. Emotions associated with speaking become more positive, and use of fluency-enhancing skills and behaviors are developed.

When attempting to modify or eliminate either a respondant or an operant behavior, clinicians should be aware that elimination of one type of behavior does not necessarily result in elimination of other behaviors that may even be in the same class. For example, eliminating a stutterer's fear of talking on the phone will not necessarily result in elimination or even reduction of his fear of speaking in front of an audience. This lack of automatic transfer requires clinicians to develop a series of sequentially ordered intervention targets for both respondant and operant behaviors.

Regardless of the form therapy takes within a two-factor approach, a critical variable for success is the need for mass therapy. Mass therapy involves intensive therapy implemented either in a clinical setting or through the use of audiotapes between sessions. Mass therapy leads to overlearning, which is required by clients so they can cope with the enivornmental and organismic stresses that contribute to their stuttering behavior.

PROLAM-GM components

Physiological Adjustments	Reduction of negative emotional reactions to sounds, words, and speech stituations through a full range of deconditioning and counterconditioning techniques.
Attitude	The stutterer's maladaptive attitudes toward speech are modified by cognitive procedures.
Operant	Use of contingencies to eliminate inappropriate instrumental behaviors and to develop fluency-enhancing skills.

Research Findings Clinical studies of technique, but not the program (Brutten, 1963, 1980). See general articles on the use of operant conditioning in stuttering therapy.

Special Features Therapy tailored and directed to the individual needs and characteristics of the client based on the results of a behavioral assessment battery.

Suggested Readings

Brutten, E.J. & Shoemaker, J.D. (1967). *The modification of stuttering.* Englewood Cliffs, N.J.: Prentice-Hall, Inc.

Brutten, E.J. (1986). The Two-Factor Theory. In G. H. Shames & H. Rubin (Eds.), *Stuttering then and now.* pp. 143–154, Columbus, OH: Charles Merrill Pub.

Brutten, E.J. (1986). The Two-Factor Theory: Postscript. In G. H. Shames & H. Rubin (Eds.), *Stuttering then and now.* pp. 155–183, Columbus, OH: Charles Merrill Pub.

Brutten, E.J. (1975). Stuttering: Topography, assessment and behavior change strategies. In J. Eisenson (Ed.) *Stuttering: A Second Symposium.* (pp. 199–262). NY: Harper & Row.

Cooper Personalized Fluency Control Therapy Revised

Person: Eugene Cooper and Crystal Cooper.

Age Range: Children and adults.

Objectives: Stuttering is the result of multiple coexisting and interacting physiological, psychological, and environmental factors. The end goal of therapy is the feeling of fluency control (Cooper & Cooper, 1985, 1993).

Summary

Cooper and Cooper (1985) define a four-stage therapy program that addresses affective, behavioral, and cognitive factors (the ABCs they perceive to comprise a stuttering syndrome). The four stages are (1) structuring, (2) targeting, (3) adjusting, and (4) regulating. During the structuring stage, speech-language pathologists assist stutterers in identifying affective, behavioral, and cognitive factors that constitute the individual's fluency disorder, and they describe how these factors will be addressed in the course of therapy. During the targeting stage, the client's affective, behavioral, and cognitive patterns that impede and facilitate therapy are targeted as the client is asked to begin altering disfluency-related behaviors, such as loss of eye contact and extraneous limb and body movements accompanying moments of disfluency. Establishment of a client-clinician relationship facilitative to modification of affective and cognitive patterns as well as behavioral patterns is the key goal of this stage of therapy.

During the adjusting stage, clinicians stress client self-reinforcement activities to strengthen the feelings, behaviors, and attitudes that enhance the feeling of fluency control. Clinicians supervise the client in the use of fluency-initiating gestures (FIGSs) during this stage. The Coopers' six "universal FIGs" are deep FIG (altering the breathing pattern), easy FIG (gentle initiation of phonation), smooth FIG (reduction in phonatory adjustments and light articulatory contacts), beat FIG (variation in prosodic features), slow FIG (altering rate of articulatory adjustments), and loud FIG (altering intensity). During the regulating stage, clinicians assist clients in developing and using strategies to maintain the feeling of fluency control in even the most difficult speaking situations. FIG-switching (altering the use of FIGs within a single speech situation) is one of the strategies that enables the client to sustain the feeling of fluency control. Termination of therapy is dependent not on the client's level of fluency, but on the client's having experienced the feeling of fluency control and on having demonstrated the ability to regain the feeling of control after having lost it.

PROLAM-GM Components

Physiological Adjustments	Altering respiratory patterns for speech production, gentle initiation of phonation, reduction in phonatory adjustments combined with light articulatory contacts, loudness control, and altering prosodic features of speech.
Rate	Use syllable by syllable reduction in rate.
Attitude	Sense of control.
Generalization	Gradual generalization of affective, behavioral, and cognitive patterns, behaviors, and situations.
Maintenance	Annual reviews.

Research Findings: Anecdotal (Cooper, 1993, Cooper and Cooper, 1985).

Special Features: Therapy kit available. Cooper, E.B. & Cooper, C.S. (1985). *Cooper Personalized Fluency Control Therapy-Revised* Allen,TX: DLM Teaching Resources

Suggested Readings

Cooper, C.S. (1991). Using collaborative/consultative service delivery models for fluency intervention and carryover. Language, Speech, and Hearing Services in Schools, 22, 152–153.

Cooper, E.B.(1984). Personalized Fluency Control Therapy: A Status Report. In M. Peins (ed.) *Contemporary Approaches in Stuttering Therapy.* Boston: Little Brown and Company.

Cooper, E.B. (1993). Red herrings, dead horses, straw men, and blind alleys: Escaping the stuttering conundrum. *Journal of Fluency disorders,* 18, 4, 375–387.

Cooper, E.B. (1993). Chronic perseverative stuttering syndrome: A harmful or helpful construct? *American Journal of Speech-Language Pathology, 3,* 11–22.

Extended Length of Utterance (ELU)

Person: Janis Costello Ingham.

Age Range: Children.

Objectives: To increase the amount of fluent speech so that it replaces stuttered speech.

Summary

The ELU program begins by using social reinforcement or redeemable tokens to reward fluent utterances of one-syllable (word) responses. It ends with the child producing a 5-minute long nonstuttered monologue. The child progresses through 20 steps, not counting branching activities that deal with failures at any given step, to reach the final 5-minute goal. Instances of stuttering are verbally punished (e.g., request to "stop" speaking, "uh oh," "oops") as soon as the moment of stuttering is recognized. Each response is recorded, and predetermined criterion levels must be met to move from one step to the next. After completion of the "basic" ELU program, specific transfer activities may be initiated if the child has not generalized fluent speech to the natural speaking environment.

If less than satisfactory results are achieved with the basic program, four "additives" are suggested. The additives are reduced speaking rate, initial utterances with gentle voice onset, simplification of linguistic complexity of utterances, and attitude modification. Rate reduction is achieved by instructing the child to slow down to an acceptable rate and only reinforcing responses that are both fluent and uttered at an acceptable rate. Prolongations to aid in phonetic transitions may also be used. When necessary, appropriate gentle onset of phonation is added to the basic program. Gentle onset usually is the result of whispered prespeech or breathy initiation of utterances. The final additives of linguistic simplification and attitude modification are employed with hesitation, and they are used only when there is compelling evidence that they are needed strategies. It is the authors' belief that all additives complicate the therapy process and should not be used routinely, especially because they may not be necessary to evoke fluency.

PROLAM-GM Components

Physiological Adjustments	Gentle onset used as an additive when needed.
Rate	Slow rate and prolongation additives used when needed.

Operant	Tokens or social reinforcement for initial fluency and response contingent verbal punishment for recognized moments of stuttering.
Length and Complexity Of Utterance	Length of fluent utterances manipulated; complexity modified only if needed.
Monitoring	Monitoring of fluent speech needed for self-reinforcement.

Research Findings: One subject described in Costello (1983a, 1984b). Large federally funded clinical efficacy research program is currently underway by Glyndon Riley.

Suggested Readings

Costello, J.M. (1983A). Current behavioral treatments for children. In D. Prins & R.J. Ingham (Eds.), *Treatment of stuttering in early childhood: Methods and issues.* San Diego: College-Hill Press.

Costello Ingham, J.M. (1993). Behavioral treatment of stuttering children. In R.F. Curlee (Ed.) *Stuttering and related disorders of fluency.* New York: Thieme-Stratton Inc.

Costello, J.M.(1984b). Treatment of the young chronic stutterer: managing fluency. In R.F. Curlee & W.H. Perkins (Eds.) *Nature and treatment of stuttering: New directions.* San Diego: College-Hill Press.

A Program for the Initial Stages of Fluency Therapy

Person: Richard Culatta and Herbert Rubin.

Age Range: Adults and children.

Objectives: Stutterers have the capacity to produce normal speech; therefore, the goal of therapy is normal speech.

Summary

One of the earliest of the fluency-based intervention strategies, this "cognitive fluency program" was the outgrowth of several theoretical articles espousing fluency as an attainable goal for stuttering clients (Culatta, 1970; Rubin and Culatta, 1971; Culatta and Rubin, 1973; Culatta, 1976). Stutterers are expected to change both the way they speak and the way they think of themselves as communicators. The initial program is divided into 11 steps that lead to fluent speech. This program stresses responsibility for and control of speaking behavior. It begins with a recognition of the concept that stutterers have the physiological ability to be fluent and that they can demonstrate this ability by utilizing the same processes that fluent speakers do when they wish to guarantee fluency, namely conscious monitoring of fluency.

The program is divided into attitudinal reorientation and performance components. Steps 1 to 6 are content-oriented, requiring that the client assume specific attitudes and vocabulary about fluency. Steps 7 to 11 require that the client perform speech acts that demonstrate the ability to control the manner of speaking. The authors believe that conceptualizing one's self as a normal speaker is a necessary component of speaking normally, and that recognizing one's ability to control the motor speech apparatus is a necessary precursor to that identity (Rubin, 1986).

After an initial reorientation period, during which clients focus on fluent behaviors, they are instructed to produce "monitored fluent speech." This deliberate, slow-normal rate of speech is expanded in clinical and extraclinical situations. The ultimate goal is to replace the fluency obtained with "monitored speech" with unmonitored speech.

PROLAM-GM Components

Rate	Initial use of slow-normal speech.
Length and Complexity Of Utterance	Increased length of monitored fluent responses.
Attitude	Reconceptualization of stutterer as potentially normal speaker. Client assumption of responsibility for manner of speech.
Monitoring	Yes.
Generalization	Use of monitored speech on assignments within and outside the clinical setting.
Maintenance	Periodic, client-initiated check-ups.

Research Findings: Data for 6 patients presented in Culatta and Rubin (1973).

Special Features: Stresses client responsibility for the development and maintenance of fluent speech.

Suggested Readings

Culatta, R. & Rubin, H. (1973). A Program For The Initial Stages Of Fluency Therapy. *JSHR, 16,* 556–567.

Rubin, H. & Culatta, R.(1971) A Point of View About Fluency. *ASHA,* 380–384.

Culatta, R.(1976). Fluency: The Other Side of the Coin. *ASHA 18.* 11.

Rubin, H.(1986). Cognitive Therapy. In Shames,G.H. & Rubin, H. (Eds.) *Stuttering: Then and Now.* Columbus: Merrill Publishing Company.

Preschool Fluency Development Program

Person: Delva M. Culp.

Age Range: Children ages 2.5 to 7.

Objectives: Fluency behavior may be modified by a cognitive program that offers alternative speech patterns and systematically uses the new pattern in increasingly difficult speaking tasks. The child learns to use an easy speech pattern in increasingly difficult speaking situations (Culp, 1984).

Summary

This program stresses early direct intervention. Both parents and their children are a part of the regimen that includes developing fluency, cognitive, and language stimulation hierarchies. Easy speech, an exaggerated, slow (80–90 words per minute) soft speech pattern in which vowels are prolonged with normal stress, intonation, and word length, is utilized initially. A fluency hierarchy evolves from single-word utterances in choral speech, to clinician-modeled tasks, to a spontaneously generated series of utterances. Single utterances are expanded via carrier phrases until fluent sentences are produced by the child. Fluency is generalized into running speech under several conditions, including storytelling, monologue, and dialogue. The cognitive hierarchy begins with clinician-modeled fluent speech and reinforcement of positive attitudes toward fluent speech, and develops into a positive attitude toward control of fluent speech. The language hierarchy begins with familiar thematic categories and proceeds to more linguistically complex tasks (Culp, 1984).

PROLAM-GM Components

Physiological Adjustments	Use of soft articulatory contacts.
Rate	Use of slow easy speech.
Length and Complexity of Utterance	Length of utterance is varied from single words to running speech. Complexity is varied via linguistic hierarchies.
Attitude	Reinforces positive attitudes toward self-generated and model-generated fluency. Reinforces self-control of fluent utterances.
Monitoring	Children self-evaluate fluent speech.
Generalization	Parent program provides for transfer to out-of-therapy environment.
Maintenance	After a 6- to 8-week period of successful speech, clinic contacts are systematically reduced. Reevaluations are scheduled 3 months after ther-

apy, and follow-up is scheduled for 2 years after therapy.

Research Findings: Data are presented for 14 children who completed the program (Culp, 1984).

Special Features: The program includes group or individual adaptations.

Suggested Readings
Culp, D.M. (1984). The Preschool Fluency Development Program: Assessment and Treatment. In M. Peins (ed.) *Contemporary Approaches to Stuttering Therapy*. Boston: Little Brown and Company.

Conversational Rate Control Therapy

Person: Richard Curlee and William Perkins.

Age Range: Adults and older children.

Objective: Establishing normal-sounding fluency in chronic stutterers is the goal.

Summary
Curlee and Perkins (1969) and later Perkins (1973 a, b, 1984) describe a program for the replacement of stuttered speech with normal-sounding speech. Initial fluency is established through the use of continuous delayed auditory feedback (DAF). This initial use of a slow articulatory rate assures fluency from the onset of therapy. To establish "fluency in slow motion," the client begins speaking under the condition of 250 msec of DAF. This slow prolonged speech is used with gradually increasing units. Along with prolongation, the stutterer learns to speak with easy vocal onset, soft articulatory contacts, a somewhat breathy voice, and sound-blending skills. The client learns all the skills, but he will rely on those that are personally the most effective to produce and to maintain fluent speech. Normal prosodic patterns are superimposed on the slow prolonged speech.

Once the skills are mastered, the client's rate of speech is increased by reducing DAF in 50-msec increments until a normal speaking rate is achieved. The client is then systematically weaned from the DAF machine. The rate of speech goal is between 150 to 200 syllables per minute, a slow normal rate. Skills are generalized by having the client utilize these fluency skills in increasingly complex speaking situations. The client is also expected to participate socially and vocationally in activities that will normalize fluent speech, and efforts are made to prepare clients for the eventuality of temporary disruptions and possible relapses.

PROLAM-GM Components

Physiological Adjustments	Initial use of easy vocal onset, soft articulatory contacts, breathy vocalization, and sound blending.
Rate	Use of prolongation.
Length and Complexity of Utterance	Length and complexity of utterances and generalization situations are systematically varied.
Attitude	Clients exert volitional control over speech.
Monitoring	Self-management is stressed throughout the program.
Generalization	Use of hierarchical speech experiences, with particular attention to disruption and relapse.

Research Findings: Report on 15 subjects in Curlee and Perkins (1969), 30 in Curlee and Perkins (1973), and 300 in Perkins (1984).

Special Features: Use of DAF device.

Suggested Readings

Curlee, R.F., & Perkins, W.H. (1969). Conversational rate control therapy for stutterers. *Journal of Speech and Hearing Disorders, 34,* 245–250.

Perkins, W.H. (1984). Techniques for establishing fluency. In W.H. Perkins (Ed.), *Stuttering disorders.* New York :Thieme-Stratton.

Perkins, W.H. (1973a). Replacement of stuttering with normal speech: I. Rational. *Journal of Speech and Hearing Disorders, 38,* 283–294.

Perkins, W.H. (1973b). Replacement of stuttering with normal speech: II Clinical procedures. *Journal of Speech and Hearing Disorders, 38,* 295–303.

Freedom of Fluency

Person: David Daly.

Age Range: Adolescents and adults.

Objectives: Fluency is an attainable goal for chronic stutterers via motor skill training and cognitive training.

Summary

Daly (1988b) devised a program that combines motor skill training (speech exercises) with a series of cognitive strategies designed to achieve and maintain fluency for chronic stutterers. The motor skill component relies on deliberate phonation, which is initially accomplished by a slow speech rate and continuous phonation. The author combines this "drone" speech with normal breathing exercises (Daly, 1992). This "stretched speech" is contrasted with normal speech in a release phase. During the release phase, a series of four hand signals are used to prompt the client to shift from prolonged speech to normally fluent utterances. Monitored and unmonitored speech are alternated, and eventually the hand signals are faded out. Cognitive strategies are introduced in a four-phased hierarchy beginning with guided relaxation exercises.

Clients are then encouraged to project a positive mental image of themselves as fluent successful speakers. Along with the mental imagery, clients utilize an affirmation training phase, during which they repeat positive statements about communication. Positive self-talk strategies, such as "each day I become more in control of my speech; at home, at work, in my mind, and in my thoughts" (Daly, 1988b), are used by clients to help maintain a positive attitude toward their control of fluent speech productions.

PROLAM-GM Components

Physiological Adjustment	Use of continuously phonated "drone" speech and breath control.
Rate	Use of slow speech.
Attitude	Use of mental imagery, affirmation training, and positive self-talk.

Research Findings: Anecdotal (Daly, 1988b).

Special Features: Therapy program and demonstration tapes available.
Daly, D.A. (1988 B) *The Freedom of Fluency: A Therapy Program for the Chronic Stutterer.* Moline Il. LinguiSystems Inc.

Suggested Readings
Daly, D.A. (1988a). A Practitioner's View of Stuttering. *ASHA, 30,* 34–35.
Daly,D.A. (1984) Treatment of the young chronic stutterer: Managing Stuttering. In Curlee,R.F. and Perkins, W.H. (Eds.) *Nature and Treatment of Stuttering: New Directions.* San Diego: College-Hill Press.

Treating the School-aged Stutterer

Person: Carl Dell.

Age Range: School-aged children.

Objectives: The key to the problem of stuttering is early intervention, which will enable growth of the disorder to be reversed and the young stutterer to be cured (Dell,1979).

Summary

Dell, who trained with Charles Van Riper, suggests treatment plans for borderline, mild, and confirmed stuttering children. Treatment for borderline clients may be indirect or directive in practice. Indirect therapy encourages conversation, and it asks clinicians to model milder forms of stuttering. More directive therapy reinforces fluent speech and provides for light contact repetition (bounce) and desensitization training. Therapy for mild stutterers begins with clinicians modeling stuttering and asking the child to also engage in pseudo-stuttering. The child is encouraged to talk about the feelings that stuttering engenders. This is followed by a self-identification phase, during which the child identifies stuttering behavior and contrasts it to normal speech. The last phase deals with the simplification of the stuttered speech. This will hopefully lead to the choice, by the child, of more fluent speech.

Therapy with a more "confirmed stutterer" begins with identifying fluent speech, "hard stuttering," and "easy stuttering." Hard stuttering is the child's typical stutter, whereas easy stuttering uses effortless prolongations or repetitions. After observing clinicians model the different types of speech, the child learns to use them. The child then learns to monitor his speech to identify any tension that will lead to stuttering. Cancellation of hard blocks and replacing them with easy blocks follows. Voluntary easy stuttering desensitizes the child to the stuttering moment. These skills are transferred into real speaking situations, which improves the attitude toward communication and builds fluency. Independence comes about by gradually fading the child from therapy and using booster sessions as needed. Counselling deals primarily with providing parents and teachers with information and encouraging parents to remind their children about easy stuttering when necessary.

PROLAM-GM Components

Physiological Adjustments	Use of purposeful pseudostuttering.
Rate	Use of easy prolongations (pull-outs) and easy repetitions (bounce).
Attitude	Acceptance of stuttering via desensitization.
Monitoring	Identification of stuttering and the tension that may lead to stuttering.
Generalization	Use of speaking situations to practice techniques.
Maintenance	Sessions gradually faded out, with booster sessions as needed.

Research Findings: None reported.

Suggested Readings

Dell, Carl (1979). Treating the school age stutterer: a guide for clinicians. Memphis: Speech Foundation of America.

Dell, Carl (1992). Treating school-age stutterers. In Richard Curlee (Ed.) *Stuttering & related disorders of fluency* (pp. 45–68). New York: Thieme Medical Publishers.

Computer-Aided Fluency Establishment Trainer (CAFET)™

Person: Martha Goebel.

Age Range: School-aged children and adults.

Objectives: To produce fluent, natural-sounding speech in children and adults.

Summary
CAFET combines the use of computer hardware and software, enabling the user to attain the speech behaviors necessary for fluent speech. The hardware consists of an internal circuit board for an Apple II or PC computer that converts microphone and transducer signals into real-time computer displays. A respiratory sensor fits around the client's chest to measure breathing patterns inferred from chest wall movement. A respiratory transducer, which converts movement to electrical signals, and a clip-on microphone are the remaining hardware items. Software consists of the programs used to establish and maintain target responses. The adult program allows the client to visualize concepts with a series of graphs and feedback screens that show attainment of skills. The child program uses computer graphics in game-like configurations to achieve similar purposes, in addition to a basic graph module.

In the adult program, there are six basic targets. Via feedback from the respiratory sensor, the client can observe the difference between diaphragmatic and upper thoracic breathing. In addition, the feedback enables the client to produce a smooth respiratory curve with a slowed expiratory phase. Prevoice exhalation is also practiced with the aid of computer feedback. Gentle onset of phonation and continuous phonation are also monitored targets. There is also a target to ensure adequate breath support for speech.

The children's program substitutes syllable-stretched speech for the gentle onset target to facilitate continuous phonation. All targets are taught in smaller components. Each target is taught at various complexity levels, beginning with vowels and progressing to monosyllabic words, bisyllabic words, controlled-length phrases, and eventually monologues and conversational speech. As the components are mastered, speech rate is targeted at 180 to 210 syllables per minute. Skills at each level are practiced first with then without visual feedback to aid in generalization. In addition, telephone and situational contracts are used. Self-monitoring of target speech is a part of the generalization process, beginning with clinician-guided group therapy. Clients are encouraged to use the CAFET programs on their own for target maintenance and further desensitization of telephone calls (e.g., during maintenance phases), as well as continued group attendance, extending to self-help group participation.

PROLAM-GM Components

Physiological Adjustments	Air flow monitoring and easy onset of phonation are part of the program.
Rate	Prolongation of the first syllable of each breath group is initially used. Overall rate reduction only if client is above 230 syllables per minute.
Operant	Reinforcement is provided for attaining various target behaviors.
Length and Complexity of Utterance	All subprograms are hierarchical in nature, initially going from isolated sounds to conversational speech.
Monitoring	The computer monitors target initially until the client assumes the responsibility. Eventually, fluent speech is monitored.
Generalization	Use of contracts and logs. Group therapy with professive tasking.
Maintenance	Periodic evaluations with access to practice sessions and continued group therapy.

Research Findings: Data on 100 adult patients, and a 7-subject experimental child study available from author.

Special Features: Requires an Apple II or PC computer. Training in the use of the computerized program is available from the Annandale Fluency Clinic, 6231 Leesburg Pike, Falls Church, VA 22044.

Suggested Readings
Blood, G.W. (1994). Efficacy of a computer-assisted voice treatment protocol. *American Journal of Speech-Language Pathology, 3,* 57–66.

Behavioral Cognitive Stuttering Therapy

Person: Stanley A. Goldberg.

Age Range: Children, adolescents, and adults.

Objectives: The development of normal fluency through the practice of specific behaviors in various settings. Clients become their own therapists through the use of a contract format, self-monitoring, and self-evaluation.

Summary

The Behavioral Cognitive Stuttering Therapy (BCST) Program contains four major components: (1) diagnostic assessment, (2) fluency shaping, (3) counselling and attitude changes, and (4) fluency maintenance. In the diagnostic assessment unit, behaviors are categorized and analyzed to gather sufficient information necessary for the development of an intervention program. Information includes perceptions, beliefs, environmental factors stutterers believe effect fluency, and various objective measures of stuttered and fluent speech.

Fluency shaping involves five steps that require a minimum of 5 hours of direct clinical contact and many hours of practice outside the clinic. The five fluency shaping steps are: (1) extensive prolongation; (2) extensive prolongation, with switching to unmonitored speech; (3) reduced prolongation; (4) reduced prolongation, with switching to unmonitored speech; and (5) slow fluent speech. The increase in rate allows for systematic approximation of a normal-speaking rate. Switching from monitored to unmonitored speech is intended to provide the stutterer with a feeling of control. Generalization of behaviors occurs at each of the five steps.

Counselling and attitude change focus on identifying those attitudes that reinforce the maintenance of stuttering and hinder the development of fluency. Clinicians begin counselling and attitude change only if the client's belief system is interfering with therapy, and only after the fluency-shaping portion of the program has been successfully completed.

During fluency maintenance, clients and their support structures assume the major responsibility for generalization of fluency. Monitoring and self-evaluation are gradually decreased during the first year. Follow-up contacts with clients occur yearly for the next 4 years.

PROLAM-GM Components

Physiological Adjustments	Continuous phonation between words.
Rate	Use of prolonged speech, gradually increased to a normal rate.
Operant	Reinforcement for achieving target behaviors.
Attitude	Examination of the role stuttering and fluency has in the life of the client. Involves both positive and negative aspects of stuttering.
Monitoring	Initial clinician monitoring, changing to client self-monitoring.
Generalization	Occurs throughout the initial stages of fluency development and continues after direct clinical contact ends.
Maintenance	Scheduled activities the client is responsible for performing; 4-year follow-up contact schedule.

Research Findings: 5-year study of 35 clients ranging in age from 7 to 42 years (Goldberg, 1981).

Special Features: Assessment and therapy kit available.

Goldberg, S.A. (1981). *Behavioral Cognitive Stuttering Therapy (BCST): The Rapid Development of Fluent Speech.* IntelliGroup Publishing, Suite 303, Taraval St., San Francisco, CA 94116.

Suggested Readings

Goldberg, S.A. (1983). The development of fluency through behavioral cognitive stuttering therapy. *Journal of Communication Disorders, 8,7,* 89–107.

Edinburgh Masker Device

Person: Herbert Goldberg.

Age Range: Adults.

Objectives: The device is designed to help adult stutterers for whom speech therapy is ineffective achieve fluent speech.

Summary

The Masker is designed to produce noise that will prevent the wearer from hearing his or her own voice when speaking. The pitch of the noise varies with the pitch variations of the speaker's voice. A contact microphone worn around the neck activates the device on phonation, and the noise is transmitted via binaural hearing–aid–type fittings to the wearer's ears.

PROLAM-GM Components

Physiological Adjustments   The stutterer hears noise on phonation that masks his ability to hear his own speech.

Research Findings: Data for 195 stammerers are reported in Dewar et al. (1979). Moore & Adams study (1985) raised questions about the masker's effectiveness.

Special Features: Requires use of Edinburgh Masker device. Distributed by the FOUNDATION FOR FLUENCY INC. 4801 West Peterson Avenue Suite 218, Chicago, Illinois 60646.

Suggested Readings

Dewar, A., Dewar, A.D., Austin, W.T.S., & Brash, H.M. (1979). The longterm use of an automatically triggered auditory feedback masking device in the treatment of stammering. *British Journal of Disorders of Communication 14,* 219–229.

Environmental Manipulation and Family Counselling

Person: Hugo Gregory and Diane Hill.

Age Range: All ages.

Objectives: *For children:* restructuring the child's environment and counseling the parents so that the young stutterer is provided with a warm, supportive structure.
   For adults: restructuring of the client's attitudes and behaviors so that speech is produced with less stress and effort.

Summary
Children. Gregory and Hill (1980) believe that one of three treatment strategies should be used, based on a differential evaluation of the child and his or her parents: (1) preventive parent counselling, (2) prescriptive parent counselling, and (3) direct therapy with the child and counselling sessions with the parents. The preventive parent counselling strategy is used when the diagnostic session reveals that the child's disfluencies are normal, but the parents are expressing concern and identifying the behavior as stuttering. Prescriptive parent counselling is conducted if the child is exhibiting borderline atypical disfluencies, which Gregory (1986a, b) defines as "the problem has existed for less than a year, and there appears to be no significant complicating speech, language, or behavioral characteristics." The last treatment strategy, which involves direct therapy and parent counselling, is selected when the child's borderline atypical disfluencies have lasted for more than 1 year.

To teach the child new, less-stressful speaking behaviors, clinicians model them for the child and the parents. These behaviors may include relaxation procedures, relaxed speech, smooth movements beginning at the word level and working up to longer utterances, slower rate, and turn-taking. Counselling involves teaching the parents how to change the child's environment, which includes their own behaviors, so the child's efforts at speaking are supported.

Adults. The approach with adults is similar to that with children (Gregory, 1968, 1986b). Efforts are made to change the stutterer's attitudes, reduce excessive bodily tension, and build new psychomotor speech patterns. Attitudes addressed include those that contribute to the stutterer's negative feelings about speech. Tension is reduced through progressive relaxation techniques and use of stuttering modification techniques, such as Van Riper's cancellations, pull-outs, preparatory sets, and substituting a less forceful stuttering pattern for a more stressful one. The new psychomotor speech patterns involve phrasing, rate, loudness, and prosodic variation.

PROLAM-GM Components
Physiological Adjustments   Any technique that reduces the amount of tension associated with the production of speech.

Rate	A normal rate of speech is emphasized.
Attitude	Changing parental attitudes to ones that are supportive of the child's effort to speak. For adults, changing negative attitudes about speaking.

Research Findings: None.

Special Features: None.

Suggested Readings

Gregory, H.H. & Hill, D. (1980). Stuttering therapy for the child. In W. Perkins (Ed.), *Strategies in stuttering therapy.* New York: Thieme-Stratton.

Gregory, H.H. (1986a). Environmental manipulation and family counseling. In G.H. Shames & H. Rubin (Eds.). *Stuttering: Then and now.* pp. 273–291. Columbus OH: Charles Merrill.

Techniques for Maintaining Fluency

Person: Roger J. Ingham.

Age Range: All ages.

Objectives: Establishment and maintenance of normal fluency.

Summary

During the establishment phase of Ingham's program, the client completes six successive speaking tasks without any stutterings. These speech tasks are performed within a specific speech rate range and evaluated by a trained clinician using an electronic button-press counter. If the clinician observes any stuttering between evaluation sessions, the previous evaluation session is disregarded and the client repeats the step. Criteria for advancement into the transfer phase requires the client to speak spontaneously in six sessions of 1,300 syllables at between 170 and 210 syllables per minute.

The transfer phase consists of approximately seven speaking tasks that clients can order in terms of complexity. To progress from one task to the next, clients must display 1,300 syllables that are stutter-free at a speaking rate of between 170 and 210 syllables per minute. Throughout the transfer phase, the clinician participates in monitoring the client's progress; however, monitoring eventually becomes the responsibility of the client.

Maintenance begins when the client completes the transfer phase and leaves the clinic. Clients initially return to the clinic after 1 week; the duration between visits can increase to 32 weeks. During each scheduled visit, syllable counts are taken. Between visits, at least one unscheduled telephone conversation is conducted. Surprise meetings may also occur without prior notice to the client.

There is no formal counseling component in this program. Ingham maintains that clients who require counseling during therapy do so largely because of difficulties independent of stuttering. Counselling is therefore neither sufficient nor even necessary for establishing fluent speech. Nevertheless, routine counseling does occur.

PROLAM-GM Components

Rate	A target rate of 170 to 210 syllables per minute is used; however, there is no attempt to systematically modify the rate of speech.
Operant	Production of fluent utterances is rewarded by advancement to the next step of therapy. Production of stutterings results in repetition of the same step or repeating a previous step.
Monitoring	Initially, both the clinician and the client are responsible for monitoring the occurrence of stutterings. Later, it becomes the responsibility of the client.
Generalization	Specific program for practicing fluent speech at the target rate outside of the clinic.
Maintenance	Scheduled and unscheduled visits to assess the extent to which the client's speech is remaining fluent.

Research Findings: Specific research conducted with the use of response contingent behavior.

Special Features: None.

Suggested Readings

Ingham, R. (1980). Modification of maintenance and generalization during stuttering treatment. *Journal of Speech and Hearing Research, 23:* 732–745.

Ingham, R. (1984). Generalization and maintenance of treatment. In R. Curlee and W. Perkins (Eds.) *Nature and treatment of stuttering: New directions.* San Diego: College-Hill Press.

Ingham, R. (1984).Techniques for maintaining fluency. In W.H. Perkins (Ed.), *Stuttering disorders.* pp. 209–221. New York: Thieme-Stratton.

An Operational Approach to Stuttering Therapy

Person: Harold Luper and Robert Mulder.

Age Range: Children.

Objectives: The goal of therapy is to achieve a change for the better in stuttering behavior.

Summary
Treatment is divided into four phases. Each phase is directed at a different developmental level of stuttering in children. Phase one deals with the modification of incipient or beginning stuttering. The primary focus is indirect, using parents and teachers along with environmental manipulation. Parents are given information about stuttering and encouraged to behave in ways that will improve the speaking environment and their interactions with the child. Phase two is concerned with modification of transitional (chronic) stuttering. The goal is to prevent the growth and development of chronic stuttering. A more directive approach than used in phase one may include desensitization of the child to fluency disruptions by providing opportunities to talk about stuttering. Conditions conducive to speaking fluently may be structured, emphasizing rhymthic speaking and choral responding. If necessary, "loose contacts" during phonation along with smooth movements by the articulators are suggested to the child.

Phase three therapy deals with direct therapy for confirmed stutterers. A confirmed stutterer is a full-fledged stutterer except for avoidances. While developing an accepting therapeutic relationship with the child, the clinician shares the goal of reducing feared situations and reducing stuttering. Checklists are developed that help the child recognize likely stuttering situations. "Loose contacts," "easy stuttering," and Van Riper's cancellation and pull-out techniques are stressed. Phase four deals with the modification of advanced stuttering, which is now a serious emotional and personal problem. Word and situational fears are dealt with in a hierarchical fashion. New attitudes are developed through experiencing enjoyable speaking situations.

PROLAM-GM Components

Physiological Adjustments	Loose articulatory contacts, easy stuttering, smooth transitions (pull-outs), and cancellations are used to manipulate stuttering.
Rate	Choral reading and rhythmic speech may be used.
Attitude	Acceptance of and desensitization to stuttering are stressed in a supportive environment.

Monitoring	Stuttering or avoidance situations are monitored.
Generalization	Use of modification techniques in daily speech.
Maintenance	Posttherapy conferences and classroom observations are scheduled.

Research Findings: None are presented.

Suggested Readings

Luper, H.L., & Mulder, R.L.(1964). *Stuttering: therapy for children.* Englewood Cliffs, N.J.: Prentice-Hall.

A Program to Establish Fluent Speech

Person: Donald E. Mowrer.

Age Range: Second grade reading level or above.

Objectives: Stuttering is a learned behavior. Thus, a client is capable of achieving fluent speech, which can be best learned by controlled presentation of specified antecedent and consequent events.

Summary

Mowrer designed this program to establish fluent speech by systematically increasing the rate, length, and complexity of fluent utterances. The author assumes that if stuttering is a learned behavior it can be manipulated by external stimuli to produce fluent speech. This is an establishment program that is divided into six subprograms. It does not provide for the maintenance of fluency once it is established. Clients begin this program by reading words following presentation of a brief tone that is presented once every 5 seconds. Fluency is also enhanced by the repeated readings of the same words. If a client anticipates stuttering on a given word, he omits that word and reads one that will be uttered fluently. By using these four conditions, there is a high expectation of fluent performance.

The first goal of the program is to establish this fluent reading skill, after which the goal is to maintain the fluency level during other speaking tasks. When a word is spoken fluently, positive verbal consequences are provided by clinicians; stuttered words are followed by a contingent "no." The single utterances read from word lists are systematically increased in length, with increasing propositionality (meaningfulness).

Once fluent speech is obtained and maintained while reading, picture stimuli are introduced following the same hierarchical format of going from single utterances to more complex ones. Lastly, topics are introduced for discussions that approximate normal conversational speech. Specific positive reinforcement, punishment contingencies, and schedules of reinforcement are detailed in the program manual. A series of "branching" steps are included for clients who experience difficulty achieving criterion levels at any given step.

PROLAM-GM Components

Physiological Adjustments	Speech rate and propositionality are reduced to initiate fluency.
Rate	A slow rate matched to a reset tone is used initially.
Operant	Positive verbal consequences for fluent words and contingent "no" from clinician following stuttered words.
Length and Complexity of Utterance	Both the complexity and the propositionality of the utterances are manipulated during the program.
Monitoring	Clients are expected to skip anticipated stuttered words initially and only produce anticipated fluent utterances.

Research Findings: None are presented with the program.

Special Features: The program is available in kit form that includes an instruction manual, stimulus tape, stimulus materials, and data sheets.

Suggested Readings
Mowrer, D.E. (1979). *A Program to Establish Fluent Speech*. Columbus: Merrill Publishing Company.

Integration of Approaches

Person: Theodore J. Peters and Barry Guitar.

Age Range: All ages.

Objectives: To provide clients with the techniques that will allow them to (1) achieve controlled fluency, (2) modify the severity of the stuttering behavior, or (3) feel comfortable with acceptable stuttering.

Summary

The authors believe that "predisposing physiological factors interact with developmental and environmental influence to produce and/or exacerbate repetitions and prolongations" (Peters and Guitar, 1991). The actual stuttering response is viewed as a classically conditioned behavior. To prevent the stuttering from occurring or to reduce its severity, the stutterer may develop other behaviors that are instrumentally reinforced. The focus of therapy is to provide clients with a sufficient number of positive and fluent speaking experiences during treatment so that fluency will generalize to nonclinical settings. For children, parent counselling is an important component of therapy.

There are a variety of speech behaviors targeted for change, including increasing the length and complexity of utterance, reducing rate, desensitization to fluency disruptors factors, and, when necessary, substituting a less severe form of stuttering for a more severe one. With children, modeling of appropriate behaviors is important. Counselling on feelings and attitudes is dependent on the age of the client and the extent it contributes to the problem. Counselling of children is usually not necessary. However, it may be useful in desensitizing children to fluency-disrupting conditions or stimuli that remain near the end of therapy. Positive reinforcement in the form of social reinforcement is provided to all clients, and token reinforcement is provided to some children.

Generalization of behaviors may involve unstructured procedures or a highly structured program involving specification of antecedent events, responses, consequent events, and criterion for advancement.

For young stutterers, monitoring or maintenance procedures are usually not necessary. Contact is maintained with the parents through periodic re-evaluations, which are systematically decreased. For older stutterers, self-monitoring and self-maintenance is important. Clients master stuttering modification and fluency-shaping techniques and learn to evaluate their own performance. Programs tend to have a loose structure and depend on clients assuming greater responsibility both for goals and activities.

PROLAM-GM Components

Physiological Adjustments	Use of light contact and repetition (bounce) of initial syllables to initial words.
Rate	Use of prolonged speech as a stuttering reduction and a fluency-enhancing technique.
Attitude	Emphasis on reducing avoidance in accepting the role of a stutterer, using feared words, and entering feared situations. Importance of functioning as one's own therapist is stressed.
Monitoring	Clients are instructed to monitor speech behaviors, including rate when fluent-sounding speech is important.

Generalization   Programs for children tend to be more struc-
                                    tured than those for adults.

Research Findings: None directly related to the approach, but substantial
amount of studies on specific components are cited in the literature.

Special Features: None.

Suggested Readings
Peters, T.J. & Guitar, B. (1991). *Stuttering: An integrated approach to its nature and
    treatment.* Baltimore, MD: Williams & Wilkins.

Stuttering Intervention Program

Person: Rebekah H. Pindzola.

Age Range: Preschool through third grade.

Objectives: The program is founded on the principles of event consequation,
physiological maneuvers, and linguistic complexity. Its objective is for young
children to utilize suggested fluency enhancement practices.

Summary
The Stuttering Intervention Program has four components: (1) evaluation of
the child, (2) parental involvement, (3) treatment, and (4) information for public school functioning. The Protocol for Differentiating the Incipient Stutterer
(Pindzola and White, 1986) and the Stuttering Severity Instrument (Riley, 1972)
are the instruments recommended for evaluation of the possibility of stuttering in children and in children who do stutter. Parental involvement begins
during evaluation of the child, and it is expected throughout the treatment
program. As treatment progresses parents have increased responsibility for
both daily practice sessions and monitoring of treatment assignments. The
treatment program consists of reinforcement of fluency, and highlighting of
instances of stuttering, and techniques for fluency enhancement.

The major fluency enhancement techniques are "slow stretched speech, soft
speech, and smooth speech." Slow stretched speech is a type of continuous
phonation that the child applies at points of "vocal initiation," which is defined
as occurring specifically at the beginning of sentences or after pauses. Soft
speaking voice decreases volume and accompanying laryngeal tension.
Smooth speech encourages blending of words in an easy onset, rhythmic,
wave-like manner. Practice sessions begin with monosyllabic words and progress through combined monosyllables to polysyllabic words, eventually lead-

ing to spontaneous speech. The final section of the program deals with public school issues, such as individualized educational program writing and information for regular and special education personnel.

PROLAM-GM Components

Physiological Adjustments	Use of decreased volume and a variant of continuous phonation.
Rate	Use of slow speech and rhythmic phonation in wave-like utterances.
Operant	Reinforcement of fluency and highlighting of stuttering.
Length and Complexity of Utterance	Systematic evolution from monosyllabic utterances to spontaneous speech.
Monitoring	Both parents and children monitor techniques outside of therapy sessions.
Generalization	Use of generalization after skills are taught.

Research Findings: Data for 3 subjects are presented in Pindzola (1987).

Special Features: Diagnostic and therapy materials available in kit form.

Suggested Readings
Pindzola, R.H. (1987). *Stuttering Intervention Program*. Austin, TX: Pro-Ed Corporation.

Managing Stuttering

Person: David Prins.

Age Range: Adolescents and adults.

Objectives: The moment of stuttering is the principal target of therapy. The person who stutters learns to speak as fluently as he is able and has the will and motivation to accomplish (Prins, 1984).

Summary
To help adolescent and adult stutterers manage their stuttering, a three-phased program of therapy is used. Phase one consists of exploring, understanding, and accepting the responsibility for stuttering, reactions, and speaking behavior generally. Phase two involves calming the stutterer and stuttering, which is

aimed at reducing the intensity of reactions during stuttering. Phase three involves replacing stuttering reactions with actions that produce fluent speech. The techniques of phase one that lead the stutterer to awareness and then responsibility include use of videotapes and mirrors to help analyze speaking behavior. Speech-language pathologists also model reactions and structure discussions about feelings and attitudes that accompany this behavior.

During phase two, calming is achieved by experiencing "high intensity" behaviors and feelings when stuttering and changing them into "low intensity" ones. Speech activities are structured in a hierarchical manner from easy to hard while maintaining a feeling of calmness. The feeling is then transferred to everyday speaking activities. During phase three, the client is taught to detect the cues that trigger stuttering reactions and then to replace these reactions with smooth, effortless speech movements that result in fluent production of the syllable or word. Self-therapy, group work, and extraclinical experiences help the client generalize behavior mastered in therapy and internalize a sense of self-efficacy regarding the ability to speak.

PROLAM-GM Components

Rate	Speech movements used to replace stuttering are done slowly and deliberately, without unneccessary effort or tension.
Length and Complexity of Utterance	Some activities are structured, from single word responses to conversational speech.
Attitude	The initial phase requires identification and description of stuttering reactions and accepting responsibility for speaking. Phase two focuses on reducing emotional reactions during stuttering. All phases emphasize cognitive change and the client's conviction self-efficacy as a speaker.
Monitoring	Throughout treatment, the client is responsible for self-evaluating behavior and changes.
Generalization	Self-therapy exercises are paired with clinician-modeled field-trip experiences to practice skills mastered within the clinic.

Research Findings: Results using the program on both adult and child clients are reported in Prins (1970), Prins and Miller (1973), and Prins and Nichols (1974).

Suggested Readings

Prins, D. (1993) Management of stuttering: Treatment of adolescents and adults. In R.F. Curlee (Ed.). Stuttering and related disorders of fluency. New York :Thieme Publishers.

A Component Model for Treating Stuttering in Children

Person: Glyndon D. Riley and Jeanna Riley.

Age Range: Children.

Objectives: Treatment of the child's stuttering based on the components that contribute to fluency breakdown.

Summary
Through the use of the Stuttering Prediction Instrument (SPI), children can be identified as having either a nonchronic or a chronic stuttering problem. Although it is anticipated that nonchronic stutterers will outgrow their problem, a fluency monitoring program is implemented that relies on the parents to monitor their child's speech. Contacts are made every 6 months for a 2-year period.

Therapy for young stutterers is based on the results of appropriate testing and clinical judgments used to identify one or more of nine different components that contributes to the development and maintenance of stuttering.

1. attending disorders
2. auditory processing disorders
3. sentence formulation disorders
4. oral motor disorders
5. high self-expectations by the child
6. manipulative stuttering
7. disruptive communication environment
8. unrealistic parental expectations
9. abnormal parental need for child to stutter

Prior to directly modifying the child's abnormal disfluencies, each of the components found to be present is treated. Only after the components have been addressed will direct work on disfluency modification occur. The older the child, the more likely direct modification will be required.

PROLAM-GM Components

Physiologial Adjustments	Use of easy onset of speech, gentle articulatory contacts, oral motor practice.
Rate	Use of reduced rate.
Operant	Use of reinforcement and punishment techniques to develop appropriate behaviors.
Length and Complexity of Utterance	Use of language programs that emphasize systematic development of linguistic competence and performance.

Attitude	Counseling of parents and children regarding the role stuttering plays in the child's life; changing parents' and children's attitudes so that positive behaviors can be developed.
Monitoring	Elaborate monitoring activities conducted by parents of nonchronic children; children's monitoring of behaviors during therapy.
Generalization	As each new behavior is stabilized in the clinic, it is generalized in nonclinic settings.

Research Findings: Studies involving 44 children enrolled in the program.

Suggested Readings
Riley, G.D. & J. Riley (1984). A component model for treating stuttering in children. In M. Peins (Ed.) Contemporary Appproaches in Stuttering Therapy. pp. 123–171, Boston: Little, Brown and Co.

Monterey Fluency Programs

Person: Bruce Ryan and Barbara Van Kirk Ryan.

Age Range: Children and adults.

Objectives: The goal of the treatment procedure is to use systematically programmed instructional techniques to obtain fluent speech.

Summary
The Monterey Programs are based on the original work of Ryan (1971), and later Ryan and Van Kirk (1978, 1974). Initially Ryan (1974b) described four procedures to establish, transfer, and maintain fluency. The first was a systematic application of symptom modification therapy (Van Riper, 1973), with addition of a final fluent phase. The second was a DAF program similar in format to those described by Goldiamond (1965) and Curlee and Perkins (1969). The third was an approach that relied on punishment, using verbal contingencies and time-out procedures. The fourth utilized a systematic approach to the Gradual Increase in the Length and Complexity of Utterance (GILCU). More recent descriptions of therapeutic procedures (Ryan, 1984) concentrate only on DAF and GILCU.

The programs have three phases. During the first phase, fluency is established in the presence of the speech-language pathologist using DAF or GILCU. The second phase involves transfer of fluent speech to environments other than the clinical setting. The third phase involves a maintenance level to establish continued use of fluency. The client performs with reading, monologue, and conversational speech. The programs are arranged in a number of steps of increasing complexity. Fluency at specified levels is required before proceeding from one step to the next. The programs feature branching possibilities that enable the client to practice failed steps, and recycling, which allows the client to re-experience failed portions of the program.

Fluency is established with GILCU or, if that approach fails, DAF. The GILCU program has 54 steps. The stutterer begins reading or speaking one fluent utterance at a time and gradually increases the length and complexity of speech until 5 minutes of fluent conversational speech are obtained. The DAF program has 26 steps and establishes a slow prolonged speech that is shaped to normal fluency. Delay begins at 250 msec, and it is decreased in steps of 50 msec, until the client is speaking independently without the use of DAF. Transfer to different speaking situations can range from 17 to 32 steps in six different settings. Fluent gains are monitored during the maintenance phase, which can last 22 months. Maintenance relies on collection and analyzing of reading samples, monologues, and conversations, in addition to teacher and parental reports for children.

PROLAM-GM Components

Rate	Reduced rate using DAF when needed.
Operant	Use of both social and token forms of reinforcement in small steps.
Length and Complexity of Utterance	The program relies on the gradual increase in length and complexity of fluent responses.
Generalization	Use of a variety of different speaking situations, audience sizes, and listeners, in addition to telephone work to transfer gains of therapy.
Maintenance	Rechecks that are gradually faded over a 22-month period, with opportunities to recycle clients who have failed to maintain fluency.

Research Findings: Data on several hundred children and adults are reported in a variety of sources, including Van Kirk and Ryan (1974), Ryan and Ryan (1983), Ryan (1985), and Rustin et al. (1987).

Special Features: Detailed descriptions of the programs are available in Ryan, B. (1974 B) Programmed Therapy for stuttering in children and adults. Springfield, Il.: Charles C. Thomas. and Ryan, B., & Van Kirk, B. (1978) Monterey fluency program. Palo Alto, Ca. Monterey Learning Systems.

Suggested Readings
Ryan, B.(1986). Operant therapy for Children. In G. Shames & H. Rubin *Stuttering Then and Now*. Columbus: Charles Merrill Publishing Company.

Ryan, B. (1981). Maintenance programs in profess-II. In E. Boberg (Ed.) *Maintenance of Fluency:* New York: Elsevier.

Ryan, B. (1985). Training the professional in E. Boberg (Ed.), *Stuttering. Part One. Seminars in Speech and Language.* New York: Thieme-Stratton, Inc.

Rustin, L., Ryan, B. & Ryan, B. (1987). Use of the Monterey programmed stuttering therapy in Great Britain. *British Journal of Disorders of Communication, 22,* 151–162.

A Modeling Approach To Stuttering Therapy For Children

Person: Herbert Seltzer and Richard Culatta.

Age Range: Young children.

Objectives: A model indulging in stuttering behavior and systematically achieving fluency can positively effect a stuttering child's speech performance and bring about fluency.

Summary

Repeated exposure to a model's reactions to a given behavior may have activating or motivating effects on an observer. Changes in model behavior can significantly effect an observers future performance (Bandura, 1969). The authors designed a three-part program based on modelling principles to be used with young stuttering children. During phase I, the child is instructed to attend to an adult model (the speech-language pathologist), who abnormally repeats or prolongs sounds on a predetermined schedule. Children are to point at the clinician and say "gotcha" contingent on the disfluencies. Identification of the model's disfluencies is the only behavior requested of the children for the entire program. During phase II, the discriminative abilities of the child are refined further. Children are now expected to respond within three repetitions or 1 second. The model smiles, says "thank you," and repeats the word fluently. After reaching criterion, the child is exposed to the third phase. During phase III, the model's speech is programmed to contain longer periods of fluency with correspondingly decreasing instances of stuttering. The model also makes evaluative statements praising the fluent speech and showing dislike for the stuttered speech. The observing child is simply requested to identify disfluencies as they are presented.

PROLAM-GM Components

Operant	Model praises self-generated fluency and punishes self-generated stuttering. Child punishes all instances of model-generated stuttering.

Attitude	Children internalize attitudes of a model who praises fluency and comments negatively about instances of stuttering.
Monitoring	Children observe a model who is aware of fluency as it occurs. Client monitors model-generated stuttering.

Research Findings: Data of the results of the program with 12 children are reported in Seltzer & Culatta (1979).

Special Features: Program can be utilized without parental involvement and may be used with reticent children or in instances where direct confrontation may not be advisable.

Suggested Readings
Seltzer, H. & Culatta, R. (1979). A Modeling Approach To Stuttering Therapy For Young Children. *Journal Of Childhood Communications Disorders, 3*, 103–110.

Vocaltech Feedback Device

Person: George Shames.

Age Range: Adults and children.

Objectives: Use of this device enhances the ability of the wearer to monitor fluent speech during initiation and generalization phases of therapy.

Summary
The device, which consists of a neck vibrator and a power source that is activated by the onset of phonation, provides vibratory stimulation to the neck area. This stimulation heightens awareness of speech patterns and fosters increased concentration on maintaining a modified speech rate.

PROLAM-GM Components

Rate	A slower rate of speech is taught and maintained by the client.
Monitoring	The device provides vibration on phonation, which assists in initial monitoring of fluent speech.
Generalization	Primary use of device is to aid in generalization of skills learned during the initial program.

Research Findings: Anecdotal reports of use with "more than 100 stutterers" and with "50 patients" have been reported in *Newsweek*, June 19, 1989 and the *Psychiatric Times*, June 1989.

Special Features: Requires use of the Vocal Feedback Device, marketed by Vocaltech Inc. 1121 Boyce Road Pittsburgh, PA 15241.

Stutter-Free Speech

Person: George Shames and Cheri Florance.

Age Range: All.

Objectives: Establishment of speech free of stuttering and a speaker who no longer perceives himself as a stutterer by combining the technologies of operant manipulation with traditional psychotherapy and counselling.

Summary

The authors designed a program wherein fluent speech is established by rate control and continuous phonation. Changed self-perceptions are a result of interactions with the clinician/counsellor. There are five phases to this program. It is suggested that phases I and II be scheduled for 1 or 2 hours a day. Scheduling for phase III can vary. Phase IV is conducted on a weekly schedule. Phase V begins on a monthly schedule, and it evolves through quarterly, semiannual, and finally annual sessions during a 5-year maintenance period. Shames (1986) reports that the program can be adapted to intensive summer camp or hospital programming.

During phase I (volitional control), stutter-free speech is instilled using a variation of DAF, wherein the client learns a continuously phonated slow rate of fluent speech. Phase II (self-reinforcement) teaches the speaker to self-regulate the stutter-free speech. A key point is that during this phase, the client rewards himself with periods of unmonitored speech. This unmonitored speech, the authors report, is an attempt to deal with the complaints of clients that monitoring speech is a tedious process not always worth the reward of fluency. Phase III (transfer) utilizes contracts written by the client that specify time, place, audience, and desired speech behavior into which the client will incorporate stutter-free speech. These contracts can be designed for within and extraclinical settings. Phase V (follow-up) is a 5-year maintenance program, during which time contracts are systematically decreased.

PROLAM-GM Components

Physiological Adjustments	Stutter-free speech is instilled with continuous phonation.

Rate	Prolongation and slow speech rates are initially used.
Operant	Client self-reinforces with unmonitored speech for monitored fluent speech.
Attitude	Self-perceptions change with speech-language pathologist's guidance.
Monitoring	Monitored and unmonitored speech are alternated.
Generalization	Use of contracts.
Maintenance	Five-year contacts scheduled.

Research Findings: Data on 152 clients are reported in Shames & Florance (1980).

Special Features: Programmed fading of monitored and unmonitored speech; use of fluency contracts; material presented in text/kit format with appropriate forms.

Suggested Readings

Shames, G.H. & Florance, C.L. (1980) *Stutter-Free Speech:A goal for Therapy.* Columbus: Merrill Publishing Company.

Shames, G.H. (1986) A Current View of Stutter-Free Speech in Shames, G.H. & Rubin H. (Eds.) *Stuttering Then and Now.* Columbus: Merrill Publishing Company.

Role Therapy

Person: Joseph G. Sheehen (reviewed by Vivian Sheehan).

Age Range: Teenagers and adults.

Objectives: (1) To help the stutterer accept the role of a stutterer, examine his behaviors, realize his responsibility for those behaviors and the power it gives him to change. (2) To achieve improvement in communication through non-avoidance and increased self-esteem in the speaker role. (3) To achieve normal speech with tolerance of normal disfluencies.

Summary:

Sheehan views stuttering as a false-role disorder: a role-specific conflict involving approach and avoidance (1958). The stutterer wishes to speak, but is afraid to. This conflict leads to the "block." Open display of stuttering reduces the fear and permits termination of the block. This cycle will continue until the conflict is resolved through elimination of avoidances by confronting fears gradually in a hierarchy of severity and going ahead rather than retreating, hiding, or pretending to be fluent. The therapy is a combination of speech therapy (to expose the learned external behaviors that are used as crutches in the attempt to speak fluently) and psychotherapy (to deal with guilt, need for fluency, and low self-esteem). Stuttering can be modified in form through an action therapy involving acceptance of stuttering and willingness to stutter in a struggle-free manner leading to normal speech. The frequency of stuttering will decrease as the struggle behaviors are eliminated. No practicings of special techniques for achieving fluency are involved—only openness and honesty and a changing role of self-acceptance as a stutterer will lead to overcoming the tyranny of stuttering in the life of the stutterer. No progress can be made in the clinic or therapy room alone. The stutterer must face this problem, talk about it, and give up his avoidances of words, people, situations, and relationships through behavior and attitudinal changes.

Sheehan lists 17 basic therapy procedures that are used in avoidance-reduction therapy (1970): (1) establishing eye contact; (2) open discussion of stuttering; (3) exploring one's own stuttering behaviors; (4) learning the language of responsibility; (5) monitoring behaviors; (6) taking the initiate in seeking out feared situations; (7) exposing the hidden aspects of stuttering; (8) focusing on successes even with stuttering; (9) stuttering openly and easily; (10) resisting time pressure; (11) using normal phrasing in proper places, not before feared words; (12) reducing struggle; (13) stuttering voluntarily on nonfeared word and on feared words later; (14) using nonreinforcement and cancellation of "tricks and crutches"; (15) tolerating disfluencies; (16) later in therapy, speaking normally without tricks; (17) accepting the new role of fluent speaker.

PROLAM-GM Components

Operant	Self-identification of those learned stuttering behaviors that may be reinforcing avoidances.
Attitude	Changing the client's attitude from avoidances of stuttering and the hiding of feelings about stuttering, to open stuttering without struggle. Frank discussion about fears of stuttering and their impact on self-esteem.
Monitoring	If behaviors and attitudes are to be changed they must be observed and monitored. The stutterer must be fully aware of what he wants to change.

Research Findings: Tangential to the approach.

Special Features: Requires knowledge and experience with stuttering and the fundamental principles of learning psychology and therapeutic techniques to change habits and attitudes.

Suggested Readings

Sheehan, J.G. (1953). Theory and Treatment of Stuttering as an approach-avoidance conflict. Journal of Psychology: 36, pp. 27–49.

Sheehan, J.G. (1970). Stuttering: Research and Therapy. New York: Harper and Row.

Sheehan, J.G. (1975). Conflict theory and avoidance reduction therapy, in J. Eisenson (Ed.), *Stuttering: A second symposium*, 97–198, New York: Harper and Row.

Systematic Fluency Training for Young Children

Person: Richard E. Shine.

Age Range: 3–12 years.

Objectives: Stuttering is a coordinative disorder resulting from a predisposing neurophysiological difference that may be genetic or the result of prenatal, natal, or neonatal complications. The predisposition may be neuromotor, neurolinguistic, or a combination of both (Shine, 1980a, 1984). The primary goal of this direct fluency training approach is to train the child to use physiological and prosodic speaking patterns that are compatible with fluency and incompatible with stuttering (Shine, 1984).

Summary

Shine (1980a) presents a program that wishes to establish speaking patterns in children that are "compatible with fluency and incompatible with stuttering" (Webster, 1979). Among the goals of this program are education of parents and significant others about stuttering (Shine, 1983). The use of pictures and other selected materials helps them establish fluency with their child in the home environment. Direct therapy with the child utilizes a number of fluency-enhancing techniques, including respiratory, phonatory, coarticulatory, stress, intonational, rate/rhythm, utterance complexity, and motor planning strategies. Fluency training is initiated with an imitated whispered speaking voice (WSV) with the primary goals of establishing understanding of the concepts of quiet and easy and developing a structured antecedent/consequent stimulus management program, in conjunction with a token economy system and verbal feedback of the correctness or incorrectness of each response. On the rare occasion that WSV training is not successful, a prolonged speaking voice is taught. The quite/easy concepts and stimulus management program are used to establish an exaggerated easy voice onset (EVO), which incorporates significantly decreased loudness and syllable duration followed by a rising intonation pattern and increased loudness on single syllable words. The EVO is transferred to establishment of an "easy speaking voice" in an 11-step program in which length and complexity of utterances are increased. The fluent ESV is generalized within each session during a series of four highly structured activities using a progressively less exaggerated EVO. Eventually the EVO is required on only the first syllable/word of a phrase or sentence with the remainder being articulated with normal rate, rhythm, intensity, and intonation.

This program does not focus on the secondary characteristics of stuttering. Attitudinal reorientation focuses on experience with fluency with the stated expectation by the SLP that the client is capable of normal-sounding speech. Generalization into the environment and establishment of fluent conversation in a variety of settings is determined by clinical judgment with regard to the appropriateness of extra therapy procedures for a given child. Maintenance sessions are scheduled with decreasing frequency for a 1-year period after dismissal.

PROLAM-GM Components

Rate	Prolongation may be used initially to establish fluency. An exaggerated slow, easy voice onset is a component of ESV.
Operant	A token system and antecedent/consequent stimulus management are recommended to reinforce fluency and to punish incorrect responses and stuttering.
Monitoring	Parents and others monitor fluent productions and make child aware of "hard" speech and stuttering.
Generalization	Clinician judgment determines generalization activities.
Maintenance	Periodic sessions for 1 year after therapy.

Research Findings: Data for 14 subjects are presented in Mason & Shine (1981) and Shine (1984), and for 9 subjects in Ammons (1993).

Special Features: Diagnostic and therapy stimuli materials are available in kit form.

Suggested Readings

Shine, R. (1988). *Systematic Fluency Training for Young Children: Third Edition.* Austin, TX: Pro-Ed.

Shine. R. (1980b). Direct Management of the Beginning Stutterer. In W. Perkins (ed.) *Strategies in Stuttering Therapy: Seminars in Speech, Language and Hearing,* New York: Thieme-Stratton.

Shine, R. (1984). Assessment and Fluency Training with the Young Stutterer. In M. Peins (ed.) *Contemporary Approached in Stuttering Therapy*, Boston: Little, Brown and Company.

Air Flow Therapy

Person: Martin F. Schwartz.

Age Range: All ages.

Objectives: Development of fluent speech by eliminating the airway dilation reflex.

Summary
Stuttering is caused by a tendency of the vocal cords to go into spasm under conditions of stress just prior to the act of speaking. The struggle to release the spasm is what is seen as stuttering; it is simply a learned reaction to the locking of the vocal cords. Consequently, the spasm rather than the stuttering is addressed. The patient is taught a new way of breathing immediately prior to speaking. This manner of breathing causes the cords to remain open and relaxed, thereby eliminating the spasm. The result is immediate aborting of the stuttering behavior.

The teaching process is segmented into two phases. The first phase is the workshop, involving concentrated treatment for 8 hours a day on 2 consecutive days. During this phase, the patient is trained in the basic principles of the airflow technique and in several techniques for reducing general stress. Each patient is given the opportunity to use the airflow technique in a variety of stressful situations, which helps the patient acquire confidence in the viability of this new technique. The second phase is designed to reinforce these techniques so they can become a habit, and it generally lasts approximately 1 year. It is performed at home and in various speaking situations. The patient is required to practice the airflow technique in specific exercises for 1 hour each day and to record samples on cassette tape. The tapes are then reviewed each week and returned to the client with comments and suggestions, with new exercise assignments. During this phase patients are gradually introduced to situations of increasing complexity and stress. They learn to apply the technique at each level before proceeding to the next. In this way, confidence is built systematically to the point where all sound, word, and situation fears become extinguished.

PROLAM-GM Components

Physiological Adjustments	Initiation of phonation only after exhalation has begun.

Attitude	Discussion of the roles of "stutterer" and "fluent speaker."
Monitoring	Clients are asked to develop their own personal method of monitoring proper breath control.
Generalization	Daily 1-hour practice sessions for 1 year.
Maintenance	Taped recorded feedback provided to the client of their performance on weekly recorded speech samples.

Research Findings: 89% success rate reported anecdotally without provision of data. Data reported using similar approach used by Azrin and Nunn (1974).

Special Features: None.

Suggested Readings
Azrin, N.H. & Nunn, R.G. (1974). A rapid method of eliminating stuttering by a regulated breathing approach. *Behavioral Research Therapy, 12,* 279–86.
Schwartz, M.F. (1991). *Stutter no more.* New York: Simon & Schuster.

Multiprocess Behavioral Approach

Person: C. Woodruff Starkweather.

Age Range: All ages.

Objectives: Development of reduced stuttering and increased fluency through the use of various stress-reducing and speech modification techniques.

Summary
Stuttering can be caused by four types of conditioning: (1) classic, (2) operant, (3) avoidance, and (4) vicarious. Therefore, improvement in the client's speech will require that the behaviors resulting from each form of conditioning be treated using specific techniques, including reversing conditioning processes that currently maintain the disorder, reducing or eliminating the avoidance behavior, modifying the actual stuttering behavior to reduce its severity, reducing the rate of speech, and self-monitoring of rate or other behaviors.

Avoidance behavior is eliminated by preventing the performance of the avoidance response in the presence of the feared stimulus. This change is accomplished through several kinds of desensitization, including pseudostuttering, and motivating clients to examine their fears. Another technique that reduces fear is the use of "freezing." "Freezing" requires the stutterer to continue stuttering on purpose after the stuttering episode begins, until the fear subsides. Another technique involves feeling and analyzing the stuttering as it is happening. Other techniques used are rate reduction and rate control. Clients are instructed to use these techniques when a fluent-sounding speech pattern is more important. A desired rate of speech is modelled, and systematic rate reduction is taught to the client. Modification of the stuttering response is accomplished by many of the techniques advocated by Van Riper, especially use of alternating between stuttering with more and less tension. Therapy therefore consists of both stuttering reduction techniques and fluency-enhancing skills.

PROLAM-GM Components

Physiological Adjustments	Rate reduction and reduction of muscular tension.
Attitude	The program stresses an acceptance of stuttering and of self, along with being less sensitive to its consequences.
Monitoring	Clients are instructed to reduce rate when fluent-sounding speech is important.

Research Finding: None presented.

Special Features: None.

Suggested Readings
Starkweather, C.E. (1987). *Fluency and stuttering.* Englewood Cliffs: Prentice Hall.
Starkweather, C.E. (1990). A multiprocess behavioral approach to stuttering therapy. *Seminars in Speech, Language and Hearing, 1,* 327–337.

Symptom Modification Therapy

Person: Charles Van Riper.

Age Range: Children and adults.

Objectives: The goals of therapy are to control and simplify stuttering.

Summary
Symptom Modification Therapy is concerned with reduction of anxiety and the deliberate modification of stuttering. The term *fluent stuttering,* or stuttering done with a minimum amount of abnormality, is the hoped-for result. There are four phases to therapy: (1) identification, (2) desensitization, (3) modification, and (4) stabilization. During the identification phase, the stutterer analyzes and classifies all overt and covert characteristics of his stutter-

ing. A symptom analysis may be performed to detail all observable stuttering behaviors. During the desensitization phase, the client is "toughened" to the realities of stuttering, and may be asked to experience a number of situations during which he is expected to stutter on purpose. These purposeful stuttering times as well as a new understanding of the anxieties and other negative emotions being felt will make the stutterer less sensitive to his disorder.

The modification phase involves modifying stuttering and lessening avoidances. Secondary characteristics may be eliminated in a piecemeal fashion while stuttering is modified using the following specific techniques. "Cancellation," wherein the client repeats a stuttered word with some successful modification of stuttering. "Bounce," whereby the stutterer simply repeats the first syllable of a stuttered word until he is ready to utter it. "Prolongation (pull-out)," which enables the client to slightly prolong the initial syllable of a stuttered word until ready to say it. Finally, "preparatory sets," wherein the stutterer attempts to place the articulators in the appropriate posture prior to initiating speech. Although taught in this order, the techniques are utilized in reverse order beginning with appropriate preparatory sets and continuing to prolongations, bounce, and finally cancellation, if all else fails. The final phase, stabilization, is designed to assist the client automatize the fluent stuttering pattern, as well as monitor his normal speech.

PROLAM-GM Components

Physiological Adjustments	Use of prolongation and repetition (bounce) of initial syllables to initial words.
Attitude	Use of "cancellation" of stuttered words. The program stresses an acceptance of stuttering along with being less sensitive to its consequences.
Monitoring	Use of "preparatory sets" and other techniques requires that the client monitor speech and anticipate moments of likely stuttering.
Generalization	Use of field trips and out-of-clinic experiences to apply techniques learned in therapy sessions.
Maintenance	Yearly follow-ups and periodic telephone contacts suggested.

Research Findings: Anecdotal reports may be found in *Stuttering Successes and Failures* (1968) published by the Speech Foundation of America and in Eisenson (1958).

Suggested Readings

Van Riper, Charles (1973). *The treatment of stuttering*. Englewood Cliffs N.J.: Prentice-Hall Inc.

Van Riper, Charles (1968). *Stuttering successes and failures. Publication #6*. Memphis: Speech Foundation of America.

Clinical Management of Childhood Stuttering

Person: Meryl Wall and Florence Myers.

Age Range: Children.

Objectives: Depending on the assessed needs of each child, the objectives of this linguistically based program are to teach fluency-enhancing techniques and techniques to modify stuttering blockage.

Summary

A three-factor model is presented for assessment and treatment of childhood stuttering. The three factors are psychosocial, physiological, and psycholinguistic characteristics of stuttering. Psychosocial factors include awareness of one's stuttering, reactions to stuttering, parental reactions to stuttering, and parent-child speech and language use. Therapy focus is on control of stuttering through manipulation of the child's environment and a language-based therapeutic approach. The physiological factor is treated by a variety of techniques, including easy onset, slowed speech rate, and, when needed, variations of Van Riper's pull-out, cancellation, and symptom analysis techniques. The psycholinguistic factor, which is based on the relationship between stuttering and speech and language, stresses the use of increasingly long and complex linguistic units in treatment along with decreasing word substitutions and circumlocutions. Generalization is structured by parent involvement, field trips, and assignments designed to practice newly acquired speech skills. Maintenance continues for a 3-year period, with 6-month check-ups.

PROLAM-GM Components

Physiological Adjustment:	Use of easy speech, loose articulatory contacts, gentle voice initiation, pull-outs, and cancellations.
Rate	Use of slow-normal rate for fluency enhancement.
Length and Complexity of Utterance	Use of gradual increase in the length of utterance.
Attitude	Role playing feared situations for appropriate ages and desensitization to stuttering are aspects of the program.
Monitoring	Children attend to use of newly learned techniques.
Generalization	Use of field trips to practice techniques.
Maintenance	Three-year follow-up in 6-month intervals.

Research Findings: Ancedotal findings.

Suggested Readings
Wall, M. & Myers, F. (1994). *Clinical Management of Childhood Stuttering*. Austin, Texas: Pro-Ed.

Precision Fluency Shaping Program

Person: Ronald Webster.

Age Range: Adults and children (10 years and older).

Objectives: Achievement of fluent speech by mastering specific target behaviors (muscle movement patterns) used by normally fluent speakers.

Summary
This program, initiated in 1968, is an intensive, 19-day long experience that is approximately 120 hours in length. Fluency is obtained by intensive practice of muscle movement patterns that generate fluent speech. At the onset of the program, prolonged speech is used to alter detailed muscle movement patterns. This prolonged "slow-motion speech" (Webster, 1980) is learned prior to training in the mastery of gentle voice productions. The skills are practiced in increasing complexity from sounds, to syllables, to words, and finally to conversational speech. An interactive computer system was designed to help provide auditory examples and visual feedback to the client concerning correct use of phonatory targets. As the stutterer masters the techniques, syllable duration are systematically reduced, use of the computer is eliminated, and new fluent speaking skills are transferred from the clinical setting to nonclinical surroundings. As of 1991, more than 3,000 patients have been treated with this program (Webster et al., 1991).

PROLAM-GM Components

Physiological Adjustments	Vocal tract stabilization, control of respiration, and gentle initiation of voicing.
Rate	Use of prolonged syllable durations, which are systematically reduced to normal syllable durations.
Length and Complexity of Utterance	Systematic progression from learning targets with isolated phonemes and words to increased speech length and complexity.

Monitoring	Initial use of computer system transferring to patient monitoring via kinesthetic feedback later in program.
Generalization	A "parallel transfer process" is used whereby all steps of the program are generalized one at a time in increasing complexity to nonclinical settings. Additional "personal contacts" and telephone calls are part of transfer.
Maintenance	Five-day refresher courses are available, but only 15% of those treated require participation.

Research Findings: Results from 200 randomly selected clients are presented in Webster (1979).

Special Features: The program is administered in an intensive residential format. The interactive computer system is an integral part of the procedure.

Suggested Readings

Webster, R.L.(1979). Empirical considerations regarding stuttering therapy. In H.H. Gregory (Ed.) *Controversies about stuttering therapy.* Baltimore: University Park Press.

Webster, R.L. (1980) Evolution of a target based behavioral therapy for stuttering. *Journal of Fluency Disorders, 5* 303–320.

Vocal Control Therapy

Person: Adeline E. Weiner.

Age Range: Children and adults.

Objectives: The two major objectives of the program are to achieve reliable fluency and to ensure its use by establishing favorable psychophysiological conditions (Weiner, 1984).

Summary

Reliable fluency is sought by retraining the client to use the vocal apparatus at its optimal level and by relieving speech anxieties through a variety of systematic desensitization techniques. There are four main components to vocal control therapy: (1) breath control through abdominal-diaphragmatic breathing, (2) easy onset of voicing, (3) voice quality control through optimal oral resonance, and (4) a technique to maintain the continuity of speech flow called vowel focus (Weiner, 1984). Breath control is taught to every client. The purpose of this breathing segment of the program is to prevent the loss of expiratory air stutterers often experience at initiation of an utterance. Easy onset of phonation is achieved through a variety of exercises and applied to increasingly complex utterances from vowels to VC, VCVC words and phrases and finally to more complex utterances.

The author believes that stuttering is a failure to maintain phonation as a result of disruption of vocal-fold reciprocal action. If vocal-fold activities could be initiated smoothly and sustained in a tension-free state, then stuttering would be prevented from occurring (Weiner, 1984). Thus, vocalization exercises are initiated and developed with increasing complexity to ensure that the client uses the "best voice" possible when speaking. "The difference between acceptable and excellent voice quality has sometimes made the difference between continued stuttering and fluency" (Weiner, 1984; p. 232). Vowel focus requires that the stutterer preset their vocal tract to properly articulate the vowel that follows consonants and sound blends that have been stuttered on previously. The belief is that the client fears the consonant sound but is really blocking in anticipation of the vowel that follows the feared consonant. The four processes are integrated via "systematic massed practice," a series of highly structured exercises that are phased into unstructured client-generated utterances. Systematic desensitization (Wolpe, 1958) techniques and role playing "behavioral rehearsals" are applied as needed prior to transfer to extraclinical settings.

PROLAM-GM Components

Physiological Adjustments   Use of a "target voice," which is found by enhanced oral resonance practice. Use of abdominal-diaphragmatic breathing with easy onset of phonation.

Length and Complexity of Utterance   General increase in length and complexity often beginning with vowels and proceeding through varied consonant blends to meaningful speech.

Monitoring   As a result of increased awareness, client monitors four learned factors that result in fluency.

Generalization   At each stage, home practice and extraclinical assignments are used as needed.

Maintenance   Sessions are scheduled monthly, decreasing to semiannually for a 3-year period with available "booster" sessions.

Research Findings: Report of results of 66 clients in Weiner (1984).

Special Features: A series of 11 videotapes, produced and directed by Warren Schloss, is available from the Temple University Media Learning Center and Office of Television Services.

Suggested Readings

Weiner, A.E. (1978). Vocal control therapy for stutterers: A trial program. *Journal of Fluency Disorders*, 3 115–126.

Weiner, A.E. (1984). Vocal Control Therapy for Stutterers. In M. Peins (Ed.) *Contemporary Approaches in Stuttering Therapy*. Boston: Little, Brown and Company.

STUDY QUESTIONS

1. In this chapter, 32 separate approaches are summarized. You should be able to identify which PROLAM-GM components are used in each approach.

2. PROLAM-GM components can be applied in various ways. For each component, identify the various ways the authors apply them.

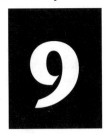

A Strategy for Constructing Intervention Protocols

As long as we don't know for sure just what stuttering is, or what the causes are, we can't be certain of the best way to treat it. So we have to use . . . whatever seems to work; we have to be pragmatic.

All things considered, I believe we are left with the inescapable realization that success in stuttering therapy results from an incredibly complex interaction among a great many variables, some known, many unknown (Perkins, 1991, p. 262).

Perkin's eloquent statements regarding the vagaries of stuttering therapy highlight the difficulties encountered by clinicians who work with stutterers. In researching this text, we found that in the past 15 years, more than 50 different approaches for the treatment of stuttering have been presented in published form. Although many of the approaches overlap, each has a distinctive twist or combination of techniques. Thus, speech-language pathologists are faced with a treatment selection decision that can be described as overwhelming, to say the least. No component of the treatment formula remains constant. Each client has different needs, and each treatment protocol presents, on the surface, different techniques. As a result, many practicing clinicians have dealt with the problem by ignoring the variability among clients. One result has been that stutterers have been historically treated as if they were a homogenous group; adherents or authors of a specific clinical techniques maintain that their techniques are applicable to all stutterers. Modifications are usually made for age variables (Goldberg, 1981; Shine, 1988), but little else. However, as diagnostic measurements become more sophisticated, it is becoming apparent that stutterers should not be viewed as a homogeneous group. Attempts, therefore, to use a single approach with all clients will most likely lead to inconsistent results. This inconsistency might help explain the data that show that every approach works with someone, but no single approach works with everyone.

THE DECISION-MAKING PROCESS

The therapy selection process that follows relies on the assessment procedures discussed in Chapter 4. The findings of the assessment procedures provide the information that clinicians must use to choose appropriate strategies and tactics. Most helpful in this task are the previously discussed diagnostic interview procedures and the Stuttering Assessment Protocol (SAP). A schematic representation of the decision-making process that incorporates both is presented in Figure 9–1.

Significant Case History Findings

The first step is to analyze any significant case history findings that speech-language pathologists may have uncovered during the interview process. Significant case history findings often help determine the direction clinicians will take in constructing or selecting an intervention protocol for a stutterer.

Analyze Baseline Data

Data derived from the SAP are divided into two sections. The first section is the Baseline Data section, which consists of measurements of frequency, duration, rate, and perceptual evaluation measures of stuttering and fluent behavior. Along with the case history, this information is critical in understanding presenting behavior prior to any behavior modifications by speech-language pathologists.

Analyze Probes of Changeability

The information derived from the probes of changeability data will be used to help select what might be the most appropriate strategies to help a given client modify their stuttering. The six available therapy strategies featured are:

1. (P) physiological adjustments of the speech mechanism,
2. (R) speech rate changes,
3. (O) application of operant controls,
4. (L) modifications in length and complexity of utterance,

5. (A) attitude changes,

6. (M) monitoring of speech.

The probes were based on these strategies and designed to help isolate the strategy or strategies that might be most helpful to a given client. This analysis is number 3 in Figure 9–1. The combination of one or more of these therapeutic intervention models with strategies for generalization of therapy gains (7; G)

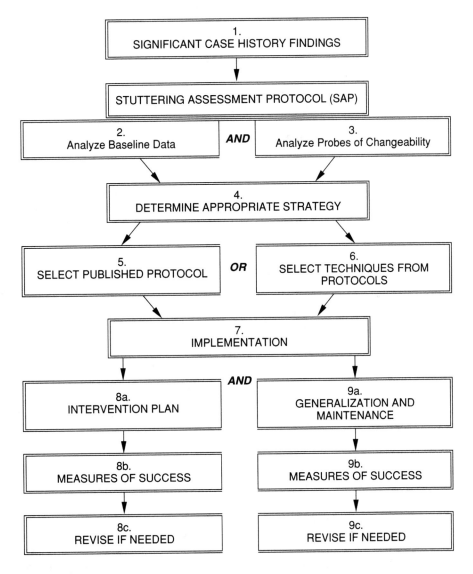

Figure 9–1
Decision-Making Process Steps

and maintenance of learned behaviors (8; M) is most likely to ensure successful intervention.

Determine Appropriate Strategy

The next step in the decision-making process is to determine just which specific strategy might be applied to a given client. This step is the culmination of the analysis of the data derived in steps 1, 2, and 3. At this point, clinicians will know what they want to do with their client. Now they must determine how they wish to accomplish their goals.

Select Published Protocols or Select Techniques From Protocols

Once the appropriate PROLAM strategy or strategies are selected, speech-language pathologists face a choice. They may select an appropriate protocol and apply it, as published, or select techniques from several protocols and weave them into an individualized treatment program (ITP). The ITP may take the form of an individualized educational program (IEP) mandated by many school systems or adapted to a format consistent with another work setting.

Implementation

In Chapter 8, the strategies and techniques used by each of the 32 protocols were summarized. Clinicians can now specify which of these techniques they will use to implement the strategies they selected. Step 7 of the plan is to detail how each procedure will be implemented.

Intervention Plan, Generalization, and Maintenance

Implementation will become the intervention, generalization, and maintenance aspects of service delivery. Client performance takes center stage at these steps (8a and 9a, respectively). The first seven steps can be accomplished in consultation with the client, but steps 8a and 9a are the testing of all the decisions made during the selection process. Their success depends on client performance. Steps 8b and 9b are efficacy measures used to determine whether a successful protocol has been designed. Revisions that might be needed are based on these measures. Thus, the final aspect of the plan is to revise, if needed, the intervention, generalization, and maintenance plans (steps 8c and 9c).

CASE HISTORY MODELS

The case study illustrations that follow provide models that might be employed with clients who bring different case histories to the evaluation session. Each of the four cases follow the decision-making process just detailed, and they illustrate why different treatment approaches might be necessary and how to select them using the PROLAM-GM model.

Selecting a Published Protocol

Client: Justin

Age: 10

Sex: Male

Step 1: Significant Case History Findings. Justin's case history interview revealed no remarkable medical problems. The educational and social problems he is currently experiencing seem directly related to his speech problems; they do not appear to be independent of communication. For example, his written work is above class average. However, he has recently refused to read aloud in class or participate in classroom discussions. Socially, although his parents report that he is popular, they also report that he refuses to participate in guessing games or other activities that require speech. He is progressing well with piano lessons, and he is an infielder in Little League baseball. He is not currently using any medications.

There is a strong family history of stuttering. Justin's paternal grandfather is a stutterer, as are two uncles and two paternal cousins. His parents report they believed his speech has been disfluent since he first began communicating in 2- and 3-word sentences at approximately age 2.5. Due to negative reports from Justin's grandfather about his experiences in speech therapy, no speech therapy was ever sought for Justin. However, the child has recently been voicing concerns about his inability to be fluent, will not recite in school, and has periodically refused to speak on the telephone. His parents say that he is fluent when he sings and joins in choral prayers at church. His teacher reports that his speech is fluent when he recites the Pledge of Allegiance.

After interviewing Justin, the speech-language pathologist felt that the combination of overt symptoms and covert attitudes he displayed placed him as a phase IV stutterer on Bloodsteins' classification system. What was particularly striking were his feelings of victimization and lack of confidence in his ability to produce fluent speech.

Step 2: Baseline Data (SAP). The analysis of the data did not reveal any significant differences between the speech Justin used with his parents and the examiners. His parents also reported that the speech heard during their interactions in the diagnostic session was typical of the speech Justin had been using for the past 6 months. Data analysis revealed stuttering on 18% of the syllables uttered during the 2-minute sample. Due to the disfluencies, he was only able to produce 100 syllables per minute (spm) when stuttering. The average duration of stuttering moments was 1.4 seconds; however, his overall speech rate when fluent was 220 spm. Justin was able to maintain fluent speech for an average of 27 seconds, during which time he spoke 315 syllables fluently.

The Perception of Speech quality rating scale was used to assess the naturalness of Justin's speech by Justin, his parents, and the speech-language pathologist. The ratings were 6, 6, and 7, respectively, of a possible 9, with 1 indicated as natural-sounding speech. However, the ratings were made for different reasons. Justin and his parents were concerned about the disfluencies, whereas the clinician was concerned about rate of utterance.

Step 3: Probes of Changeability (SAP). The greatest changes in Justin's speech were brought about using whispered speech (tactic 2), prolonged speech (tactic 4), and single word responses (tactic 7). Less effective were verbal punishment (tactic 5) and reduced rate (tactic 3). Attitude probes (tactic 10 and 11) revealed that Justin believed stuttering was neither curable nor modifiable, because it was something that "just happens to me when I try to talk." He reported that he would "do anything" the therapist told him to do that would help him speak better.

Step 4: Strategy Selection. After studying the significant case history findings and SAP results, several factors began to emerge as important for treatment selection. The child's rapid rate of fluent speech when combined with the overt symptomatology were the most visible symptoms. However, the symptoms virtually disappeared during prolonged speech. In addition, during the fluent whispering that resulted when the probe was administered, speech rate was markedly slower than 220 spm, dropping to 180 spm. Thus, one factor that appeared important was rate control. The second major theme appeared to center on Justin's negative attitudes about his ability to modify his speech. He appeared surprised, but he provided no comments when his fluent whispered speech and prolonged speech was played back for him to hear. Therefore, in the clinicians' judgment, attitude shift was felt to be of importance. Thus, the two initial strategies to be selected were rate control and attitude manipulation.

Step 5: Protocol Options. Several of the published protocols seemed appropriate for consideration because they concentrated on rate reduction and attitude manipulation. In this illustration, speech-language pathologists had access to four: Freedom of Fluency (Daly, 1988b), Behavioral Cognitive Stuttering Therapy (Goldberg, (1981), Stutter-Free Speech (Shames and Florance 1980), and Systematic Fluency Training for Children (Shine, 1988).

Step 7: Implementation. Due to familiarity with the techniques involved, previous success with the protocol, and its emphasis on attitude manipulation, the Behavioral Cognitive Stuttering Therapy protocol was selected.

Step 8a: Intervention Plan, and Step 9a: Generalization and Maintenance. It was decided to run this program in its entirety from initial instillation of fluency using prolonged speech, through its attitudinal manipulation phases and generalization via the use of behavioral contracts.

Step 8b and 9b: Measures of Success. At each step of this program, criterion measures are provided so that the speech-language pathologist might determine whether the part of the protocol she is using is being successfully mastered. These suggestions continue through the generalization and maintenance phases of the protocol.

Discussion. Using the SAP and the PROLAM model, the speech-language pathologist was led to a logical selection of therapy intervention strategies based on the client's behavior. Data, clinical intuition, available materials, work setting, client schedules, and many other factors will all affect the final decision-making process. Differences in any of these variables might shift the choice from one program to another. Regardless of the system or logic used, there can never be a substitution for clinical intuition.

Selecting Techniques from Various Protocols

Name: Elizabeth

Age: 32

Sex: Female

Step 1: Significant Case History Findings. Elizabeth's medical, educational, and social history revealed no significant information. She reports that she has stuttered all of her life, and that the problem was first diagnosed by her second grade teacher. She successfully completed college and the first year of graduate training in architectural studies before leaving school to enter a partnership in an interior design firm 10 years ago. She reports a sporadic history of speech therapy, stating that she has been "cured" several times but it never seems "to stick" after she leaves the speech clinic. She could not recall any attempts that were ever made at generalization or maintenance other than several unscheduled follow-up surveys from one university clinic she attended as a student. She reports that she was always too embarrassed to go back to a therapist because she knew her failures were her own fault. She is not currently using medications other than the occasional use of over-the-counter pain relievers. She reports that although she is always aware of her speech, especially with clients, stuttering has not impeded her professional or social life. An article in the local newspaper describing recent advances in stuttering therapy motivated her to try "one more time" to speak without worrying about stuttering.

Step 2: Baseline Data (SAP). Baseline data were analyzed from samples of speech recorded during the diagnostic session. The frequency of occurrence of stuttering was slightly under 2%. Despite disfluent utterances, her speech rate was 165 spm. Each moment of stuttering took the form of a slight hesitation that was no longer than a fraction of a second. Her overall stutter-free speech rate was 178 spm. She was fluent for one 5-minute period during the diagnostic session, but she averaged 3 minutes and 25 seconds for stutter-free utterances, during which time she spoke at 165 spm. She reported that the speech she was displaying during the diagnostic interview was consistent with her usual performance. Perceptual ratings of speech quality differed as measured on The Perception of Speech quality rating scale. The clinician rated Elizabeth's speech as natural sounding "2," and the client rating her own speech as more unnatural "6," noting that her voice sounded "flat" and that she was "stuttering a lot."

Step 3: Probes of Changability. All the probes resulted in complete fluency. Elizabeth remarked that by having clinicians help her focus attention on speech she became much more fluent, but she knew the tricks would not last. She did not appear impressed with her fluent performances. In response to the attitude probes, she replied that "I would like to believe that stuttering is curable, but I can't believe it right now." She felt her role in therapy was to apply what she might learn to her "real life" talking.

Step 4: Strategy Selection. Analysis of the diagnostic interview and SAP data led the clinician into the following train of thought. Elizabeth presented with very mild overt characteristics that she could apparently control when they were brought to her attention by the clinician. Also, she had been "cured" several times but never brought the behavior outside of the clinical setting with any success. In addition she had never experienced, as she reported, any systematic work on generalization and maintenance. It appeared logical that the following series of therapeutic strategies might be effective. First, some combination of monitoring fluent speech and a more aggressive attitude toward achieving and maintaining fluency needed to be instilled. Then Elizabeth had to be prepared to take the new attitude and skills out of the clinical setting in a structured format. Finally, she had to be prepared to deal with any relapse or set-backs that might occur.

Step 5: Select Published Protocol. Although many protocols dealt with some of the strategies envisioned, none provided the plan outlined. Thus, the clinician decided to select techniques from several programs that might contribute to the ITP that was most suited to Elizabeth's needs.

Step 6: Selected Techniques. The techniques selected came from several sources. The philosophy that fluency was an attainable goal that might be aggressively pursued was incorporated from *A Program for the Initial Stages of Fluency Therapy* (Culatta and Rubin, 1971); the conscious monitoring techniques that would be used to bring purposeful fluency to a conscious level were derived from *Stutter-Free Speech* (Shames and Florance, 1980). The visualization techniques that would be used prior to leaving the clinical setting came from *Freedom of Fluency* (Daly 1988b); the methodology that would go into the field experiences that would generalize fluency from the clinic to the real world environment would be taken from the contracting aspects of the

Behavioral Cognitive Stuttering Therapy protocol (Goldberg, 1981) and the counseling needed to prepare her for possible relapse would rely on the suggestions of techniques for establishing fluency (Perkins, 1984). In addition, when appropriate, a strict maintenance program similar to that suggested in the *Gradual Increase in the Length and Complexity of Utterance program* (Ryan and Van Kirk, 1971) would be implemented.

Step 7: Implementation. Thus, pulling this whole package together, the clinician visualized a step-by-step process whereby Elizabeth would go from being exposed to a philosophy that stressed her aggressively pursuing fluency and stressing that only purposefully monitored fluent speech would be acceptable in the clinic, to learning how to reinforce herself with unmonitored speech as a reward for purposeful fluency. She would then use visualization exercises in the clinic where she might see herself successfully accomplishing the goal of purposefully being fluent outside of the clinic in specific situations. Contracts would be developed for her to actually experience these situations. If successful, she would be placed on a strictly monitored maintenance program with the understanding that relapse was a possibility and that she should contact the clinic if she ever became unsure of her fluency abilities.

Step 8b: Measures of Success. Each of the strategies described comes with suggestions in the original protocols for measuring attainment of the objectives. Whether analyzing the content of responses to attest to a more positive attitude toward fluency or discussing the criteria for successfully completing an out-of-clinic contract, clinicians will be certain the client has met criteria before going on to the next step in the program or branching to find other ways to meet objectives.

Discussion. It should be evident from this case history that a published program may not always meet the needs of given clients. However, it should not be impossible to map out what those needs might be and to construct an ITP that is both logical and accountable. The modifications that might be necessary along the road to success cannot be preordained; However, the plan can remain internally consistent.

Using All PROLAM Strategies

Client: Richard

Age: 15

Sex: Male

Step 1: Significant Case History Findings. Richard's medical, educational, and social history revealed no significant information. His parents report that they first noticed an unusual number of repetitions when he was approximately 3 years old. These easy repetitions developed during a 6-month period into unusually long pauses and struggle to articulate words. They report that until the first grade, there were periodic remissions in the disfluent speech. However, each cycle appeared to be shorter than the last. By age 6, the disfluencies were less severe but highly consistent. Richard has an uncle who stutters, and his father remembers stuttering as a child, but he no longer feels he has a problem.

Richard was enrolled in a school group therapy program during the latter part of the second grade and the beginning of the third grade. He remembers "stretching" out his words in class but he has no other recollections. His parents remember that he was in therapy, but that they were not involved in the process. They did not report any significant change in his speech during the therapy. Richard is not currently using medications of any sort. Although he is aware of his stuttering and "would like to do something about it," he did not believe that change was possible. He reports that he "switches" words around so he can say "easy ones." He feels that all sounds that "you keep on saying, like /s/ or /f/" are particularly difficult.

Secondary characteristics observed during the interview included inappropriate eye blinks, averted gaze, pill rolling finger movements, and occasional head jerks at termination of a stuttering moment. A chance encounter with his second grade speech-language pathologist who commented disfavorably about his speech led him to ask his parents to schedule the current evaluation.

Step 2: Baseline Data (SAP). Baseline data were analyzed from recordings made during the diagnostic interview and parental observation sections of the evaluation. His parents reported that the speech sample taken during their interactions were typical of Richard's speech with them at home. Analysis of the tape samples of speech with his parents and the clinician were not significantly different. The frequency of occurrence of stuttering was 8.3%. His speech rate was approximately 150 spm. A variety of stuttering behaviors were exhibited as previously described. The longest stuttering moment was 3 seconds in duration; most blocks were 1-second long or shorter. His overall stutter-free speech rate was 180 spm. His longest stutter-free period was 48 seconds, whereas the average was less than 24 seconds. He felt the speech he used for the examiner was "pretty much normal." Both Richard and the examiner rated his speech a 5 in terms of naturalness.

Step 3: Probes of Changeability (SAP). All of the probes were somewhat effective, but no one probe was noticeably more effective than another. Richard did not express a preference, but he was surprised that his speech could change under different conditions. Several of the probes affected specific aspects of the stuttering pattern, but not others. For example, the light contact probe brought about cessation of the effortful aspects of articulatory contact, but it did not affect secondary characteristics. Whispering had a similar effect.

Thus, the data collected did not reflect the changes that the clinician observed. Slow rate of speech did reduce stuttering, as did continuously phonated prolonged speech. However, during the sample, Richard found it difficult to maintain the condition, which required the clinician to provide a large number of prompts, thereby making the data collected suspect. Both punishment of stuttering moments and reinforcement of fluency brought about a 3% decrement in frequency of occurrence. Single word responses brought about a 4% reduction, which dropped to only a 2% reduction in both concrete and abstract response probes.

Attitudinal probes revealed that Richard was surprised that his stuttering could be changed. He reported that he always believed that there was nothing to do about stuttering. He reported that he would be willing to try suggestions the therapist made during his sessions. Attempts at monitoring brought about a reduction comparable to the operant control probes; however, his recognition of moments of stuttering was not consistent with the speech-language pathologist's, either for frequency or specific word identification.

Step 4: Strategy Selection. Observations, analysis of the clinical interview, and SAP data did not provide any clear-cut information about a specific protocol or strategy that the speech-language pathologist might feel comfortable emphasizing. Each of the PROLAM strategies appeared somewhat effective, but none came to the forefront as being particularly powerful. In contrast, none appeared weak or ineffective enough to discard. Although it is hoped that a strategy or strategies might eventually arise that would be most effective, this did not seem to be initially the case. As a result, the speech-language pathologist decided to begin with a treatment program that emphasized all the PROLAM components. Therapy sessions would be divided into 8 to 10 minute segments using tactics derived from programs that emphasized each of the strategies. Data analysis results and client and clinician judgments would hopefully evolve a more focused treatment plan over time.

Step 6: Selected Techniques. For Richard, the speech-language pathologist developed the following initial treatment plan that would encompass the PROLAM aspects of treatment. The light articulatory contact drills presented by Cooper and Cooper (1985) in their *Personalized Fluency Control Therapy Revised* protocol, although a bit on the juvenile side, presented the ideal tactics for Richard. The clinician, with only slight modifications, was able to adopt them for her needs. *The Symptom Modification Therapy* program outlined by Van Riper (1973) provides suggestions for modification of the secondary characteristics that Richard displayed during the interview. The fact that they did not disappear during probe conditions that brought about more fluent speech led the clinician to include the "symptom analysis" aspect of *Symptom Modification Therapy* into the treatment program.

Rate reduction and continuous phonation experiences will be provided by two different feedback machines. The first will use the computerized programs of the *Computer-Aided Fluency Establishment Trainer* (CAFET©) program by Goebel (1994) to instill the prolonged speech experiences. It was felt that Richard's interest in computers, along with the visual as well as auditory feedback of this system, might be helpful. A back-up approach would be derived from the *Conversational Rate Control* protocol of Curlee and Perkins (1969), which uses DAF to help establish stutter-free speech beginning with continuously prolonged reduced rate speech. *A Program to Establish Fluent Speech* (Mowrer, 1979) combines both length and complexity of utterance experiences with operant controls, and it appears to be matched to the client's needs. Instilling and developing more positive attitudes toward fluent speech might be accomplished by using the techniques and exercises suggested by Culatta and Rubin (1973) in their *Program for the Initial Stages of Fluency Therapy.* Finally, the monitoring techniques offered by Shames and Florance in the Stutter-Free Speech program (1980) not only provide a methodology for insuring monitoring, but also instill a self-evaluational component that appeared to be a weakness during the evaluation.

Step 9a: Generalization and Maintenance.   Generalization and maintenance will be attempted using the contracting format discussed by Goldberg (1981) in his *Behavioral Cognitive Stuttering Therapy* protocol. The adult series of contract forms seem to be most appropriate. The clinician will also incorporate the visualization techniques discussed by Daly (1988b) in *Freedom of Fluency.* The listed components, not necessarily presented in order each session, will comprise Richard's individualized treatment program.

Step 8b: Measures of Success.   The goals of each subcomponent will be measured to see if the client is accomplishing the task at hand, whether it is light contacts, stuttering without secondary characteristics, or completion of contracts. Suggestions for how to measure performance are provided by most of the authors. If they are not, clinicians will have to devise their own assessment procedure to see if the tasks are being accomplished. In addition, speech naturalness and frequency of occurrence data will be collected during the use of each technique, to determine which is most effective.

Discussion.   This lengthy and complex program is obviously not the plan of choice for all clients. It is hoped that the majority of clients might be treated by carefully selecting a published protocol that closely meets their needs with only minor modifications. When this approach is not feasible, clinicians can usually select from the PROLAM components that appear most potent for a given client. This illustration is for that small number of clients who do not show a clear preference. This cumbersome process appears to be the most logical and defensible way to construct a program for these clients. This multifaceted approach at least provides the client with the opportunity to develop prerequisite skills needed to modify speech.

Disfluency Pattern that Is Not Stuttering

Client: Jessica

Age: 11

Sex: Female

Step 1: Significant Case History Findings. Jessica was referred by her psychologist who was concerned about the severity of her "stuttering." Jessica began to speak disfluently quite suddenly. The disfluent speech began within 1 month of her eleventh birthday, and soon after she experienced the San Francisco earthquake and resultant fires in October of 1990. Although neither she nor any member of her family were injured, the family home and most possessions were destroyed in a spectacular fire that was replayed repeatedly on television. Jessica is experiencing vivid dreams of the event. Her parents report that she is more withdrawn, listless, and now emotionally labile. Speech screenings in her public school did not indicate a communication disorder of any type. There is no history of stuttering on either side of her family.

Her parents report that the disfluency came "all at once." They report no concern about her speech prior to this incident. She is not currently being medicated, and she has no significant medical history or a history of injuries. Her psychologist reports no injuries from the earthquake other than "just a real good scare." Her parents report that Jessica speaks in all situations, and she does not appear to be terribly concerned about her speech. They report that the speech recorded during their observed interaction during the diagnostic is typical of her new disfluent speech pattern.

Step 2: Baseline Data (SAP). Baseline data were derived from recordings made during the clinical interview. The frequency of occurrence of disfluencies was unusually high: 63% of the total syllables attempted during a 2-minute sample (82 syllables stuttered of 130 attempted). She was disfluent on the initial sounds or syllables of almost all the words she attempted to say. Disfluencies took the form of repetitions of extremely brief duration. It was difficult to measure her overall fluent speech rate because there were so few instances of fluent speech to measure. However, it appeared that her fluent speech was articulated at expected rates. The naturalness of her speech was evaluated using the Perception of Speech quality rating scale. The high rate of rapidly produced speech seemed unnatural to clinicians (a 7 rating) and to her parents (an 8 rating). Jessica declined to rate her speech, protesting that she did not understand what the clinician wanted her to do.

Step 3: Probes of Changeability (SAP). The probes were not effective in changing Jessica's speech. She maintained the same frequency and pattern of disfluency during all the probes attempted as she did during the baseline data tapes. Additional probes, such as using white noise while she spoke and asking her to sing, also proved ineffective. Her replies to the attitude questions were "I don't know."

Step 4: Strategy Selection.   The case history data as well as the baseline and probe data all point toward the same conclusion. The speech-language pathologist felt that although Jessica was highly disfluent, she was not a stutterer. The sudden onset as well as the significant identifiable trauma she experienced pointed toward emotionally based disfluency. This diagnosis was further strengthened by the lack of family history, the lack of concern the child evidenced about speaking, her willingness to speak in all situations, a pattern of initial repetitions, and an absence of any secondary characteristics. The failure of the probes of changeability to modify her disfluency pattern was characteristic of nonstuttering disfluency. As a result, clinicians did not recommend that Jessica be enrolled in speech therapy. The reasons for this lack of referral was explained to the parents and subsequently to the psychologist. The speech-language pathologist did request that the psychologist pay particular attention to the child's disfluencies during continued counselling. It was anticipated that the disfluency rate would drop significantly with the help of psychotherapy to better understand her fears.

Step 8b: Measures of Success.   Successful psychotherapy should bring about a decrease in disfluency rates.

Discussion.   Jessica's evaluation illustrates how attempting to treat a disfluency other than stuttering with stuttering therapy methodology would not be successful. It is critical at such a time for clinicians to not be seduced by the obvious disfluency symptomatology and as a result attempt to provide inappropriate service.

SUMMARY

The goal of this chapter was to provide examples of the utility of the PROLAM-GM model and how it might be used clinically to determine the best treatment package for a given client. Guidelines and examples were presented of how speech-language pathologists might go about constructing an individualized therapy program for a variety of clients. We illustrated how baseline data and the probes of changeability of the SAP can help guide this selection. We also presented guidelines and illustrations to help apply the PROLAM model to cases that are not clearly susceptible to any given published protocol. The chapter ended with a case report of a client who displayed a fluency disorder other than stuttering.

STUDY QUESTIONS

The decision making process for using PROLAM-GM components is very specific. Construct hypothetical cases to exemplify the steps in your decision making from the use of the SAP to the revision of the intervention plan. You should construct hypothetical cases (child, adolescent, adult) for each of the following decisions:

1. Selection of a published protocol.
2. Selection of specific techniques from various protocols.
3. Selection of all PROLAM-GM strategies using various protocols.
4. Decision not to use any PROLAM-GM strategies.

Challenge for the Future

Our journey is both over and just beginning. We began our trip by defining stuttering and tracing its study in modern times. A tutorial on the different possibilities for disfluency in speech warned us not to mistake all disfluent behavior for stuttering. Prior to discussing diagnosis and treatment issues, we considered the process by which we might most effectively obtain the information needed to diagnose stuttering. Armed with a methodology for delving into stuttering and the families it affects, we shared assessment and measurement techniques that can lead to the construction of valid intervention programs. A side trip was taken to highlight how different work settings might change our treatment approaches. We also stopped to understand how, in a multicultural society, sensitivity to ethnic, racial, and gender differences are not a luxury, but rather a necessary skill for the success of our culturally diverse clients. We then presented a model that might tie together the work of all the dedicated researchers and research clinicians who are trying to understand and eliminate stuttering and then presented an in-depth sampling of the works of these researchers. We made suggestions for selecting the most effective ways to treat stutterers. Our trip ended with a discussion of several fundamental clinical issues that must be addressed by every clinician. These issues go beyond just knowing the techniques of modifying behavior. They are related to the very core of the therapeutic process. That is where we have been. This epilogue is concerned with where we need to go. We have interpreted the past and explained the present as best as we could. Now we need to challenge the future. We need to learn if there might be bedrock strategies and techniques that should be as much a part of each therapy plan as antiseptic techniques are to the operating room. Should operant techniques with their reliance on objective measures be part of every protocol regardless of its objectives? Do all adults need to monitor their fluency before success might be achieved? What are the constant cross categorical needs with which all stutterers must deal before treatment will be able to succeed? What are the differences that stutterers bring to speech pathologists that challenge the notion that they are a homogeneous population? And finally, and possibly most important, where does stuttering occur in the mind? Will answers to these and other critical questions challenge the models we have presented in this text? We certainly hope so. We have come so far. Far from pebbles in the mouth and the surgical mutilation of the tongue, in our efforts to cure stuttering. Far from fearful warnings not to intervene with the young to data based pleas for early intervention. Far from viewing stuttering as a life long curse of which to be ashamed to a puzzling human behavior to be understood, controlled, and even eliminated. We have journeyed far from being stumped because we did not know how to deal with stuttering behavior to being stumped because our cures do not seem to last. We may not have very much further to go.

Appendix

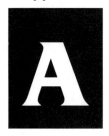

Research Bibliography

A profession advances with the accumulation of new knowledge. And new knowledge is acquired through careful and relevant research. In the area of stuttering, The PsycLIT Database lists over 1400 articles that have been written on the subject over the last 23 years. This number reflects only those articles that are contained in the journals for which it provides abstracts. Obviously, many more articles exist throughout the world. We have attempted in this section to provide the reader with a categorization of the 1400 articles. The combined articles had 840 locator words listed. These locator words were grouped into appropriate semantic categories. For example, articles containing the locator words "assertiveness" and "assertiveness training", were grouped together. We then examined the categories to determine if further collapsing could be accomplished. The primary focus in this effort was to group the articles into logical categories that would aide the researcher in becoming familiar with the research in relevant areas.

This resulted in 26 article categories. Many articles appear in multiple categories since their topics were diverse. When deciding where an article should be placed, judgement calls were necessary. We apologize to those authors who believe that their work is misrepresented. The concise placement of over 1400 articles becomes a mixture of knowledge, individual preferences and educated guesses.

A number of excellent articles are published in journals outside of the United States. Some are published in English while for others, only English abstracts are available. All of these articles are contained in the 26 categories. We thought that for some researchers, it would be interesting to see the type of research being conducted in various parts of the world. Articles published outside of the U.S. are also grouped into 10 geographic categories.

Aggression/Assertiveness   278
Anxiety   279
Articulation/Phonology/Rate   282

Attitudes/Subjective Judgements   286
Audition   290
Biochemistry   296
Cognition/Learning Disabilities   297
Culture   298
Demographics   300
Diagnostics/Assessment   300
Drugs   305
Efficacy   307
Etiology   311
Family   313
Genetics   316
Group Therapy   318
Hyponosis   318
Language   319
Motor Speech   324
Neurology   329
Neurogenic Disfluencies   338
Operant Conditioning/
   Behavioral Management   340
Physiology   345
Psychological Issues   349
Psychogenic Disfluencies   356
Research/Methodological Issues   356
Self-Evaluation   361
Therapaeutic Strategies   364
Voice/Laryngeal Behaviors   377
Australia/New Zealand   382
British Isles   382
Canada   385
China   385
Europe (Eastern)   385
Europe (Western)   389
India   394
Japan   395
Latin America   396
Middle East/Africa   397

Aggression and Assertiveness

Ablon, Steven L. Psychoanalysis of a stuttering boy. Special Issue: Psychoanalysis of children. International Review of Psycho-Analysis; 1988 Vol 15 (1) 83–91

Antonucci, Gianfranco; de Rosa, Emilia. La balbuzie: evoluzione dei concetti e prospettive per una comprensione psicodinamica del sintomo. (Stuttering: Evolution of its conceptualizations and prospects for a psychodynamic understanding of this symptom.) Archivio di Psicologia, Neurologia e Psichiatria; 1986 Oct–Dec Vol 47 (4) 451–476

Attanasio, Joseph S. The dodo was Lewis Carroll, you see: Reflections and speculations. Journal of Fluency Disorders; 1987 Apr Vol 12(2) 107–118

Azrin, Nathan, H. A strategy for applied research: Learning based but outcome oriented. American Psychologist; 1977 Feb Vol 32(2) 140–149

Berkowitz, Leonard; Frodi, Ann. Reactions to a child's mistakes as affected by her/his looks and speech. Social Psychology Quarterly; 1979 Dec Vol 42(4) 420–425

Bounes, Marika. Test de Rorschach avant et apres traitement de relaxation chez l'enfant. (Rorschach test before and after relaxation treatment of a child.) 11th International Congress on the Rorschach and Projective Methods (1984, Barcelona, Spain). Bulletin de Psychologie; 1986 Jun–Aug Vol 39(11–15) 651–654

D'Onofrio, Angelo. Occhio per occhio, dente per dente. / An eye for an eye, a tooth for a tooth. Centro Ricerche Biopsichiche, Padova; 1987–88 Vol 30–31 17–23

Dalali, Isobel D.; Sheehan, Joseph G. Stuttering and assertion training. Journal of Communication Disorders; 1974 Jun Vol 7(2) 97–111

Dolto, Francoise. L'agressivite chez le jeune enfant. (Aggressiveness in the young child.) Pratique des Mots; 1982 Mar No 38 19–25

Floyd, Nathaniel M. Billy Budd: A psychological autopsy. American Imago; 1977 Spr Vol 34(1) 28–49

Guy, Nina. Stuttering as an expression of aggression: Transferential and countertransferential aspects: A case study. Israel Journal of Psychiatry and Related Sciences; 1987 Vol 24(3) 211–221

Ibanez Ramirez, Manuel. Tratamiento de un caso de tartamudez. / Treatment of a stuttering case. Analisis y Modificacion de Conducta; 1985 Vol 11(30) 605–611

Lavkai, I. Yu. On personality deviations in stuttering adolescents. Defektologiya; 1976 Feb No 2 16–18

Mempel, Sigurd. Therapiemotivation bei Kindern: Ergebnisse einer empirischen Untersuchung. / Children's motivation for treatment. Praxis der Kinderpsychologie und Kinderpsychiatrie; 1989 May–Jun Vol 38(5) 146–151

Mizumachi, Toshiro. Assertiveness in stutterers—with reference to within-group differences. Japanese Journal of Special Education; 1985 Mar Vol 22(4) 1–9

Mizumachi, Toshiro. Study on the assertiveness in stutterers. Japanese Journal of Behavior Therapy; 1987 Mar Vol 12(2) 50–58

Petrunik, Michael; Shearing, Clifford D. Fragile facades: Stuttering and the strategic manipulation of awareness. Social Problems; 1983 Dec Vol 31(2) 125–138

Samuel Lajeunesse, B.; Degleris, N.; Brouri, R.; Agathon, M. Appreciation des effets des techniques assertives en groupe en milieu psychiatrie. (Group training in assertive techniques in a psychiatric milieu.) Annales Medico Psychologiques; 1985 May Vol 143(5) 458–464

Schloss, Patrick J.; Espin, Christine A.; Smith, Maureen A.; Suffolk, Debra R. Developing assertiveness during employment interviews with young adults who stutter. Journal of Speech and Hearing Disorders; 1987 Feb Vol 52(1) 30–36

Schloss, Patrick J.; Freeman, Catherine A.; Smith, Maureen A.; Espin, Christine A. Influence of assertiveness training of the stuttering rates exhibited by three young adults. Journal of Fluency Disorders; 1987 Oct Vol 12(5) 333–353

Scopazzo, Maurizio. (Rosenzweig Picture Frustration Study and EEG features in an adolescent stuttering group.) Lavoro Neuropsichiatrico; 1974 Jan–Jun Vol 54(1–3) 49–60

Silverman, Lloyd H. An experimental method for the study of unconscious conflict: A progress report. British Journal of Medical Psychology; 1975 Dec Vol 48(4) 291–298

Tkaczenko, Oleh G. Tiefenpsychologische Aspekte des Stotterns. / The depth psychological aspects of stuttering. Zeitschrift fur Individualpsychologie; 1990 Vol 15(4) 298–306

Wagner, Alejandro M. Acera de la tartamudez: Introduccion a la patologia del acto. (Stuttering: An introduction to the pathology of the act.) Revista de Psicoanalisis; 1988 Mar–Apr Vol 45(2) 391–417

Weiss, Amy L.; Zebrowski, Patricia M. Patterns of assertiveness and responsiveness in parental interactions with stuttering and fluent children. Journal of Fluency Disorders; 1991 Vol 16(2–3) 125–141

Wendlandt, Wolfgang. (Self-assertive training: A behavioral therapeutic phase in the treatment of adult stutterers.) Zeitschrift fur Klinische Psychologie und Psychotherapie; 1974 Vol 22(3) 236–246

Zielinski, Joseph J.; Williams, Leslie J. Situational determinants of stuttering in assertive contexts: A case study. Behavior Therapist; 1979 May–Jun Vol 2(3) 13

Anxiety

Ablon, Steven L. Psychoanalysis of a stuttering boy. Special Issue: Psychoanalysis of children. International Review of Psycho Analysis; 1988 Vol 15(1) 83–91

Aguilar, Guido. Ansiedad y comportamiento de tartamudeo. / Anxiety and stuttering behavior. Avances en Psicologia Clinica Latinoamericana; 1982 Vol 1 33–60

Alarcia, J.; Pinard, Gilbert; Serrano, M.; Tetreault, L. Etude comparative de trois traitements du begaiement: relaxation, desensibilisation, reeducation. (A comparative study of three treatments for stuttering: Relaxation, desensitization, reeducation.) Revue de Psychologie Appliquee; 1982 Vol 32(1) 1–25

Arkin, Arthur M.; et al. Behavior modification: Present status in psychiatry. New York State Journal of Medicine; 1976 Feb Vol 76(2) 190–196

Attanasio, Joseph S. Research design issues in relationships between anxiety and stuttering: Comments on Craig. Journal of Speech and Hearing Research; 1991 Oct Vol 34(5) 1079–1080

Azorin, Jean Michel; Pringuey, Dominique; Samuelian, Jean Claude; Benychou, Michele. Les Nouvelles benzodiazepines. / The new benzodiazepines. XXth Psychiatric Meeting (1986, Marseille, France). Psychologie Medicale; 1987 Mar Vol 19(3) 363–365

Bounes, Marika. Test de Rorschach avant et apres traitement de relaxation chez l'enfant.

(Rorschach test before and after relaxation treatment of a child.) 11th International Congress on the Rorschach and Projective Methods (1984, Barcelona, Spain). Bulletin de Psychologie; 1986 Jun–Aug Vol 39(11–15) 651–654

Burgraff, Roger I. The efficacy of systematic desensitization via imagery as a therapeutic technique with stutterers. British Journal of Disorders of Communication; 1974 Oct Vol 9(2) 134–139

Costa, D.; Pop, A.; Dumitriu, L.; Marinescu, Luzia; et al. Serum immunoreactive parathormone levels correlate with depression and anxiety in hypocalcemic stutterers. Activitas Nervosa Superior; 1986 Vol 28(2) 155–156

Craig, Ashley. An investigation into the relationship between anxiety and stuttering. Journal of Speech and Hearing Disorders; 1990 May Vol 55(2) 290–294

Craig, Ashley. "Research design issues in relationships between anxiety and stuttering: Comments on Craig": Reply. Journal of Speech and Hearing Research; 1991 Oct Vol 34(5) 1080–1081

Dabul, Barbara; Perkins, William H. The effects of stuttering on systolic blood pressure. Journal of Speech and Hearing Research; 1973 Dec Vol. 16(4) 586–591

de Rosa, E.; Antonucci, G.; Rinaldi, L. Balbuzie, complesso edipico e angosce primitive: Osservazioni su un caso clinico. / Stuttering, Oedipus complex and earliest anxieties: Some observations on a clinical case. Archivio di Psicologia, Neurologia e Psichiatria; 1987 Vol 48(3) 327–335

Fink, Hans; Niebergall, Gerhard. An attempt to measure anxieties in children who stutter. Heilpadagogik; 1975 Sep Vol 44(3) 220–227

Florin, Irmela. Stuttering: Theoretical approaches, experimental research results, suggestions for therapy. European Journal of Behavioural Analysis and Modification; 1976 Nov Vol 3(1) 189–200

Gerstman, Hubert L. The concatenation of stuttering to negative behavioral events: A clinical insight. Journal of Fluency Disorders; 1983 Jun Vol 8(2) 169–173

Gonzalez Valenzuela, M. Jose. Evaluacion y Tratamiento cognitivo-conductual de un caso de tartamudez. / Evaluation and cognitive-behavioral treatment in a severe stuttering case. Analisis y Modificacion de Conducta; 1990 Vol 16(47) 137–148

Ham, Richard E. Clinician preparation: Experiences with pseudostuttering: "It was the longest day of my life." Journal of Fluency Disorders; 1990 Oct–Dec Vol 15(5–6) 305–315

Hegde, M. N. The effect of shock on stuttering. Journal of the All India Institute of Speech and Hearing; 1971 Jan Vol. 2 104–110

Horovitz, Linda J.; et al. Stapedial reflex and anxiety in fluent and disfluent speakers. Journal of Speech and Hearing Research; 1978 Dec Vol 21(4) 762–767

Ikezuki, Makoto; Harano, Kotaro; Yamaguchi, Shoji. (Research on the effect of reciprocal inhibition elicited with kinetic response.) Japanese Journal of Behavior Therapy; 1989 Vol 15(1) 56–61

Janssen, Peggy; Kraaimaat, Floor. Angst als predictor van het behandelingsresultaat bij stotteren. / Anxiety as a predictor in the outcome of stuttering therapy. Gedragstherapie; 1986 Sep Vol 19(3) 161–170

Kalyagin, V. A. Characteristics of attention in stutterers. Soviet Neurology and Psychiatry; 1985–86 Win Vol 18(4) 85–88

Kelemen, Z. Hypno-behavioural therapy for the treatment of stuttering. Australian Journal of Clinical Hypnotherapy; 1980 Mar Vol 1(1) 17–23

Khavin, Aleksandr B. Individual-psychological factors in prediction of help to stutterers. Voprosy Psikhologii; 1985 Mar–Apr No 2 133–135

Kondas, Ondrej. Emocionalne a situacne premenne pri reci balbutikov. / Emotional and situational variables in the speech of stutterers. Zbornik Univerzity Komenskeho Psychologica; 1982 Vol 26–27 197–208

Kotbi, Naser; Farag, Safwat; Yousif, Mahmoud; Baraka, Mohamed et al. A comparison between stutterers and non-stutterers in intelligence, self-concept, anxiety and depression. Derasat Nafseyah; 1992 2(2) 37–349

Kraaimaat, Floor; Janssen, Peggy; Brutten, Gene J. The relationship between stutterers' cognitive and autonomic anxiety and therapy outcome. Journal of Fluency Disorders; 1988 Apr Vol 13(2) 107–113

Kraaimaat, Floor W.; Janssen, Peggy. Een werkmodel voor een differentiele diagnostiek en behandeling van stotteren. (A working model for the differential diagnosis and treatment of stuttering.) Gedragstherapie; 1983 Dec Vol 16(4) 299–309

Kraaimaat, Floor W.; Janssen, Peggy; Van Dam Baggen, Rien. Social anxiety and stuttering. Perceptual and Motor Skills; 1991 Jun Vol 72(3, Pt 1) 766

Leith, William R.; Timmons, Jack L. The stutterer's reaction to the telephone as a speaking situation. Journal of Fluency Disorders; 1983 Sep Vol 8(3) 233–243

McDonough, Alanna N.; Quesal, Robert W. Locus of control orientation of stutterers and nonstutterers. Journal of Fluency Disorders; 1988 Apr Vol 13(2) 97–106

Miller, Susan; Watson, Ben C. The relationship between communication attitude, anxiety, and depression in stutterers and nonstutterers. Journal of Speech and Hearing Research; 1992 Aug Vol 35(4) 789–798

Moleski, Richard; Tosi, Donald J. Comparative psychotherapy: Rational-emotive therapy versus systematic desensitization in the treatment of stuttering. Journal of Consulting and Clinical Psychology; 1976 Apr Vol 44(2) 309–311

Muckenhoff, Elisabeth. Modell zur Genese und Manifestation des Stotterns auf lerntheoretischer Basis. (A learning theory model of the origins of stuttering and stuttering behavior.) Vierteljahresschrift fur Heilpadagogik und ihre Nachbargebiete; 1976 Dec Vol 45(4) 341–346

Murray, K. S.; Empson, J. A.; Weaver, S. M. Rehearsal and preparation for speech in stutterers: A psychophysiological study. British Journal of Disorders of Communication; 1987 Aug Vol 22(2) 145–150

Neiman, Gary S.; Rubin, Rebecca B. Changes in communication apprehension, satisfaction, and competence in foreign dialect and stuttering clients. Journal of Communication Disorders; 1991 Oct–Dec Vol 24(5–6) 353–366

Nekrasova, Yuliya B. Dynamics of psychological states in stutterers in the process of logopsychotherapy. Voprosy Psikhologii; 1985 Mar–Apr No 2 127–133

Ohashi, Yoshiko; Hagiwara, Sachiko. The onset and development of stuttering problems: Discussion of self-acceptance of stuttering in adolescence. Japanese Journal of Child and Adolescent Psychiatry; 1982 Vol 23(5) 287–299

Petermann, Franz. Aktuelle Trends bei der Verhaltensmodifikation mit Kindern. (Current trends in behavior modification with children.) Psychologische Rundschau; 1981 Oct Vol 32(4) 250–266

Peters, Herman F.; Hulstijn, Wouter. Stuttering and anxiety: The difference between stutterers and nonstutterers in verbal apprehension and physiologic arousal during the anticipation of speech and non-speech tasks. Journal of Fluency Disorders; 1984 Feb Vol 9(1) 67–84

Pukacova, Marianna. (Psychological characteristics of stuttering children.) Psychologia a Patopsychologia Dietata; 1973 Vol. 8(3) 233–238

Rudmin, Floyd. Parent's report of stress and articulation oscillation as factors in a preschooler's dysfluencies. Journal of Fluency Disorders; 1984 Feb Vol 9(1) 85–87

Still, A. W.; Griggs, S. Changes in the probability of stuttering following a stutter: A test of some recent models. Journal of Speech and Hearing Research; 1979 Sep Vol 22(3) 565–571

Still, A. W.; Sherrard, Carol A. Formalizing theories of stuttering. British Journal of Mathematical and Statistical Psychology; 1976 Nov Vol 29(2) 129–138

Tyre, Timothy E.; Maisto, Stephen A.; Companik, Paul J. The use of systematic desensitization in the treatment of chronic stuttering behavior. Journal of Speech and Hearing Disorders; 1973 Nov Vol. 38(4) 514–519

Young, Martin A. Increasing the frequency of stuttering. Journal of Speech and Hearing Research; 1985 Jun Vol 28(2) 282–293

Articulation/Phonology/Rate

Adams, Martin R. Voice onsets and segment durations of normal speakers and beginning stutterers. Journal of Fluency Disorders; 1987 Apr Vol 12(2) 133–139

Andrews, Gavin J.; Howie, Pauline M.; Dozsa, Melinda; Guitar, Barry E. Stuttering: Speech pattern characteristics under fluency-inducing conditions. Journal of Speech and Hearing Research; 1982 Jun Vol 25(2) 208–216

Aram, Dorothy M.; Meyers, Susan C.; Ekelman, Barbara L. Fluency of conversational speech in children with unilateral brain lesions. Brain and Language; 1990 Jan Vol 38(1) 105–121

Baken, R. J.; McManus, Devin A.; Cavallo, Stephen A. Prephonatory chest wall posturing in stutterers. Journal of Speech and Hearing Research; 1983 Sep Vol 26(3) 444–450

Beliakova, L. I.; Kumalia, I. (Comparative analysis of motor and speech-motor functions in preschool stutterers.) Defektologiya; 1985 No 1 69–74

Bergmann, Gunther. Studies in stuttering as a prosodic disturbance. Journal of Speech and Hearing Research; 1986 Sep Vol 29(3) 290–300

Berkowitz, Leonard; Frodi, Ann. Reactions to a child's mistakes as affected by her/his looks and speech. Social Psychology Quarterly; 1979 Dec Vol 42(4) 420–425

Bishop, Judith H.; Williams, Harriet G.; Cooper, William A. Age and task complexity variables in motor performance of children with articulation-disordered, stuttering, and normal speech. Journal of Fluency Disorders; 1991 Vol 16(4) 219–228

Blood, Gordon W.; Seider, Robin. The concomitant problems of young stutterers. Journal of Speech and Hearing Disorders; 1981 Feb Vol 46(1) 31–33

Bloodstein, Oliver; Grossman, Marcia. Early stutterings: Some aspects of their form and distribution. Journal of Speech and Hearing Research; 1981 Jan Vol 24(2) 298–302

Boehmler, R. M.; Boehmler, S. I. The cause of stuttering: What's the question? Journal of Fluency Disorders; 1989 Dec Vol 14(6) 447–450

Bosshardt, Hans Georg; Nandyal, Indira. Reading rates of stutterers and nonstutterers during silent and oral reading. Journal of Fluency Disorders; 1988 Dec Vol 13(6) 407–420

Brown, C. J.; Zimmermann, G. N.; Linville, R. N.; Hegmann, J. P. Variations in self-paced behaviors in stutterers and nonstutterers. Journal of Speech and Hearing Research; 1990 Jun Vol 33(2) 317–323

Byrd, Kathryn; Cooper, Eugene B. Apraxic speech characteristics in stuttering, developmentally apraxic, and normal speaking children. Journal of Fluency Disorders; 1989 Jun Vol 14(3) 215–229

Cantwell, Dennis P.; Baker, Lorian. Psychiatric and learning disorders in children with speech and language disorders: A descriptive analysis. Advances in Learning and Behavioral Disabilities; 1985 Vol 4 29–47

Cross, Douglas E.; Olson, Patricia L. Articulatory-laryngeal interaction in stutterers and normal speakers: Effects of a bite-block on rapid voice initiation. Journal of Fluency Disorders; 1987 Dec Vol 12(6) 407–418

Freedman, Morris; Alexander, Michael P.; Naeser, Margaret A. Anatomic basis of transcortical motor aphasia. Neurology; 1984 Apr Vol 34(4) 409–417

Fukawa, Teruyo; Kato, Noriaki. Identification thresholds of nonsense syllables by stutterers. Perceptual and Motor Skills; 1986 Oct Vol 63(2, Pt 1) 592–594

Gagnon, Mireille; Ladouceur, Robert. Defining clinically significant changes in the treatment of child stutterers. Perceptual and Motor Skills; 1991 Oct Vol 73(2) 375–378

Griggs, S.; Still, A. W. An analysis of individual differences in words stuttered. Journal of Speech and Hearing Research; 1979 Sep Vol 22(3) 572–580

Guitar, Barry; Guitar, Carroll; Neilson, Peter; O'Dwyer, Nicholas; et al. Onset sequencing of selected lip muscles in stutterers and nonstutterers. Journal of Speech and Hearing Research; 1988 Mar Vol 31(1) 28–35

Guitar, Barry; Schaefer, Helen K.; Donahue-Kilburg, Gail; Bond, Lynne. Parent verbal interactions and speech rate: A case study in stuttering. Journal of Speech and Hearing Research; 1992 Aug Vol 35(4) 742–754

Harbison, Dan C.; Porter, Robert J.; Tobey, Emily A. Shadowed and simple reaction times in stutterers and nonstutterers. Journal of the Acoustical Society of America; 1989 Oct Vol 86(4) 1277–1284

Harrington, Jonathan. Stuttering, delayed auditory feedback, and linguistic rhythm. Journal of Speech and Hearing Research; 1988 Mar Vol 31(1) 36–47

Healey, E. Charles. Fundamental frequency contours of stutterers' vowels following fluent stop consonant productions. Folia Phoniatrica; 1984 May–Jun Vol 36(3) 145–151

Homzie, Marvin J.; Lindsay, Jean S.; Simpson, Joanne; Hasenstab, Suzanne. Concomitant speech, language, and learning problems in adult stutterers and in members of their families. Journal of Fluency Disorders; 1988 Aug Vol 13(4) 261–277

Horii, Yoshiyuki. Phonatory initiation, termination, and vocal frequency change reaction times of stutterers. Journal of Fluency Disorders; 1984 May Vol 9(2) 115–124

Howell, Peter; Powell, David J. Hearing your voice through bone and air: Implications for explanations of stuttering behavior from studies of normal speakers. Journal of Fluency Disorders; 1984 Dec Vol 9(4) 247–263

Howell, Peter; Wingfield, Trudie. Perceptual and acoustic evidence for reduced fluency in the vicinity of stuttering episodes. Language and Speech; 1990 Jan–Mar Vol 33(1) 31–46

Hubbard, Carol P.; Prins, David. Word familiarity, syllabic stress pattern, and stuttering. Journal of Speech and Hearing Research; 1994 37(3) 564–572

Hutchinson, John M.; Watkin, Kenneth L. Jaw mechanics during release of the stuttering moment: Some initial observations and interpretations. Journal of Communication Disorders; 1976 Dec Vol 9(4) 269–279

Ingham, Roger J.; Packman, Ann. A further evaluation of the speech of stutterers during chorus- and nonchorus-reading conditions. Journal of Speech and Hearing Research; 1979 Dec Vol 22(4) 784–817

Janssen, Peggy; Wieneke, George; Vaane, Eveline. Variability in the initiation of articulatory movements in the speech of stutterers and normal speakers. Journal of Fluency Disorders; 1983 Dec Vol 8(4) 341–358

Jayaram, M. Phonetic influences on stuttering in monolingual and bilingual stutterers. Journal of Communication Disorders; 1983 Jul Vol 16(4) 287–297

Jayaram, M. Relationship of stuttering to word information value in a phonemic clause. Journal of the All India Institute of Speech and Hearing; 1982 Vol 13 1–6

Kalveram, Karl T.; Jancke, Lutz. Vowel duration and voice onset time for stressed and nonstressed syllables in stutterers under delayed auditory feedback condition. Folia Phoniatrica; 1989 Jan–Feb Vol 41(1) 30–42

Kent, Ray D. Some comments on "Articulatory dynamics of fluent utterances of stutterers and nonstutterers." Journal of Speech and Hearing Research; 1983 Jun Vol 26(2) 319–320

Klich, Richard J.; May, Gaylene M. Spectrographic study of vowels in stutterers' fluent speech. Journal of Speech and Hearing Research; 1982 Sep Vol 25(3) 364–370

Kooman, E. A. Speech disturbance under delayed acoustic feedback and stuttering. Defektologiya; 1975 Jun No 6 27–33

Krikorian, Carol M.; Runyan, Charles M. A perceptual comparison: Stuttering and nonstuttering children's nonstuttered speech. Journal of Fluency Disorders; 1983 Dec Vol 8(4) 283–290

Lebrun, Yvan; Van Borsel, John. Final sound repetitions. Journal of Fluency Disorders; 1990 Apr Vol 15(2) 107–113

Lewis, Barbara A. Pedigree analysis of children with phonology disorders. Journal of Learning Disabilities; 1992 Nov Vol 25(9) 586–597

Louko, Linda J.; Edwards, Mary L.; Conture, Edward G. Phonological characteristics of young stutterers and their normally fluent peers: Preliminary observations. Journal of Fluency Disorders; 1990 Aug Vol 15(4) 191–210

Lutz, Konnie C.; Mallard, A. R. Disfluencies and rate of speech in young adult nonstutterers. Journal of Fluency Disorders; 1986 Dec Vol 11(4) 307–316

Mallard, A. R.; Westbrook, J. B. Vowel duration in stutterers participating in precision fluency shaping. Journal of Fluency Disorders; 1985 Sep Vol 10(3) 221–228

Manning, Walter H.; Reinsche, Linda. Auditory assembly abilities of stuttering and nonstuttering children. Journal of Speech and Hearing Research; 1976 Dec Vol 19(4) 777–783

Martens, Colleen F.; Engel, Dean C. Measurement of the sound-based word avoidance of persons who stutter. Journal of Fluency Disorders; 1986 Sep Vol 11(3) 241–250

McClean, Michael D.; Goldsmith, Howard; Cerf, Ann. Lower-lip EMG and displacement during bilabial disfluencies in adult stutterers. Journal of Speech and Hearing Research; 1984 Sep Vol 27(3) 342–349

McFarlane, Stephen C.; Prins, David. Neural response time of stutterers and nonstutterers in selected oral motor tasks. Journal of Speech and Hearing Research; 1978 Dec Vol 21(4) 768–778

McMillan, Marcia O.; Pindzola, Rebekah H. Temporal disruptions in the "accurate" speech of articulatory defective speakers and stutterers. Journal of Motor Behavior; 1986 Sep Vol 18(3) 279–286

Meyers, Susan C.; Freeman, Frances J. Mother and child speech rates as a variable in stuttering and disfluency. Journal of Speech and Hearing Research; 1985 Sep Vol 28(3) 436–444

Meyers, Susan C.; Hughes, Larry F.; Schoeny, Zahrl G. Temporal-phonemic processing skills in adult stutterers and nonstutterers. Journal of Speech and Hearing Research; 1989 Jun Vol 32(2) 274–280

Montgomery, Allen A.; Cooke, Paul A. Perceptual and acoustic analysis of repetitions in stuttered speech. Journal of Communication Disorders; 1976 Dec Vol 9(4) 317–330

Mowrer, Donald E. Repetition of final consonants in the speech of a young child. Journal of Speech and Hearing Disorders; 1987 May Vol 52(2) 174–178

Mowrer, Donald E.; Fairbank, Carlene. A case report of within-vowel glottal stop insertion in the speech of an adult male. Journal of Fluency Disorders; 1991 Feb Vol 16(1) 55–69

Nippold, Marilyn A. Concomitant speech and language disorders in stuttering children: A critique of the literature. Journal of Speech and Hearing Disorders; 1990 Feb Vol 55(1) 51–60

Onslow, Mark; Van Doorn, Janis; Newman, Denis. Variability of acoustic segment durations after prolonged-speech treatment for stuttering. Journal of Speech and Hearing Research; 1992 Jun Vol 35(3) 529–536

Perkins, William H. Implications of scientific research for treatment of stuttering: A lecture. Journal of Fluency Disorders; 1981 Jun Vol 6(2) 155–162

Perkins, William H.; Bell, Jody; Johnson, Linda; Stocks, Janice. Phone rate and the effective planning time hypothesis of stuttering. Journal of Speech and Hearing Research; 1979 Dec Vol 22(4) 747–755

Perkins, William H.; Kent, Raymond D.; Curlee, Richard F. A theory of neuropsycholinguistic function in stuttering. Journal of Speech and Hearing Research; 1991 Aug Vol 34(4) 734–752

Perkins, William; Rudas, Joanna; Johnson, Linda; Bell, Jody. Stuttering: Discoordination of phonation with articulation and respiration. Journal of Speech and Hearing Research; 1976 Sep Vol 19(3) 509–522

Peters, Herman F.; Boves, Louis. Coordination of aerodynamic and phonatory processes in fluent speech utterances of stutterers. Journal of Speech and Hearing Research; 1988 Sep Vol 31(3) 352–361

Pindzola, Rebekah H. Acoustic evidence of aberrant velocities in stutterers' fluent speech. Perceptual and Motor Skills; 1986 Apr Vol 62(2) 399–405

Platt, L. Jay; Basili, Annamaria. Jaw tremor during stuttering block: An electromyographic study. Journal of Communication Disorders; 1973 Jun Vol. 6(2) 102–109

Prins, David; Hubbard, Carol P.; Krause, Michelle. Syllabic stress and the occurrence of stuttering. Journal of Speech and Hearing Research; 1991 Oct Vol 34(5) 1011–1016

Prosek, Robert A.; Montgomery, Allen A.; Walden, Brian E. Constancy of relative timing for stutterers and nonstutterers. Journal of Speech and Hearing Research; 1988 Dec Vol 31(4) 654–658

Prosek, Robert A.; Montgomery, Allen A.; Walden, Brian E.; Hawkins, David B. Formant frequencies of stuttered and fluent vowels. Journal of Speech and Hearing Research; 1987 Sep Vol 30(3) 301–305

Prosek, Robert A.; Runyan, Charles M. Effects of segment and pause manipulations on the identification of treated stutterers. Journal of

Speech and Hearing Research; 1983 Dec Vol 26(4) 510–516

Prosek, Robert A.; Runyan, Charles M. Temporal characteristics related to the discrimination of stutterers' and nonstutterers' speech samples. Journal of Speech and Hearing Research; 1982 Mar Vol 25(1) 29–33

Ramig, Peter R. Rate changes in the speech of stutterers after therapy. Journal of Fluency Disorders; 1984 Dec Vol 9(4) 285–294

Rastatter, Michael; Dell, Carl W. Simple motor and phonemic processing reaction times of stutterers. Perceptual and Motor Skills; 1985 Oct Vol 61(2) 463–466

Rudmin, Floyd. Parent's report of stress and articulation oscillation as factors in a preschooler's dysfluencies. Journal of Fluency Disorders; 1984 Feb Vol 9(1) 85–87

Runyan, Charles M.; Bonifant, Debra C. A perceptual comparison: All-voiced versus typical reading passage read by children. Journal of Fluency Disorders; 1981 Sep Vol 6(3) 247–255

Ryan, Bruce P. Articulation, language, rate, and fluency characteristics of stuttering and nonstuttering preschool children. Journal of Speech and Hearing Research; 1992 Apr Vol 35(2) 333–342

Schwartz, Martin F. The core of the stuttering block. Journal of Speech and Hearing Disorders; 1974 May Vol. 39(2) 169–177

Silverman, Ellen Marie. Effect of selected word attributes on preschoolers' speech disfluency: Initial phoneme and length. Journal of Speech and Hearing Research; 1975 Sep Vol 18(3) 430–434

Silverman, Franklin H.; Hummer, Kathy. Spastic dysphonia: A fluency disorder? Journal of Fluency Disorders; 1989 Aug Vol 14(4) 285–291

Silverman, Franklin H.; Umberger, Forrest G. Effect of pacing speech with a miniature electronic metronome on the frequency and duration of selected disfluency behaviors in the spontaneous speech of adult stutterers. Behavior Therapy; 1974 May Vol. 5(3) 410–414

St. Louis, Kenneth O.; Hinzman, Audrey R. A descriptive study of speech, language, and hearing characteristics of school-aged stutterers. Journal of Fluency Disorders; 1988 Oct Vol 13(5) 331–355

St. Louis, Kenneth O.; Hinzman, Audrey R.; Hull, Forrest M. Studies of cluttering: Disfluency and language measures in young possible clutterers and stutterers. Journal of Fluency Disorders; 1985 Sep Vol 10(3) 151–172

St. Louis, Kenneth O.; Murray, Cheryl D.; Ashworth, Melanie S. Coexisting communication disorders in a random sample of school-aged stutterers. Journal of Fluency Disorders; 1991 Feb Vol 16(1) 13–23

Stephenson-Opsal, Deborah; Bernstein-Ratner, Nan. Maternal speech rate modification and childhood stuttering. Annual Convention of the American Speech Language and Hearing Association (1986, Detroit, Michigan). Journal of Fluency Disorders; 1988 Feb Vol 13(1) 49–56

Throneburg, Rebecca Niermann; Yairi, Ehud; Paden, Elaine P. Relation between phonologic difficulty and the occurrence of disfluencies in the early stage of stuttering. Journal of Speech and Hearing Research; 1994 37(3) 504–510

Till, James A.; Reich, Alan; Dickey, Stanley; Seiber, James. Phonatory and manual reaction times of stuttering and nonstuttering children. Journal of Speech and Hearing Research; 1983 Jun Vol 26(2) 171–180

Vankatagiri, Horabail S. Reaction time for /s/ and /z/ in stutterers and nonstutterers: A test of discoordination hypothesis. Journal of Communication Disorders; 1982 Jan Vol 15(1) 55–62

Viswanath, N. S. Global- and local-temporal effects of a stuttering event in the context of a clausal utterance. Journal of Fluency Disorders; 1989 Aug Vol 14(4) 245–269

Weiner, Adeline E. Stuttering and syllable stress. Journal of Fluency Disorders; 1984 Dec Vol 9(4) 301–305

Wells, G. B. A feature analysis of stuttered phonemes. Journal of Fluency Disorders; 1983 Jun Vol 8(2) 119–124

Wijnen, Frank; Boers, Inge. Phonological priming effects in stutterers. Journal of Fluency Disorders; 1994 19(1) 1–21

Zebrowski, Patricia M. Duration of sound prolongation and sound/syllable repetition in children who stutter: Preliminary observations. Journal of Speech and Hearing Research; 1994 37(2), 254–264

Zebrowski, Patricia M. Duration of the speech disfluencies of beginning stutterers. Journal of Speech and Hearing Research; 1991 Jun Vol 34(3) 483–491

Zebrowski, Patricia M.; Conture, Edward G.; Cudahy, Edward A. Acoustic analysis of young stutterers' fluency: Preliminary observations. Journal of Fluency Disorders; 1985 Sep Vol 10(3) 173–192

Zimmermann, Gerald. Articulatory behaviors associated with stuttering: A cinefluorographic analysis. Journal of Speech and Hearing Research; 1980 Mar Vol 23(1) 108–121

Zimmermann, Gerald. Articulatory dynamics of fluent utterances of stutterers and nonstutterers. Journal of Speech and Hearing Research; 1980 Mar Vol 23(1) 95–107

Zimmermann, Gerald N.; Hanley, J. M. A cinefluorographic investigation of repeated fluent productions of stutterers in an adaptation procedure. Journal of Speech and Hearing Research; 1983 Mar Vol 26(1) 35–42

Attitudes and Subjective Judgements

Andrews, Gavin; Craig, Ashley. Prediction of outcome after treatment for stuttering. British Journal of Psychiatry; 1988 Aug Vol 153 236–240

Andrews, Gavin; Cutler, Jeffrey. Stuttering therapy: The relation between changes in symptom level and attitudes. Journal of Speech and Hearing Disorders; 1974 Aug Vol 39(3) 312–319

Andrews, Moya L.; Smith, Raymond G. Perceptions of auditory components of stuttered speech. Journal of Communication Disorders; 1976 Jun Vol 9(2) 121–128

Atkins, Carolyn P. Perceptions of speakers with minimal eye contact: Implications for stutterers. Journal of Fluency Disorders; 1988 Dec Vol 13(6) 429–436

Black, James A. A comparative study of the perception of freedom-in-leisure between stuttering and nonstuttering individuals. Journal of Fluency Disorders: 1987 Aug Vol 12(4) 239–248

Bubenickova, Milena. The stuttering child's relation to school. Psychologia a Patopsychologia Dietata; 1977 Vol 12(6) 535–545

Burley, Peter M.; Rinaldi, Wendy. Effects of sex of listener and of stutterer on ratings of stuttering speakers. Journal of Fluency Disorders; 1986 Dec Vol 11(4) 329–333

Bushey, Tahirih; Martin, Richard. Stuttering in children's literature. Language, Speech, and Hearing Services in Schools; 1988 Jul Vol 19(3) 235–250

Campbell, Michel; Boudreau, Leonce; Ladouceur, Robert. L'influence d'interlocuteurs sur l'evaluation du begaiement. (The influence of speakers on the evaluation of stuttering.) Revue de Modification du Comportement; 1984 Vol 14(3) 112–122

Cooper, Eugene B.; Cooper, Crystal S. Clinician attitudes toward stuttering: A decade of change (1973–1983). Journal of Fluency Disorders; 1985 Mar Vol 10(1) 19–33

Cooper, Eugene B.; Rustin, Lena. Clinician attitudes toward stuttering in the United States and Great Britain: A cross-cultural study. Journal of Fluency Disorders; 1985 Mar Vol 10(1) 1–17

Cox, Nancy J.; Seider, Robin A.; Kidd, Kenneth K. Some environmental factors and hypotheses for stuttering in families with several stutterers. Journal of Speech and Hearing Research; 1984 Dec Vol 27(4) 543–548

Crowe, Thomas A.; Cooper, Eugene B. Parental attitudes toward and knowledge of stuttering. Journal of Communication Disorders; 1977 Jun Vol 10(4) 343–357

Crowe, Thomas A.; Walton, Julie H. Teacher attitudes toward stuttering. Journal of Fluency Disorders; 1981 Jun Vol 6(2) 163–174

Culatta, Richard A.; Bader, Julie; McCaslin, Anita; Thomason, Nancy. Primary-school stutterers: Have attitudes changed? Journal of Fluency Disorders; 1985 Jun Vol 10(2) 87–91

de Nil, Luc F.; Brutten, Gene J. Speech-associated attitudes of stuttering and nonstuttering children. Journal of Speech and Hearing Research; 1991 Feb Vol 34(1) 60–66

de Nil, Luc F.; Brutten, Gene J. Speech-associated attitudes: Stuttering, voice disordered, articulation disordered, and normal speaking children. Journal of Fluency Disorders; 1990 Apr Vol 15(2) 127–134

DeJoy, Daniel A.; Jordan, William J. Listener reactions to interjections in oral reading versus spontaneous speech. Journal of Fluency Disorders; 1988 Feb Vol 13(1) 11–25

Devore, Jon E.; Nandur, Mallika S.; Manning, Walter H. Projective drawings and children who stutter. Journal of Fluency Disorders; 1984 Sep Vol 9(3) 217–226

Floyd, Susan; Perkins, William H. Early syllable dysfluency in stutterers and nonstutterers: A preliminary report. Journal of Communication Disorders; 1974 Sep Vol 7(3) 279–282

Fransella, Fay. The development of attitudes to prejudice: A personal construct psychology view. Educational and Child Psychology; 1985 Vol 2(3) 150–156

Gagnon, Mireille; Ladouceur, Robert. Behavioral treatment of child stutterers: Replication and extension. Behavior Therapy; 1992 Win Vol 23(1) 113–129

Gonzalez-Ochoa, A. M.; Parra-Parra, M. L.; Rodriguez-Carrillo, P. R. Actitudes y tartamudez II. (Attitudes and stuttering: II.) Revista de Psicologia General y Aplicada; 1990 Jul 43(3) 393–400

Grzybowska, Aldona; Lapinska, Irena; Michalska, Roza. Postawy nauczycieli wobec jakania. / Teachers' attitudes to stuttering. Psychologia Wychowawcza; 1991 Mar–Apr Vol 34(2) 139–150

Guitar, Barry. Pretreatment factors associated with the outcome of stuttering therapy. Journal of Speech and Hearing Research; 1976 Sep Vol 19(3) 590–600

Guitar, Barry; Bass, Colin. Stuttering therapy: The relation between attitude change and long-term outcome. Journal of Speech and Hearing Disorders; 1978 Aug Vol 43(3) 392–400

Ham, Richard E. Clinician preparation: Experiences with pseudostuttering: "It was the longest day of my life" Journal of Fluency Disorders; 1990 Oct–Dec Vol 15(5–6) 305–315

Ham, Richard E. What is stuttering: Variations and stereotypes. Journal of Fluency Disorders; 1990 Oct–Dec Vol 15(5–6) 259–273

Hirasawa, Hajima; Ohashi, Yoshiko; Hagiwara, Sachiko. (Listeners' attitudes toward stuttering—a study on some illustrative cases in literary works.) Japanese Journal of Special Education; 1982 Feb Vol 19(3) 39–46

Horsley, Irmgarde A.; Fitzgibbon, Carol T. Stuttering children: Investigation of a stereotype. British Journal of Disorders of Communication; 1987 Apr Vol 22(1) 19–35

Hulit, Lloyd M. A stutterer like me. Journal of Fluency Disorders; 1989 Jun Vol 14(3) 209–214

Hurst, Melanie I.; Cooper, Eugene B. Employer attitudes toward stuttering. Journal of Fluency Disorders; 1983 Mar Vol 8(1) 1–12

Hurst, Michele A.; Cooper, Eugene B. Vocational rehabilitation counselors' attitudes toward stuttering. Journal of Fluency Disorders; 1983 Mar Vol 8(1) 13–27

James, Jack E.; Ingham, Roger J. The influence of stutterer's expectancies of improvement upon response to time-out. Journal of Speech and Hearing Research; 1974 Mar Vol. 17(1) 86–93

Johnson, Gerald F. A clinical study of Porky Pig cartoons. Journal of Fluency Disorders; 1987 Aug Vol 12(4) 235–238

Kalinowski, Joseph; Noble, Sandra; Armson, Joy; Stuart Andrew. Pretreatment and posttreatment speech naturalness ratings of adults with mild and severe stuttering. American Journal of Speech-Language Pathology; 1994 3(1) 61–67

Khavin, A. B. (Personality reactions to a communication disorder.) Defektologiya; 1974 Vol 1 26–29

Klinger, Herbert. Effects of pseudostuttering on normal speakers' self-ratings of beauty. Journal of Communication Disorders; 1987 Aug Vol 20(4) 353–358

Kulas, Henryk. Sytuacja szkolna dzieci jakajacych sie. / The school situation of stuttering children. Psychologia Wychowawcza; 1990 Nov–Dec Vol 33(5) 331–344

Ladouceur, Robert; Saint-Laurent, Lise. Stuttering: A multidimensional treatment and evaluation package. Journal of Fluency Disorders; 1986 Jun Vol 11(2) 93–103

Ladouceur, Robert; Caron, Chantal; Caron, Guylaine. Stuttering severity and treatment outcome. Journal of Behavior Therapy and

Experimental Psychiatry; 1989 Mar Vol 20(1) 49–56

Lankford, Sally D.; Cooper, Eugene B. Recovery from stuttering as viewed by parents of self-diagnosed recovered stutterers. Journal of Communication Disorders; 1974 Jun Vol 7(2) 171–180

Lass, Norman J.; Ruscello, Dennis M.; Schmitt, John F.; Pannbacker, Mary D.; et al. Teachers' perceptions of stutterers. Language, Speech, and Hearing Services in Schools; 1992 Jan Vol 23(1) 78–81

Lass, Norman J.; Ruscello, Dennis M.; Pannbacker, Mary; Schmitt, John F.; Kiser, Angela Marsh; Mussa, Ashraf M.; Lockhart, Mary Jo. School administrators' perceptions of people who stutter. Language, Speech and Hearing Services in the Schools; 1994 25(2) 90–94

Lass, Norman J.; Ruscello, Dennis M.; Pannbacker, Mary D.; Schmitt, John F.; et al. Speech-language pathologists' perceptions of child and adult female and male stutterers. Journal of Fluency Disorders; 1989 Apr Vol 14(2) 127–134

Lawson, R.; Pring, T.; Fawcus, M. The effects of short courses in modifying the attitudes of adult and adolescent stutterers to communication. European Journal of Disorders of Communication; 1993 Vol 28(3) 299–308

Lechta, Viktor; Vanhara, Ladislav. Analyza postojov uciteliek a matiek k zajakavemu diet'at'u. / Analysis of attitudes of teachers and mothers towards a stammering child. Jednotna Skola; 1985 Apr Vol 37(4) 357–362

Madison, Lynda S.; Budd, Karen S.; Itzkowitz, Judy S. Changes in stuttering in relation to children's locus of control. Journal of Genetic Psychology; 1986 Jun Vol 147(2) 233–240

Mallard, A. R.; Westbrook, J. B. Vowel duration in stutterers participating in precision fluency shaping. Journal of Fluency Disorders; 1985 Sep Vol 10(3) 221–228

Manning, Walter H.; Dailey, Deborah; Wallace, Sue. Attitude and personality characteristics of older stutterers. Journal of Fluency Disorders; 1984 Sep Vol 9(3) 207–215

McCabe, Robert B.; McCollum, Judith D. The personal reactions of a stuttering adult to delayed auditory feedback. Journal of Speech and Hearing Disorders; 1972 Nov Vol. 37(4) 536–541

McKinnon, Shauna L.; Hess, Carla W.; Landry, Richard G. Reactions of college students to speech disorders. Journal of Communication Disorders; 1986 Feb Vol 19(1) 75–82

Mempel, Sigurd. Therapiemotivation bei Kindern: Ergebnisse einer empirischen Untersuchung. / Children's motivation for treatment. Praxis der Kinderpsychologie und Kinderpsychiatrie; 1989 May-Jun Vol 38(5) 146–151

Miller, Susan; Watson, Ben C. The relationship between communication attitude, anxiety, and depression in stutterers and nonstutterers. Journal of Speech and Hearing Research; 1992 Aug Vol 35(4) 789–798

Mizumachi, Toshiro. An experimental study of listeners' attitudes toward stuttering children: I. The influence different encounter modes in the stuttering situation exercise on listeners' attitude changes. Japanese Journal of Special Education; 1983 Jun Vol 21(1) 21–26

Mizumachi, Toshiro. (Assessment of the results of stuttering therapy—from the behavior therapeutic point of view.) Japanese Journal of Special Education; 1981 Oct Vol 19(2) 48–55

Mizumachi, Toshiro. (The factor analytic study on listeners' attitudes toward stuttering children.) Japanese Journal of Special Education; 1982 Jul Vol 20(1) 27–33

Moore, Margaret; Nystul, Michael S. Parent-child attitudes and communication processes in families with stutterers and families with non-stutterers. British Journal of Disorders of Communication; 1979 Dec Vol 14(3) 173–180

Nekrasova, Yuliya B. The teacher and the psychological atmosphere in the classroom. Soviet Psychology; 1987–88 Win Vol 26(2) 79–83

Patterson, J.; Pring, T. Listeners' attitudes to stuttering speakers: No evidence for a gender difference. Journal of Fluency Disorders; 1991 Vol 16(4) 201–205

Peutelschmiedova, Alzbeta; Rauerova, Martina. Profesionalni orientace balbutiku. (Vocational orientation of stutterers.) Psychologia a Patopsychologia Dietata; 1990 Vol 25(5) 405–416

Quesal, Robert W. Stuttering research: Have we forgotten the stutterer? Journal of Fluency Disorders; 1989 Jun Vol 14(3) 153–164

Ragsdale, J. Donald; Ashby, Jon K. Speech-language pathologists' connotations of stuttering. Journal of Speech and Hearing Research; 1982 Mar Vol 25(1) 75–80

Ralston, Lenore D. Stammering: A stress index in Caribbean classrooms. Journal of Fluency Disorders; 1981 Jun Vol 6(2) 119–133

Rodriguez, Pedro R. Actitudes y conductas de los maestros de educacion primaria hacia la tartamudez. (Attitudes and behaviors of primary school teachers toward stuttering.) Revista Intercontinental de Psicologia y Educacion; 1988 Dec Vol 1(2) 165–183

Rodriguez, Pedro R. Actitudes y tartamudez. (Attitudes and stuttering.) Revista de Psicologia General y Aplicada; 1986 Vol 41(6) 1229–1252

Rodriguez, Pedro R.; Silva, Celia. Perfil de la tartamudez y del tartamudo. (Profile of stuttering and the stutterer.) Revista Latinoamericana de Psicologia; 1985 Vol 17(1) 87–112

Santacreu-Mas, Jose. El condicionamiento ante determinadas palabras en la tartamudez. (Conditioning before some words in stuttering.) Revista de Psicologia General y Aplicada; 1984 Vol 39(6) 1115–1129

Scheidegger, Ursula. Spieltherapie mit stotternden Kindern: Ein Erfahrungsbericht. / Play therapy with stuttering children: Practical experiences. Vierteljahresschrift fur Heilpadagogik und ihre Nachbargebiete; 1987 Dec Vol 56(4) 619–629

Schliesser, Herbert F. Psychological scaling of speech by students in training compared to that by experienced speech-language pathologists. Perceptual and Motor Skills; 1985 Dec Vol 61(3, Pt 2) 1299–1302

Sheehan, Joseph G. Level of aspiration in female stutterers: Changing times? Journal of Speech and Hearing Disorders; 1979 Nov Vol 44(4) 479–486

Sheehan, Joseph G.; Lyon, Martha A. Role perception in stuttering. Journal of Communication Disorders; 1974 Jun Vol 7(2) 113–125

Silverman, Ellen Marie. Communication attitudes of women who stutter. Journal of Speech and Hearing Disorders; 1980 Nov Vol 45(4) 533–539

Silverman, Franklin H. Are professors likely to report having "beliefs" about the intelligence and competence of students who stutter? Journal of Fluency Disorders; 1990 Oct–Dec Vol 15(5–6) 319–321

Silverman, Franklin H. Impact of a T-shirt message on stutterer stereotypes. Journal of Fluency Disorders; 1988 Aug Vol 13(4) 279–281

Silverman, Franklin H.; Marik, Judith H. "Teachers' perceptions of stutterers": A replication. Language, Speech, and Hearing Services in Schools; 1993 Apr Vol 24(2) 108

Silverman, Franklin H.; Paynter, Kathryn K. Impact of stuttering on perception of occupational competence. Journal of Fluency Disorders; 1990 Apr Vol 15(2) 87–91

St. Louis, Kenneth O.; Atkins, Carolyn P. Nonstutterers' perceptions of stuttering and speech difficulty. Journal of Fluency Disorders; 1988 Dec Vol 13(6) 375–384

Stewart, Trudy M. The relationship of attitudes and intentions to behave to the acquisition of fluent speech behaviour by stammerers. British Journal of Disorders of Communication; 1982 Sep Vol 17(2) 3–13

Tatchell, R. H.; Van den Berg, S.; Lerman, J. W. Fluency and eye contact as factors influencing observers' perceptions of stutterers. Journal of Fluency Disorders; 1983 Sep Vol 8(3) 221–231

Turnbaugh, Karen; Guitar, Barry; Hoffman, Paul. The attribution of personality traits: The stutterer and nonstutterer. Journal of Speech and Hearing Research; 1981 Jan Vol 24(2) 288–291

Turnbaugh, Karen R.; Guitar, Barry E.; Hoffman, Paul R. Speech clinicians' attribution of personality traits as a function of stuttering severity. Journal of Speech and Hearing Research; 1979 Mar Vol 22(1) 37–45

Watson, Jennifer B. A comparison of stutterers' and nonstutterers' affective, cognitive, and behavioral self-reports. Journal of Speech and Hearing Research; 1988 Sep Vol 31(3) 377–385

Watson, Jennifer B. Profiles of stutterers' and nonstutterers' affective, cognitive, and behavioral communication attitudes. Journal of Fluency Disorders; 1987 Dec Vol 12(6) 389–405

Watson, Jennifer B.; Gregory, Hugo H.; Kistler, Doris J. Development and evaluation of an inventory to assess adult stutterers' communication attitudes. Journal of Fluency Disorders; 1987 Dec Vol 12(6) 429–450

Watts, Fraser. Mechanisms of fluency control in stutterers. British Journal of Disorders of Communication; 1973 Oct Vol. 8(2) 131–138

Wertheim, Eleanor S. Ego dysfunction in stuttering and its relationship to the subculture of the nuclear family: A predictive study based on the bio-adaptive theory of stuttering: II. British Journal of Medical Psychology; 1973 Jun Vol. 46(2) 155–180

White, Peter A.; Collins, Sara R. Stereotype formation by inference: A possible explanation for the "stutterer" stereotype. Journal of Speech and Hearing Research; 1984 Dec Vol 27(4) 567–570

Woods, C. Lee. Does the stigma shape the stutterer? Journal of Communication Disorders; 1978 Dec Vol 11(6) 483–487

Woods, C. Lee. Teachers' predictions of the social position and speaking competence of stuttering students. Language, Speech and Hearing Services in the Schools; 1975 Oct Vol 6(4) 177–182

Woods, C. Lee; Williams, Dean E. Traits attributed to stuttering and normally fluent males. Journal of Speech and Hearing Research; 1976 Jun Vol 19(2) 267–278

Yeakle, Mary K.; Cooper, Eugene B. Teacher perceptions of stuttering. Journal of Fluency Disorders; 1986 Dec Vol 11(4) 345–359

Young, Martin A. A reanalysis of "Stuttering therapy: The relation between attitude change and long-term outcome." A reanalysis of stuttering therapy: The relationship between attitude change and long-term outcome. Journal of Speech and Hearing Disorders; 1981 46, 2, 221–222.

Audition

Adamczyk, Bogdan; Kuniszyk Jozkowiak, Wieslawa. Effect of echo and reverberation of a restricted information capacity on the speech process. Folia Phoniatrica; 1987 Jan–Feb Vol 39(1) 9–17

Adams, Martin R.; Hutchinson, John. The effects of three levels of auditory masking on selected vocal characteristics and the frequency of disfluency of adult stutterers. Journal of Speech and Hearing Research; 1974 Dec Vol 17(4) 682–688

Altrows, Irwin F. Anomalous auditory feedback delays and stuttering. Journal of Speech and Hearing Research; 1982 Dec Vol 25(4) 631–632

Altrows, Irwin F.; Bryden, M. P. Temporal factors in the effects of masking noise on fluency of stutterers. Journal of Communication Disorders; 1977 Jun Vol 10(4) 315–329

Anderson, Jill M.; Hood, Stephen B.; Sellers, Dan E. Central auditory processing abilities of adolescent and preadolescent stuttering and nonstuttering children. Journal of Fluency Disorders; 1988 Jun Vol 13(3) 199–214

Andrews, Gavin. Stuttering: A tutorial. Australian and New Zealand Journal of Psychiatry; 1981 Jun Vol 15(2) 105–109

Andrews, Gavin J.; Howie, Pauline M.; Dozsa, Melinda; Guitar, Barry E. Stuttering: Speech pattern characteristics under fluency-inducing conditions. Journal of Speech and Hearing Research; 1982 Jun Vol 25(2) 208–216

Aoki, Tsuyoshi. (Delayed auditory feedback and stuttering.) Japanese Journal of Educational Psychology; 1974 Sep Vol 22(3) 186–191

Berezhkovskaya, E. L.; Golod, V. I.; Turovskaya, Z. G. Sensory asymmetry in stutterers and normal individuals. Voprosy Psikhologii; 1980 No 1 57–63

Blood, Gordon W. Laterality differences in child stutterers: Heterogeneity, severity levels, and statistical treatments. Journal of Speech and Hearing Disorders; 1985 Feb Vol 50(1) 66–72

Blood, Gordon W.; Blood, Ingrid M. Central auditory function in young stutterers. Perceptual and Motor Skills; 1984 Dec Vol 59(3) 699–705

Blood, Gordon W.; Blood, Ingrid M. Laterality preferences in adult female and male stutterers. Journal of Fluency Disorders; 1989 Feb Vol 14(1) 1–10

Blood, Gordon W.; Blood, Ingrid M. Multiple data analyses of dichotic listening advantages of stutterers. Journal of Fluency Disorders; 1989 Apr Vol 14(2) 97–107

Blood, Gordon W.; Blood, Ingrid M.; Hood, Stephen B. The development of ear preferences in stuttering and nonstuttering children: A longitudinal study. Journal of Fluency Disorders; 1987 Apr Vol 12(2) 119–131

Blood, Gordon W.; Blood, Ingrid M.; Newton, Karen R. Effect of directed attention on cerebral asymmetries in stuttering adults. Perceptual and Motor Skills; 1986 Apr Vol 62(2) 351–355

Blood, Ingrid M.; Blood, Gordon W. Relationship between specific disfluency variables and dichotic listening in stutterers. Perceptual and Motor Skills; 1986 Feb Vol 62(1) 337–338

Blood, Ingrid M.; Blood, Gordon W. Relationship between stuttering severity and brain-stem-evoked response testing. Perceptual and Motor Skills; 1984 Dec Vol 59(3) 935–938

Bonin, Betsy; Ramig, Peter; Prescott, Thomas. Performance differences between stuttering and nonstuttering subjects on a sound fusion task. Journal of Fluency Disorders; 1985 Dec Vol 10(4) 291–300

Brady, John P.; Berson, Janet. Stuttering, dichotic listening, and cerebral dominance. Archives of General Psychiatry; 1975 Nov Vol 32(11) 1449–1452

Brayton, Evelyn R.; Conture, Edward G. Effects of noise and rhythmic stimulation on the speech of stutterers. Journal of Speech and Hearing Research; 1978 Jun Vol 21(2) 285–294

Brown, T.; Sambrooks, J. E.; MacCulloch, M. J. Auditory thresholds and the effect of reduced auditory feedback on stuttering. Acta Psychiatrica Scandinavica; 1975 Jun Vol 51(5) 297–311

Burke, Bryan D. Variables affecting stutterer's initial reactions to delayed auditory feedback. Journal of Communication Disorders; 1975 Jun Vol 8(2) 141–155

Carpenter, Mary; Sommers, Ronald K. Unisensory and bisensory perceptual and memory processing in stuttering adults and normal speakers. Journal of Fluency Disorders; 1987 Aug Vol 12(4) 291–304

Cimorell Strong, Jacqueline M.; Gilbert, Harvey R.; Frick, James V. Dichotic speech perception: A comparison between stuttering and non-stuttering children. Journal of Fluency Disorders; 1983 Mar Vol 8(1) 77–91

Code, Chris. Dichotic listening with the communicatively impaired: Results from trials of a short British-English dichotic word test. Journal of Phonetics; 1981 Oct Vol 9(4) 375–383

Code, Christopher; Muller, David. Comments on paper: The long-term use of an automatically triggered masking device in the treatment of stammering. British Journal of Disorders of Communication; 1980 Sep Vol 15(2) 141–142

Cohen, Melvin S.; Hanson, Marvin L. Intersensory processing efficiency of fluent speakers and stutterers. British Journal of Disorders of Communication; 1975 Oct Vol 10(2) 111–122

Conture, Edward G. Some effects of noise on the speaking behavior of stutterers. Journal of Speech and Hearing Research; 1974 Dec Vol 17(4) 714–723

Conture, Edward G.; Brayton, Evelyn R. The influence of noise on stutterers' different disfluency types. Journal of Speech and Hearing Research; 1975 Jun Vol 18(2) 381–384

Conture, Edward G.; Colton, Raymond H.; Gleason, John R. Selected temporal aspects of coordination during fluent speech of young stutterers. Journal of Speech and Hearing Research; 1988 Dec Vol 31(4) 640–653

Conture, Edward G.; Wingate, M. E. Comment on "Effect on stuttering of changes in audition." Journal of Speech and Hearing Research; 1973 Dec Vol. 16(4) 753–754

Costa, D.; Antoniac, Maria; Berghianu, S.; Marinescu, Rodica; et al. Clinical and paraclinical aspects of tetany in stuttering. Activitas Nervosa Superior; 1986 Vol 28(2) 156–158

Costa, D.; et al. Clinical and paraclinical aspects of tetany in stuttering. Revue Roumaine de Neurologie et Psychiatrie; 1983 Jul Sep Vol 21(3) 277–279

Cox, Nancy J.; Kidd, Kenneth K. Can recovery from stuttering be considered a genetically milder subtype of stuttering? Behavior Genetics; 1983 Mar Vol 13(2) 129–139

Cross, Douglas E. Comparison of reaction time and accuracy measures of laterality for stutterers and normal speakers. Journal of Fluency Disorders; 1987 Aug Vol 12(4) 271–286

Cross, Douglas E.; Luper, Harold L. Relation between finger reaction time and voice reaction time in stuttering and nonstuttering children and adults. Journal of Speech and Hearing Research; 1983 Sep Vol 26(3) 356–361

Cullinan, Walter L.; Springer, Mark T. Voice initiation and termination times in stuttering and nonstuttering children. Journal of Speech and Hearing Research; 1980 Jun Vol 23(2) 344–360

Curlee, Richard F.; Perkins, William H. Effectiveness of a DAF conditioning program for adolescent and adult stutterers. Behaviour Research and Therapy; 1973 Nov Vol. 11(4) 395–401

Dewar, A. D. Influence of auditory feedback masking on stammering and its use in treatment. International Journal of Rehabilitation Research; 1984 Vol 7(3) 341–342

Dorman, M. F.; Porter, R. J. Hemispheric lateralization for speech perception in stutterers. Cortex; 1975 Jun Vol 11(2) 181–185

Ferrand, Carole T.; Gilbert, Harvey R.; Blood, Gordon W. Selected aspects of central processing and vocal motor function in stutterers and nonstutterers. Journal of Fluency Disorders; 1991 Vol 16(2–3) 101–115

Fitch, James L.; Batson, Elizabeth A. Hemispheric asymmetry of alpha wave suppression in stutterers and nonstutterers. Journal of Fluency Disorders; 1989 Feb Vol 14(1) 47–55

Fucci, Donald; Petrosino, Linda; Gorman, Peter; Harris, Daniel. Vibrotactile magnitude production scaling: A method for studying sensory-perceptual responses of stutterers and fluent speakers. Journal of Fluency Disorders; 1985 Mar Vol 10(1) 69–75

Fucci, Donald J.; Petrosino, Linda; Schuster, Susan; Belch, Marianne. Lingual vibrotactile threshold shift differences between stutterers and normal speakers during magnitude-estimation scaling. Perceptual and Motor Skills; 1991 Aug Vol 73(1) 55–62

Fukawa, Teruyo; Kato, Noriaki. Identification thresholds of nonsense syllables by stutterers. Perceptual and Motor Skills; 1986 Oct Vol 63(2, Pt 1) 592–594

Fukawa, Teruyo; Yoshioka, Hirohide; Ozawa, Emi; Yoshida, Shigeru. Difference of susceptibility to delayed auditory feedback between stutterers and nonstutterers. Journal of

Speech and Hearing Research; 1988 Sep Vol 31(3) 475–479

Garber, Sharon F.; Martin, Richard R. Effects of noise and increased vocal intensity on stuttering. Journal of Speech and Hearing Research; 1977 Jun Vol 20(2) 233–240

Garber, Sharon F.; Martin, Richard R. The effects of white noise on the frequency of stuttering. Journal of Speech and Hearing Research; 1974 Mar Vol. 17(1) 73–79

Gibney, Noel J. Delayed auditory feedback: Changes in the volume intensity and the delay interval as variables affecting the fluency of stutterers' speech. British Journal of Psychology; 1973 Feb Vol. 64(1) 55–63

Gruber, L.; Powell, R. L. Responses of stuttering and non-stuttering children to a dichotic listening task. Perceptual and Motor Skills; 1974 Feb Vol. 38(1) 263–264

Hageman, Carlin F.; Greene, Penny N. Auditory comprehension of stutterers on a competing message task. Journal of Fluency Disorders; 1989 Apr Vol 14(2) 109–120

Hall, James W.; Jerger, James. Central auditory function in stutterers. Journal of Speech and Hearing Research; 1978 Jun Vol 21(2) 324–337

Hall, James W.; Jerger, James. Central auditory function in stutterers. Journal of Speech and Hearing Research; 1978 Jun Vol 21(2) 324–337

Hand, C. Rebekah; Haynes, William O. Linguistic processing and reaction time differences in stutterers and nonstutterers. Journal of Speech and Hearing Research; 1983 Jun Vol 26(2) 181–185

Haney, R. R. Modification of oral reading disfluency by a paced reading procedure: II. An experimental evaluation. American Corrective Therapy Journal; 1976 May Jun Vol 30(3) 75–79

Harbison, Dan C.; Porter, Robert J.; Tobey, Emily A. Shadowed and simple reaction times in stutterers and nonstutterers. Journal of the Acoustical Society of America; 1989 Oct Vol 86(4) 1277–1284

Harrington, Jonathan. Stuttering, delayed auditory feedback, and linguistic rhythm. Journal of Speech and Hearing Research; 1988 Mar Vol 31(1) 36–47

Harris, Daniel; Fucci, Donald; Petrosino, Linda. Magnitude estimation and cross-modal matching of auditory and lingual vibrotactile sensation by normal speakers and stutterers. Journal of Speech and Hearing Research; 1991 Feb Vol 34(1) 177–182

Hayden, Paul A.; Adams, Martin R.; Jordahl, Nanette. The effects of pacing and masking on stutterers' and nonstutterers' speech initiation times. Journal of Fluency Disorders; 1982 Mar Vol 7(1–1) 9–19

Hayden, Paul A.; Jordahl, Nanette; Adams, Martin R. Stutterers' voice initiation times during conditions of novel stimulation. Journal of Fluency Disorders; 1982 Mar Vol 7(1–1) 1–7

Healey, E. Charles; Howe, Susan W. Speech shadowing characteristics of stutterers under diotic and dichotic conditions. Journal of Communication Disorders; 1987 Dec Vol 20(6) 493–506

Healey, E. Charles; Ramig, Peter R. Acoustic measures of stutterers' and nonstutterers' fluency in two speech contexts. Journal of Speech and Hearing Research; 1986 Sep Vol 29(3) 325–331

Horovitz, Linda J.; et al. Stapedial reflex and anxiety in fluent and disfluent speakers. Journal of Speech and Hearing Research; 1978 Dec Vol 21(4) 762–767

Howell, Peter. Changes in voice level caused by several forms of altered feedback in fluent speakers and stutterers. Language and Speech; 1990 Oct–Dec Vol 33(4) 325–338

Howell, Peter; El Yaniv, Nirit. The effects of presenting a click in syllable-initial position on the speech of stutterers: Comparison with a metronome click. Journal of Fluency Disorders; 1987 Aug Vol 12(4) 249–256

Howell, Peter; Powell, David J. Hearing your voice through bone and air: Implications for explanations of stuttering behavior from studies of normal speakers. Journal of Fluency Disorders; 1984 Dec Vol 9(4) 247–263

Howell, Peter; Wingfield, Trudie. Perceptual and acoustic evidence for reduced fluency in the vicinity of stuttering episodes. Language and Speech; 1990 Jan–Mar Vol 33(1) 31–46

Howell, Peter; Williams, Mark. The contribution of the excitatory source to the perception of neutral vowels in stuttered speech. Journal of the Acoustical Society of America; 1988 Jul Vol 84(1) 80–89

Hutchinson, John M.; Burk, Kenneth W. An investigation of the effects of temporal alterations in auditory feedback upon stutterers and clutterers. Journal of Communication Disorders; 1973 Sep Vol. 6(3) 193–205

Hutchinson, John M.; Burk, Kenneth W. An investigation of the effects of temporal alterations in auditory feedback upon stutterers and clutterers. Journal of Communication Disorders; 1973 Sep Vol. 6(3) 193–205

Ingham, Roger J.; Southwood, Helen; Horsburgh, Gay. Some effects of the Edinburgh Masker on stuttering during oral reading and spontaneous speech. Journal of Fluency Disorders; 1981 Jun Vol 6(2) 135–154

Jancke, Lutz; Kalveram, Karl T. Kontrolle von on-time (Phonationsdauer) und voice-onset-time bei rechts- bzw. linksohrig dargebotener auditiver Ruckmeldungen: Unterschiedliche Lateralisierung bei stotternden und nichtstotternden Personen? (Control of on-time (phonation duration) and voice-onset time with right- or left-ear auditory feedback: Different lateralization in stutterers and nonstutterers?) Zeitschrift fur Experimentelle und Angewandte Psychologie; 1987 Vol 34(1) 54–63

Kalveram, Karl T.; Jancke, Lutz. Vowel duration and voice onset time for stressed and nonstressed syllables in stutterers under delayed auditory feedback condition. Folia Phoniatrica; 1989 Jan–Feb Vol 41(1) 30–42

Kelly, Ellen M.; Conture, Edward G. Acoustic and perceptual correlates of adult stutterers' typical and imitated stutterings. Journal of Fluency Disorders; 1988 Aug Vol 13(4) 233–252

Klouda, Gayle V.; Cooper, William E. Syntactic clause boundaries, speech timing, and stuttering frequency in adult stutterers. Language and Speech; 1987 Jul–Sep Vol 30(3) 263–276

Kooman, E. A. Speech disturbance under delayed acoustic feedback and stuttering. Defektologiya; 1975 Jun No 6 27–33

Kramer, Mitchell B.; Green, Deborah; Guitar, Barry. A comparison of stutterers and non-stutterers on masking level differences and synthetic sentence identification tasks. Journal of Communication Disorders; 1987 Oct Vol 20(5) 379–390

Kuz'min, Yu. I.; Dmitrieva, E. S.; Zaitseva, K. A. Functional asymmetry of the brain in stuttering children during perception of emotions. Human Physiology; 1989 Mar Apr Vol 15(2) 129–131

Lechner, Barbara K. The effects of delayed auditory feedback and masking on the fundamental frequency of stutterers and nonstutterers. Journal of Speech and Hearing Research; 1979 Jun Vol 22(2) 343–353

Liebetrau, R. Mark; Daly, David A. Auditory processing and perceptual abilities of "organic" and "functional" stutterers. Journal of Fluency Disorders; 1981 Sep Vol 6(3) 219–231

Macioszek, Gisela. (On delayed auditory feedback in stutterers with various levels of stuttering severity.) Zeitschrift fur Klinische Psychologie; 1973 Vol 2(4) 278–299

Mallard, A. R.; Webb, W. G. The effects of auditory and visual "distractors" on the frequency of stuttering. Journal of Communication Disorders; 1980 May Vol 13(3) 207–212

Manning, Walter H.; Coufal, Kathy J. The frequency of disfluencies during phonatory transitions in stuttered and nonstuttered speech. Journal of Communication Disorders; 1976 Mar Vol 9(1) 75–81

Manning, Walter H.; Reinsche, Linda. Auditory assembly abilities of stuttering and nonstuttering children. Journal of Speech and Hearing Research; 1976 Dec Vol 19(4) 777–783

Marshall, Robert C.; Neuburger, Sandra I. Effects of delayed auditory feedback on acquired stuttering following head injury. Journal of Fluency Disorders; 1987 Oct Vol 12(5) 355–365

Martin, Richard; Haroldson, Samuel K. Effects of five experimental treatments on stuttering. Journal of Speech and Hearing Research; 1979 Mar Vol 22(1) 132–146

Martin, Richard R.; Johnson, Linda J.; Siegel, Gerald M.; Haroldson, Samuel K. Auditory stimulation, rhythm, and stuttering. Journal of Speech and Hearing Research; 1985 Dec Vol 28(4) 487–495

Martin, Richard R.; Siegel, Gerald M.; Johnson, Linda J.; Haroldson, Samuel K. Sidetone amplification, noise, and stuttering. Journal of Speech and Hearing Research; 1984 Dec Vol 27(4) 518–527

McCabe, Robert B.; McCollum, Judith D. The personal reactions of a stuttering adult to delayed auditory feedback. Journal of Speech and Hearing Disorders; 1972 Nov Vol. 37(4) 536–541

McCormick, Barry. Therapeutic and diagnostic applications of delayed auditory feedback. British Journal of Disorders of Communication; 1975 Oct Vol 10(2) 98–110

McLean Muse, Ann; Larson, Charles R.; Gregory, Hugo H. Stutterers' and nonstutterers' voice fundamental frequency changes in response to auditory stimuli. Journal of Speech and Hearing Research; 1988 Dec Vol 31(4) 549–555

Meshcherskaya, L. N. Use of external acoustic influence for correction of stuttering. Defektologiya; 1985 No 3 14–19

Meyers, Susan C.; Ghatak, Lila R.; Woodford, Lee L. Case descriptions of nonfluency and loci: Initial and follow-up conversations with three preschool children. Journal of Fluency Disorders; 1989 Dec Vol 14(6) 383–397

Meyers, Susan C.; Hughes, Larry F.; Schoeny, Zahrl G. Temporal-phonemic processing skills in adult stutterers and nonstutterers. Journal of Speech and Hearing Research; 1989 Jun Vol 32(2) 274–280

Morozov, V. P.; Kuz'min, Yu. I.; Zaitseva, K. A.; Dmitrieva, E. S. Hemispheric functional asymmetry in stuttering. Human Physiology; 1988 May Jun Vol 14(3) 188–194

Nandur, V. U. Effect of binaural masking noise on stuttering: A spectographic analysis. Journal of the All India Institute of Speech and Hearing; 1982 Vol 13 164–169

Nataraja, N. P.; Rajkumar, P.; Ramesh, M. V. Disfluencies in normals under DAF—in reading combined and voiced passages. Hearing Aid Journal; 1983 Jul–Dec Vol 4(1) 23–26

Newman, Parley W.; Bunderson, Karin; Brey, Robert H. Brain stem electrical responses of stutterers and normals by sex, ears, and re-covery. Journal of Fluency Disorders; 1985 Mar Vol 10(1) 59–67

Newton, Karen R.; Blood, Gordon W.; Blood, Ingrid M. Simultaneous and staggered dichotic word and digit tests with stutterers and nonstutterers. Journal of Fluency Disorders; 1986 Sep Vol 11(3) 201–216

Pinsky, Seth D.; McAdam, Dale W. Electroencephalographic and dichotic indices of cerebral laterality in stutterers. Brain and Language; 1980 Nov Vol 11(2) 374–397

Rastatter, Michael P.; Loren, Catherine; Colcord, Roger. Visual coding strategies and hemisphere dominance characteristics of stutterers. Journal of Fluency Disorders; 1987 Oct Vol 12(5) 305–315

Robb, Michael P.; Lybolt, John T.; Price, Harold A. Acoustic measures of stutterers' speech following an intensive therapy program. Journal of Fluency Disorders; 1985 Dec Vol 10(4) 269–279

Rosenfield, David B.; Goodglass, Harold. Dichotic testing of cerebral dominance in stutterers. Brain and Language; 1980 Sep Vol 11(1) 170–180

Ryan, Bruce P.; Van Kirk, Barbara. The establishment, transfer, and maintenance of fluent speech in 50 stutterers using delayed auditory feedback and operant procedures. Journal of Speech and Hearing Disorders; 1974 Feb Vol. 39(1) 3–10

Shurgaya, German G.; Korolyova, Inna V.; Kuzmin, Urii I.; Sakhnovskaya, Oksana S. Interhemispheric asymmetry at the perception of speech signals in stutterers. Psikologicheskii Zhurnal; 1987 Jul–Aug Vol 8(4) 80–91

Silverman, Franklin H.; Trotter, William D. Bibliography related to use of instrumental aids in stuttering therapy: Supplement 2. Perceptual and Motor Skills; 1974 Jun Vol 38(3, Pt 2) 1329–1330

Slorach, Neil; Noehr, Bonnie. Dichotic listening in stuttering and dyslalic children. Cortex; 1973 Sep Vol. 9(3) 295–300

Smith, K. M.; Blood, I. M.; Blood, Gorden W. Auditory brainstem responses of stutterers and nonstutterers during speech production.

Journal of Fluency Disorders; 1990 Aug Vol 15(4) 211–222

Sommers, Ronald K.; Brady, William A.; Moore, W. H. Dichotic ear preferences of stuttering children and adults. Perceptual and Motor Skills; 1975 Dec Vol 41(3) 931–938

St. Louis, Kenneth O.; Hinzman, Audrey R. A descriptive study of speech, language, and hearing characteristics of school-aged stutterers. Journal of Fluency Disorders; 1988 Oct Vol 13(5) 331–355

Stager, Sheila V. Heterogeneity in stuttering: Results from auditory brainstem response testing. American Speech Language Hearing Association Convention (1982, Toronto, Canada). Journal of Fluency Disorders; 1990 Feb Vol 15(1) 9–19

Stephen, Simon C.; Haggard, Mark P. Acoustic properties of masking/delayed feedback in the fluency of stutterers and controls. Journal of Speech and Hearing Research; 1980 Sep Vol 23(3) 527–538

Stephen, Simon C.; Haggard, Mark P. Critical feedback variables in stuttering: A reply to Irwin Altrows. Journal of Speech and Hearing Research; 1982 Dec Vol 25(4) 632–633

Strub, Richard L.; Black, F. William; Naeser, Margaret A. Anomalous dominance in sibling stutterers: Evidence from CT scan asymmetries, dichotic listening, neuropsychological testing, and handedness. Brain and Language; 1987 Mar Vol 30(2) 338–350

Sussman, Harvey M.; MacNeilage, Peter F. Studies of hemispheric specialization for speech production. Brain and Language; 1975 Apr Vol 2(2) 131–151

Timmons, Beverly A. Physiological factors related to delayed auditory feedback and stuttering: A review. Perceptual and Motor Skills; 1982 Dec Vol 55(3, Pt 2) 1179–1189

Timmons, Beverly A.; Boudreau, James P. Auditory feedback as a major factor in stuttering. Journal of Speech and Hearing Disorders; 1972 Nov Vol. 37(4) 476–484

Timmons, Beverly A.; Boudreau, James P. Delayed auditory feedback and the speech of stuttering and non-stuttering children. Perceptual and Motor Skills; 1978 Apr Vol 46(2) 551–555

Timmons, Beverly A.; Boudreau, James P. Speech disfluencies and delayed auditory feedback reactions of stuttering and non-stuttering children. Perceptual and Motor Skills; 1978 Dec Vol 47(3, Pt 1) 859–862

Toscher, Mark M.; Rupp, Ralph R. A study of the central auditory processes in stutterers using the Synthetic Sentence Identification (SSI) Test battery. Journal of Speech and Hearing Research; 1978 Dec Vol 21(4) 779–792

Trotter, William D.; Silverman, Franklin H. Experiments with the Stutter Aid. Perceptual and Motor Skills; 1973 Jun Vol. 36(3, Pt. 2) 1129–1130

Tsunoda, Tadanobu; Moriyama, Haruyuki. Specific patterns of cerebral dominance for various sounds in adult stutterers. Journal of Auditory Research; 1972 Jul Vol 12(3) 216–227

Van Borsel, J. Imperceptivity in stutterers. Communication and Cognition; 1987 Vol 20(4) 383–390

Venkatagiri, Horabail S. A comparison of DAF-induced disfluencies with stuttering. Journal of Communication Disorders; 1982 Sep Vol 15(5) 385–393

Venkatagiri, Horabail S. Reaction time for /s/ and /z/ in stutterers and nonstutterers: A test of discoordination hypothesis. Journal of Communication Disorders; 1982 Jan Vol 15(1) 55–62

von Deuster, C. Untersuchungen zur Hemispharendominanz und Handigkeit bei stammelnden Kindern mit normaler und gestorter auditiver Wahrnehmung. / Studies of hemisphere dominance and handedness of stammering children with normal and disturbed auditory perception. Folia Phoniatrica; 1983 Nov–Dec Vol 35(6) 265–272

Watson, Ben C.; Alfonso, Peter J. Foreperiod and stuttering severity effects on acoustic laryngeal reaction time. Journal of Fluency Disorders; 1983 Sep Vol 8(3) 183–205

Watson, Ben C.; Pool, Kenneth D.; Devous, Michael D.; Freeman, Frances J.; et al. Brain blood flow related to acoustic laryngeal reaction time in adult developmental stutterers. Journal of Speech and Hearing Research; 1992 Jun Vol 35(3) 555–561

Wynne, Michael K.; Boehmler, Richard M. Central auditory function in fluent and disfluent normal speakers. Journal of Speech and Hearing Research; 1982 Mar Vol 25(1) 54–57

Yairi, Ehud. Effects of binaural and monaural noise on stuttering. Journal of Auditory Research; 1976 Apr Vol 16(2) 114–119

Zebrowski, Patricia M.; Conture, Edward G.; Cudahy, Edward A. Acoustic analysis of young stutterers' fluency: Preliminary observations. Journal of Fluency Disorders; 1985 Sep Vol 10(3) 173–192

Biochemistry

Costa, D.; Antoniac, Maria; Berghianu, S.; Marinescu, Rodica; et al. Clinical and paraclinical aspects of tetany in stuttering. Activitas Nervosa Superior; 1986 Vol 28(2) 156–158

Costa, D.; et al. Clinical and paraclinical aspects of tetany in stuttering. Revue Roumaine de Neurologie et Psychiatrie; 1983 Jul–Sep Vol 21(3) 277–279

Costa, D.; Pop, A.; Dumitriu, L.; Marinescu, Luzia; et al. Serum immunoreactive parathormone levels correlate with depression and anxiety in hypocalcemic stutterers. Activitas Nervosa Superior; 1986 Vol 28(2) 155–156

Dabul, Barbara; Perkins, William H. The effects of stuttering on systolic blood pressure. Journal of Speech and Hearing Research; 1973 Dec Vol. 16(4) 586–591

Geschwind, Norman. Biological associations of left-handedness. Annals of Dyslexia; 1983 Vol 33 29–40

Lagutina, T. S.; Lovchikova, N. N.; Obukhovskii, N. G. Electrophysiological study of patients with logoneuroses. Soviet Neurology and Psychiatry; 1985 Fal Vol 18(3) 53–61

Raisova, Vera; Hyanek, J. Speech disorders associated with histidinemia and other hereditary disorders of amino acid metabolism. Folia Phoniatrica; 1986 Jan–Feb Vol 38(1) 43–48

Rastatter, Michael P.; Harr, Robert. Measurements of plasma levels of adrenergic neurotransmitters and primary amino acids in five stuttering subjects: A preliminary report (biochemical aspects of stuttering). Journal of Fluency Disorders; 1988 Apr Vol 13(2) 127–139

Scheiber, Stephen C.; Ziesat, Harold. Clinical and psychological test findings in cerebral dyspraxia associated with hemodialysis. Journal of Nervous and Mental Disease; 1976 Mar Vol 162(3) 212–214

Silverman, Ellen Marie; Zimmer, Catherine H.; Silverman, Franklin H. Variability of stutterers' speech disfluency: The menstrual cycle. Perceptual and Motor Skills; 1974 Jun Vol 38(3, Pt 2) 1037–1038

Steidl, Ladislav; Pesak, Josef; Chytilova, Hana. Stuttering and tetanic syndrome. Folia Phoniatrica; 1991 Jan–Feb Vol 43(1) 7–12

Watson, Ben C.; Pool, Kenneth D.; Devous, Michael D.; Freeman, Frances J.; et al. Brain blood flow related to acoustic laryngeal reaction time in adult developmental stutterers. Journal of Speech and Hearing Research; 1992 Jun Vol 35(3) 555–561

Weber, Christine M.; Smith, Anne. Autonomic correlates of stuttering and speech assessed in a range of experimental tasks. Journal of Speech and Hearing Research; 1990 Dec Vol 33(4) 690–706

Wood, Frank; et al. Patterns of regional cerebral blood flow during attempted reading aloud by stutterers both on and off haloperidol medication: Evidence for inadequate left frontal activation during stuttering. Brain and Language; 1980 Jan Vol 9(1) 141–144

Cognition and Learning Disabilities

Baker, Lorian; Cantwell, Dennis P. Psychiatric and learning disorders in children with speech and language disorders: A critical review. Advances in Learning and Behavioral Disabilities; 1985 Vol 4 1–28

Banjac Karovic, Milena; Povse Ivkic, Violica; Bojanin, Svetomir. Inhibicija govora i mucanje. (Speech inhibition and stuttering.) Psihijatrija Danas; 1990 Vol 22(1) 99–104

Boberg, Einer. Stuttering in the retarded: I. Review of prevalence literature. Mental Retardation Bulletin; 1977 Vol 5(3) 90–100

Boberg, Einer; et al. Stuttering in the retarded: II. Prevalence of stuttering in EMR and TMR children. Mental Retardation Bulletin; 1978 Vol 6(2) 67–76

Cantwell, Dennis P.; Baker, Lorian. Psychiatric and learning disorders in children with speech and language disorders: A descriptive analysis. Advances in Learning and Behavioral Disabilities; 1985 Vol 4 29–47

Carpenter, Mary; Sommers, Ronald K. Unisensory and bisensory perceptual and memory processing in stuttering adults and normal speakers. Journal of Fluency Disorders; 1987 Aug Vol 12(4) 291–304

Chapman, Ann H.; Cooper, Eugene B. Nature of stuttering in a mentally retarded population. American Journal of Mental Deficiency; 1973 Sep Vol. 78(2) 153–157

Devenny, Darlynne A.; Silverman, W.; Balgley, H.; Wall, M. J.; et al. Specific motor abilities associated with speech fluency in Down's syndrome. Journal of Mental Deficiency Research; 1990 Oct Vol 34(5) 437–443

Gotestam, K. Olof; Coates, Tom J.; Ekstrand, Maria. Handedness, dyslexia and twinning in homosexual men. International Journal of Neuroscience; 1992 Apr Vol 63(3–4) 179–186

Homzie, Marvin J.; Lindsay, Jean S.; Simpson, Joanne; Hasenstab, Suzanne. Concomitant speech, language, and learning problems in adult stutterers and in members of their families. Journal of Fluency Disorders; 1988 Aug Vol 13(4) 261–277

Kastelova, Darina; Szenteova, Iveta. Socialna interakcia recovo narusenych deti (vo vol'nom case mimo skoly). / Social interaction of speech disordered children (out of school—in their leisure time). Psychologia a Patopsychologia Dietata; 1990 Vol 25(6) 551–557

Kaubish, V. K.; Linskaia, L. N. Characteristics of neurosislike states and their treatment in children with retarded mental development. Soviet Neurology and Psychiatry; 1991 Fal Vol 24(3) 38–42

Kerbeshian, Jacob; et al. Gilles de la Tourette disease in multiply disabled children. Special Issue: Children with multiple disabilities. Rehabilitation Literature; 1985 Sep–Oct Vol 46(9–10) 255–258

Kraaimaat, Floor; Janssen, Peggy; Brutten, Gene J. The relationship between stutterers' cognitive and autonomic anxiety and therapy out-come. Journal of Fluency Disorders; 1988 Apr Vol 13(2) 107–113

Kramer, Josefine. Wesen, Haufigkeit, Ursachen und Erscheinungsformen der geistigen Behinderung: II. (Nature, frequency, causes, and forms of mental retardation: II.) Vierteljahresschrift fur Heilpadagogik und ihre Nachbargebiete; 1976 Sep Vol 45(3) 270–283

Liles, Betty Z.; Lerman, Jay; Christensen, Lisa; St. Ledger, Joy. A case description of verbal and signed disfluencies of a 10-year-old boy who is retarded. Language, Speech, and Hearing Services in Schools; 1992 Apr Vol 23(2) 107–112

Lindsay, Jean S. Relationship of developmental disfluency and episodes of stuttering to the emergence of cognitive stages in children. Journal of Fluency Disorders; 1989 Aug Vol 14(4) 271–284

Newman, Parley W.; Fawcett, Kerilynn D.; Russon, Karen V. Cognitive processing in stuttering as related to translating slurvian. Journal of Fluency Disorders; 1986 Sep Vol 11(3) 251–256

Nippold, Marilyn A.; Schwarz, Ilsa E. Reading disorders in stuttering children. Journal of Fluency Disorders; 1990 Jun Vol 15(3) 175–189

Pauls, David L.; Leckman, James F.; Cohen, Donald J. Familial relationship between Gilles de la Tourette's syndrome, attention deficit disorder, learning disabilities, speech disorders, and stuttering. Journal of the American Academy of Child and Adolescent Psychiatry; 1993 Sep Vol 32(5) 1044–1050

Pennington, Bruce F.; Smith, Shelley D. Genetic influences on learning disabilities and speech and language disorders. Child Development; 1983 Apr Vol 54(2) 369–387

Peterson, John M. Some comments on Gotestam's (1990) "Lefthandedness among students of architecture and music." Perceptual and Motor Skills; 1990 Jun Vol 70(3, Pt 2) 1345–1346

Preus, Alf. Treatment of mentally retarded stutterers. Journal of Fluency Disorders; 1990 Aug Vol 15(4) 223–233

Rosenfield, David B.; Freeman, Frances J. Stuttering onset after laryngectomy. Journal

of Fluency Disorders; 1983 Sep Vol 8(3) 265–268

Segalowitz, Sidney J.; Brown, Deborah. Mild head injury as a source of developmental disabilities. Journal of Learning Disabilities; 1991 Nov Vol 24(9) 551–559

Silliman, Elaine R.; Leslie, Susan P. Social and cognitive aspects of fluency in the instructional setting. Topics in Language Disorders; 1983 Dec Vol 4(1) 61–74

Stansfield, Jois. Stuttering and cluttering in the mentally handicapped population: A review of the literature. British Journal of Mental Subnormality; 1988 Jan Vol 34(1)(66) 54–61

Stansfield, J. Prevalence of stuttering and cluttering in adults with mental handicaps. Journal of Mental Deficiency Research; 1990 Aug Vol 34(4) 287–307

Steffen, Hartmut; Seidel, Christa. Perceptive and cognitive school and social behavior of children with language and speech disorders. Zeitschrift fur Kinder und Jugendpsychiatrie; 1976 Vol 4(3) 216–232

Van Strien, Jan W.; Bouma, Anke; Bakker, Dirk J. Birth stress, autoimmune diseases, and handedness. Journal of Clinical and Experimental Neuropsychology; 1987 Dec Vol 9(6) 775–780

Vekassy, Laszlo. Idegrendszeri es pszichologiai vizsgalatok dadogoknal. (Psychological and nervous system examination with stutterers.) Magyar Pszichologiai Szemle; 1981 Vol 38(5) 481–494

Watson, Jennifer B. A comparison of stutterers' and nonstutterers' affective, cognitive, and behavioral self-reports. Journal of Speech and Hearing Research; 1988 Sep Vol 31(3) 377–385

Webster, William G. Rapid letter transcription performance by stutterers. Neuropsychologia; 1987 Vol 25(5) 845–847

Culture

Bebout, Linda; Arthur, Bradford. Cross-cultural attitudes toward speech disorders. Journal of Speech and Hearing Research; 1992 Feb Vol 35(1) 45–52

Bergmann, Gunther. Studies in stuttering as a prosodic disturbance. Journal of Speech and Hearing Research; 1986 Sep Vol 29(3) 290–300

Brady, William A.; Hall, Donald E. The prevalence of stuttering among school-age children. Language, Speech and Hearing Services in the Schools; 1976 Apr Vol 7(2) 75–81

Cooper, Eugene B.; Rustin, Lena. Clinician attitudes toward stuttering in the United States and Great Britain: A cross-cultural study. Journal of Fluency Disorders; 1985 Mar Vol 10(1) 1–17

Fitzgerald, Hiram E.; Djurdjic, Slavoljub D.; Maguin, Eugene. Assessment of sensitivity to interpersonal stress in stutterers. Journal of Communication Disorders; 1992 Mar Vol 25(1) 31–42

Jayaram, M. Distribution of stuttering in sentences: Relationship to sentence length and clause position. Journal of Speech and Hearing Research; 1984 Sep Vol 27(3) 338–341

Jayaram, M. Grammatical context of stuttered and nonstuttered words. NIMHANS-Journal; 1989 Jan Vol 7(1) 55–63

Jayaram, M. Phonetic influences on stuttering in monolingual and bilingual stutterers. Journal of Communication Disorders; 1983 Jul Vol 16(4) 287–297

Jayaram, M. Relationship of stuttering to word information value in a phonemic clause. Journal of the All India Institute of Speech and Hearing; 1982 Vol 13 1–6

Jehle, Peter; Boberg, Einer. Intensivbehandlung fur jugendliche und erwachsene Stotternde von Boberg und Kully. / Intensive treatment for adolescent and adult stutterers by Boberg and Kully. Folia Phoniatrica; 1987 Sep–Oct Vol 39(5) 256–268

Kirk, Lorraine. Stuttering and quasi-stuttering in Ga. Journal of Communication Disorders; 1977 Mar Vol 10(1–2) 109–126

Leith, William R.; Mims, Howard A. Cultural influences in the development and treatment of stuttering: A preliminary report on the Black stutterer. Journal of Speech and Hearing Disorders; 1975 Nov Vol 40(4) 459–466

Leith, William R.; Timmons, Jack L. The stutterer's reaction to the telephone as a speaking situation. Journal of Fluency Disorders; 1983 Sep Vol 8(3) 233–243

Mallard, A. R.; Westbrook, J. B. Variables affecting stuttering therapy in school settings. Language, Speech, and Hearing Services in Schools; 1988 Oct Vol 19(4) 362–370

Neiman, Gary S.; Rubin, Rebecca B. Changes in communication apprehension, satisfaction, and competence in foreign dialect and stuttering clients. Journal of Communication Disorders; 1991 Oct–Dec Vol 24(5–6) 353–366

Nwokah, Evangeline E. The imbalance of stuttering behavior in bilingual speakers. Journal of Fluency Disorders; 1988 Oct Vol 13(5) 357–373

Pill, Jaan. A comparison between two treatment programs for stuttering: A personal account. Journal of Fluency Disorders; 1988 Dec Vol 13(6) 385–398

Ralston, Lenore D. Stammering: A stress index in Caribbean classrooms. Journal of Fluency Disorders; 1981 Jun Vol 6(2) 119–133

Ratner, Nan B.; Benitez, Mercedes. Linguistic analysis of a bilingual stutterer. Journal of Fluency Disorders; 1985 Sep Vol 10(3) 211–219

Rustin, Lena; Ryan, Bruce P.; Ryan, Barbara V. Use of the Monterey programmed stuttering therapy in Great Britain. British Journal of Disorders of Communication; 1987 Aug Vol 22(2) 151–162

Shames, George H. Stuttering: An RFP for a cultural perspective. Journal of Fluency Disorders; 1989 Feb Vol 14(1) 67–77

Stewart, Joseph L. Cross-cultural studies and linguistic aspects of stuttering. Journal of the All India Institute of Speech and Hearing; 1971 Jan Vol. 2 1–6

Stewart, Joseph L. Stuttering Indians: A reply to Zimmermann et al. Journal of Speech and Hearing Research; 1985 Jun Vol 28(2) 313–315

Thompson, Julia. Update: School-age stutterers. Journal of Fluency Disorders; 1984 Sep Vol 9(3) 199–206

Zimmermann, Gerald N. The Bannock Shoshoni still have terms for it: Whither Stewart. Journal of Speech and Hearing Research; 1985 Jun Vol 28(2) 315–316

Zimmermann, Gerald N.; Liljeblad, Sven; Frank, Arthur; Cleeland, Charlotte. The Indians have many terms for it: Stuttering among the Bannock-Shoshoni. Journal of Speech and Hearing Research; 1983 Jun Vol 26(2) 315–318

Demographics

Brady, William A.; Hall, Donald E. The prevalence of stuttering among school-age children. Language, Speech and Hearing Services in the Schools; 1976 Apr Vol 7(2) 75–81

Dellatolas, Georges; Annesi, Isabella; Jallon, Pierre; Chavance, Michel; et al. An epidemiological reconsideration of the Geschwind-Galaburda theory of cerebral lateralization. Archives of Neurology; 1990 Jul Vol 47(7) 778–782

Franke, Ulrike. Zur Frage de mannlichen Disposition fur Kommunikationsstorungen. / Predisposition of males for communication disorders. Folia Phoniatrica; 1985 Jan–Feb Vol 37(1) 36–43

Geschwind, Norman. Biological associations of left-handedness. Annals of Dyslexia; 1983 Vol 33 29–40

Gillespie, Susan K.; Cooper, Eugene B. Prevalence of speech problems in junior and senior high schools. Journal of Speech and Hearing Research; 1973 Dec Vol. 16(4) 739–743

Leung, Alexander K.; Robson, W. Lane. Stuttering. Clinical Pediatrics; 1990 Sep Vol 29(9) 498–502

Montgomery, Brenda M.; Fitch, James L. The prevalence of stuttering in the hearing-impaired school age population. Journal of Speech and Hearing Disorders; 1988 May Vol 53(2) 131–135

Ohashi, Yoshiko. The development of stuttering in children: A cross-sectional study. Japanese Journal of Child Psychiatry; 1976 Dec–Feb Vol 17(1) 57–68

Porfert, Alan R.; Rosenfield, David B. Prevalence of stuttering. Journal of Neurology, Neurosurgery and Psychiatry; 1978 Oct Vol 41(10) 954–956

Stansfield, J. Prevalence of stuttering and cluttering in adults with mental handicaps. Journal of Mental Deficiency Research; 1990 Aug Vol 34(4) 287–307

Steffen, Hartmut; Seidel, Christa. Perceptive and cognitive school and social behavior of children with language and speech disorders. Zeitschrift fur Kinder und Jugendpsychiatrie; 1976 Vol 4(3) 216–232

Wagner, Cynthia O.; Gray, Laurie L.; Potter, Robert E. Communicative disorders in a group of adult female offenders. Journal of Communication Disorders; 1983 Jul Vol 16(4) 269–277

Wingate, Marcel E. Speaking unassisted: Comments on a paper by Andrews et al. Journal of Speech and Hearing Disorders; 1983 Aug Vol 48(3) 255–263

Yairi, Ehud. Epidemiologic and other considerations in treatment efficacy research with preschool age children who stutter. Journal of Fluency Disorders; 1993 18(2–3) 197–219

Yairi, Ehud. Longitudinal studies of disfluencies in two-year-old children. Journal of Speech and Hearing Research; 1982 Mar Vol 25(1) 155–160

Diagnostics and Assessment

Adams, Martin R.; Runyan, Charles M. Stuttering and fluency: Exclusive events or points on a continuum? Journal of Fluency Disorders; 1981 Sep Vol 6(3) 197–218

Adams, Martin R.; Webster, L. Michael. Case selection strategies with children "at risk" for stuttering. Journal of Fluency Disorders; 1989 Feb Vol 14(1) 11–16

Aguilar, Guido; de Aguilar, Maria T.; de Berganza, Maria R. El tartamudeo y su deteccion temprana. / Stuttering and its early detection. 5th Latin American Congress of Behavior Analysis and Behavior Modification: Applied behavior analysis (1986, Caracas, Venezuela). Avances en Psicologia Clinica Latinoamericana; 1988 Vol 6 41–51

Andrews, Gavin. Stuttering: A tutorial. Australian and New Zealand Journal of Psychiatry; 1981 Jun Vol 15(2) 105–109

Andrews, Gavin; Harvey, Robin. Regression to the mean in pretreatment measures of stuttering. Journal of Speech and Hearing Disorders; 1981 May Vol 46(2) 204–207

Aram, Dorothy M.; Meyers, Susan C.; Ekelman, Barbara L. Response to Cordes, Gow, and Ingham: On valid and reliable identification of normal disfluencies and stuttering disfluencies: A response to Aram, Meyers, and Ekelman (1990). Brain and Language; 1991 Feb Vol 40(2) 287–292

Bakker, Klaas; Brutten, Gene J. Speech-related reaction times of stutterers and nonstutterers: Diagnostic implications. Journal of Speech and Hearing Disorders; 1990 May Vol 55(2) 295–299

Blood, Gordon W.; Seider, Robin. The concomitant problems of young stutterers. Journal of Speech and Hearing Disorders; 1981 Feb Vol 46(1) 31–33

Bloodstein, Oliver. Verification of stuttering in a suspected malingerer. Journal of Fluency Disorders; 1988 Apr Vol 13(2) 83–88

Bojanin, Svetomir; Vuletic Peco, Aleksandra; Radojkovic, Dejan. Porodica dece sa razvojnim hiperkinetskim sindromom, tikovima i mucanjem. (Families of children with developing hyperkinetic syndrome, tics, and stuttering.) Psihijatrija Danas; 1991 Vol 23(1–2) 37–48

Bounes, Marika. Test de Rorschach avant et apres traitement de relaxation chez l'enfant. (Rorschach test before and after relaxation treatment of a child.) 11th International Congress on the. Rorschach and Projective Methods (1984, Barcelona, Spain). Bulletin de Psychologie; 1986 Jun–Aug Vol 39(11–15) 651–654

Burley, Peter M.; Rinaldi, Wendy. Effects of sex of listener and of stutterer on ratings of stuttering speakers. Journal of Fluency Disorders; 1986 Dec Vol 11(4) 329–333

Byrd, Kathryn; Cooper, Eugene B. Apraxic speech characteristics in stuttering, developmentally apraxic, and normal speaking children. Journal of Fluency Disorders; 1989 Jun Vol 14(3) 215–229

Campbell, Michel; Boudreau, Leonce; Ladouceur, Robert. L'influence d'interlocuteurs sur l'evaluation du begaiement. (The influence of speakers on the evaluation of stuttering.) Revue de Modification du Comportement; 1984 Vol 14(3) 112–122

Cheveliova, N. A. Toward the problem of stuttering in children. Defektologiya; 1977 Jan No 1 20–23

Code, Chris. Dichotic listening with the communicatively impaired: Results from trials of a short British-English dichotic word test. Journal of Phonetics; 1981 Oct Vol 9(4) 375–383

Colcord, Roger D.; Gregory, Hugo H. Perceptual analyses of stuttering and nonstuttering children's fluent speech productions. Journal of Fluency Disorders; 1987 Jun Vol 12(3) 185–195

Conture, Edward G. Youngsters who stutter: Diagnosis, parent counseling, and referral. Journal of Developmental and Behavioral Pediatrics; 1982 Sep Vol 3(3) 163–169

Conture, Edward G.; Brayton, Evelyn R. The influence of noise on stutterers' different disfluency types. Journal of Speech and Hearing Research; 1975 Jun Vol 18(2) 381–384

Cooper, Eugene B. Case-selection procedures for school-aged disfluent children. Language, Speech and Hearing Services in the Schools; 1977 Oct Vol 8(4) 264–269

Cooper, Eugene B. The chronic perseverative stuttering syndrome: Incurable stuttering. Journal of Fluency Disorders; 1987 Dec Vol 12(6) 381–388

Cooper, Eugene B. The development of a stuttering chronicity prediction checklist: A preliminary report. Journal of Speech and Hearing Disorders; 1973 May Vol. 38(2) 215–223

Cordes, Anne K.; Gow, Merrilyn L.; Ingham, Roger J. On valid and reliable identification of normal disfluencies and stuttering disfluencies: A response to Aram, Meyers, and Ekelman (1990). Brain and Language; 1991 Feb Vol 40(2) 282–286

Cox, Nancy J.; Seider, Robin A.; Kidd, Kenneth K. Some environmental factors and hypotheses for stuttering in families with several stutterers. Journal of Speech and Hearing Research; 1984 Dec Vol 27(4) 543–548

Craig, Ashley R.; Franklin, J. A.; Andrews, Gavin. A scale to measure locus of control of behaviour. British Journal of Medical Psychology; 1984 Jun Vol 57(2) 173–180

Crowe, Thomas A.; Cooper, Eugene B. Parental attitudes toward and knowledge of stuttering. Journal of Communication Disorders; 1977 Jun Vol 10(4) 343–357

Cullinan, Walter L. Consistency measures revisited. Journal of Fluency Disorders; 1988 Feb Vol 13(1) 1–9

Dembowski, James; Watson, Ben C. An instrumented method for assessment and remediation of stuttering: A single-subject case study. Journal of Fluency Disorders; 1991 Vol 16(5–6) 241–273

Dickson, Stanley. An application of the Blacky Test to a study of the psychosexual development of stutterers. International Journal of Social Psychiatry; 1974 Fal-Win Vol 20(3–4) 269–273

Ecker, Willi; Meyer, Victor. Individualized behavioural treatment of severe stuttering. Behavioural Psychotherapy; 1991 Vol 19(4) 347–357

Emrich, H. M.; Eilert, P. Evaluation of speech and language in neuropsychiatric disorders. Archiv fur Psychiatrie und Nervenkrankheiten; 1978 Vol 225(3) 209–221

Gonzalez Valenzuela, M. Jose. Evaluacion y Tratamiento cognitivo-conductual de un caso de tartamudez. / Evaluation and cognitive-behavioral treatment in a severe stuttering case. Analisis y Modificacion de Conducta; 1990 Vol 16(47) 137–148

Gottinger, Werner. A concept for the guidance of stutterers. Praxis der Kinderpsychologie und Kinderpsychiatrie; 1980 Feb–Mar Vol 29(2) 55–62

Gottwald, Sheryl R.; Goldbach, Peggy; Isack, Audrey H. Stuttering: Prevention and detection. Young Children; 1985 Nov Vol 41(1) 9–14

Gregory, Hugo H. Stuttering: A contemporary perspective. XXth Congress of the International Association of Logopedics and Phoniatrics (1986, Tokyo, Japan). Folia Phoniatrica; 1986 Mar–Aug Vol 38(2–4) 89–120

Helm, Nancy A.; Butler, Russell B.; Benson, D. Frank. Acquired stuttering. Neurology; 1978 Nov Vol 28(1) 1159–1165

Horsley, Irmgarde A.; FitzGibbon, Carol T. Stuttering children: Investigation of a stereotype. British Journal of Disorders of Communication; 1987 Apr Vol 22(1) 19–35

Howell, Peter; El Yaniv, Nirit. The effects of presenting a click in syllable-initial position on the speech of stutterers: Comparison with a metronome click. Journal of Fluency Disorders; 1987 Aug Vol 12(4) 249–256

Ingham, Roger J.; Southwood, Helen; Horsburgh, Gay. Some effects of the Edinburgh Masker on stuttering during oral reading and spontaneous speech. Journal of Fluency Disorders; 1981 Jun Vol 6(2) 135–154

Ingham, Roger J.; et al. Modification of listener-judged naturalness in the speech of stutterers. Journal of Speech and Hearing Research; 1985 Dec Vol 28(4) 495–504

Ingham, Roger J.; Carroll, Philippa J. Listener judgment of differences in stutterers' nonstuttered speech during chorus- and nonchorus-reading conditions. Journal of Speech and Hearing Research; 1977 Jun Vol 20(2) 293–302

Ivanova, G. A.; Lapa, A. Z.; Lokhov, M. I.; Movsisyants, S. A. EEG features in stammering pre-school children. Zhurnal Nevropatologii i Psikhiatrii imeni S. S. Korsakova; 1990 Vol 90(3) 78–81

Ivanova, G. A.; Lapa, A. Z.; Lokhov, M. I.; Movsisyants, S. A. Features of stuttering pre-school children. Neuroscience and Behavioral Physiology; 1991 May–Jun Vol 21(3) 284–287

Janssen, Peggy; Kraaimaat, Floor; Brutten, Gene. Relationship between stutterers' genetic history and speech-associated variables. Journal of Fluency Disorders; 1990 Feb Vol 15(1) 39–48

Jehle, Peter; Boberg, Einer. Intensivbehandlung fur jugendliche und erwachsene Stotternde von Boberg und Kully./Intensive treatment for adolescent and adult stutterers by Boberg and Kully. Folia Phoniatrica; 1987 Sep–Oct Vol 39(5) 256–268

Kraaimaat, Floor W., Janssen, Peggy. Eeen wekmodel voor een differntiele diagnostiek en behandeling van stotteren. (A working model for the differential diagnosis and treatment of stuttering.) Gedragstherapie; 1983 Dec Vol 16(4) 299–309.

Kripke, D. F.; Lavie, P.; Hernandez, J. Polygraphic evaluation of ethchlorvynol (14 days). Psychopharmacology; 1978 Vol 56(2) 221–223

Kroll, Robert M.; Hood, Stephen B. Differences in stuttering adaptation between oral reading and spontaneous speech. Journal of Communication Disorders; 1974 Sep Vol 7(3) 227–237

Kroll, Robert M.; Hood, Stephen B. The influence of task presentation and information load on the adaptation effect in stutterers and normal speakers. Journal of Communication Disorders; 1976 Jun Vol 9(2) 95–110

Kroll, Robert M.; O'Keefe, Bernard M. Molecular self-analyses of stuttered speech via speech time expansion. Journal of Fluency Disorders; 1985 Jun Vol 10(2) 93–105

Kully, Deborah; Boberg, Einer. An investigation of interclinic agreement in the identification of fluent and stuttered syllables. Journal of Fluency Disorders; 1988 Oct Vol 13(5) 309–318

Ladouceur, Robert; Saint Laurent, Lise. Stuttering: A multidimensional treatment and evaluation package. Journal of Fluency Disorders; 1986 Jun Vol 11(2) 93–103

Lankford, Sally D.; Cooper, Eugene B. Recovery from stuttering as viewed by parents of self-diagnosed recovered stutterers. Journal of Communication Disorders; 1974 Jun Vol 7(2) 171–180

Legewie, H.; Cleary, P.; Rackensperger, W. EMG-recording and biofeedback in the diagnosis and therapy of stuttering: A case study. European Journal of Behavioural Analysis and Modification; 1975 Dec Vol 1(2) 137–143

Leith, William R.; Timmons, Jack L. The stutterer's reaction to the telephone as a speaking situation. Journal of Fluency Disorders; 1983 Sep Vol 8(3) 233–243

Leung, Alexander K.; Robson, W. Lane. Stuttering. Clinical Pediatrics; 1990 Sep Vol 29(9) 498–502

Mahr, Greg; Leith, William. Psychogenic stuttering of adult onset. Journal of Speech and Hearing Research; 1992 Apr Vol 35(2) 283–286

Market, Karen E.; Montague, James C.; Buffalo, M. D.; Drummond, Sakina S. Acquired stuttering: Descriptive data and treatment outcome. Journal of Fluency Disorders; 1990 Feb Vol 15(1) 21–33

Martin, Richard R.; Haroldson, Samuel K.; Woessner, Garry L. Perceptual scaling of stuttering severity. Journal of Fluency Disorders; 1988 Feb Vol 13(1) 27–47

Meyers, Susan C. Qualitative and quantitative differences and patterns of variability in dis-fluencies emitted by preschool stutterers and nonstutterers during dyadic conversations. Journal of Fluency Disorders; 1986 Dec Vol 11(4) 293–306

Meyers, Susan C.; Ghatak, Lila R.; Woodford, Lee L. Case descriptions of nonfluency and loci: Initial and follow-up conversations with three preschool children. Journal of Fluency Disorders; 1989 Dec Vol 14(6) 383–397

Minderaa, R. B.; Van Gemert, T. M.; Van de Wetering, B. J. Onverwachte presentatiewijzen van het syndroom van Gilles de la Tourette. / Unexpected types of presentation of Gilles de la Tourette's syndrome. Tijdschrift voor Psychiatrie; 1988 Vol 30(4) 246–254

Mizumachi, Toshiro. (Assessment of the results of stuttering therapy—from the behavior therapeutic point of view.) Japanese Journal of Special Education; 1981 Oct Vol 19(2) 48–55

Myers, Florence L.; Wall, Meryl J. Issues to consider in the differential diagnosis of normal childhood nonfluencies and stuttering. Journal of Fluency Disorders; 1981 Sep Vol 6(3) 189–195

Myers, Florence L.; Wall, Meryl J. Toward an integrated approach to early childhood stuttering. Journal of Fluency Disorders; 1982 Mar Vol 7(1–1) 47–54

Nekrasov, Y. B. (Diagnosis and prognosis of stutterers: I. A discussion of esting during the preparatory phases of stutterers' social rehabilitation) Novye Issledovaniya v Psikhologii; 1981 No 1(24) 85–89

Pindzola, Rebekah H.; White, Dorenda T. A protocol for differentiating the incipient stutterer. Language, Speech, and Hearing Services in Schools; 1986 Jan Vol 17(1) 2–15

Poulos, Marie G.; Webster, William G. Family history as a basis for subgrouping people who stutter. Journal of Speech and Hearing Research; 1991 Feb Vol 34(1) 5–10

Preus, Alf. Treatment of mentally retarded stutterers. Journal of Fluency Disorders; 1990 Aug Vol 15(4) 223–233

Prins, David; Beaudet, Rudolph. Defense preference and stutterers' speech disfluencies: Implications for the nature of the disorder. Journal of Speech and Hearing Research; 1980 Dec Vol 23(4) 757–768

Prosek, Robert A.; Runyan, Charles M. Effects of segment and pause manipulations on the identification of treated stutterers. Journal of Speech and Hearing Research; 1983 Dec Vol 26(4) 510–516

Riley, Glyndon D.; Riley, Jeanna. Physician's screening procedure for children who may stutter. Journal of Fluency Disorders; 1989 Feb Vol 14(1) 57–66

Roth U., Erick; Aguilar S., Guido G. Speech therapy: A comparative study of the stutterer. Aprendizaje y Comportamiento; 1979 Vol 2(1–2) 93–108

Schliesser, Herbert F. Psychological scaling of speech by students in training compared to that by experienced speech language pathologists. Perceptual and Motor Skills; 1985 Dec Vol 61(3, Pt 2) 1299–1302

Schultheis, Josef R. Modern theories of stuttering. Praxis der Kinderpsychologie und Kinderpsychiatrie; 1978 Apr Vol 27(3) 83–87

Schwartz, Howard D.; Conture, Edward G. Subgrouping young stutterers: Preliminary behavioral observations. Journal of Speech and Hearing Research; 1988 Mar Vol 31(1) 62–71

Seidel, Christa; Biesalski, P. (Psychological and clinical experiences with the Frostig Test and the Frostig therapy in speech-impaired children.) Praxis der Kinderpsychologie und Kinderpsychiatrie; 1973 Jan Vol. 22(1) 3–15

Seider, Robin A.; Gladstien, Keith L.; Kidd, Kenneth K. Language onset and concomitant speech and language problems in subgroups of stutterers and their siblings. Journal of Speech and Hearing Research; 1982 Dec Vol 25(4) 482–486

Seymour, Charlena M.; Ruggiero, Alisa; McEneaney, Joseph. The identification of stuttering: Can you look and tell. Journal of Fluency Disorders; 1983 Sep Vol 8(3) 215–220

Sheehan, Joseph G.; Tanaka, Jeffrey S. Prognostic validity of the Rorschach. Journal of Personality Assessment; 1983 Oct Vol 47(5) 462–465

Shirkey, Edward A. Forensic verification of stuttering. Journal of Fluency Disorders; 1987 Jun Vol 12(3) 197–203

Silverman, Franklin H. The stuttering problem profile: A task that assists both client and clinician in defining therapy goals. Journal of Speech and Hearing Disorders; 1980 Feb Vol 45(1) 119–123

Starkweather, C. Woodruff. Current trends in therapy for stuttering children and suggestions for future research. ASHA-Reports Series American Speech Language Hearing Association; 1990 Apr No 18 82–90

Still, A. W.; Griggs, S. Changes in the probability of stuttering following a stutter: A test of some recent models. Journal of Speech and Hearing Research; 1979 Sep Vol 22(3) 565–571

Strub, Richard L.; Black, F. William; Naeser, Margaret A. Anomalous dominance in sibling stutterers: Evidence from CT scan asymmetries, dichotic listening, neuropsychological testing, and handedness. Brain and Language; 1987 Mar Vol 30(2) 338–350

Thompson, A. H. A test of the distraction explanation of disfluency modification in stuttering. Journal of Fluency Disorders; 1985 Mar Vol 10(1) 35–50

Thompson, Julia. Update: School-age stutterers. Journal of Fluency Disorders; 1984 Sep Vol 9(3) 199–206

Toscher, Mark M.; Rupp, Ralph R. A study of the central auditory processes in stutterers using the Synthetic Sentence Identification (SSI) Test battery. Journal of Speech and Hearing Research; 1978 Dec Vol 21(4) 779–792

Traugott, N. N.; Onopriychuk, E. I. EEG peculiarities of different clinical types of stuttering in preschoolers. Defektologiya; 1985 No 4 79–83

Ward, David. Voice-onset time and electroglottographic dynamics in stutterers' speech: Implications for a differential diagnosis. British Journal of Disorders of Communication; 1990 Apr Vol 25(1) 93–104

Watson, Jennifer B.; Gregory, Hugo H.; Kistler, Doris J. Development and evaluation of an inventory to assess adult stutterers' communication attitudes. Journal of Fluency Disorders; 1987 Dec Vol 12(6) 429–450

Watson, Peter; Guitar, Barry. Respiratory stuttering? A case history. Journal of Fluency Disorders; 1986 Jun Vol 11(2) 165–173

Wertheim, Eleanor S. Ego dysfunction in stuttering and its relationship to the subculture of the nuclear family: A predictive study based on the bio-adaptive theory of stuttering: II.

British Journal of Medical Psychology; 1973 Jun Vol. 46(2) 155–180

Wexler, Karin B. Developmental disfluency in 2-, 4-, and 6-year-old boys in neutral and stress situations. Journal of Speech and Hearing Research; 1982 Jun Vol 25(2) 229–234

Wingate, Marcel E. Adaptation, consistency and beyond: II. An integral account. Journal of Fluency Disorders; 1986 Mar Vol 11(1) 37–53

Wingate, Marcel E. Fluency, disfluency, dysfluency, and stuttering. Journal of Fluency Disorders; 1984 May Vol 9(2) 163–168

Wynne, Michael K.; Boehmler, Richard M. Central auditory function in fluent and disfluent normal speakers. Journal of Speech and Hearing Research; 1982 Mar Vol 25(1) 54–57

Yairi, Ehud. Subtyping child stutterers for research purposes. ASHA-Reports Series American Speech Language Hearing Association; 1990 Apr No 18 50–57

Yastrebova, A. V.; Voronova, G. G. Examination of stuttering students. Defektologiya; 1980 No 5 51–57

Young, Martin A. Comparison of stuttering frequencies during reading and speaking. Journal of Speech and Hearing Research; 1980 Mar Vol 23(1) 216–217

Zebrowski, Patricia M. Duration of the speech disfluencies of beginning stutterers. Journal of Speech and Hearing Research; 1991 Jun Vol 34(3) 483–491

Zivkovic, Momcilo. Validity and reliability of Initial Letter Word Association Test. Perceptual and Motor Skills; 1979 Oct Vol 49(2) 366

Drugs

Andronova, L. Z.; Lokhov, M. I. Use of methods of destabilization of a stable pathological state in the investigation and treatment of stuttering. Human Physiology; 1984 Jul Vol 9(5) 377–381

Azorin, Jean Michel; Pringuey, Dominique; Samuelian, Jean Claude; Benychou, Michele. Les Nouvelles benzodiazepines. / The new benzodiazepines. XXth Psychiatric Meeting (1986, Marseille, France). Psychologie Medicale; 1987 Mar Vol 19(3) 363–365

Becker, H. Ungewohnliche Sprechstorungen bei der endogenen Depression. / Unusual speech disorders in endogenous depression. Nervenarzt; 1989 Dec Vol 60(12) 757–758

Bhatnagar, Subhash C.; Andy, Orlando J. Alleviation of acquired stuttering with human centremedian thalamic stimulation. Journal of Neurology, Neurosurgery and Psychiatry; 1989 Oct Vol 52(10) 1182–1184

Brady, John P. The pharmacology of stuttering: A critical review. American Journal of Psychiatry; 1991 Oct Vol 148(10) 1309–1316

Brady, John P.; McAllister, Thomas W.; Price, Trevor R. Verapamil in stuttering. Biological Psychiatry; 1990 Mar Vol 27(6) 680–681

Brady, John P.; Price, Trevor R.; McAllister, Thomas W.; Dietrich, Kimberly. A trial of verapamil in the treatment of stuttering in adults. Biological Psychiatry; 1989 Mar Vol 25(5) 630–633

Burd, Larry; Kerbeshian, Jacob. Stuttering and stimulants. Journal of Clinical Psychopharmacology; 1991 Feb Vol 11(1) 72–73

Burns, David; Brady, John P.; Kuruvilla, Kurien. The acute effect of haloperidol and apomorphine on the severity of stuttering. Biological Psychiatry; 1978 Apr Vol 13(2) 255–264

Cocores, James A.; Dackis, Charles A.; Davies, Robert K.; Gold, Mark S. Propranolol and stuttering. American Journal of Psychiatry; 1986 Aug Vol 143(8) 1071–1072

Costa, Daniel. Antidepressants and the treatment of stuttering. American Journal of Psychiatry; 1992 Sep Vol 149(9) 1281

Costa, D.; et al. Clinical and paraclinical aspects of tetany in stuttering. Revue Roumaine de Neurologie et Psychiatrie; 1983 Jul Sep Vol 21(3) 277–279

Costa, D.; Pop, A.; Dumitriu, L.; Marinescu, Luzia; et al. Serum immunoreactive parathormone levels correlate with depression and anxiety in hypocalcemic stutterers. Activitas Nervosa Superior; 1986 Vol 28(2) 155–156

Frankl, Viktor E. The first published cases of paradoxical intention. International Forum for Logotherapy; 1992 15(1) 2–6

Friedman, Ernest H. Fluoxetine and stuttering. Journal of Clinical Psychiatry; 1990 Jul Vol 51(7) 310–311

Goldstein, Jay A. Carbamazepine treatment for stuttering. Journal of Clinical Psychiatry; 1987 Jan Vol 48(1) 39

Guthrie, Sally; Grunhaus, Leon. Fluoxetine-induced stuttering. Journal of Clinical Psychiatry; 1990 Feb Vol 51(2) 85

Harvey, Jan E.; Culatta, Richard; Halikas, James A.; Sorenson, Jackie; et al. The effects of carbamazepine on stuttering. Journal of Nervous and Mental Disease; 1992 Jul Vol 180(7) 451–457

Hutchinson, John M.; Ringel, Robert L. The effect of oral sensory deprivation on stuttering behavior. Journal of Communication Disorders; 1975 Sep Vol 8(3) 249–258

Kampman, Kyle; Brady, John P. Bethanechol in the treatment of stuttering. Journal of Clinical Psychopharmacology; 1993 Aug Vol 13(4) 284–285

Kripke, D. F.; Lavie, P.; Hernandez, J. Polygraphic evaluation of ethchlorvynol (14 days). Psychopharmacology; 1978 Vol 56(2) 221–223

Lokhov, M. I.; Vartanyan, G. A. Stammering: New therapeutic approaches. Zhurnal Nevropatologii i Psikhiatrii imeni S. S. Korsakova; 1989 Vol 89(3) 68–73 1989

Lomachenkov, A. S.; Martsinkevich, N. E. Maladjustment in children in the form of masked depressions. Trudy Leningradskogo Nauchno Issledovatel'skogo Psikhonevrologicheskogo Instituta i m V M Bekhtereva; 1988 Vol 119 38–42

Ludlow, Christy L.; Braun, Allen. Research evaluating the use of neuropharmacological agents for treating stuttering: Possibilities and problems. Journal of Fluency Disorders, 1993 18(2–3) 169–182

McClean, Michael D.; McLean, Alvin. Case report of stuttering acquired in association with phenytoin use for post-head-injury seizures. Journal of Fluency Disorders; 1985 Dec Vol 10(4) 241–255

Menkes, David B.; Ungvari, Gabor S. Adult-onset stuttering as a presenting feature of schizophrenia: Restoration of fluency with trifluoperazine. Journal of Nervous and Mental Disease; 1993 Jan Vol 181(1) 64–65

Mokrovskaya, A. A. Therapeutic and corrective work with stammering preschool children in conditions of a day-time semi-hospital institution. Zhurnal Nevropatologii i Psikhiatrii imeni S. S. Korsakova; 1986 Vol 86(10) 1565–1569

Mouren Simeoni, M. C.; Bouvard, M. P. Les indications des neuroleptiques chez l'enfant. / Neuroleptic indications in children. Encephale; 1990 Mar Apr Vol 16(2) 133–141

Murray, T. J.; Kelly, Patrick; Campbell, Lynda; Stefanik, Kathy. Haloperidol in the treatment of stuttering. British Journal of Psychiatry; 1977 Apr Vol 130 370–373

Nurnberg, H. George; Greenwald, Blaine. Stuttering: An unusual side effect of phenothiazines. American Journal of Psychiatry; 1981 Mar Vol 138(3) 386–387

Oberlander, Eryn; Schneier, Franklin R.; Liebowitz, Michael R. Treatment of stuttering with phenelzine. American Journal of Psychiatry; 1993 Feb Vol 150(2) 355

Oganesian, E. V. (Study of the effectiveness of speech correction within the context of a complex approach to the treatment of stuttering in adults in specialized hospital departments.) Defektologiya; 1985 No 4 23–28

Pimental, Patricia A.; Gorelick, Philip B. Aphasia, apraxia and neurogenic stuttering as complications of metrizamide myelography: Speech deficits following myelography. Acta Neurologica Scandinavica; 1985 Nov Vol 72(5) 481–488

Prins, David; Mandelkorn, Theodore; Cerf, F. Ann. Principal and differential effects of haloperidol and placebo treatments upon speech disfluencies in stutterers. Journal of Speech and Hearing Research; 1980 Sep Vol 23(3) 614–629

Raisova, Vera; Hyanek, J. Speech disorders associated with histidinemia and other hereditary disorders of amino acid metabolism. Folia Phoniatrica; 1986 Jan Feb Vol 38(1) 43–48

Rastatter, Michael P.; Harr, Robert. Measurements of plasma levels of adrenergic neurotransmitters and primary amino acids in five stuttering subjects: A preliminary report (biochemical aspects of stuttering). Journal of Fluency Disorders; 1988 Apr Vol 13(2) 127–139

Rentschler, Gary J.; Driver, Lynn E.; Callaway, Elizabeth A. The onset of stuttering following drug overdose. Journal of Fluency Disorders; 1984 Dec Vol 9(4) 265–284

Rosenberger, Peter B.; Wheelden, Julie A.; Kalotkin, Madeline. The effect of haloperidol on stuttering. American Journal of Psychiatry; 1976 Mar Vol 133(3) 331–334

Schultheis, Josef R. Modern theories of stuttering. Praxis der Kinderpsychologie und Kinderpsychiatrie; 1978 Apr Vol 27(3) 83–87

Schultheis, Josef R. Stottern in historischer und "komplexer" Hinsicht. (Stuttering: Historical and complex perpectives.) Vierteljahresschrift fur Heilpadagogik und ihre Nachbargebiete; 1979 Jun Vol 48(2) 125–138

Swift, W. J.; Swift, E. W.; Arellano, Max. Haloperidol as a treatment for adult stuttering. Comprehensive Psychiatry; 1975 Jan Feb Vol 16(1) 61–67

Tozman, Seymour; Kramer, Steven S. A speech deficit syndrome associated with addictive drug use. British Journal of Addiction; 1977 Mar Vol 72(1) 37–40

Vink, H. J.; Althaus, M.; Goorhuis Brouwer, S. M.; Minderaa, R. B. Clonidine and stuttering. American Journal of Psychiatry; 1992 May Vol 149(5) 717–718

Wood, Frank; et al. Patterns of regional cerebral blood flow during attempted reading aloud by stutterers both on and off haloperidol medication: Evidence for inadequate left frontal activation during stuttering. Brain and Language; 1980 Jan Vol 9(1) 141–144

Efficacy

Adams, Martin R. Learning from negative outcomes in stuttering therapy: I. Getting off on the wrong foot. Journal of Fluency Disorders; 1983 Jun Vol 8(2) 147–153

Adams, Martin R. Stuttering theory, research, and therapy: A five-year retrospective and look ahead. Journal of Fluency Disorders; 1984 May Vol 9(2) 103–113

Alarcia, J.; Pinard, Gilbert; Serrano, M.; Tetreault, L. Etude comparative de trois traitements du begaiement: relaxation, desensibilisation, reeducation. (A comparative study of three treatments for stuttering: Relaxation, desensitization, reeducation.) Revue de Psychologie Appliquee; 1982 Vol 32(1) 1–25

Andrews, Gavin; Craig, Ashley. Prediction of outcome after treatment for stuttering. British Journal of Psychiatry; 1988 Aug Vol 153 236–240

Andrews, Gavin; Feyer, Anne Marie. Does behavior therapy still work when the experimenters depart? An analysis of a behavioral treatment program for stuttering. Behavior Modification; 1985 Oct Vol 9(4) 443–457

Andrews, Gavin; Guitar, Barry; Howie, Pauline M. Meta-analysis of the effects of stuttering treatment. Journal of Speech and Hearing Disorders; 1980 Aug Vol 45(3) 287–307

Andrews, Gavin J.; Howie, Pauline M.; Dozsa, Melinda; Guitar, Barry E. Stuttering: Speech pattern characteristics under fluency-inducing conditions. Journal of Speech and Hearing Research; 1982 Jun Vol 25(2) 208–216

Andrews, Gavin; Tanner, Susan. Stuttering treatment: An attempt to replicate the regulated-breathing method. Journal of Speech and Hearing Disorders; 1982 May Vol 47(2) 138–140

Atkinson, Leslie. Rational-emotive therapy versus systematic desensitization: A comment on Moleski and Tosi. Journal of Consulting and Clinical Psychology; 1983 Oct Vol 51(5) 776–778

Azrin, Nathan H.; Nunn, Robert G.; Frantz, Sharmon E. Comparison of regulated-breathing versus abbreviated desensitization on reported stuttering episodes. Journal of Speech and Hearing Disorders; 1979 Aug Vol 44(3) 331–339

Becker, Peter; Kessler, Bernd; Fuchsgruber, Konrad. (A comparative therapeutic experiment on the theory and the efficiency of operant methods of treatment of stutterers.) Archiv fur Psychologie; 1975 Vol 127(1–2) 78–92

Blood, Gordon. Treatment efficacy in adults who stutter: Review and recommendations. Journal of Fluency Disorders; 1993 18(2–3) 303–318

Burgraff, Roger I. The efficacy of systematic desensitization via imagery as a therapeutic technique with stutterers. British Journal of Disorders of Communication; 1974 Oct Vol 9(2) 134–139

Caron, Chantal; Ladouceur, Robert. Multidimensional behavioral treatment for child stutterers. Behavior Modification; 1989 Apr Vol 13(2) 206–215

Conture, Edward, G.; Guitar, Barry E. Evaluating efficacy of treatment of stuttering: School-age children. Journal of Fluency Disorders; 1993 18(2–3) 253–287

Cox, Nancy J.; Kidd, Kenneth K. Can recovery from stuttering be considered a genetically milder subtype of stuttering? Behavior Genetics; 1983 Mar Vol 13(2) 129–139

Craig, A. R.; Calver, P. Following up on treated stutterers: Studies of perceptions of fluency and job status. Journal of Speech and Hearing Research; 1991 Apr Vol 34(2) 279–284

Craig, Ashley; Andrews, Gavin. The prediction and prevention of relapse in stuttering: The value of self-control techniques and locus of control measures. Behavior Modification; 1985 Oct Vol 9(4) 427–442

Curlee, Richard F.; Perkins, William H. Effectiveness of a DAF conditioning program for adolescent and adult stutterers. Behaviour Research and Therapy; 1973 Nov Vol. 11(4) 395–401

Curlee, Richard F. Evaluating treatment efficacy for adults: Assessment of stuttering disability. Journal of Fluency Disorders; 1993 18(2–3) 319–331

Dugas, Michel; Ladouceur, Robert. Traitement multidimensionnel et progressif des begues severes. (Multidimensional and progressive treatment of severe stuttering.) Science et Comportement; 1988 Win Vol 18(4) 221–232

Falkowski, Glenn L.; Guilford, Arthur M.; Sandler, Jack. Effectiveness of a modified version of airflow therapy: Case studies. Journal of Speech and Hearing Disorders; 1982 May Vol 47(2) 160–164

Fosnot, Susan M. Research design for examining treatment efficacy in fluency disorders. Journal of Fluency Disorders; 1993 18(2–3) 221–251

Gagnon, Mireille; Ladouceur, Robert. Behavioral treatment of child stutterers: Replication and extension. Behavior Therapy; 1992 Win Vol 23(1) 113–129

Gagnon, Mireille; ert. Defining clinically signif he treatment of child stutte and Motor Skills; 1991 Oct

Garcia Moreno, J ca de dos alternativas terap miento de la tartamudez. (C f two therapeutic alternat nent of stuttering.) Revist General y Aplicada; 1984 13

Grzybowska, A aline teorie jakania. / Beh of stuttering. Przeglad Psycl Vol 30(1) 71–80

Guitar, Barry; B ring therapy: The relation l change and long-term out Speech and Hearing Disorders; 1978 Aug Vol 43(3) 392–400

Hayden, Paul A.; Adams, Martin R.; Jordahl, Nanette. The effects of pacing and masking on stutterers' and nonstutterers' speech initiation times. Journal of Fluency Disorders; 1982 Mar Vol 7(1–1) 9–19

Howell, Peter. An investigation of interclinic agreement in the identification of fluent and stuttered syllables. Journal of Fluency Disorders; 1988 Oct Vol 13(5) 309–318

Howie, Pauline M.; Tanner, Susan; Andrews, Gavin. Short- and long-term outcome in an intensive treatment program for adult stutterers. Journal of Speech and Hearing Disorders; 1981 Feb Vol 46(1) 104–109

Ingham, Roger J. Stuttering treatment efficacy: Paradigm dependent or independent? Journal of Fluency Disorders; 1993 18(2–3) 133–149

Ingham, Roger J.; et al. Modification of listener-judged naturalness in the speech of stutterers. Journal of Speech and Hearing Research; 1985 Dec Vol 28(4) 495–504

Ingham, Roger J.; Adams, Susan; Reynolds, Glenda. The effects on stuttering of self-recording the frequency of stuttering or the word "the." Journal of Speech and Hearing Research; 1978 Sep Vol 21(3) 459–469

Ingham, Roger J.; Packman, Ann C. Perceptual assessment of normalcy of speech following stuttering therapy. Journal of Speech and Hearing Research; 1978 Mar Vol 21(1) 63–73

James, Jack E. Behavioral self-control of stuttering using time-out from speaking. Journal of Applied Behavior Analysis; 1981 Spr Vol 14(1) 25–37

James, Jack E.; Ingham, Roger J. The influence of stutterer's expectancies of improvement upon response to time-out. Journal of Speech and Hearing Research; 1974 Mar Vol. 17(1) 86–93

James, Jack E.; Ricciardelli, Lina A.; Hunter, Christine E.; Rogers, Peter. Relative efficacy of intensive and spaced behavioral treatment of stuttering. Behavior Modification; 1989 Jul Vol 13(3) 376–395

Kalinowski, Joseph; Noble, Sandra; Armson, Joy; Stuart Andrew. Pretreatment and post-treatment speech naturalness ratings of adults with mild and severe stuttering. American Journal of Speech-Language Pathology; 1994 3(1) 61–67.

Kraaimaat, Floor; Janssen, Peggy; Brutten, Gene J. The relationship between stutterers' cognitive and autonomic anxiety and therapy outcome. Journal of Fluency Disorders; 1988 Apr Vol 13(2) 107–113

Kuhr, Armin; Rustin, Lena. The maintenance of fluency after intensive in-patient therapy: Long-term follow-up. Journal of Fluency Disorders; 1985 Sep Vol 10(3) 229–236

Kully, Deborah; Boberg, Einer. An investigation of interclinic agreement in the identification of fluent and stuttered syllables. Journal of Fluency Disorders; 1988 Oct Vol 13(5) 309–318

Kurman, Paula. Research: An aerial view. Etc.; 1977 Sep Vol 34(3) 265–276

Ladouceur, Robert; Caron, Chantal; Caron, Guy-laine. Stuttering severity and treatment outcome. Journal of Behavior Therapy and Experimental Psychiatry; 1989 Mar Vol 20(1) 49–56

Ladouceur, Robert; Cote, Christiane; Leblond, Georges; Bouchard, Leandre. Evaluation of regulated-breathing method and awareness training in the treatment of stuttering. Journal of Speech and Hearing Disorders; 1982 Nov Vol 47(4) 422–426

Ladouceur, Robert; Saint Laurent, Lise. Stuttering: A multidimensional treatment and evaluation package. Journal of Fluency Disorders; 1986 Jun Vol 11(2) 93–103

Lankford, Sally D.; Cooper, Eugene B. Recovery from stuttering as viewed by parents of self-diagnosed recovered stutterers. Journal of Communication Disorders; 1974 Jun Vol 7(2) 171–180

Lees, Roberta M. Some thoughts on the use of hypnosis in the treatment of stuttering. British Journal of Experimental and Clinical Hypnosis; 1990 Jun Vol 7(2) 109–114

Madison, Lynda S.; Budd, Karen S.; Itzkowitz, Judy S. Changes in stuttering in relation to children's locus of control. Journal of Genetic Psychology; 1986 Jun Vol 147(2) 233–240

Manning, Walter H.; Dailey, Deborah; Wallace, Sue. Attitude and personality characteristics of older stutterers. Journal of Fluency Disorders; 1984 Sep Vol 9(3) 207–215

Manschreck, Theo C.; Kalotkin, Madeline; Jacobson, Alan M. Utility of electromyographic biological feedback in chronic stuttering: A clinical study with follow-up. Perceptual and Motor Skills; 1980 Oct Vol 51(2) 535–540

Market, Karen E.; Montague, James C.; Buffalo, M. D.; Drummond, Sakina S. Acquired stuttering: Descriptive data and treatment outcome. Journal of Fluency Disorders; 1990 Feb Vol 15(1) 21–33

Martin, Richard R.; Haroldson, Samuel K. Stuttering and speech naturalness: Audio and audiovisual judgements. Journal of Speech and Hearing Research; 1992 Jun Vol 35(3) 521–528

Mizumachi, Toshiro. (Assessment of the results of stuttering therapy—from the behavior therapeutic point of view.) Japanese Journal of Special Education; 1981 Oct Vol 19(2) 48–55

Moore, Mary S.; Adams, Martin R. The Edinburgh Masker: A clinical analog study. Journal of Fluency Disorders; 1985 Dec Vol 10(4) 281–290

Nurnberger, John I.; Hingtgen, Joseph N. Is symptom substitution an important issue in behavior therapy? Biological Psychiatry; 1973 Dec Vol. 7(3) 221–236

Oganesian, E. V. On unification of registration and assessment of rehabilitation effects in adult stutterers. Defektologiya; 1986 No 4 75–78

Ornstein, Amy F.; Manning, Walter H. Self-efficacy scaling by adult stutterers. Journal of Communication Disorders; 1985 Aug Vol 18(4) 313–320

Orta Rodriguez, Martha; Gallegos B., Xochitl. Una evaluacion de tres tecnicas conductuales en el tratamiento de la tartamudez. (An evaluation of 3 behavioral techniques used to treat stuttering.) Revista Mexicana de Psicologia; 1986 Jul-Dec Vol 3(2) 168–173

Perkins, William H.; et al. Replacement of stuttering with normal speech: III. Clinical effectiveness. Journal of Speech and Hearing Disorders; 1974 Nov Vol 39(4) 416–428

Pill, Jaan. A comparison between two treatment programs for stuttering: A personal account. Journal of Fluency Disorders; 1988 Dec Vol 13(6) 385–398

Prins, David. Stutterers' perceptions of therapy improvement and of posttherapy regression: Effects of certain program modifications. Journal of Speech and Hearing Disorders; 1976 Nov Vol 41(4) 452–463

Prins, David. Models for treatment efficacy studies of adult stutters. Journal of Fluency Disorders; 1993 18(2–3) 333–349

Prins, David; Nichols, Anne. Client impressions of the effectiveness of stuttering therapy: A comparison of two programs. British Journal of Disorders of Communication; 1974 Oct Vol 9(2) 123–133

Ramig, Peter R. Rate changes in the speech of stutterers after therapy. Journal of Fluency Disorders; 1984 Dec Vol 9(4) 285–294

Roth U. Erick; Aguilar, S.; Guido, G. Speech therapy: A comparative study of the stutterer. Aprendizaje y Comportamiento; 1979 Vol 2(1–2) 93–108

Rudolf, Sharon R.; Manning, Walter H.; Sewell, William R. The use of self-efficacy scaling in training student clinicians: Implications for working with stutterers. Journal of Fluency Disorders; 1983 Mar Vol 8(1) 55–75

Runyan, Charles M.; Hames, Patricia E.; Prosek, Robert A. A perceptual comparison between paired stimulus and single stimulus methods of presentation of the fluent utterances of stutterers. Journal of Fluency Disorders; 1982 Mar Vol 7(1–1) 71–77

Saint Laurent, Lise; Ladouceur, Robert. Analyse des traitements behavioraux du begaiement. (Analyses of behavioral treatments for stuttering.) Canadian Psychology; 1987 Jul Vol 28(3) 239–250

Saint Laurent, Lise; Ladouceur, Robert. Massed versus distributed application of the regulated-breathing method for stutterers and its long-term effect. Behavior Therapy; 1987 Win Vol 18(1) 38–50

Schwartz, Arthur H.; Daly, David A. Elicited imitation in language assessment: A tool for formulating and evaluating treatment programs. Journal of Communication Disorders; 1978 Feb Vol 11(1) 25–35

Shenker, Rosalee C.; Finn, Patrick. An evaluation of the effects of supplemental "fluency" training during maintenance. Journal of Fluency Disorders; 1985 Dec Vol 10(4) 257–267

Stocker, Beatrice; Gerstman, Louis J. A comparison of the Probe technique and conventional therapy for young stutterers. Journal of Fluency Disorders; 1983 Dec Vol 8(4) 331–339

Strang, Harold R.; Meyers, Susan C. A microcomputer simulation to evaluate and train effective intervention techniques in listening partners of preschool stutterers. Journal of Fluency Disorders; 1987 Jun Vol 12(3) 205–215

Waterloo, Knut K.; Gotestam, K. Gunnar. The regulated-breathing method for stuttering: An experimental evaluation. Journal of Behavior Therapy and Experimental Psychiatry; 1988 Mar Vol 19(1) 11–19

Watts, Fraser. Mechanisms of fluency control in stutterers. British Journal of Disorders of Communication; 1973 Oct Vol. 8(2) 131–138

Wolak, Krzysztof. Zasstosowanie techniki biofeedback w terapii osab jakajacych sie./Biofeedback technique in stuttering therapy. Psychologia Wychowawcza; 1988 Jan-Feb Vol 31(1) 56–69

Yairi, Ehud. Epidemiologic and other considerations in treatment efficacy research with preschool age children who stutter. Journal of Fluency Disorders; 1993 18(2–3) 197–219

Etiology

Adams, Martin R. The demands and capacities model: I. Theoretical elaborations. Journal of Fluency Disorders; 1990 Jun Vol 15(3) 135–141

Adams, Martin R. Stuttering theory, research, and therapy: A five-year retrospective and look ahead. Journal of Fluency Disorders; 1984 May Vol 9(2) 103–113

Andrews, Gavin. Stuttering: A tutorial. Australian and New Zealand Journal of Psychiatry; 1981 Jun Vol 15(2) 105–109

Andrews, Gavin; et al. Stuttering: A review of research findings and theories circa 1982. Journal of Speech and Hearing Disorders; 1983 Aug Vol 48(3) 226–246

Antonucci, Gianfranco; de Rosa, Emilia. La balbuzie: evoluzione dei concetti e prospettive per una comprensione psicodinamica del sintomo. (Stuttering: Evolution of its conceptualizations and prospects for a psychodynamic understanding of this symptom.) Archivio di Psicologia, Neurologia e Psichiatria; 1986 Oct Dec Vol 47(4) 451–476

Anzieu, Annie. Essai sur le corps fantasmatique du begue. (Essay on the phantasmatic body of the stutterer.) Pratique des Mots; 1982 Sep No 40 14–18

Bloodstein, Oliver; Grossman, Marcia. Early stutterings: Some aspects of their form and distribution. Journal of Speech and Hearing Research; 1981 Jan Vol 24(2) 298–302

Bloom, Leon. Notes for a history of speech pathology: An addendum. Folia Phoniatrica; 1982 Nov-Dec Vol 34(6) 296–299

Boehmler, R. M.; Boehmler, S. I. The cause of stuttering: What's the question? Journal of Fluency Disorders; 1989 Dec Vol 14(6) 447–450

Christensen, John M. Did primitive man really talk like an ape? Journal of Speech and Hearing Research; 1992 Aug Vol 35(4) 805

Christensen, John M.; Sacco, Pat R. Association of hair and eye color with handedness and stuttering. Journal of Fluency Disorders; 1989 Feb Vol 14(1) 37–45

Cox, Nancy J.; Seider, Robin A.; Kidd, Kenneth K. Some environmental factors and hypothe-ses for stuttering in families with several stutterers. Journal of Speech and Hearing Research; 1984 Dec Vol 27(4) 543–548

de Hirsch, Katrina. Cluttering and stuttering. Bulletin of the Orton Society; 1975 Vol 25 57–68

Elbers, L. Ontwikkelingsstotteren: Wat ontwikkelt? / The development of stuttering in young children. Gedrag Tijdschrift voor Psychologie; 1983 Vol 11(1) 28–43

Franke, Ulrike. Zur Frage de mannlichen Disposition fur Kommunikationsstorungen. / Predisposition of males for communication disorders. Folia Phoniatrica; 1985 Jan-Feb Vol 37(1) 36–43

Gamelli, Ralph J. Classification of child stuttering: I. Transient developmental, neurogenic acquired, and persistent child stuttering. Child Psychiatry and Human Development; 1982 Sum Vol 12(4) 220–253

Grempel, Franz. Stuttering as a crisis in achieving adult status: Contribution to the etiology and therapy of a stutterer. Praxis der Psychotherapie; 1976 Feb Vol 21(1) 29–41

Howie, Pauline M. Concordance for stuttering in monozygotic and dizygotic twin pairs. Journal of Speech and Hearing Research; 1981 Sep Vol 24(3) 317–321

Ivanova, G. A.; Lapa, A. Z.; Lokhov, M. I.; Movsisyants, S. A. EEG features in stammering pre-school children. Zhurnal Nevropatologii i Psikhiatrii imeni S. S. Korsakova; 1990 Vol 90(3) 78–81

Leung, Alexander K.; Robson, W. Lane. Stuttering. Clinical Pediatrics; 1990 Sep Vol 29(9) 498–502

Muckenhoff, Elisabeth. Modell zur Genese und Manifestation des Stotterns auf lerntheoretischer Basis. (A learning theory model of the origins of stuttering and stuttering behavior.) Vierteljahresschrift fur Heilpadagogik und ihre Nachbargebiete; 1976 Dec Vol 45(4) 341–346

Muhs, Aribert; Schepank, Heinz. Aspekte des Verlaufs und der geschlectsspezifischen Pravalenz psychogener Erkrankungen bei Kindern und Erwachsenen unter dem Einfluss von Erb- und Umweltfaktoren. (Aspects of development of the incidence of psychogenic disorders in children and adults under the influence of hereditary and environmental factors.) Zeitschrift fur Psychosomatische Medizin und Psychoanalyse; 1991 Vol 37(2) 194–206

Myers, Florence L.; Wall, Meryl J. Toward an integrated approach to early childhood stuttering. Journal of Fluency Disorders; 1982 Mar Vol 7(1–1) 47–54

Nemes, Livia. Die klinische Bedeutung der Anklammerungstheorie von Imre Hermann. (The clinical significance of Imre Hermann's theory of clinging.) Zeitschrift fur Psychoanalytische Theorie und Praxis; 1990 Vol 5(2) 112–121

Oganesyan, E. V. (Different rhythmic speech therapy exercises for adolescent and adult stutterers.) Defektologiya; 1983 No 1 60–63

Ohashi, Yoshiko. The development of stuttering in children: A cross-sectional study. Japanese Journal of Child Psychiatry; 1976 Dec-Feb Vol 17(1) 57–68

Ohashi, Yoshiko; Hagiwara, Sachiko. The onset and development of stuttering problems: Discussion of self-acceptance of stuttering in adolescence. Japanese Journal of Child and Adolescent Psychiatry; 1982 Vol 23(5) 287–299

Perkins, William H.; Kent, Raymond D.; Curlee, Richard F. A theory of neuropsycholinguistic function in stuttering. Journal of Speech and Hearing Research; 1991 Aug Vol 34(4) 734–752

Peters, Herman F.; Starkweather, C. Woodruff. The interaction between speech motor coordination and language processes in the development of stuttering: Hypotheses and suggestions for research. Journal of Fluency Disorders; 1990 Apr Vol 15(2) 115–125

Poulos, Marie G.; Webster, William G. Family history as a basis for subgrouping people who stutter. Journal of Speech and Hearing Research; 1991 Feb Vol 34(1) 5–10

Ralston, Lenore D. Stammering: A stress index in Caribbean classrooms. Journal of Fluency Disorders; 1981 Jun Vol 6(2) 119–133

Ryan, Bruce P.; Ryan, Barbara V. Additions to Andrews, Craig, Feyer, Hoddinott, Howie, and Neilson (1983) and to Andrews, Guitar, and Howie (1980). Journal of Speech and Hearing Disorders; 1984 Nov Vol 49(4) 429

Schultheis, Josef R. Modern theories of stuttering. Praxis der Kinderpsychologie und Kinderpsychiatrie; 1978 Apr Vol 27(3) 83–87

Schultheis, Josef R. Stottern in historischer und "komplexer" Hinsicht. (Stuttering: Historical and complex perpectives.) Vierteljahresschrift fur Heilpadagogik und ihre Nachbargebiete; 1979 Jun Vol 48(2) 125–138

Schulze, Hartmut; Johannsen, H. S. Importance of parent-child interaction in the genesis of stuttering. Folia Phoniatrica; 1991 May Jun Vol 43(3) 133–143

Seider, Robin A.; Gladstien, Keith L.; Kidd, Kenneth K. Language onset and concomitant speech and language problems in subgroups of stutterers and their siblings. Journal of Speech and Hearing Research; 1982 Dec Vol 25(4) 482–486

Smith, Anne. "A theory of neuropsycholinguistic function in stuttering": Commentary. Journal of Speech and Hearing Research; 1992 Aug Vol 35(4) 805–809

Smith, Anne. Factors in the etiology of stuttering. ASHA-Reports Series American Speech Language Hearing Association; 1990 Apr No 18 39–47

Snyder, Murry A. A psychodynamic approach to the theory and therapy of stuttering. Journal of Communication Disorders; 1977 Mar Vol 10(1–2) 85–88

Staffolani, Giuseppe. La balbuzie infantile. / Childhood stuttering. Rivista Internazionale di Psicologia e Ipnosi; 1984 Jan-Mar Vol 25(1) 37–41

Stansfield, Jois. Stuttering and cluttering in the mentally handicapped population: A review of the literature. British Journal of Mental Subnormality; 1988 Jan Vol 34(1)(66) 54–61

Tarkowski, Zbigniew; Jaworska, Malgorzata. Gielkot: Stan i perspektywy badan. / Disorderly speech: State and perspectives of research. Psychologia Wychowawcza; 1987 Sep-Oct Vol 30(4) 440–447

Travis, Lee E. Neurophysiological dominance. Journal of Speech and Hearing Disorders; 1978 Aug Vol 43(3) 275–277

Virag, Terez. Gyermekkori neurotikus allapotok, magatartaszavarok tortenelmi hattere. /

The historical background of neurotic states and conduct disorders in childhood. Magyar Pszichologiai Szemle; 1987–88 Vol 44(3) 227–244

Wagner, Alejandro M. Acera de la tartamudez: Introduccion a la patologia del acto. (Stuttering: An introduction to the pathology of the act.) Revista de Psicoanalisis; 1988 Mar-Apr Vol 45(2) 391–417

Wakaba, Yoko. The process of onset of stuttering: A survey of male children who started to stutter in the first six months of the third year. RIEEC-Report; 1990 Feb Vol 39 35–41

Wingate, Marcel E. The immediate source of stuttering: An integration of evidence. Journal of Communication Disorders; 1977 Mar Vol 10(1–2) 45–51

Wolff, Tore. En teori om hur stamning uppkommer. (A theory about the cause of stuttering.) Psykisk Halsa; 1989 Vol 30(1) 45–49

Yairi, Ehud. Longitudinal studies of disfluencies in two-year-old children. Journal of Speech and Hearing Research; 1982 Mar Vol 25(1) 155–160

Yairi, Ehud; Ambrose, Nicoline. A longitudinal study of stuttering in children: A preliminary report. Journal of Speech and Hearing Research; 1992 Aug Vol 35(4) 755–760

Yairi, Ehud. The onset of stuttering in two- and three-year-old children: A preliminary report. Journal of Speech and Hearing Disorders; 1983 May Vol 48(2) 171–177

Yairi, Ehud; Ambrose, Nicoline. Onset of stuttering in preschool children: Selected factors. Journal of Speech and Hearing Research; 1992 Aug Vol 35(4) 782–788

Yairi, Ehud; Lewis, Barbara. Disfluencies at the onset of stuttering. Journal of Speech and Hearing Research; 1984 Mar Vol 27(1) 154–159

Yanagawa, Mitsuaki. On the etiology of stuttering and personality tendencies in mothers and children. Japanese Journal of Child Psychiatry; 1973–74 Dec-Feb Vol 15(1) 22–28

Family

Ananthamurthy, H. S.; Parameswaran, T. M. Management of speech problems. Child Psychiatry Quarterly; 1978 Jan Vol 11(1) 10–13

Andrews, Gavin; Morris-Yates, Allen; Howie, Pauline; Martin, Nicholas. Genetic factors in stuttering confirmed. Archives of General Psychiatry; 1991 Nov Vol 48(11) 1034–1035

Antonucci, Gianfranco; de Rosa, Emilia. La balbuzie: evoluzione dei concetti e prospettive per una comprensione psicodinamica del sintomo. (Stuttering: Evolution of its conceptualizations and prospects for a psychodynamic understanding of this symptom.) Archivio di Psicologia, Neurologia e Psichiatria; 1986 Oct–Dec Vol 47(4) 451–476

Boberg, Julia M.; Boberg, Einer. The other side of the block: The stutterer's spouse. Journal of Fluency Disorders; 1990 Feb Vol 15(1) 61–75

Bojanin, Svetomir; Vuletic Peco, Aleksandra; Radojkovic, Dejan. Porodica dece sa razvojnim hiperkinetskim sindromom, tikovima i mucanjem. (Families of children with developing hyperkinetic syndrome, tics, and stuttering.) Psihijatrija Danas; 1991 Vol 23(1–2) 37–48

Budd, Karen S.; Madison, Lynda S.; Itzkowitz, Judy S.; George, Catherine H.; et al. Parents and therapists as allies in behavioral treatment of children's stuttering. Behavior Therapy; 1986 Nov Vol 17(5) 538–553

Conture, Edward G.; Kelly, Ellen M. Young stutterers' nonspeech behaviors during stuttering. Journal of Speech and Hearing Research; 1991 Oct Vol 34(5) 1041–1056

Conture, Edward G. Youngsters who stutter: Diagnosis, parent counseling, and referral. Journal of Developmental and Behavioral Pediatrics; 1982 Sep Vol 3(3) 163–169

Cox, Nancy J.; Seider, Robin A.; Kidd, Kenneth K. Some environmental factors and hypotheses for stuttering in families with several stutterers. Journal of Speech and Hearing Research; 1984 Dec Vol 27(4) 543–548

Crowe, Thomas A.; Cooper, Eugene B. Parental attitudes toward and knowledge of stuttering. Journal of Communication Disorders; 1977 Jun Vol 10(4) 343–357

Daly, David A. Use of the home VCR to facilitate transfer of fluency. Journal of Fluency Disorders; 1987 Apr Vol 12(2) 103–106

de Vries, Ursula. "Laut—langsam—deutlich"—eine Phase aus der Therapie stotternder Schuler. / "Loudly—slowly—intelligibly":

One phase of the therapy for children who stutter. Vierteljahresschrift fur Heilpadagogik und ihre Nachbargebiete; 1990 Mar Vol 59(1) 60–72

DiGiuseppe, Ray; Wilner, R. Stefanie. An eclectic view of family therapy: When is family therapy the treatment of choice? When is it not? Journal of Clinical Child Psychology; 1980 Spr Vol 9(1) 70–72

Dorgan, Barbara J.; Dorgan, Richard E. A theoretical rationale for total family therapy with stutterers. British Journal of Social Psychiatry and Community Health; 1972–1973 Vol. 6(3) 214–222

Dorgan, Barbara J.; Dorgan, Richard E. A theoretical rationale for total family therapy with stutterers. British Journal of Social Psychiatry and Community Health; 1972–1973 Vol. 6(3) 214–222

Feldman, Ronald L. Self-disclosure in parents of stuttering children. Journal of Communication Disorders; 1976 Sep Vol 9(3) 227–234

Ferreiro-Diaz, M. D.; Dominguez, M. Dolores; Rodriguez, A. Psicoterapis de grupos infantiles: la madre co-terapeuta. (Group psychotherapy for children: The mother as co-therapist.) Clinica y Analisis Grupal; 1990 May–Aug Vol 12(2) 291–313

Filimoshkina, N. M.; Timchenko, V. A. (Counsel for parents of a stuttering child.) Defektologiya; 1982 Vol 5 69–72

Gotestam, K. Olof; Coates, Tom J.; Ekstrand, Maria. Handedness, dyslexia and twinning in homosexual men. International Journal of Neuroscience; 1992 Apr Vol 63(3–4) 179–186

Gottwald, Sheryl R.; Goldbach, Peggy; Isack, Audrey H. Stuttering: Prevention and detection. Young Children; 1985 Nov Vol 41(1) 9–14

Guitar, Barry; Schaefer, Helen K.; Donahue Kilburg, Gail; Bond, Lynne. Parent verbal interactions and speech rate: A case study in stuttering. Journal of Speech and Hearing Research; 1992 Aug Vol 35(4) 742–754

Homzie, Marvin J.; Lindsay, Jean S.; Simpson, Joanne; Hasenstab, Suzanne. Concomitant speech, language, and learning problems in adult stutterers and in members of their families. Journal of Fluency Disorders; 1988 Aug Vol 13(4) 261–277

Janssen, Peggy; Kraaimaat, Floor; Brutten, Gene. Relationship between stutterers' genetic history and speech-associated variables. Journal of Fluency Disorders; 1990 Feb Vol 15(1) 39–48 1990

Krause, Matthias P. Stottern als Beziehungsstorung—Psychotherapeutische Arbeit mit Eltern stotternder Kinder. / Stuttering as an expression of disturbed parent-child relationship. Praxis de   ogie und Kinderpsychiatrie;   ) 15–18

Krause, Rainer. Non   behavior in stutterers and th   ers. Psychologie Schweize   fur Psychologie und ihre   1978 Vol 37(3) 177–201.

Ladouceur, Robert;   e. Evaluation of regulated-   with and without parental   treatment of child stutterers   vior Therapy and Experim   1982 Dec Vol 13(4) 301–306

Langlois, Aimee; H   .; Inouye, Lynn L. A compar   s between stuttering childre   children, and their mother   ncy Disorders; 1986 Sep Vo

Langlois, Aimee; L   model for teaching parents   nt speech. Journal of Fluency Disorders; 1988 Jun Vol 13(3) 163–172

Lankford, Sally D.; Cooper, Eugene B. Recovery from stuttering as viewed by parents of self-diagnosed recovered stutterers. Journal of Communication Disorders; 1974 Jun Vol 7(2) 171–180

LaSalle, Lisa R.; Conture, Edward G. Eye contact between young stutterers and their mothers. Journal of Fluency Disorders; 1991 Vol 16(4) 173–199

Lasogga, Frank; Wedemeyer, Marina. The childrearing practices of parents of stuttering children. Zeitschrift fur Klinische Psychologie. Forschung und Praxis; 1979 Vol 8(4) 270–282

Lechta, Viktor; Vanhara, Ladislav. Analyza postojov uciteliek a matiek k zajakavemu diet'at'u. / Analysis of attitudes of teachers and mothers towards a stammering child. Jednotna Skola; 1985 Apr Vol 37(4) 357–362

Levina, R. Ye. On emociogenic factors of stuttering which arise in the course of formation of voluntary speech. Defektologiya; 1981 Jan No 1 7–13

Lucas, Tina. Communication therapy. Journal of Adolescence; 1982 Sep Vol 5(3) 285–299

Madison, Lynda S.; Budd, Karen S.; Itzkowitz, Judy S. Changes in stuttering in relation to children's locus of control. Journal of Genetic Psychology; 1986 Jun Vol 147(2) 233–240

Meyers, Susan C. Qualitative and quantitative differences and patterns of variability in disfluencies emitted by preschool stutterers and nonstutterers during dyadic conversations. Journal of Fluency Disorders; 1986 Dec Vol 11(4) 293–306

Meyers, Susan C.; Freeman, Frances J. Are mothers of stutterers different? An investigation of social-communicative interaction. Journal of Fluency Disorders; 1985 Sep Vol 10(3) 193–209

Meyers, Susan C. Verbal behaviors of preschool stutterers and conversational partners: Observing reciprocal relationships. Journal of Speech and Hearing Disorders; 1990 Nov Vol 55(4) 706–712

Meyers, Susan C. Nonfluencies of preschool stutterers and conversational partners: Observing reciprocal relationships. Journal of Speech and Hearing Disorders; 1989 Feb Vol 54(1) 106–112

Meyers, Susan C.; Freeman, Frances J. Interruptions as a variable in stuttering and disfluency. Journal of Speech and Hearing Research; 1985 Sep Vol 28(3) 428–435

Meyers, Susan C.; Freeman, Frances J. Mother and child speech rates as a variable in stuttering and disfluency. Journal of Speech and Hearing Research; 1985 Sep Vol 28(3) 436–444

Meyers, Susan C.; Ghatak, Lila R.; Woodford, Lee L. Case descriptions of nonfluency and loci: Initial and follow-up conversations with three preschool children. Journal of Fluency Disorders; 1989 Dec Vol 14(6) 383–397

Moore, Margaret; Nystul, Michael S. Parent-child attitudes and communication processes in families with stutterers and families with non-stutterers. British Journal of Disorders of Communication; 1979 Dec Vol 14(3) 173–180

Mowrer, Donald E. Repetition of final consonants in the speech of a young child. Journal of Speech and Hearing Disorders; 1987 May Vol 52(2) 174–178

Neils, Jean; Aram, Dorothy M. Family history of children with developmental language disorders. Perceptual and Motor Skills; 1986 Oct Vol 63(2, Pt 1) 655–658

Nemes, Livia. Die klinische Bedeutung der Anklammerungstheorie von Imre Hermann. (The clinical significance of Imre Hermann's theory of clinging.) Zeitschrift fur Psychoanalytische Theorie und Praxis; 1990 Vol 5(2) 112–121

Onslow, Mark; Costa, Leanne; Rue, Stephen. Direct early intervention with stuttering: Some preliminary data. Journal of Speech and Hearing Disorders; 1990 Aug Vol 55(3) 405–416

Pollack, Janet; Lubinski, Rosemary; Weitzner Lin, Barbara. A pragmatic study of child dysfluency. Journal of Fluency Disorders; 1986 Sep Vol 11(3) 231–239

Quarrington, Bruce. The parents of stuttering children: The literature re-examined. Canadian Psychiatric Association Journal; 1974 Feb Vol 19(1) 103–110

Ratner, Nan B. Measurable outcomes of instructions to modify normal parent-child verbal interactions: Implications for indirect stuttering therapy. Journal of Speech and Hearing Research; 1992 Feb Vol 35(1) 14–20

Reich, Gunter. Stotternde Kinder und ihre Familien. / Stuttering children and their families. Praxis der Kinderpsychologie und Kinderpsychiatrie; 1987 Jan Vol 36(1) 16–22

Roden, Rudolph G.; Roden, Michelle M. Children of Holocaust survivors. Adolescent Psychiatry; 1982 Vol 10 66–72

Rudmin, Floyd. Parent's report of stress and articulation oscillation as factors in a preschooler's dysfluencies. Journal of Fluency Disorders; 1984 Feb Vol 9(1) 85–87

Schulze, Hartmut; Johannsen, H. S. Importance of parent-child interaction in the genesis of stuttering. Folia Phoniatrica; 1991 May–Jun Vol 43(3) 133–143

Seider, Robin A.; Gladstien, Keith L.; Kidd, Kenneth K. Recovery and persistence of stuttering among relatives of stutterers. Journal of Speech and Hearing Disorders; 1983 Nov Vol 48(4) 402–409

Steffen, Hartmut; Seidel, Christa. Perceptive and cognitive school and social behavior of children with language and speech disorders. Zeitschrift fur Kinder und Jugendpsychiatrie; 1976 Vol 4(3) 216–232

Stephenson Opsal, Deborah; Bernstein-Ratner, Nan. Maternal speech rate modification and childhood stuttering. Annual Convention of the American Speech Language and Hearing Association (1986, Detroit, Michigan). Journal of Fluency Disorders; 1988 Feb Vol 13(1) 49–56

Tkaczenko, Oleh G. Tiefenpsychologische Aspekte des Stotterns. / The depth psychological aspects of stuttering. Zeitschrift fur Individualpsychologie; 1990 Vol 15(4) 298–306

Virag, Terez. Gyermekkori neurotikus allapotok, magatartaszavarok tortenelmi hattere. / The historical background of neurotic states and conduct disorders in childhood. Magyar Pszichologiai Szemle; 1987–88 Vol 44(3) 227–244

Wagner, Alejandro M. Acera de la tartamudez: Introduccion a la patologia del acto. (Stuttering: An introduction to the pathology of the act.) Revista de Psicoanalisis; 1988 Mar–Apr Vol 45(2) 391–417

Wakaba, Yoko. Research on mother-child interaction of stuttering children: Preliminary observation. RIEEC-Report; 1987 Feb Vol 36 29–37

Weiss, Amy L.; Zebrowski, Patricia M. Patterns of assertiveness and responsiveness in parental interactions with stuttering and fluent children. Journal of Fluency Disorders; 1991 Vol 16(2–3) 125–141

Wertheim, Eleanor S. Ego dysfunction in stuttering and its relationship to the subculture of the nuclear family: A predictive study based on the bio-adaptive theory of stuttering: II. British Journal of Medical Psychology; 1973 Jun Vol. 46(2) 155–180

Yairi, Ehud. Item analysis for parental behavior rated by stutterers and nonstutterers. Perceptual and Motor Skills; 1973 Apr Vol. 36(2) 451–452

Yanagawa, Mitsuaki. On the etiology of stuttering and personality tendencies in mothers and children. Japanese Journal of Child Psychiatry; 1973–74 Dec–Feb Vol 15(1) 22–28

Zebrowski, Patricia M.; Conture, Edward G. Judgments of disfluency by mothers of stuttering and normally fluent children. Journal of Speech and Hearing Research; 1989 Sep Vol 32(3) 625–634

Genetics

Andrews, Gavin; et al. Stuttering: A review of research findings and theories circa 1982. Journal of Speech and Hearing Disorders; 1983 Aug Vol 48(3) 226–246

Andrews, Gavin; Yates-Morris, Allen; Howie, Pauline; Martin, Nicholas. Genetic factors in stuttering confirmed. Archives of General Psychiatry; 1991 Nov Vol 48(11) 1034–1035

Borden, Gloria J. Subtyping adult stutterers for research purposes. ASHA Reports Series American Speech Language Hearing Association; 1990 Apr No 18 58–62

Buyanov, M. I.; Bogdanova, E. V.; Subbotina, R. A.; Trebuleva, V. N. On heredity in stuttering. Defektologiya; 1987 No 3 20–22

Cox, N., Kramer, P., Kidd, K. Segregation analyses of stuttering. Genetic Epidemiology; 1984 1, 245–253.

Cox, Nancy J.; Kidd, Kenneth K. Can recovery from stuttering be considered a genetically milder subtype of stuttering? Behavior Genetics; 1983 Mar Vol 13(2) 129–139

Andrews, Gavin; Yates-Morris, Allen; Howie, Pauline; Martin, Nicholas. Genetic factors in stuttering confirmed. Archives of General Psychiatry; 1991 Nov Vol 48(11) 1034–1035

Craven, Duane C.; Ryan, Bruce P. The use of a portable delayed auditory feedback unit in stuttering therapy. Journal of Fluency Disorders; 1984 Sep Vol 9(3) 237–243

Gladstien, Keith L.; Seider, Robin A.; Kidd, Kenneth K. Analysis of the sibship patterns of stutterers. Journal of Speech and Hearing Research; 1981 Sep Vol 24(3) 460–462

Gotestam, K. Olof. Lefthandedness among students of architecture and music. Perceptual and Motor Skills; 1990 Jun Vol 70(3, Pt 2) 1323–1327

Gotestam, K. Olof; Coates, Tom J.; Ekstrand, Maria. Handedness, dyslexia and twinning in homosexual men. International Journal of Neuroscience; 1992 Apr Vol 63(3–4) 179–186

Hays, Peter; Field, L. Leigh. Postulated genetic linkage between manic-depression and stuttering. Journal of Affective Disorders; 1989 Jan–Feb Vol 16(1) 37–40

Homzie, Marvin J.; Lindsay, Jean S.; Simpson, Joanne; Hasenstab, Suzanne. Concomitant speech, language, and learning problems in adult stutterers and in members of their families. Journal of Fluency Disorders; 1988 Aug Vol 13(4) 261–277

Howie, Pauline M. Concordance for stuttering in monozygotic and dizygotic twin pairs. Journal of Speech and Hearing Research; 1981 Sep Vol 24(3) 317–321

Howie, Pauline M. Intrapair similarity in frequency of disfluency in monozygotic and dizygotic twin pairs containing stutterers. Behavior Genetics; 1981 May Vol 11(3) 227–238

Janssen, Peggy; Kraaimaat, Floor; Brutten, Gene. Relationship between stutterers' genetic history and speech-associated variables. Journal of Fluency Disorders; 1990 Feb Vol 15(1) 39–48

Kidd, K. A genetic perspective on stuttering. Journal of Fluency Disorders; 1977 2 259–269

Kidd, K. Genetic models of stuttering. Journal of Fluency Disorders; 1980 5, 187– 201.

Kidd, Kenneth K.; et al. Familial stuttering patterns are not related to one measure of severity. Journal of Speech and Hearing Research; 1980 Sep Vol 23(3) 539–545

Kidd, K, Heimbuch, R., & Records, M. Vertical transmission of susceptibility to stuttering with sex-modified expression. Proceedings of the National Academy of Science; 1981 78, 606–610.

Lewis, Barbara A. Pedigree analysis of children with phonology disorders. Journal of Learning Disabilities; 1992 Nov Vol 25(9) 586–597

Ludlow, C., & Dooman, A. Genetic aspects of idiopathic speech and language disorders. Molecular Biology and Genetics; 1992 25, 979–991.

MacFarlane, Wendy B.; Hanson, Marvin; Walton, Wendel; Mellon, Charles D. Stuttering in five generations of a single family: A preliminary report including evidence supporting a sex-modified mode of transmission. Journal of Fluency Disorders; 1991 Vol 16(2–3) 117–123

Muhs, Aribert; Schepank, Heinz. Aspekte des Verlaufs und der geschlectsspezifischen Pravalenz psychogener Erkrankungen bei Kindern und Erwachsenen unter dem Einfluss von Erb- und Umweltfaktoren. (Aspects of development of the incidence of psychogenic disorders in children and adults under the influence of hereditary and environmental factors.) Zeitschrift fur Psychosomatische Medizin und Psychoanalyse; 1991 Vol 37(2) 194–206

Neils, Jean; Aram, Dorothy M. Family history of children with developmental language disorders. Perceptual and Motor Skills; 1986 Oct Vol 63(2, Pt 1) 655–658

Pauls, David L. A review of the evidence for genetic factors in stuttering. ASHA Reports Series American Speech Language Hearing Association; 1990 Apr No 18 34–38

Pauls, David L.; Kidd, Kenneth K. Genetic strategies for the analysis of childhood behavioral traits. Schizophrenia Bulletin; 1982 Vol 8(2) 253–266

Pennington, Bruce F.; Smith, Shelley D. Genetic influences on learning disabilities and speech and language disorders. Child Development; 1983 Apr Vol 54(2) 369–387

Poulos, Marie G.; Webster, William G. Family history as a basis for subgrouping people who stutter. Journal of Speech and Hearing Research; 1991 Feb Vol 34(1) 5–10

Seider, Robin A.; Gladstien, Keith L.; Kidd, Kenneth K. Language onset and concomitant speech and language problems in subgroups of stutterers and their siblings. Journal of Speech and Hearing Research; 1982 Dec Vol 25(4) 482–486

Sheehan, Joseph G.; Costley, Marian S. A reexamination of the role of heredity in stuttering. Journal of Speech and Hearing Disorders; 1977 Feb Vol 42(1) 47–59

Strub, Richard L.; Black, F. William; Naeser, Margaret A. Anomalous dominance in sibling stutterers: Evidence from CT scan asymmetries, dichotic listening, neuropsychological testing, and handedness. Brain and Language; 1987 Mar Vol 30(2) 338–350

Group Therapy

Buchta, Herbert. Hypnotherapie und Stottern Eine Falldarstellung. (Hypnotherapy and stuttering: A case report.) Experimentelle und Klinische Hypnose; 1987 Vol 3(2) 143–148

Caron, Chantal; Dugas, Michel; Ladouceur, Robert. Le traitement individuel et en groupe de begues adultes. (Individual and group treatment of adult stutterers.) Science et Comportement; 1990 Vol 20(3–4) 185–193

Ferreiro-Diaz, M. D.; Dominguez, M. Dolores; Rodriguez, A. Psicoterapis de grupos infantiles: la madre co-terapeuta. (Group psychotherapy for children: The mother as co-therapist.) Clinica y Analisis Grupal; 1990 May–Aug Vol 12(2) 291–313

Khavin, A. B.; Diakova, E. A. (Characteristics of communication impairments in adult stutterers and effectiveness of medical-rehabilitation work.) Defektologiya; 1988 No 3 20–24

Lasogga, Frank; Kondring, Irmgard. Stotterer in Selbsthilfegruppen und in Einzeltherapie. (Stutterers in self-help groups and in individual therapy.) Zeitschrift fur Klinische Psychologie. Forschung und Praxis; 1982 Vol 11(3) 201–214

Leahy, Margaret M.; Collins, Geraldine. Therapy for stuttering: Experimenting with experimenting. Irish Journal of Psychological Medicine; 1991 Mar Vol 8(1) 37–39

Leahy, M.; O'Sullivan, B. Psychological change and fluency therapy: A pilot project. British Journal of Disorders of Communication; 1987 Dec Vol 22(3) 245–251

Nekrasova, Julia B. Wiederherstellung einer gestorten Kommunikation (am Beispiel einer Logoneurose). / Repair of disturbed communication in logoneurosis. Dynamische-Psychiatrie; 1989 Vol 22(114–115) 37–50

Nekrasova, Y. B. Psychotherapy sessions and some mental states of stutterers. Voprosy Psikhologii; 1980 Sep–Oct No 5 32–40

Nekrasova, Yuliya B. (Group emotional and stress psychotherapy to correct mental states of stutterers.) Voprosy Psikhologii; 1984 Mar–Apr No 2 75–82

Ojha, K. N.; Bettagere, R. N. Group psychotherapy with stutterers. Indian Journal of Clinical Psychology; 1982 Sep Vol 9(2) 125–129

Polaino-Lorente, Aquilino M. Experiences in the treatment of childhood stuttering. Revista de Psicologia General y Aplicada; 1976 Mar–Apr Vol 31(139) 171–183

Raou, Ye. Y. Dynamics of some characteristics of stutterer's personality in the process of psychotherapy. Voprosy Psikhologii; 1984 May–Jun Vol 3 67–72

Samuel Lajeunesse, B.; Degleris, N.; Brouri, R.; Agathon, M. Appreciation des effets des techniques assertives en groupe en milieu psychiatrie. (Group training in assertive techniques in a psychiatric milieu.) Annales Medico Psychologiques; 1985 May Vol 143(5) 458–464

Shklovskii, Viktor M.; Krol, Leonid M.; Mikhailova, Ekaterina L. The psychotherapy of stuttering: On the model of stuttering patients' psychotherapy group. Soviet Journal of Psychiatry and Psychology Today; 1988 Vol 1(1) 130–141

Shklovsky, V. M.; Krol, L. M.; Mikhailova, E. L. Specificity of group psychotherapy in stammering. Trudy Leningradskogo Nauchno Issledovatel'skogo Psikhonevrologicheskogo Instituta i m V M Bekhtereva; 1988 Vol 121 112–117

Shklovsky, Victor M.; Kroll, Leonid M.; Mikhailova, Ekaterina L. Group psychotherapy: Problems of theory and practical application. Psikologicheskii Zhurnal; 1985 May–Jun Vol 6(3) 100–110

Srivastava, K. Indira. Socio-psychological factors of stammering and the problem of rehabilitation of stammerers. Indian Psychological Review; 1985 Vol 29(Spec Iss) 24–34

Stewart, Trudy M. The relationship of attitudes and intentions to behave to the acquisition of fluent speech behaviour by stammerers. British Journal of Disorders of Communication; 1982 Sep Vol 17(2) 3–13

Wakaba, Yoko Y. Group play therapy for Japanese children who stutter. Journal of Fluency Disorders; 1983 Jun Vol 8(2) 93–118

Hypnosis and Stuttering

Buchta, Herbert. Hypnotherapie und Stottern Eine Falldarstellung. (Hypnotherapy and stuttering: A case report.) Experimentelle und Klinische Hypnose; 1987 Vol 3(2) 143–148

Cassar, Mary C. Hypnosis and stuttering intervention. Australian Journal of Clinical Hypnotherapy and Hypnosis; 1987 Mar Vol 8(1) 37–49

Cassar, Mary C. Stuttering and hypnosis: Processes of cortical control. Australian Journal of Clinical Hypnotherapy and Hypnosis; 1988 Sep Vol 9(2) 49–65

Dempsey, George L.; Granich, Marina. Hypnobehavioral therapy in the case of a traumatic stutterer: A case study. International Journal of Clinical and Experimental Hypnosis; 1978 Jul Vol 26(3) 125–133

Doughty, Patricia. Case study: The use of hypnosis with a stammerer. British Journal of Experimental and Clinical Hypnosis; 1990 Feb Vol 7(1) 65–67

Francis, J. G. Stopping stuttering starting with hypnosis. Australian Journal of Clinical and Experimental Hypnosis; 1984 May Vol 12(1) 9–21

Kelemen, Z. Hypno-behavioural therapy for the treatment of stuttering. Australian Journal of Clinical Hypnotherapy; 1980 Mar Vol 1(1) 17–23

Lees, Roberta M. Some thoughts on the use of hypnosis in the treatment of stuttering. British Journal of Experimental and Clinical Hypnosis; 1990 Jun Vol 7(2) 109–114

Lockhart, Myra S.; Robertson, Alan W. Hypnosis and speech therapy as a combined therapeutic approach to the problem of stammering: A study of thirty patients. British Journal of Disorders of Communication; 1977 Oct Vol 12(2) 97–108

London, Ray W. International perspectives on pediatric hypnosis. Australian Journal of Clinical Hypnotherapy and Hypnosis; 1983 Sep Vol 4(2) 83–91

Pesci, Guido. Nuove modalita diagnostiche e ipnoterapeutiche per ridurre o annullare la balbuzie. / New diagnostic methods and hypnotherapy in the reduction or cure of stammering. 2nd National Hypnotherapy and Handwriting Psychology Convention (1985, Milan, Italy). Rivista Internazionale di Psicologia e Ipnosi; 1985 Apr–Sep Vol 26(2–3) 181–188

Sanders, Shirley. Hypnotic dream utilization in hypnotherapy. American Journal of Clinical Hypnosis; 1982 Jul Vol 25(1) 62–67

Silber, Samuel. Fairy tales and symbols in hypnotherapy of children with certain speech disorders. International Journal of Clinical and Experimental Hypnosis; 1973 Oct Vol. 21(4) 272–283

Silverman, Lloyd H. Psychoanalytic theory: "The reports of my death are greatly exaggerated." American Psychologist; 1976 Sep Vol 31(9) 621–637

Tarkowski, Zbigniew. Psychoterapia osob jakajacych sie. / Psychotherapy of stutterers. Psychologia Wychowawcza; 1987 Mar–Apr Vol 30(2) 184–192

Language

Abeleva, I. Yu. (Psychology of stuttering in adults during various phases of verbal communication.) Voprosy Psikhologii; 1974 Jul–Aug No 4 144–149

Alarcia, J.; Pinard, Gilbert; Serrano, M.; Tetreault, L. Etude comparative de trois traitements du begaiement: relaxation, desensibilisation, reeducation. (A comparative study of three treatments for stuttering: Relaxation, desensitization, reeducation.) Revue de Psychologie Appliquee; 1982 Vol 32(1) 1–25

Andrews, Gavin J.; Howie, Pauline M.; Dozsa, Melinda; Guitar, Barry E. Stuttering: Speech pattern characteristics under fluency-inducing conditions. Journal of Speech and Hearing Research; 1982 Jun Vol 25(2) 208–216

Baker, Lorian; Cantwell, Dennis P. Psychiatric and learning disorders in children with speech and language disorders: A critical review. Advances in Learning and Behavioral Disabilities; 1985 Vol 4 1–28

Barblan, Leo. Therapeutique du langage: Science ou intuition? (Therapeutics of language: Science or intuition?) Pratique des Mots; 1983 Sep No 44 23–36

Belyakova, Lidiya I.; Matanova, Vanya. Psycholinguistic characteristics of stammering preschoolers' speech. Voprosy Psikhologii; 1990 Jul–Aug No 4 61–67

Blood, Gordon W.; Seider, Robin. The concomitant problems of young stutterers. Journal of Speech and Hearing Disorders; 1981 Feb Vol 46(1) 31–33

Blood, Gordon W. Laterality differences in child stutterers: Heterogeneity, severity levels, and statistical treatments. Journal of Speech and Hearing Disorders; 1985 Feb Vol 50(1) 66–72

Bloodstein, Oliver. The rules of early stuttering. Journal of Speech and Hearing Disorders; 1974 Nov Vol 39(4) 379–394

Bloodstein, Oliver; Grossman, Marcia. Early stutterings: Some aspects of their form and distribution. Journal of Speech and Hearing Research; 1981 Jan Vol 24(2) 298–302

Bosshardt, Hans Georg; Nandyal, Indira. Reading rates of stutterers and nonstutterers during silent and oral reading. Journal of Fluency Disorders; 1988 Dec Vol 13(6) 407–420

Brundage, Shelley B.; Ratner, Nan B. Measurement of stuttering frequency in children's speech. Journal of Fluency Disorders; 1989 Oct Vol 14(5) 351–358

Byrd, Kathryn; Cooper, Eugene B. Apraxic speech characteristics in stuttering, developmentally apraxic, and normal speaking children. Journal of Fluency Disorders; 1989 Jun Vol 14(3) 215–229

Byrd, Kathryn; Cooper, Eugene B. Expressive and receptive language skills in stuttering children. Journal of Fluency Disorders; 1989 Apr Vol 14(2) 121–126

Cantwell, Dennis P.; Baker, Lorian. Psychiatric and learning disorders in children with speech and language disorders: A descriptive analysis. Advances in Learning and Behavioral Disabilities; 1985 Vol 4 29–47

Cheveliova, N. A. Toward the problem of stuttering in children. Defektologiya; 1977 Jan No 1 20–23

Crowe, Kathryn M.; Kroll, Robert M. Response latency and response class for stutterers and nonstutterers as measured by a word-association task. Journal of Fluency Disorders; 1991 Feb Vol 16(1) 35–54

Danzger, Miriam; Halpern, Harvey. Relation of stuttering to word abstraction, part of speech, word length, and word frequency. Perceptual and Motor Skills; 1973 Dec Vol. 37(3) 959–962

Friedman, Silvia. Fluencia, disfluencia, gagueira. / Fluency, disfluency, stuttering. Revista Interamericana de Psicologia; 1991 Vol 25(1) 83–92

Gaines, Natalie D.; Runyan, Charles M.; Meyers, Susan C. A comparison of young stutterers' fluent versus stuttered utterances on measures of length and complexity. Journal of Speech and Hearing Research; 1991 Feb Vol 34(1) 37–42

Gordon, Pearl A.; Luper, Harold L. Speech disfluencies in nonstutterers: Syntactic complexity and production task effects. Journal of Fluency Disorders; 1989 Dec Vol 14(6) 429–445

Griggs, S.; Still, A. W. An analysis of individual differences in words stuttered. Journal of Speech and Hearing Research; 1979 Sep Vol 22(3) 572–580

Guitar, Barry; Schaefer, Helen K.; Donahue Kilburg, Gail; Bond, Lynne. Parent verbal interactions and speech rate: A case study in stuttering. Journal of Speech and Hearing Research; 1992 Aug Vol 35(4) 742–754

Hand, C. Rebekah; Haynes, William O. Linguistic processing and reaction time differences in stutterers and nonstutterers. Journal of Speech and Hearing Research; 1983 Jun Vol 26(2) 181–185

Helmreich, Helaine G.; Bloodstein, Oliver. The grammatical factor in childhood disfluency in relation to the continuity hypothesis. Journal of Speech and Hearing Research; 1973 Dec Vol. 16(4) 731–738

Homzie, M. J.; Lindsay, Jean S. Language and the young stutterer: A new look at old theories and findings. Brain and Language; 1984 Jul Vol 22(2) 232–252

Homzie, Marvin J.; Lindsay, Jean S.; Simpson, Joanne; Hasenstab, Suzanne. Concomitant speech, language, and learning problems in adult stutterers and in members of their families. Journal of Fluency Disorders; 1988 Aug Vol 13(4) 261–277

Hubbard, Carol P.; Prins, David. Word familiarity, syllabic stress pattern, and stuttering. Journal of Speech and Hearing Research; 1994 37(3) 564–572

Hulit, Lloyd M. Effects of nonfluencies on comprehension. Perceptual and Motor Skills; 1976 Jun Vol 42(3, Pt 2) 1119–1122

Janssen, Peggy; Kraaimaat, Floor; Van der Meulen, Sjoeke. Reading ability and disfluency in stuttering and nonstuttering elementary school children. Journal of Fluency Disorders; 1983 Mar Vol 8(1) 39–53

Jayaram, M. Distribution of stuttering in sentences: Relationship to sentence length and clause position. Journal of Speech and Hearing Research; 1984 Sep Vol 27(3) 338–341

Jayaram, M. Grammatical context of stuttered and nonstuttered words. NIMHANS Journal; 1989 Jan Vol 7(1) 55–63

Jayaram, M. Phonetic influences on stuttering in monolingual and bilingual stutterers. Journal of Communication Disorders; 1983 Jul Vol 16(4) 287–297

Jayaram, M. Relationship of stuttering to word information value in a phonemic clause. Journal of the All India Institute of Speech and Hearing; 1982 Vol 13 1–6

Jensen, Paul J.; Markel, Norman N.; Beverung, John W. Evidence of conversational disrhythmia in stutterers. Journal of Fluency Disorders; 1986 Sep Vol 11(3) 183–200

Kalveram, Karl T.; Jancke, Lutz. Vowel duration and voice onset time for stressed and nonstressed syllables in stutterers under delayed auditory feedback condition. Folia Phoniatrica; 1989 Jan–Feb Vol 41(1) 30–42

Klouda, Gayle V.; Cooper, William E. Syntactic clause boundaries, speech timing, and stuttering frequency in adult stutterers. Language and Speech; 1987 Jul–Sep Vol 30(3) 263–276

Kooman, E. A. Speech disturbance under delayed acoustic feedback and stuttering. Defektologiya; 1975 Jun No 6 27–33

Leith, William R.; Timmons, Jack L. The stutterer's reaction to the telephone as a speaking situation. Journal of Fluency Disorders; 1983 Sep Vol 8(3) 233–243

Liles, Betty Z.; Lerman, Jay; Christensen, Lisa; St. Ledger, Joy. A case description of verbal and signed disfluencies of a 10-year-old boy who is retarded. Language, Speech, and Hearing Services in Schools; 1992 Apr Vol 23(2) 107–112

Long, Karen M.; Pindzola, Rebekah H. Manual reaction time to linguistic stimuli in child stutterers and nonstutterers. Journal of Fluency Disorders; 1985 Jun Vol 10(2) 143–149

Lucke, Herman H. Treatment of language fluency disorders by a procedure combining several techniques. Revista Latinoamericana de Psicologia; 1977 Vol 9(3) 437–441

Martin, Richard; Parlour, Susan F.; Haroldson, Samuel. Stuttering and level of linguistic demand: The Stocker Probe. Journal of Fluency Disorders; 1990 Apr Vol 15(2) 93–106

McLaughlin, Scott F.; Cullinan, Walter L. Disfluencies, utterance length, and linguistic complexity in nonstuttering children. Journal of Fluency Disorders; 1989 Feb Vol 14(1) 17–36

McMillan, Marcia O.; Pindzola, Rebekah H. Temporal disruptions in the "accurate" speech of articulatory defective speakers and stutterers. Journal of Motor Behavior; 1986 Sep Vol 18(3) 279–286

Moore, W. H. Hemispheric alpha asymmetries of stutterers and nonstutterers for the recall and recognition of words and connected reading passages: Some relationships to severity of stuttering. Journal of Fluency Disorders; 1986 Mar Vol 11(1) 71–89

Myers, Florence L.; Wall, Meryl J. Toward an integrated approach to early childhood stuttering. Journal of Fluency Disorders; 1982 Mar Vol 7(1–1) 47–54

Neils, Jean; Aram, Dorothy M. Family history of children with developmental language disorders. Perceptual and Motor Skills; 1986 Oct Vol 63(2, Pt 1) 655–658

Newman, Parley W.; Fawcett, Kerilynn D.; Russon, Karen V. Cognitive processing in stuttering as related to translating slurvian. Journal of Fluency Disorders; 1986 Sep Vol 11(3) 251–256

Nicolaidis, Nicos; Papilloud, Janine. Une langue privee pour combler le manque. (A private language to fill a gap.) 47th Congress of Romance Languages Psychoanalysts (1987, Paris, France). Revue Francaise de Psychanalyse; 1988 Mar–Apr Vol 52(2) 523–531

Nippold, Marilyn A.; Schwarz, Ilsa E. Reading disorders in stuttering children. Journal of Fluency Disorders; 1990 Jun Vol 15(3) 175–189

Nippold, Marilyn A.; Schwarz, Ilsa E.; Jescheniak, Jorg Dieter. Narrative ability in school-age stuttering boys: A preliminary investigation. Journal of Fluency Disorders; 1991 Vol 16(5–6) 289–308

Nippold, Marilyn A. Concomitant speech and language disorders in stuttering children: A critique of the literature. Journal of Speech and Hearing Disorders; 1990 Feb Vol 55(1) 51–60

Nwokah, Evangeline E. The imbalance of stuttering behavior in bilingual speakers. Journal of Fluency Disorders; 1988 Oct Vol 13(5) 357–373

Palen, Chet; Peterson, Jodi M. Word frequency and children's stuttering: The relationship to sentence structure. Journal of Fluency Disorders; 1982 Mar Vol 7(1–1) 55–62

Perkins, William H.; Kent, Raymond D.; Curlee, Richard F. A theory of neuropsycholinguistic function in stuttering. Journal of Speech and Hearing Research; 1991 Aug Vol 34(4) 734–752

Peters, Herman F.; Starkweather, C. Woodruff. The interaction between speech motor coordination and language processes in the development of stuttering: Hypotheses and suggestions for research. Journal of Fluency Disorders; 1990 Apr Vol 15(2) 115–125

Peters, Herman F.; Starkweather, C. Woodruff. Development of stuttering throughout life. Journal of Fluency Disorders; 1989 Oct Vol 14(5) 303–321

Pollack, Janet; Lubinski, Rosemary; Weitzner Lin, Barbara. A pragmatic study of child dysfluency. Journal of Fluency Disorders; 1986 Sep Vol 11(3) 231–239

Rastatter, Michael P.; Dell, Carl W. Reading reaction times of stuttering and nonstuttering subjects to unilaterally presented concrete and abstract words. Journal of Fluency Disorders; 1988 Oct Vol 13(5) 319–329

Rastatter, Michael P.; Dell, Carl W. Simple visual versus lexical decision vocal reaction times of stuttering and normal subjects. Journal of Fluency Disorders; 1987 Feb Vol 12(1) 63–69

Rastatter, Michael P.; Dell, Carl. Vocal reaction times of stuttering subjects to tachistoscopically presented concrete and abstract words: A closer look at cerebral dominance and language processing. Journal of Speech and Hearing Research; 1987 Sep Vol 30(3) 306–310

Rastatter, Michael P.; Loren, Catherine A. Visual coding dominance in stuttering: Some evidence from central tachistoscopic stimulation (tachistoscopic viewing and stuttering). Journal of Fluency Disorders; 1988 Apr Vol 13(2) 89–95

Rastatter, Michael P.; McGuire, Richard A.; Loren, Catherine. Linguistic encoding dominance in stuttering: Some evidence for temporal and qualitative hemispheric processing differences. Journal of Fluency Disorders; 1988 Jun Vol 13(3) 215–224

Ratner, Nan B. Measurable outcomes of instructions to modify normal parent-child verbal interactions: Implications for indirect stuttering therapy. Journal of Speech and Hearing Research; 1992 Feb Vol 35(1) 14–20

Ratner, Nan B.; Sih, Catherine C. Effects of gradual increases in sentence length and complexity on children's dysfluency. Journal of Speech and Hearing Disorders; 1987 Aug Vol 52(3) 278–287

Riley, Glyndon D.; Riley, Jeanna. Motoric and linguistic variables among children who stutter: A factor analysis. Journal of Speech and Hearing Disorders; 1980 Nov Vol 45(4) 504–514

Ronson, Irwin. Word frequency and stuttering: The relationship to sentence structure. Journal of Speech and Hearing Research; 1976 Dec Vol 19(4) 813–819

Rosenfield, David B.; Goodglass, Harold. Dichotic testing of cerebral dominance in stutterers. Brain and Language; 1980 Sep Vol 11(1) 170–180

Ryan, Bruce P. Articulation, language, rate, and fluency characteristics of stuttering and nonstuttering preschool children. Journal of Speech and Hearing Research; 1992 Apr Vol 35(2) 333–342

Santacreu Mas, Jose. El condicionamiento ante determinadas palabras en la tartamudez. (Conditioning before some words in stuttering.) Revista de Psicologia General y Aplicada; 1984 Vol 39(6) 1115–1129

Santacreu Mas, Jose. Respuestas psicofisiologicas de sujetos tartamudos durante la pronunciacion de palabras. (Psychophysiological responses of stutterers during pronunciation of words.) Revista de Psicologia General y Aplicada; 1985 Vol 40(2) 221–242

Schultheis, Josef R. Stottern in historischer und "komplexer" Hinsicht. (Stuttering: Historical and complex perpectives.) Vierteljahresschrift fur Heilpadagogik und ihre Nachbargebiete; 1979 Jun Vol 48(2) 125–138

Schwartz, Arthur H.; Daly, David A. Elicited imitation in language assessment: A tool for formulating and evaluating treatment programs. Journal of Communication Disorders; 1978 Feb Vol 11(1) 25–35

Seidel, Christa; Biesalski, P. (Psychological and clinical experiences with the Frostig Test and the Frostig therapy in speech-impaired children.) Praxis der Kinderpsychologie und Kinderpsychiatrie; 1973 Jan Vol. 22(1) 3–15

Seider, Robin A.; Gladstien, Keith L.; Kidd, Kenneth K. Language onset and concomitant speech and language problems in subgroups of stutterers and their siblings. Journal of Speech and Hearing Research; 1982 Dec Vol 25(4) 482–486

Silverman, Ellen Marie. Effect of selected word attributes on preschoolers' speech disfluency: Initial phoneme and length. Journal of Speech and Hearing Research; 1975 Sep Vol 18(3) 430–434

Silverman, Ellen Marie. Word position and grammatical function in relation to preschoolers' speech disfluency. Perceptual and Motor Skills; 1974 Aug Vol 39(1) 267–272

Silverman, Franklin H. Do elementary-school stutterers talk less than their peers? Language, Speech and Hearing Services in the Schools; 1976 Apr Vol 7(2) 90–92

Silverman, Franklin H.; Umberger, Forrest G. Effect of pacing speech with a miniature electronic metronome on the frequency and duration of selected disfluency behaviors in the spontaneous speech of adult stutterers. Behavior Therapy; 1974 May Vol. 5(3) 410–414

Silverman, Lloyd H. An experimental method for the study of unconscious conflict: A progress report. British Journal of Medical Psychology; 1975 Dec Vol 48(4) 291–298

Smith, Anne. "A theory of neuropsycholinguistic function in stuttering": Commentary. Journal of Speech and Hearing Research; 1992 Aug Vol 35(4) 805–809

St. Louis, Kenneth O.; Hinzman, Audrey R. A descriptive study of speech, language, and hearing characteristics of school-aged stutterers. Journal of Fluency Disorders; 1988 Oct Vol 13(5) 331–355

St. Louis, Kenneth O.; Hinzman, Audrey R.; Hull, Forrest M. Studies of cluttering: Disfluency and language measures in young possible clutterers and stutterers. Journal of Fluency Disorders; 1985 Sep Vol 10(3) 151–172

St. Louis, Kenneth O.; Murray, Cheryl D.; Ashworth, Melanie S. Coexisting communication disorders in a random sample of school-aged stutterers. Journal of Fluency Disorders; 1991 Feb Vol 16(1) 13–23

Starkweather, C. Woodruff; Hirschman, Paula; Tannenbaum, Robert S. Latency of vocalization onset: Stutterers versus nonstutterers. Journal of Speech and Hearing Research; 1976 Sep Vol 19(3) 481–492

Stephenson-Opsal, Deborah; Bernstein-Ratner, Nan. Maternal speech rate modification and childhood stuttering. Annual Convention of the American Speech Language and Hearing Association (1986, Detroit, Michigan). Journal of Fluency Disorders; 1988 Feb Vol 13(1) 49–56

Sussman, Harvey M. Contrastive patterns of intrahemispheric interference to verbal and spatial concurrent tasks in right-handed, left-handed and stuttering populations. Neuropsychologia; 1982 Vol 20(6) 675–684

Tornick, Gaye B.; Bloodstein, Oliver. Stuttering and sentence length. Journal of Speech and Hearing Research; 1976 Dec Vol 19(4) 651–654

Van Jaarsveld, Pieter E.; du Plessis, Wynand F. Audio-psycho-phonology at Potchefstroom: A review. South African Journal of Psychology; 1988 Dec Vol 18(4) 136–143

Wall, Meryl J.; Myers, Florence L. A review of linguistic factors associated with early childhood stuttering. Journal of Communication Disorders; 1982 Nov Vol 15(6) 441–449

Watson, Ben C.; Freeman, Frances J.; Chapman, Sandra B.; Miller, Susan; et al. Linguistic performance deficits in stutterers: Relation to laryngeal reaction time profiles. Journal of Fluency Disorders; 1991 Vol 16(2–3) 85–100

Weiss, Amy, L.; Zebrowski, Patricia M. The narrative productions of children who stutter: A preliminary view. Journal of Fluency Disorders; 1994 19(1) 39–63

Wells, Betsy G.; Moore, W. H. EEG alpha asymmetries in stutterers and non-stutterers: Effects of linguistic variables on hemispheric processing and fluency. Neuropsychologia; 1990 Vol 28(12) 1295–1305

Westby, Carol E. Language performance of stuttering and nonstuttering children. Journal of Communication Disorders; 1979 Apr Vol 12(2) 133–145

Wingate, Marcel E. The first three words. Journal of Speech and Hearing Research; 1979 Sep Vol 22(3) 604–612

Wingate, Marcel E. The immediate source of stuttering: An integration of evidence. Journal of Communication Disorders; 1977 Mar Vol 10(1–2) 45–51

Wingate, Marcel E. The loci of stuttering: Grammar or prosody? Journal of Communication Disorders; 1979 Jul Vol 12(4) 283–290

Wingate, Marcel E. Stutter events and linguistic stress. Journal of Fluency Disorders; 1984 Dec Vol 9(4) 285–300

Yairi, Ehud. Longitudinal studies of disfluencies in two-year-old children. Journal of Speech and Hearing Research; 1982 Mar Vol 25(1) 155–160

Zivkovic, Momcilo. Validity and reliability of Initial Letter Word Association Test. Perceptual and Motor Skills; 1979 Oct Vol 49(2) 366

Motor Speech

Andronova, L. Z.; Arutiunyan, M. A.; Aleksandrovskaya, A. S. On the influence of singing on stuttering. Defektologiya; 1987 No 4 58–60

Beliakova, L. I.; Kumalia, I. (Comparative analysis of motor and speech-motor functions in preschool stutterers.) Defektologiya; 1985 No 1 69–74

Bishop, Judith H.; Williams, Harriet G.; Cooper, William A. Age and task complexity variables in motor performance of children with articulation-disordered, stuttering, and normal speech. Journal of Fluency Disorders; 1991 Vol 16(4) 219–228

Borden, Gloria J. Initiation versus execution time during manual and oral counting by stutterers. Journal of Speech and Hearing Research; 1983 Sep Vol 26(3) 389–396

Brutten, Gene J.; Trotter, Alice C. A dual-task investigation of young stutterers and nonstutterers. Journal of Fluency Disorders; 1986 Dec Vol 11(4) 275–284

Brutten, Gene J.; Trotter, Alice C. Hemispheric interference: A dual-task investigation of youngsters who stutter. Journal of Fluency Disorders; 1985 Jun Vol 10(2) 77–85

Byrd, Kathryn; Cooper, Eugene B. Apraxic speech characteristics in stuttering, developmentally apraxic, and normal speaking children. Journal of Fluency Disorders; 1989 Jun Vol 14(3) 215–229

Caruso, Anthony J.; Conture, Edward G.; Colton, Raymond H. Selected temporal parameters of coordination associated with stuttering in children. Journal of Fluency Disorders; 1988 Feb Vol 13(1) 57–82

Conture, Edward G.; Colton, Raymond H.; Gleason, John R. "Comment on Conture et al. (1988) and Prosek et al. (1988)": Reply. Journal of Speech and Hearing Research; 1990 Jun Vol 33(2) 404–406

Conture, Edward G.; Colton, Raymond H.; Gleason, John R. Selected temporal aspects of coordination during fluent speech of young stutterers. Journal of Speech and Hearing Research; 1988 Dec Vol 31(4) 640–653

Conture, Edward G.; Kelly, Ellen M. Young stutterers' nonspeech behaviors during stuttering. Journal of Speech and Hearing Research; 1991 Oct Vol 34(5) 1041–1056

Conture, Edward G.; Rothenberg, Martin; Molitor, Richard D. Electroglottographic observations of young stutterers' fluency. Journal of Speech and Hearing Research; 1986 Sep Vol 29(3) 384–393

Cooper, Margaret H.; Allen, George D. Timing control accuracy in normal speakers and stutterers. Journal of Speech and Hearing Research; 1977 Mar Vol 20(1) 55–71

Cross, Douglas E. Comparison of reaction time and accuracy measures of laterality for stutterers and normal speakers. Journal of Fluency Disorders; 1987 Aug Vol 12(4) 271–286

Cross, Douglas E.; Olson, Patricia. Interaction between jaw kinematics and voice onset for stutterers and nonstutterers in a VRT task. Journal of Fluency Disorders; 1987 Oct Vol 12(5) 367–380

Cross, Douglas E.; Olson, Patricia L. Articulatory-laryngeal interaction in stutterers and normal speakers: Effects of a bite-block on rapid voice initiation. Journal of Fluency Disorders; 1987 Dec Vol 12(6) 407–418

Crowe, Kathryn M.; Kroll, Robert M. Response latency and response class for stutterers and nonstutterers as measured by a word-association task. Journal of Fluency Disorders; 1991 Feb Vol 16(1) 35–54

Devenny, Darlynne A.; Silverman, W.; Balgley, H.; Wall, M. J.; et al. Specific motor abilities associated with speech fluency in Down's syndrome. Journal of Mental Deficiency Research; 1990 Oct Vol 34(5) 437–443

DiSimoni, Frank. Comment on Conture et al. (1988) and Prosek et al. (1988). Journal of Speech and Hearing Research; 1990 Jun Vol 33(2) 402–404

Ferrand, Carole T.; Gilbert, Harvey R.; Blood, Gordon W. Selected aspects of central processing and vocal motor function in stutterers and nonstutterers. Journal of Fluency Disorders; 1991 Vol 16(2–3) 101–115

Forster, David C.; Webster, William G. Concurrent task interference in stutterers: Dissociating hemispheric specialization and activation. Canadian Journal of Psychology; 1991 Sep Vol 45(3) 321–335

Geschwind, Norman. Biological associations of left-handedness. Annals of Dyslexia; 1983 Vol 33 29–40

Goldsmith, Howard. Some comments on "Articulatory dynamics of fluent utterances of stutterers and nonstutterers." Journal of Speech and Hearing Research; 1983 Jun Vol 26(2) 319–320

Gregory, Hugo H. Stuttering: A contemporary perspective. XXth Congress of the International Association of Logopedics and Phonia-trics (1986, Tokyo, Japan). Folia Phoniatrica; 1986 Mar-Aug Vol 38(2–4) 89–120

Greiner, Jay R.; Fitzgerald, Hiram E.; Cooke, Paul A. Speech fluency and hand performance on a sequential tapping task in left- and right-handed stutterers and nonstutterers. Journal of Fluency Disorders; 1986 Mar Vol 11(1) 55–69

Guitar, Barry. Reduction of stuttering frequency using analog electromyographic feedback. Journal of Speech and Hearing Research; 1975 Dec Vol 18(4) 672–685

Guitar, Barry; Guitar, Carroll; Neilson, Peter; O'Dwyer, Nicholas; et al. Onset sequencing of selected lip muscles in stutterers and nonstutterers. Journal of Speech and Hearing Research; 1988 Mar Vol 31(1) 28–35

Hand, C. Rebekah; Haynes, William O. Linguistic processing and reaction time differences in stutterers and nonstutterers. Journal of Speech and Hearing Research; 1983 Jun Vol 26(2) 181–185

Harbison, Dan C.; Porter, Robert J.; Tobey, Emily A. Shadowed and simple reaction times in stutterers and nonstutterers. Journal of the Acoustical Society of America; 1989 Oct Vol 86(4) 1277–1284

Harrington, Jonathan. Stuttering, delayed auditory feedback, and linguistic rhythm. Journal of Speech and Hearing Research; 1988 Mar Vol 31(1) 36–47

Healey, E. Charles; Adams, Martin R. Speech timing skills of normally fluent and stuttering children and adults. Journal of Fluency Disorders; 1981 Sep Vol 6(3) 233–246

Howell, Peter; El Yaniv, Nirit. The effects of presenting a click in syllable-initial position on the speech of stutterers: Comparison with a metronome click. Journal of Fluency Disorders; 1987 Aug Vol 12(4) 249–256

Hulstijn, Wouter; Summers, Jeffery J.; Van Lieshout, Pascal H.; Peters, Herman F. Timing in finger tapping and speech: A comparison between stutterers and fluent speakers. Special Issue: Sequencing and timing of human movement. Human Movement Science; 1992 Feb Vol 11(1–2) 113–124

Hurford, David P.; Webster, Ronald L. Decreases in simple reaction time as a function of stutterers' participation in a behavioral therapy. Journal of Fluency Disorders; 1985 Dec Vol 10(4) 301–310

Hutchinson, John M.; Watkin, Kenneth L. Jaw mechanics during release of the stuttering moment: Some initial observations and interpretations. Journal of Communication Disorders; 1976 Dec Vol 9(4) 269–279

Ikezuki, Makoto; Harano, Kotaro; Yamaguchi, Shoji. (Research on the effect of reciprocal inhibition elicited with kinetic response.) Japanese Journal of Behavior Therapy; 1989 Vol 15(1) 56–61

Janssen, Peggy; Kraaimaat, Floor. Onset and termination of accessory facial movements during stuttering. Perceptual and Motor Skills; 1986 Aug Vol 63(1) 11–17

Janssen, Peggy; Kraaimaat, Floor; Brutten, Gene. Relationship between stutterers' genetic history and speech-associated variables. Journal of Fluency Disorders; 1990 Feb Vol 15(1) 39–48

Kalotkin, Madeline; Manschreck, Theo C.; O'Brien, Donna. Electromyographic tension levels in stutterers and normal speakers. Perceptual and Motor Skills; 1979 Aug Vol 49(1) 109–110

Kalveram, K. A neural-network model enabling sensorimotor learning: Application to the control of arm movements and some implications for speech motor control and stuttering. Psychological Research/Psychologische Forschung; 1993 55(4) 299–314

Klouda, Gayle V.; Cooper, William E. Syntactic clause boundaries, speech timing, and stuttering frequency in adult stutterers. Language and Speech; 1987 Jul-Sep Vol 30(3) 263–276

Kraaimaat, Floor; Janssen, Peggy. Are the accessory facial movements of the stutterer learned behaviours? Perceptual and Motor Skills; 1985 Feb Vol 60(1) 11–17

Long, Karen M.; Pindzola, Rebekah H. Manual reaction time to linguistic stimuli in child stutterers and nonstutterers. Journal of Fluency Disorders; 1985 Jun Vol 10(2) 143–149

MacKenzie, Catherine. Aphasic articulatory defect and aphasic phonological defect. British Journal of Disorders of Communication; 1982 Apr Vol 17(1) 27–46

McClean, Michael D. Neuromotor aspects of stuttering: Levels of impairment and disability. ASHA Reports Series American Speech Language Hearing Association; 1990 Apr No 18 64–71

McClean, Michael D. Surface EMG recording of the perioral reflexes: Preliminary observations on stutterers and nonstutterers. Journal of Speech and Hearing Research; 1987 Jun Vol 30(2) 283–287

McClean, Michael D.; Goldsmith, Howard; Cerf, Ann. Lower-lip EMG and displacement during bilabial disfluencies in adult stutterers. Journal of Speech and Hearing Research; 1984 Sep Vol 27(3) 342–349

McClean, Michael D.; Kroll, Robert M.; Loftus, Nirit S. Kinematic analysis of lip closure in stutterers' fluent speech. Journal of Speech and Hearing Research; 1990 Dec Vol 33(4) 755–760

McFarlane, Stephen C.; Prins, David. Neural response time of stutterers and nonstutterers in selected oral motor tasks. Journal of Speech and Hearing Research; 1978 Dec Vol 21(4) 768–778

McFarlane, Stephen C.; Prins, David. Neural response time of stutterers and nonstutterers in selected oral motor tasks. Journal of Speech and Hearing Research; 1978 Dec Vol 21(4) 768–778

Mesalam, Linda. The power of communication. Cognitive Rehabilitation; 1988 May-Jun Vol 6(3) 32–36

Moore, Walter H. Pathophysiology of stuttering: Cerebral activation differences in stutterers vs. nonstutterers. ASHA Reports Series American Speech Language Hearing Association; 1990 Apr No 18 72–80

Newman, Parley W.; Channell, Ron; Palmer, Mary L. A comparative study of the independence of unilateral ocular motor control in stutterers and nonstutterers. Journal of Fluency Disorders; 1986 Jun Vol 11(2) 105–116

Nudelman, H. B.; Herbrich, K. E.; Hoyt, B. D.; Rosenfield, D. B. A neuroscience model of stuttering. Journal of Fluency Disorders; 1989 Dec Vol 14(6) 399–427

Oganesian, Ye. V.; Beliakova, L. I. The rationale for principles of differential application of logopaedic rhythmics in remediation of adult stutterers. Defektologiya; 1982 No 1 3–12

Oganesyan, E. V. (Analysis of interrelations among some aspects of the motor sphere and speech in adult stutterers.) Defektologiya; 1983 No 3 16–20

Parry, William D. Stuttering and the Valsalva mechanism: A hypothesis in need of investigation. Journal of Fluency Disorders; 1985 Dec Vol 10(4) 317–324

Perkins, William H. Implications of scientific research for treatment of stuttering: A lecture. Journal of Fluency Disorders; 1981 Jun Vol 6(2) 155–162

Perkins, William H.; Bell, Jody; Johnson, Linda; Stocks, Janice. Phone rate and the effective planning time hypothesis of stuttering. Journal of Speech and Hearing Research; 1979 Dec Vol 22(4) 747–755

Perkins, William H.; Kent, Raymond D.; Curlee, Richard F. A theory of neuropsycholinguistic function in stuttering. Journal of Speech and Hearing Research; 1991 Aug Vol 34(4) 734–752

Perkins, William; Rudas, Joanna; Johnson, Linda; Bell, Jody. Stuttering: Discoordination of phonation with articulation and respiration. Journal of Speech and Hearing Research; 1976 Sep Vol 19(3) 509–522

Peters, Herman F.; Boves, Louis. Coordination of aerodynamic and phonatory processes in fluent speech utterances of stutterers. Journal of Speech and Hearing Research; 1988 Sep Vol 31(3) 352–361

Peters, Herman F.; Hulstijn, Wouter; Starkweather, C. Woodruff. Acoustic and physiological reaction times of stutterers and nonstutterers. Journal of Speech and Hearing Research; 1989 Sep Vol 32(3) 668–680

Peters, Herman F.; Starkweather, C. Woodruff. The interaction between speech motor coordination and language processes in the development of stuttering: Hypotheses and suggestions for research. Journal of Fluency Disorders; 1990 Apr Vol 15(2) 115–125

Platt, L. Jay; Basili, Annamaria. Jaw tremor during stuttering block: An electromyographic study. Journal of Communication Disorders; 1973 Jun Vol. 6(2) 102–109

Postma, Albert; Kolk, Herman; Povel, Dirk Jan. Speech planning and execution in stutterers. Journal of Fluency Disorders; 1990 Feb Vol 15(1) 49–59

Prescott, John. Event-related potential indices of speech motor programming in stutterers and non-stutterers. Biological Psychology; 1988 Dec Vol 27(3) 259–273

Prosek, Robert A.; Montgomery, Allen A.; Walden, Brian E. Constancy of relative timing for stutterers and nonstutterers. Journal of Speech and Hearing Research; 1988 Dec Vol 31(4) 654–658

Rastatter, Michael; Dell, Carl W. Simple motor and phonemic processing reaction times of stutterers. Perceptual and Motor Skills; 1985 Oct Vol 61(2) 463–466

Reich, Alan; Till, James A.; Goldsmith, Howard. Laryngeal and manual reaction times of stuttering and nonstuttering adults. Journal of Speech and Hearing Research; 1981 Jan Vol 24(2) 192–196

Riley, Glyndon; Riley, Jeanna. Oral motor discoordination among children who stutter. Journal of Fluency Disorders; 1986 Dec Vol 11(4) 335–344

Riley, Glyndon D.; Riley, Jeanna. Motoric and linguistic variables among children who stutter: A factor analysis. Journal of Speech and Hearing Disorders; 1980 Nov Vol 45(4) 504–514

Rychkova, N. A. State of voluntary motor activity and speech in preschool children with neurotic and pseudo-neurotic forms of stuttering. Defektologiya; 1981 No 6 73–77

Scheiber, Stephen C.; Ziesat, Harold. Clinical and psychological test findings in cerebral dyspraxia associated with hemodialysis. Journal of Nervous and Mental Disease; 1976 Mar Vol 162(3) 212–214

Schultheis, Josef R. Modern theories of stuttering. Praxis der Kinderpsychologie und Kinderpsychiatrie; 1978 Apr Vol 27(3) 83–87

Schultheis, Josef R. Stottern in historischer und "komplexer" Hinsicht. (Stuttering: Historical and complex perpectives.) Vierteljahresschrift fur Heilpadagogik und ihre Nachbargebiete; 1979 Jun Vol 48(2) 125–138

Smith, Anne. Neural drive to muscles in stuttering. Journal of Speech and Hearing Research; 1989 Jun Vol 32(2) 252–264

Smith, Anne; Luschei, Erich S. Assessment of oral-motor reflexes in stutterers and normal speakers: Preliminary observations. Journal of Speech and Hearing Research; 1983 Sep Vol 26(3) 322–328

Starkweather, C. Woodruff; Franklin, Sharon; Smigo, Therese M. Vocal and finger reaction times in stutterers and nonstutterers: Differences and correlations. Journal of Speech and Hearing Research; 1984 Jun Vol 27(2) 193–196

Sussman, Harvey M. Contrastive patterns of intrahemispheric interference to verbal and spatial concurrent tasks in right-handed, left-handed and stuttering populations. Neuropsychologia; 1982 Vol 20(6) 675–684

Till, James A.; Reich, Alan; Dickey, Stanley; Seiber, James. Phonatory and manual reaction times of stuttering and nonstuttering children. Journal of Speech and Hearing Research; 1983 Jun Vol 26(2) 171–180

Vekassy, Laszlo. Dadogok oral-praxia es oral stereognosis vizsgalata. / Oral praxia and oral stereognosis examinations in stutterers. Magyar Pszichologiai Szemle; 1987–88 Vol 44(4) 291–304

Venkatagiri, Horabail S. Reaction time for voiced and whispered /a/ in stutterers and nonstutterers. Journal of Fluency Disorders; 1981 Sep Vol 6(3) 265–271

Weber, Christine M.; Smith, Anne. Autonomic correlates of stuttering and speech assessed in a range of experimental tasks. Journal of Speech and Hearing Research; 1990 Dec Vol 33(4) 690–706

Webster, William G. Evidence in bimanual finger-tapping of an attentional component to stuttering. Behavioural Brain Research; 1990 Mar Vol 37(2) 93–100

Webster, William G. Motor performance of stutterers: A search for mechanisms. Journal of Motor Behavior; 1990 Dec Vol 22(4) 553–571

Webster, William G. Neural mechanisms underlying stuttering: Evidence from bimanual handwriting performance. Brain and Language; 1988 Mar Vol 33(2) 226–244

Webster, William G. Neuropsychological models of stuttering: I. Representation of sequential response mechanisms. Neuropsychologia; 1985 Vol 23(2) 263–267

Webster, William G. Neuropsychological models of stuttering: II. Interhemispheric interference. Neuropsychologia; 1986 Vol 24(5) 737–741

Webster, William G. Rapid letter transcription performance by stutterers. Neuropsychologia; 1987 Vol 25(5) 845–847

Webster, William G. Response sequence organization and reproduction by stutterers. Neuropsychologia; 1986 Vol 24(6) 813–821

Webster, William G. Sequence initiation performance by stutterers under conditions of response competition. Brain and Language; 1989 Feb Vol 36(2) 286–300

Webster, William G.; Ryan, C. Lynne. Task complexity and manual reaction times in people who stutter. Journal of Speech and Hearing Research; 1991 Aug Vol 34(4) 708–714

Winkler, Lisa E.; Ramig, Peter. Temporal characteristics in the fluent speech of child stutterers and nonstutterers. Journal of Fluency Disorders; 1986 Sep Vol 11(3) 217–229

Zimmermann, Gerald. Articulatory behaviors associated with stuttering: A cinefluorographic analysis. Journal of Speech and Hearing Research; 1980 Mar Vol 23(1) 108–121

Zimmermann, Gerald. Stuttering: A disorder of movement. Journal of Speech and Hearing Research; 1980 Mar Vol 23(1) 122–136

Zimmermann, Gerald. Articulatory dynamics of fluent utterances of stutterers and nonstutterers. Journal of Speech and Hearing Research; 1980 Mar Vol 23(1) 95–107

Zimmermann, Gerald N. In agreement with Goldsmith. Journal of Speech and Hearing Research; 1983 Jun Vol 26(2) 320

Zimmermann, Gerald N.; Hanley, J. M. A cinefluorographic investigation of repeated fluent productions of stutterers in an adaptation procedure. Journal of Speech and Hearing Research; 1983 Mar Vol 26(1) 35–42

Zimmermann, Gerald N.; Smith, Anne; Hanley, John M. Stuttering: In need of a unifying conceptual framework. Journal of Speech and Hearing Research; 1981 Mar Vol 24(1) 25–31

Neurology

Abeleva, I. Yu. Respiration dynamics during speech production in stuttering adults. Defektologiya; 1976 Jan No 1 17–20

Ananthamurthy, H. S.; Parameswaran, T. M. Management of speech problems. Child Psychiatry Quarterly; 1978 Jan Vol 11(1) 10–13

Andrews, Gavin; Tanner, Susan. Stuttering treatment: An attempt to replicate the regulated-breathing method. Journal of Speech and Hearing Disorders; 1982 May Vol 47(2) 138–140

Andy, Orlando J.; Bhatnagar, Subhash C. Stuttering acquired from subcortical pathologies and its alleviation from thalamic perturbation. Brain and Language; 1992 May Vol 42(4) 385–401

Andy, Orlando J.; Bhatnagar, Subhash C. Thalamic-induced stuttering (surgical observations). Journal of Speech and Hearing Research; 1991 Aug Vol 34(4) 796–800

Aram, Dorothy M.; Meyers, Susan C.; Ekelman, Barbara L. Fluency of conversational speech in children with unilateral brain lesions. Brain and Language; 1990 Jan Vol 38(1) 105–121

Ardila, Alfredo; Lopez, Maria V. Severe stuttering associated with right hemisphere lesion. Brain and Language; 1986 Mar Vol 27(2) 239–246

Arends, Nico; Povel, Dirk Jan; Kolk, Herman. Stuttering as an attentional phenomenon. Journal of Fluency Disorders; 1988 Apr Vol 13(2) 141–151

Azrin, Nathan H.; Nunn, Robert G.; Frantz, Sharmon E. Comparison of regulated-breathing versus abbreviated desensitization on reported stuttering episodes. Journal of Speech and Hearing Disorders; 1979 Aug Vol 44(3) 331–339

Ballesteros, Rocio F.; Mas, Jose S.; Carrobles, Jose A. Relaciones entre respuestas psicofisiologicas y autoinformes. / Relationships between psychophysiological responses and self-reports. Analisis y Modificacion de Conducta; 1984 Vol 10(25) 299–311

Becker, H. Ungewohnliche Sprechstorungen bei der endogenen Depression. / Unusual speech disorders in endogenous depression. Nervenarzt; 1989 Dec Vol 60(12) 757–758

Berezhkovskaya, E. L.; Golod, V. I.; Turovskaya, Z. G. Sensory asymmetry in stutterers and normal individuals. Voprosy Psikhologii; 1980 No 1 57–63

Bhatnagar, Subhash C.; Andy, Orlando J. Alleviation of acquired stuttering with human centremedian thalamic stimulation. Journal of Neurology, Neurosurgery and Psychiatry; 1989 Oct Vol 52(10) 1182–1184

Blood, Gordon W. Laterality differences in child stutterers: Heterogeneity, severity levels, and statistical treatments. Journal of Speech and Hearing Disorders; 1985 Feb Vol 50(1) 66–72

Blood, Gordon W.; Blood, Ingrid M. Central auditory function in young stutterers. Perceptual and Motor Skills; 1984 Dec Vol 59(3) 699–705

Blood, Gordon W.; Blood, Ingrid M.; Newton, Karen R. Effect of directed attention on cerebral asymmetries in stuttering adults. Perceptual and Motor Skills; 1986 Apr Vol 62(2) 351–355

Blood, Gordon W.; Blood, Ingrid M. Laterality preferences in adult female and male stutterers. Journal of Fluency Disorders; 1989 Feb Vol 14(1) 1–10

Blood, Gordon W.; Blood, Ingrid M.; Hood, Stephen B. The development of ear preferences in stuttering and nonstuttering children: A longitudinal study. Journal of Fluency Disorders; 1987 Apr Vol 12(2) 119–131

Blood, Ingrid M.; Blood, Gordon W. Relationship between stuttering severity and brainstem-evoked response testing. Perceptual and Motor Skills; 1984 Dec Vol 59(3) 935–938

Bloom, Leon. Notes for a history of speech pathology. Psychoanalytic Review; 1978 Fal Vol 65(3) 433–463

Boberg, Einer; Yeudall, Lorne T.; Schopflocher, Donald; Bo Lassen, Peter. The effect of an intensive behavioral program on the distribution of EEG alpha power in stutterers during the processing of verbal and visuospatial information. Journal of Fluency Disorders; 1983 Sep Vol 8(3) 245–263

Bojanin, Svetomir; Vuletic Peco, Aleksandra; Radojkovic, Dejan. Porodica dece sa razvojnim hiperkinetskim sindromom, tikovima i mucanjem. (Families of children with developing hyperkinetic syndrome, tics, and stuttering.) Psihijatrija Danas; 1991 Vol 23(1–2) 37–48

Borden, Gloria J. Initiation versus execution time during manual and oral counting by stutterers. Journal of Speech and Hearing Research; 1983 Sep Vol 26(3) 389–396

Boudreau, Leonce; Ladouceur, Robert. L'influence de l'aide sociale associee a la respiration regularisee sur le traitement du begaiement. / The influence of social help associated with regularized respiration on the treatment of stuttering. Technologie et Therapie du Comportement; 1985 Fal Vol 8(2) 125–151

Brady, John P.; Berson, Janet. Stuttering, dichotic listening, and cerebral dominance. Archives of General Psychiatry; 1975 Nov Vol 32(11) 1449–1452

Brutten, Gene J.; Trotter, Alice C. A dual-task investigation of young stutterers and nonstutterers. Journal of Fluency Disorders; 1986 Dec Vol 11(4) 275–284

Brutten, Gene J.; Trotter, Alice C. Hemispheric interference: A dual-task investigation of youngsters who stutter. Journal of Fluency Disorders; 1985 Jun Vol 10(2) 77–85

Burd, Larry; Kerbeshian, Jacob. Stuttering and stimulants. Journal of Clinical Psychopharmacology; 1991 Feb Vol 11(1) 72–73

Byrd, Kathryn; Cooper, Eugene B. Apraxic speech characteristics in stuttering, developmentally apraxic, and normal speaking children. Journal of Fluency Disorders; 1989 Jun Vol 14(3) 215–229

Campbell, Michel; Boudreau, Leonce; Ladouceur, Robert. L'influence d'interlocuteurs sur l'evaluation du begaiement. (The influence of speakers on the evaluation of stuttering.) Revue de Modification du Comportement; 1984 Vol 14(3) 112–122

Caron, Chantal; Ladouceur, Robert. Multidimensional behavioral treatment for child stutterers. Behavior Modification; 1989 Apr Vol 13(2) 206–215

Carpenter, Mary; Sommers, Ronald K. Unisensory and bisensory perceptual and memory processing in stuttering adults and normal speakers. Journal of Fluency Disorders; 1987 Aug Vol 12(4) 291–304

Caruso, Anthony J.; Conture, Edward G.; Colton, Raymond H. Selected temporal parameters of coordination associated with stuttering in children. Journal of Fluency Disorders; 1988 Feb Vol 13(1) 57–82

Cassar, Mary C. Stuttering and hypnosis: Processes of cortical control. Australian Journal of Clinical Hypnotherapy and Hypnosis; 1988 Sep Vol 9(2) 49–65

Christensen, John M. Did primitive man really talk like an ape? Journal of Speech and Hearing Research; 1992 Aug Vol 35(4) 805

Cimorell-Strong, Jacqueline M.; Gilbert, Harvey R.; Frick, James V. Dichotic speech perception: A comparison between stuttering and nonstuttering children. Journal of Fluency Disorders; 1983 Mar Vol 8(1) 77–91

Code, Chris. Dichotic listening with the communicatively impaired: Results from trials of a short British-English dichotic word test. Journal of Phonetics; 1981 Oct Vol 9(4) 375–383

Conture, Edward G.; Colton, Raymond H.; Gleason, John R. Selected temporal aspects of coordination during fluent speech of young stutterers. Journal of Speech and Hearing Research; 1988 Dec Vol 31(4) 640–653

Cooper, Eugene B. A brain-stem contusion and fluency: Vicki's story. Journal of Fluency Disorders; 1983 Sep Vol 8(3) 269–274

Cordes, Anne K.; Gow, Merrilyn L.; Ingham, Roger J. On valid and reliable identification of normal disfluencies and stuttering disfluencies: A response to Aram, Meyers, and Ekelman (1990). Brain and Language; 1991 Feb Vol 40(2) 282–286

Costa, D.; Antoniac, Maria; Berghianu, S.; Marinescu, Rodica; et al. Clinical and paraclinical aspects of tetany in stuttering. Activitas Nervosa Superior; 1986 Vol 28(2) 156–158

Costa, D.; Pop, A.; Dumitriu, L.; Marinescu, Luzia; et al. Serum immunoreactive parathormone levels correlate with depression and anxiety in hypocalcemic stutterers. Activitas Nervosa Superior; 1986 Vol 28(2) 155–156

Cote, Christiane; Ladouceur, Robert. Effects of social aids and the regulated breathing method in the treatment of stutterers. Journal of Consulting and Clinical Psychology; 1982 Jun Vol 50(3) 450

Cross, Douglas E. Comparison of reaction time and accuracy measures of laterality for stutterers and normal speakers. Journal of Fluency Disorders; 1987 Aug Vol 12(4) 271–286

Crowe, Kathryn M.; Kroll, Robert M. Response latency and response class for stutterers and nonstutterers as measured by a word-association task. Journal of Fluency Disorders; 1991 Feb Vol 16(1) 35–54

Cullinan, Walter L.; Springer, Mark T. Voice initiation and termination times in stuttering and nonstuttering children. Journal of Speech and Hearing Research; 1980 Jun Vol 23(2) 344–360

Dellatolas, Georges; Annesi, Isabella; Jallon, Pierre; Chavance, Michel; et al. An epidemiological reconsideration of the Geschwind Galaburda theory of cerebral lateralization. Archives of Neurology; 1990 Jul Vol 47(7) 778–782

Devenny, Darlynne A.; Silverman, W.; Balgley, H.; Wall, M. J.; et al. Specific motor abilities associated with speech fluency in Down's syndrome. Journal of Mental Deficiency Research; 1990 Oct Vol 34(5) 437–443

Dorman, M. F.; Porter, R. J. Hemispheric lateralization for speech perception in stutterers. Cortex; 1975 Jun Vol 11(2) 181–185

Dugas, Michel; Ladouceur, Robert. Traitement multidimensionnel et progressif des begues severes. (Multidimensional and progressive treatment of severe stuttering.) Science et Comportement; 1988 Win Vol 18(4) 221–232

Emrich, H. M.; Eilert, P. Evaluation of speech and language in neuropsychiatric disorders. Archiv fur Psychiatrie und Nervenkrankheiten; 1978 Vol 225(3) 209–221

Falkowski, Glenn L.; Guilford, Arthur M.; Sandler, Jack. Effectiveness of a modified version of airflow therapy: Case studies. Journal of Speech and Hearing Disorders; 1982 May Vol 47(2) 160–164

Farmer, Alvirda. Stuttering repetitions in aphasic and nonaphasic brain damaged adults. Cortex; 1975 Dec Vol 11(4) 391–396

Ferrand, Carole T.; Gilbert, Harvey R.; Blood, Gordon W. Selected aspects of central processing and vocal motor function in stutterers and nonstutterers. Journal of Fluency Disorders; 1991 Vol 16(2–3) 101–115

Fitch, James L.; Batson, Elizabeth A. Hemispheric asymmetry of alpha wave suppression in stutterers and nonstutterers. Journal of Fluency Disorders; 1989 Feb Vol 14(1) 47–55

Fitzgerald, Hiram E.; Cooke, Paul A.; Greiner, Jay R. Speech and bimanual hand organization in adult stutterers and nonstutterers. Journal of Fluency Disorders; 1984 Feb Vol 9(1) 51–65

Fleet, W. Shepherd; Heilman, Kenneth M. Acquired stuttering from a right hemisphere lesion in a right-hander. Neurology; 1985 Sep Vol 35(9) 1343–1346

Forster, David C.; Webster, William G. Concurrent task interference in stutterers: Dissociating hemispheric specialization and activation. Canadian Journal of Psychology; 1991 Sep Vol 45(3) 321–335

Franke, Ulrike. Zur Frage de mannlichen Disposition fur Kommunikationsstorungen. / Predisposition of males for communication disorders. Folia Phoniatrica; 1985 Jan–Feb Vol 37(1) 36–43

Freedman, Morris; Alexander, Michael P.; Naeser, Margaret A. Anatomic basis of transcortical motor aphasia. Neurology; 1984 Apr Vol 34(4) 409–417

Fucci, Donald; Petrosino, Linda; Gorman, Peter; Harris, Daniel. Vibrotactile magnitude production scaling: A method for studying sensory-perceptual responses of stutterers and fluent speakers. Journal of Fluency Disorders; 1985 Mar Vol 10(1) 69–75

Fucci, Donald J.; Petrosino, Linda; Schuster, Susan; Belch, Marianne. Lingual vibrotactile threshold shift differences between stutterers and normal speakers during magnitude-estimation scaling. Perceptual and Motor Skills; 1991 Aug Vol 73(1) 55–62

Garcia-Moreno, Juan. Tratamiento de la tartamudez por el metodo de la regulacion de la respiracion. (Treatment of stuttering by the regulated-breathing method.) Informes de Psicologia; 1985 Vol 4(1–2) 67–72

Goldstein, Jay A. Carbamazepine treatment for stuttering. Journal of Clinical Psychiatry; 1987 Jan Vol 48(1) 39

Gregory, Hugo H. Stuttering: A contemporary perspective. XXth Congress of the International Association of Logopedics and

Phoniatrics (1986, Tokyo, Japan). Folia Phoniatrica; 1986 Mar–Aug Vol 38(2–4) 89–120

Greiner, Jay R.; Fitzgerald, Hiram E.; Cooke, Paul A. Speech fluency and hand performance on a sequential tapping task in left- and right-handed stutterers and nonstutterers. Journal of Fluency Disorders; 1986 Mar Vol 11(1) 55–69

Gruber, L.; Powell, R. L. Responses of stuttering and non-stuttering children to a dichotic listening task. Perceptual and Motor Skills; 1974 Feb Vol. 38(1) 263–264

Hall, James W.; Jerger, James. Central auditory function in stutterers. Journal of Speech and Hearing Research; 1978 Jun Vol 21(2) 324–337

Hand, C. Rebekah; Haynes, William O. Linguistic processing and reaction time differences in stutterers and nonstutterers. Journal of Speech and Hearing Research; 1983 Jun Vol 26(2) 181–185

Harbison, Dan C.; Porter, Robert J.; Tobey, Emily A. Shadowed and simple reaction times in stutterers and nonstutterers. Journal of the Acoustical Society of America; 1989 Oct Vol 86(4) 1277–1284

Harris, Daniel; Fucci, Donald; Petrosino, Linda. Magnitude estimation and cross-modal matching of auditory and lingual vibrotactile sensation by normal speakers and stutterers. Journal of Speech and Hearing Research; 1991 Feb Vol 34(1) 177–182

Hasbrouck, Jon M.; Lowry, Fran. Elimination of stuttering and maintenance of fluency by means of airflow, tension reduction, and discriminative stimulus control procedures. Journal of Fluency Disorders; 1989 Jun Vol 14(3) 165–183

Helm, Nancy A.; Butler, Russell B.; Benson, D. Frank. Acquired stuttering. Neurology; 1978 Nov Vol 28(1) 1159–1165

Helm-Estabrooks, Nancy; Yeo, Ronald; Geschwind, Norman; Freedman, Morris; et al. Stuttering: Disappearance and reappearance with acquired brain lesions. Neurology; 1986 Aug Vol 36(8) 1109–1112

Helm-Estabrooks, Nancy; Yeo, Ronald; Geschwind, Norman; Freedman, Morris; et al. Anomalous dominance in sibling stutterers: Evidence from CT scan asymmetries, dichotic listening, neuropsychological testing, and handedness.

Horner, Jennifer; Massey, E. Wayne. Progressive dysfluency associated with right hemisphere disease. Brain and Language; 1983 Jan Vol 18(1) 71–85

Horovitz, Linda J.; et al. Stapedial reflex and anxiety in fluent and disfluent speakers. Journal of Speech and Hearing Research; 1978 Dec Vol 21(4) 762–767

Ivanova, G. A.; Lapa, A. Z.; Lokhov, M. I.; Movsisyants, S. A. EEG features in stammering pre-school children. Zhurnal Nevropatologii i Psikhiatrii imeni S.S. Korsakova; 1990 Vol 90(3) 78–81

Ivanova, G. A.; Lapa, A. Z.; Lokhov, M. I.; Movsisyants, S. A. Features of stuttering pre-school children. Neuroscience and Behavioral Physiology; 1991 May–Jun Vol 21(3) 284–287

Jancke, Lutz; Kalveram, Karl T. Kontrolle von on-time (Phonationsdauer) und voice-onset-time bei rechts- bzw. linksohrig dargebotener auditiver Ruckmeldungen: Unterschiedliche Lateralisierung bei stotternden und nichtstotternden Personen? (Control of on-time (phonation duration) and voice-onset time with right- or left-ear auditory feedback: Different lateralization in stutterers and nonstutterers?) Zeitschrift fur Experimentelle und Angewandte Psychologie; 1987 Vol 34(1) 54–63

Johannsen, Helge S.; Victor, Claudia. Visual information processing in the left and right hemispheres during unilateral tachistoscopic stimulation of stutterers. Journal of Fluency Disorders; 1986 Dec Vol 11(4) 285–291

Jones, R. Barrie. Modified regulated-breathing in treatment of a single case of stuttering. Perceptual and Motor Skills; 1981 Feb Vol 52(1) 130

Joseph, Anthony B. Transient stuttering in catatonic bipolar patients. Behavioural Neurology; 1991 Win Vol 4(4) 265–269

Kent, Ray D. Facts about stuttering: Neuropsychologic perspectives. Journal of Speech and Hearing Disorders; 1983 Aug Vol 48(3) 249–255

Klepel, Helene; Kuhne, Gert Eberhard; Mackerodt, Gerd. Untersuchungen zur Haufigkeit elektroenzephalographischer Befunde bei Kindern mit Stottern im Vergleich zu gesunden Gleichaltrigen. / Studies on the frequency of encephalographic findings in stuttering children in comparison to healthy children of the same age group. Psychiatrie, Neurologie und medizinische Psychologie; 1982 Aug Vol 34(8) 488–492

Kraaimaat, Floor; Janssen, Peggy; Brutten, Gene J. The relationship between stutterers' cognitive and autonomic anxiety and therapy outcome. Journal of Fluency Disorders; 1988 Apr Vol 13(2) 107–113

Kramer, Josefine. Wesen, Haufigkeit, Ursachen und Erscheinungsformen der geistigen Behinderung: II. (Nature, frequency, causes, and forms of mental retardation: II.) Vierteljahresschrift fur Heilpadagogik und ihre Nachbargebiete; 1976 Sep Vol 45(3) 270–283

Kuz'min, Yu. I.; Dmitrieva, E. S.; Zaitseva, K. A. Functional asymmetry of the brain in stuttering children during perception of emotions. Human Physiology; 1989 Mar–Apr Vol 15(2) 129–131

Ladouceur, Robert; Boudreau, Leonce; Theberge, Sylvie. Awareness training and regulated-breathing method in modification of stuttering. Perceptual and Motor Skills; 1981 Aug Vol 53(1) 187–194

Ladouceur, Robert; Cote, Christiane; Leblond, Georges; Bouchard, Leandre. Evaluation of regulated-breathing method and awareness training in the treatment of stuttering. Journal of Speech and Hearing Disorders; 1982 Nov Vol 47(4) 422–426

Ladouceur, Robert; Saint Laurent, Lise. Stuttering: A multidimensional treatment and evaluation package. Journal of Fluency Disorders; 1986 Jun Vol 11(2) 93–103

Lagutina, T. S.; Lovchikova, N. N.; Obukhovskii, N. G. Electrophysiological study of patients with logoneuroses. Soviet Neurology and Psychiatry; 1985 Fal Vol 18(3) 53–61

Lara-Cantu, Maria A. Pilot study on electromyographic biofeedback for the treatment of stuttering. Ensenanza e Investigacion en Psicologia; 1978 Jul Dec Vol 4(2) 259–265

Lebrun, Yvan; Bijleveld, Henny; Rousseau, Jean Jacques. A case of persistent neurogenic stuttering following a missile wound. Journal of Fluency Disorders; 1990 Oct–Dec Vol 15(5–6) 251–258

Lebrun, Yvan; Leleux, Chantal. Acquired stuttering following right brain damage in dextrals. Journal of Fluency Disorders; 1985 Jun Vol 10(2) 137–141

Lebrun, Yvan; Leleux, Chantal; Rousseau, Jean Jacques; Devreux, Francoise. cquired stuttering. Journal of Fluency Disorders; 1983 Dec Vol 8(4) 323–330

Lebrun, Yvan; Retif, Jean; Kaiser, Gudrun. Acquired stuttering as a forerunner of motorneuron disease. Journal of Fluency Disorders; 1983 Jun Vol 8(2) 161–167

Lebrun, Yvan; Van Borsel, John. Final sound repetitions. Journal of Fluency Disorders; 1990 Apr Vol 15(2) 107–113

Liebetrau, R. Mark; Daly, David A. Auditory processing and perceptual abilities of "organic" and "functional" stutterers. Journal of Fluency Disorders; 1981 Sep Vol 6(3) 219–231

Lokhov, M. I. Interhemispheric asymmetry in mechanisms of nonaphasic speech disturbances. Human Physiology; 1988 Jan–Feb Vol 14(1) 27–31

Lussenhop, Alfred J.; Boggs, John S.; LaBorwit, Louis J.; Walle, Eugene L. Cerebral dominance in stutterers determined by Wada testing. Neurology; 1973 Nov Vol. 23(11) 1190–1192

MacKenzie, Catherine. Aphasic articulatory defect and aphasic phonological defect. British Journal of Disorders of Communication; 1982 Apr Vol 17(1) 27–46

Mallard, A. R.; Hicks, Douglas M.; Riggs, Donald E. A comparison of stutterers and nonstutterers in a task of controlled voice onset. Journal of Speech and Hearing Research; 1982 Jun Vol 25(2) 287–290

Manders, Eric; Bastijns, Paul. Sudden recovery from stuttering after an epileptic attack: A case report. Journal of Fluency Disorders; 1988 Dec Vol 13(6) 421–425

Marshall, Robert C.; Neuburger, Sandra I. Effects of delayed auditory feedback on acquired stuttering following head injury. Journal of Fluency Disorders; 1987 Oct Vol 12(5) 355–365

Martin, Richard R.; Lawrence, Barbara A.; Haroldson, Samuel K.; Gunderson, Donna. Stuttering and oral stereognosis. Perceptual and Motor Skills; 1981 Aug Vol 53(1) 155–162

McClean, Michael D. Neuromotor aspects of stuttering: Levels of impairment and disability. ASHA Reports Series American Speech Language Hearing Association; 1990 Apr No 18 64–71

McClean, Michael D. Surface EMG recording of the perioral reflexes: Preliminary observations on stutterers and nonstutterers. Journal of Speech and Hearing Research; 1987 Jun Vol 30(2) 283–287

McClean, Michael D.; McLean, Alvin. Case report of stuttering acquired in association with phenytoin use for post-head-injury seizures. Journal of Fluency Disorders; 1985 Dec Vol 10(4) 241–255

McFarlane, Stephen C.; Prins, David. Neural response time of stutterers and nonstutterers in selected oral motor tasks. Journal of Speech and Hearing Research; 1978 Dec Vol 21(4) 768–778

McKnight, Roxanne C.; Cullinan, Walter L. Subgroups of stuttering children: Speech and voice reaction times, segmental durations, and naming latencies. Journal of Fluency Disorders; 1987 Jun Vol 12(3) 217–233

McLean-Muse, Ann; Larson, Charles R.; Gregory, Hugo H. Stutterers' and nonstutterers' voice fundamental frequency changes in response to auditory stimuli. Journal of Speech and Hearing Research; 1988 Dec Vol 31(4) 549–555

Mesalam, Linda. The power of communication. Cognitive Rehabilitation; 1988 May–Jun Vol 6(3) 32–36

Meyers, Susan C.; Hall, Nancy E.; Aram, Dorothy M. Fluency and language recovery in a child with a left hemisphere lesion. Journal of Fluency Disorders; 1990 Jun Vol 15(3) 159–173

Miller, Aaron E. Cessation of stuttering with progressive multiple sclerosis. Neurology; 1985 Sep Vol 35(9) 1341–1343

Minderaa, R. B.; Van Gemert, T. M.; Van de Wetering, B. J. Onverwachte presentatiewijzen van het syndroom van Gilles de la Tourette. / Unexpected types of presentation of Gilles de la Tourette's syndrome. Tijdschrift voor Psychiatrie; 1988 Vol 30(4) 246–254

Moore, W. H. Bilateral tachistoscopic word perception of stutterers and normal subjects. Brain and Language; 1976 Jul Vol 3(3) 434–442

Moore, W. H. Hemispheric alpha asymmetries of stutterers and nonstutterers for the recall and recognition of words and connected reading passages: Some relationships to severity of stuttering. Journal of Fluency Disorders; 1986 Mar Vol 11(1) 71–89

Moore, Walter H. Hemispheric alpha asymmetries during an electromyographic biofeedback procedure for stuttering: A single-subject experimental design. Journal of Fluency Disorders; 1984 May Vol 9(2) 143–162

Moore, Walter H. Pathophysiology of stuttering: Cerebral activation differences in stutterers vs. nonstutterers. ASHA Reports Series American Speech Language Hearing Association; 1990 Apr No 18 72–80

Moore, W. H.; Craven, Duane C.; Faber, Michele M. Hemispheric alpha asymmetries of words with positive, negative, and neutral arousal values preceding tasks of recall and recognition: Electrophysiological and behavioral results from stuttering males and nonstuttering males and females. Brain and Language; 1982 Nov Vol 17(2) 211–224

Moore, W. H.; Haynes, William O. Alpha hemispheric asymmetry and stuttering: Some support for a segmentation dysfunction hypothesis. Journal of Speech and Hearing Research; 1980 Jun Vol 23(2) 229–247

Moore, W. H.; Lang, Mary K. Alpha asymmetry over the right and left hemispheres of stutterers and control subjects preceding massed oral readings: A preliminary investigation. Perceptual and Motor Skills; 1977 Feb Vol 44(1) 223–230

Morozov, V. P.; Kuz'min, Yu. I.; Zaitseva, K. A.; Dmitrieva, E. S. Hemispheric functional asymmetry in stuttering. Human Physiology; 1988 May–Jun Vol 14(3) 188–194

Murdoch, Bruce E.; Killin, Heather; McCaul, Annette. A kinematic analysis of respiratory function in a group of stutterers pre- and posttreatment. Journal of Fluency Disorders; 1989 Oct Vol 14(5) 323–350

Myers, Florence L.; Wall, Meryl J. Issues to consider in the differential diagnosis of normal childhood nonfluencies and stuttering. Journal of Fluency Disorders; 1981 Sep Vol 6(3) 189–195

Myers, Florence L.; Wall, Meryl J. Toward an integrated approach to early childhood stuttering. Journal of Fluency Disorders; 1982 Mar Vol 7(1–1) 47–54

Newman, Parley W.; Bunderson, Karin; Brey, Robert H. Brain stem electrical responses of stutterers and normals by sex, ears, and recovery. Journal of Fluency Disorders; 1985 Mar Vol 10(1) 59–67

Nowack, William J.; Stone, R. Edward. Acquired stuttering and bilateral cerebral disease. Journal of Fluency Disorders; 1987 Apr Vol 12(2) 141–146

Nudelman, H. B.; Herbrich, K. E.; Hoyt, B. D.; Rosenfield, D. B. A neuroscience model of stuttering. Journal of Fluency Disorders; 1989 Dec Vol 14(6) 399–427

Orta-Rodriguez, Martha; Gallegos B., Xochitl. Una evaluacion de tres tecnicas conductuales en el tratamiento de la tartamudez. (An evaluation of 3 behavioral techniques used to treat stuttering.) Revista Mexicana de Psicologia; 1986 Jul–Dec Vol 3(2) 168–173

Parry, William D. Stuttering and the Valsalva mechanism: A hypothesis in need of investigation. Journal of Fluency Disorders; 1985 Dec Vol 10(4) 317–324

Pennington, Bruce F.; Smith, Shelley D. Genetic influences on learning disabilities and speech and language disorders. Child Development; 1983 Apr Vol 54(2) 369–387

Perkins, William H. Implications of scientific research for treatment of stuttering: A lecture. Journal of Fluency Disorders; 1981 Jun Vol 6(2) 155–162

Perkins, William H.; Bell, Jody; Johnson, Linda; Stocks, Janice. Phone rate and the effective planning time hypothesis of stuttering. Journal of Speech and Hearing Research; 1979 Dec Vol 22(4) 747–755

Perkins, William H.; Kent, Raymond D.; Curlee, Richard F. A theory of neuropsycholinguistic

function in stuttering. Journal of Speech and Hearing Research; 1991 Aug Vol 34(4) 734–752

Perkins, William; Rudas, Joanna; Johnson, Linda; Bell, Jody. Stuttering: Discoordination of phonation with articulation and respiration. Journal of Speech and Hearing Research; 1976 Sep Vol 19(3) 509–522

Peters, M. The view of learning theory. Zeitschrift fur Kinder und Jugendpsychiatrie; 1976 Vol 4(2) 104–112

Peters, Herman F.; Boves, Louis. Coordination of aerodynamic and phonatory processes in fluent speech utterances of stutterers. Journal of Speech and Hearing Research; 1988 Sep Vol 31(3) 352–361

Petrosino, Linda; Fucci, Donald; Gorman, Peter; Harris, Daniel. Midline and off-midline tongue and right- and left-hand vibrotactile thresholds of stutterers and normal-speaking individuals. Perceptual and Motor Skills; 1987 Aug Vol 65(1) 253–254

Pimental, Patricia A.; Gorelick, Philip B. Aphasia, apraxia and neurogenic stuttering as complications of metrizamide myelography: Speech deficits following myelography. Acta Neurologica Scandinavica; 1985 Nov Vol 72(5) 481–488

Pinsky, Seth D.; McAdam, Dale W. Electroencephalographic and dichotic indices of cerebral laterality in stutterers. Brain and Language; 1980 Nov Vol 11(2) 374–397

Prescott, John; Andrews, Gavin. Early and late components of the contingent negative variation prior to manual and speech responses in stutterers and non-stutterers. International Journal of Psychophysiology; 1984 Nov Vol 2(2) 121–130

Quinn, P. T.; Andrews, Gavin. Neurological stuttering—a clinical entity? Journal of Neurology, Neurosurgery and Psychiatry; 1977 Jul Vol 40(7) 699–701

Rastatter, Michael; Dell, Carl W. Simple motor and phonemic processing reaction times of stutterers. Perceptual and Motor Skills; 1985 Oct Vol 61(2) 463–466

Rastatter, Michael P.; Dell, Carl W. Reaction times of moderate and severe stutterers to monaural verbal stimuli: Some implications for neurolinguistic organization. Journal of

Speech and Hearing Research; 1987 Mar Vol 30(1) 21–27

Rastatter, Michael P.; Dell, Carl W. Simple visual versus lexical decision vocal reaction times of stuttering and normal subjects. Journal of Fluency Disorders; 1987 Feb Vol 12(1) 63–69

Rastatter, Michael P.; Dell, Carl. Vocal reaction times of stuttering subjects to tachistoscopically presented concrete and abstract words: A closer look at cerebral dominance and language processing. Journal of Speech and Hearing Research; 1987 Sep Vol 30(3) 306–310

Rastatter, Michael P.; Dell, Carl W. Reading reaction times of stuttering and nonstuttering subjects to unilaterally presented concrete and abstract words. Journal of Fluency Disorders; 1988 Oct Vol 13(5) 319–329

Rastatter, Michael P.; Loren, Catherine A. Visual coding dominance in stuttering: Some evidence from central tachistoscopic stimulation (tachistoscopic viewing and stuttering). Journal of Fluency Disorders; 1988 Apr Vol 13(2) 89–95

Rastatter, Michael P.; Loren, Catherine; Colcord, Roger. Visual coding strategies and hemisphere dominance characteristics of stutterers. Journal of Fluency Disorders; 1987 Oct Vol 12(5) 305–315

Rastatter, Michael P.; McGuire, Richard A.; Loren, Catherine. Linguistic encoding dominance in stuttering: Some evidence for temporal and qualitative hemispheric processing differences. Journal of Fluency Disorders; 1988 Jun Vol 13(3) 215–224

Reed, Charles G.; Lingwall, James B. Some relationships between punishment, stuttering, and galvanic skin responses. Journal of Speech and Hearing Research; 1976 Jun Vol 19(2) 197–205

Rentschler, Gary J.; Driver, Lynn E.; Callaway, Elizabeth A. The onset of stuttering following drug overdose. Journal of Fluency Disorders; 1984 Dec Vol 9(4) 265–284

Rosenfield, David B.; Goodglass, Harold. Dichotic testing of cerebral dominance in stutterers. Brain and Language; 1980 Sep Vol 11(1) 170–180

Scopazzo, Maurizio. (Rosenzweig Picture Frustration Study and EEG features in an adolescent stuttering group.) Lavoro Neuropsichiatrico; 1974 Jan–Jun Vol 54(1–3) 49–60

Seider, Robin A.; Gladstien, Keith L.; Kidd, Kenneth K. Recovery and persistence of stuttering among relatives of stutterers. Journal of Speech and Hearing Disorders; 1983 Nov Vol 48(4) 402–409

Silverman, Franklin H.; Hummer, Kathy. Spastic dysphonia: A fluency disorder? Journal of Fluency Disorders; 1989 Aug Vol 14(4) 285–291

Smith, Anne. "A theory of neuropsycholinguistic function in stuttering": Commentary. Journal of Speech and Hearing Research; 1992 Aug Vol 35(4) 805–809

Smith, Anne. Neural drive to muscles in stuttering. Journal of Speech and Hearing Research; 1989 Jun Vol 32(2) 252–264

Smith, Barry D.; Meyers, Marilyn B.; Kline, Robert. For better or for worse: Left-handedness, pathology, and talent. Journal of Clinical and Experimental Neuropsychology; 1989 Dec Vol 11(6) 944–959

Smith, K. M.; Blood, I. M.; Blood, Gorden W. Auditory brainstem responses of stutterers and nonstutterers during speech production. Journal of Fluency Disorders; 1990 Aug Vol 15(4) 211–222

Souvorova, V. V.; Matova, M. A.; Tourovskaya, Z. G. Binocular reproductive images under conditions of atypical interhemispheric relations (in stutterers). Voprosy Psikhologii; 1984 Jan–Feb No 1 105–110

Steffen, Hartmut; Seidel, Christa. Perceptive and cognitive school and social behavior of children with language and speech disorders. Zeitschrift fur Kinder und Jugendpsychiatrie; 1976 Vol 4(3) 216–232

Stewart, Cheryl; Evans, W. Bryce; Fitch, James L. Oral form perception skills of stuttering and nonstuttering children measured by stereognosis. Journal of Fluency Disorders; 1985 Dec Vol 10(4) 311–316

Stigora, Joseph A.; DiSimoni, Frank G. Resolution of opposing forces: An approach to the understanding and clinical management of stuttering. Journal of Fluency Disorders; 1989 Aug Vol 14(4) 293–302

Strub, Richard L.; Black, F. William; Naeser, Margaret A. Anomalous dominance in sibling stutterers: Evidence from CT scan asymmetries, dichotic listening, neuropsychological testing, and handedness. Brain and Language; 1987 Mar Vol 30(2) 338–350

Sussman, Harvey M. Contrastive patterns of intrahemispheric interference to verbal and spatial concurrent tasks in right-handed, left-handed and stuttering populations. Neuropsychologia; 1982 Vol 20(6) 675–684

Sussman, Harvey M.; MacNeilage, Peter F. Hemispheric specialization for speech production and perception in stutterers. Neuropsychologia; 1975 Jan Vol 13(1) 19–26

Sussman, Harvey M.; MacNeilage, Peter F. Studies of hemispheric specialization for speech production. Brain and Language; 1975 Apr Vol 2(2) 131–151

Szelag, Elzbieta; Garwarska-Kolek, Dantua; Heerman, Anna; Stasiek, Janina. Brain lateralization and severity of stuttering in children. Acta Neurobiologiae Experimentalis; 1993 Vol 53(1) 263–267

Toscher, Mark M.; Rupp, Ralph R. A study of the central auditory processes in stutterers using the Synthetic Sentence Identification (SSI) Test battery. Journal of Speech and Hearing Research; 1978 Dec Vol 21(4) 779–792

Traugott, N. N.; Onopriychuk, E. I. EEG peculiarities of different clinical types of stuttering in preschoolers. Defektologiya; 1985 No 4 79–83

Travis, Lee E. The cerebral dominance theory of stuttering: 1931–1978. Journal of Speech and Hearing Disorders; 1978 Aug Vol 43(3) 278–281

Travis, Lee E. Neurophysiological dominance. Journal of Speech and Hearing Disorders; 1978 Aug Vol 43(3) 275–277

Tsunoda, Tadanobu; Moriyama, Haruyuki. Specific patterns of cerebral dominance for various sounds in adult stutterers. Journal of Auditory Research; 1972 Jul Vol 12(3) 216–227

von Deuster, C. Untersuchungen zur Hemispharendominanz und Handigkeit bei stammelnden Kindern mit normaler und gestorter auditiver Wahrnehmung. / Studies of hemisphere dominance and handedness of stammering children with normal and disturbed auditory perception. Folia Phoniatrica; 1983 Nov–Dec Vol 35(6) 265–272

Watson, Ben C.; Pool, Kenneth D.; Devous, Michael D.; Freeman, Frances J.; et al. Brain blood flow related to acoustic laryngeal reaction time in adult developmental stutterers. Journal of Speech and Hearing Research; 1992 Jun Vol 35(3) 555–561

Watson, Ben C.; Alfonso, Peter J. Physiological bases of acoustic LRT in nonstutterers, mild stutterers, and severe stutterers. Journal of Speech and Hearing Research; 1987 Dec Vol 30(4) 434–447

Webster, William G. Evidence in bimanual finger-tapping of an attentional component to stuttering. Behavioural Brain Research; 1990 Mar Vol 37(2) 93–100

Webster, William G. Motor performance of stutterers: A search for mechanisms. Journal of Motor Behavior; 1990 Dec Vol 22(4) 553–571

Webster, William G. Neural mechanisms underlying stuttering: Evidence from bimanual handwriting performance. Brain and Language; 1988 Mar Vol 33(2) 226–244

Webster, William G. Neuropsychological models of stuttering: I. Representation of sequential response mechanisms. Neuropsychologia; 1985 Vol 23(2) 263–267

Webster, William G. Neuropsychological models of stuttering: II. Interhemispheric interference. Neuropsychologia; 1986 Vol 24(5) 737–741

Webster, William G. Sequence reproduction deficits in stutterers tested under nonspeeded response conditions. Journal of Fluency Disorders; 1989 Apr Vol 14(2) 79–86

Wells, Betsy G.; Moore, W. H. EEG alpha asymmetries in stutterers and non-stutterers: Effects of linguistic variables on hemispheric processing and fluency. Neuropsychologia; 1990 Vol 28(12) 1295–1305

Wilkins, Candace; Webster, Ronald L.; Morgan, Bryant T. Cerebral lateralization of visual stimulus recognition in stutterers and fluent speakers. Journal of Fluency Disorders; 1984 May Vol 9(2) 131–141

Zaitseva, K. A.; Miroshnikov, D. B.; Dmitrieva, E. S. Principle of parallel processing by brain of various kinds of speech information. Sensory Systems; 1991 Jul–Sep Vol 5(3) 254–260

Zimmermann, Gerald N.; Knott, J. R. Slow potentials of the brain related to speech processing in normal speakers and stutterers. Electroencephalography and Clinical Neurophysiology; 1974 Dec Vol 37(6) 599–607

Neurogenic Disfluencies

Andy, Orlando J.; Bhatnagar, Subhash C. Stuttering acquired from subcortical pathologies and its alleviation from thalamic perturbation. Brain and Language; 1992 May Vol 42(4) 385–401

Andy, Orlando J.; Bhatnagar, Subhash C. Thalamic-induced stuttering (surgical observations). Journal of Speech and Hearing Research; 1991 Aug Vol 34(4) 796–800

Aram, Dorothy M.; Meyers, Susan C.; Ekelman, Barbara L. Fluency of conversational speech in children with unilateral brain lesions. Brain and Language; 1990 Jan Vol 38(1) 105–121

Ardila, Alfredo; Lopez, Maria V. Severe stuttering associated with right hemisphere lesion. Brain and Language; 1986 Mar Vol 27(2) 239–246

Becker, H. Ungewohnliche Sprechstorungen bei der endogenen Depression. / Unusual speech disorders in endogenous depression. Nervenarzt; 1989 Dec Vol 60(12) 757–758

Bhatnagar, Subhash C.; Andy, Orlando J. Alleviation of acquired stuttering with human centremedian thalamic stimulation. Journal of Neurology, Neurosurgery and Psychiatry; 1989 Oct Vol 52(10) 1182–1184

Buyanov, M. I.; et al. Follow-up data on quasi-neurotic stuttering. Defektologiya; 1981 No 5 10–13

Byrd, Kathryn; Cooper, Eugene B. Apraxic speech characteristics in stuttering, developmentally apraxic, and normal speaking children. Journal of Fluency Disorders; 1989 Jun Vol 14(3) 215–229

Byrne, Alan; Byrne, Mary K.; Zibin, Terry O. Transient neurogenic stuttering. International Journal of Eating Disorders; 1993 14(4) 511–514

Cooper, Eugene B. A brain-stem contusion and fluency: Vicki's story. Journal of Fluency Disorders; 1983 Sep Vol 8(3) 269–274

Emrich, H. M.; Eilert, P. Evaluation of speech and language in neuropsychiatric disorders. Archiv fur Psychiatrie und Nervenkrankheiten; 1978 Vol 225(3) 209–221

Farmer, Alvirda. Stuttering repetitions in aphasic and nonaphasic brain damaged adults. Cortex; 1975 Dec Vol 11(4) 391–396

Fleet, W. Shepherd; Heilman, Kenneth M. Acquired stuttering from a right hemisphere lesion in a right-hander. Neurology; 1985 Sep Vol 35(9) 1343–1346

Floyd, Susan; Perkins, William H. Early syllable dysfluency in stutterers and nonstutterers: A preliminary report. Journal of Communication Disorders; 1974 Sep Vol 7(3) 279–282

Freedman, Morris; Alexander, Michael P.; Naeser, Margaret A. Anatomic basis of transcortical motor aphasia. Neurology; 1984 Apr Vol 34(4) 409–417

Gamelli, Ralph J. Classification of child stuttering: I. Transient developmental, neurogenic acquired, and persistent child stuttering. Child Psychiatry and Human Development; 1982 Sum Vol 12(4) 220–253

Halpern, Harvey. Stuttering therapy for nonfluent psychiatric adults. Perceptual and Motor Skills; 1990 Dec Vol 71(3, Pt 1) 914

Halpern, Harvey; McCartin Clark, Marguerite; Wallack, Wendy. The nonfluencies of eight psychiatric adults. Journal of Communication Disorders; 1989 Aug Vol 22(4) 233–241

Helm, Nancy A.; Butler, Russell B.; Benson, D. Frank. Acquired stuttering. Neurology; 1978 Nov Vol 28(1) 1159–1165

Helm Estabrooks, Nancy; Yeo, Ronald; Geschwind, Norman; Freedman, Morris; et al. Stuttering: Disappearance and reappearance with acquired brain lesions. Neurology; 1986 Aug Vol 36(8) 1109–1112

Horner, Jennifer; Massey, E. Wayne. Progressive dysfluency associated with right hemisphere disease. Brain and Language; 1983 Jan Vol 18(1) 71–85

Lebrun, Yvan; Retif, Jean; Kaiser, Gudrun. Acquired stuttering as a forerunner of motor-neuron disease. Journal of Fluency Disorders; 1983 Jun Vol 8(2) 161–167

Lebrun, Yvan; Leleux, Chantal. Acquired stuttering following right brain damage in dextrals. Journal of Fluency Disorders; 1985 Jun Vol 10(2) 137–141

Lebrun, Yvan; Bijleveld, Henny; Rousseau, Jean Jacques. A case of persistent neurogenic stuttering following a missile wound. Journal of Fluency Disorders; 1990 Oct-Dec Vol 15(5–6) 251–258

MacKenzie, Catherine. Aphasic articulatory defect and aphasic phonological defect. British Journal of Disorders of Communication; 1982 Apr Vol 17(1) 27–46

Manders, Eric; Bastijns, Paul. Sudden recovery from stuttering after an epileptic attack: A case report. Journal of Fluency Disorders; 1988 Dec Vol 13(6) 421–425

Market, Karen E.; Montague, James C.; Buffalo, M. D.; Drummond, Sakina S. Acquired stuttering: Descriptive data and treatment outcome. Journal of Fluency Disorders; 1990 Feb Vol 15(1) 21–33

Marshall, Robert C.; Neuburger, Sandra I. Effects of delayed auditory feedback on acquired stuttering following head injury. Journal of Fluency Disorders; 1987 Oct Vol 12(5) 355–365

McClean, Michael D.; McLean, Alvin. Case report of stuttering acquired in association with phenytoin use for post-head-injury seizures. Journal of Fluency Disorders; 1985 Dec Vol 10(4) 241–255

Mesalam, Linda. The power of communication. Cognitive Rehabilitation; 1988 May-Jun Vol 6(3) 32–36

Meyers, Susan C.; Hall, Nancy E.; Aram, Dorothy M. Fluency and language recovery in a child with a left hemisphere lesion. Journal of Fluency Disorders; 1990 Jun Vol 15(3) 159–173

Miller, Aaron E. Cessation of stuttering with progressive multiple sclerosis. Neurology; 1985 Sep Vol 35(9) 1341–1343

Minderaa, R. B.; Van Gemert, T. M.; Van de Wetering, B. J. Onverwachte presentatiewijzen van het syndroom van Gilles de la Tourette. / Unexpected types of presentation of Gilles de la Tourette's syndrome. Tijdschrift voor Psychiatrie; 1988 Vol 30(4) 246–254

Nowack, William J.; Stone, R. Edward. Acquired stuttering and bilateral cerebral disease. Journal of Fluency Disorders; 1987 Apr Vol 12(2) 141–146

Nurnberg, H. George; Greenwald, Blaine. Stuttering: An unusual side effect of phenothiazines. American Journal of Psychiatry; 1981 Mar Vol 138(3) 386–387

Oganesian, Ye. V.; Beliakova, L. I. The rationale for principles of differential application of logopaedic rhythmics in remediation of adult stutterers. Defektologiya; 1982 No 1 3–12

Pimental, Patricia A.; Gorelick, Philip B. Aphasia, apraxia and neurogenic stuttering as complications of metrizamide myelography: Speech deficits following myelography. Acta Neurologica Scandinavica; 1985 Nov Vol 72(5) 481–488

Poulos, Marie G.; Webster, William G. Family history as a basis for subgrouping people who stutter. Journal of Speech and Hearing Research; 1991 Feb Vol 34(1) 5–10

Quinn, P. T.; Andrews, Gavin. Neurological stuttering—a clinical entity? Journal of Neurology, Neurosurgery and Psychiatry; 1977 Jul Vol 40(7) 699–701

Rentschler, Gary J.; Driver, Lynn E.; Callaway, Elizabeth A. The onset of stuttering following drug overdose. Journal of Fluency Disorders; 1984 Dec Vol 9(4) 265–284

Rosenbek, John; Messert, Bernard; Collins, Michael; Wertz, Robert T. Stuttering following brain damage. Brain and Language; 1978 Jul Vol 6(1) 82–96

Rosenfield, David B.; Freeman, Frances J. Stuttering onset after laryngectomy. Journal of Fluency Disorders; 1983 Sep Vol 8(3) 265–268

Rosenfield, David B.; Jones, Barbara P.; Liljestrand, James S. Effects of right hemisphere damage in an adult stutterer. Journal of Fluency Disorders; 1981 Jun Vol 6(2) 175–179

Rousey, Carol G.; Arjunan, K. N.; Rousey, Clyde L. Successful treatment of stuttering following closed head injury. Journal of Fluency Disorders; 1986 Sep Vol 11(3) 257–261

Segalowitz, Sidney J.; Brown, Deborah. Mild head injury as a source of developmental disabilities. Journal of Learning Disabilities; 1991 Nov Vol 24(9) 551–559

Silverman, Franklin H.; Hummer, Kathy. Spastic dysphonia: A fluency disorder? Journal of

Fluency Disorders; 1989 Aug Vol 14(4) 285–291

Soroker, N.; Bar Israel, Y.; Schechter, I.; Solzi, P. Stuttering as a manifestation of right-hemispheric subcortical stroke. European Neurology; 1990 Sep-Oct Vol 30(5) 268–270

Traugott, N. N.; Onopriychuk, E. I. EEG peculiarities of different clinical types of stuttering in preschoolers. Defektologiya; 1985 No 4 79–83

Wagaman, Joel R.; Miltenberger, Raymond G.; Arndorfer, Richard E Analysis of a simplified treatment for stuttering in children.. Journal of Applied Behavior Analysis; 1993 Spr Vol 26(1) 53–61

Wood, Frank; et al. Patterns of regional cerebral blood flow during attempted reading aloud by stutterers both on and off haloperidol medication: Evidence for inadequate left frontal activation during stuttering. Brain and Language; 1980 Jan Vol 9(1) 141–144

Operant Conditioning/
Behavioral Management

Adams, Martin R.; Hotchkiss, John. Some reactions and responses of stutterers to a miniaturized metronome and metronome-conditioning therapy: Three case reports. Behavior Therapy; 1973 Jul Vol. 4(4) 565–569

Andrews, Gavin J.; Howie, Pauline M.; Dozsa, Melinda; Guitar, Barry E. Stuttering: Speech pattern characteristics under fluency-inducing conditions. Journal of Speech and Hearing Research; 1982 Jun Vol 25(2) 208–216

Arkin, Arthur M.; et al. Behavior modification: Present status in psychiatry. New York State Journal of Medicine; 1976 Feb Vol 76(2) 190–196

Arkin, Arthur M.; et al. Behavior modification: Present status in psychiatry. New York State Journal of Medicine; 1976 Feb Vol 76(2) 190–196

Azrin, Nathan, H. A strategy for applied research: Learning based but outcome oriented. American Psychologist; 1977 Feb Vol 32(2) 140–149

Ballesteros, Rocio F.; Mas, Jose S.; Carrobles, Jose A. Relaciones entre respuestas psicofisi-

ologicas y autoinformes. / Relationships between psychophysiological responses and self-reports. Analisis y Modificacion de Conducta; 1984 Vol 10(25) 299–311

Beattie, Michael S. A behaviour therapy programme for stuttering. British Journal of Disorders of Communication; 1973 Oct Vol. 8(2) 120–130

Beaty, David T. A multimodal approach to elimination of stuttering. Perceptual and Motor Skills; 1980 Feb Vol 50(1) 51–55

Becker, Peter; Kessler, Bernd; Fuchsgruber, Konrad. (A comparative therapeutic experiment on the theory and the efficiency of operant methods of treatment of stutterers.) Archiv fur Psychologie; 1975 Vol 127(1–2) 78–92

Berecz, John M. Cognitive conditioning therapy in the treatment of stuttering. Journal of Communication Disorders; 1976 Dec Vol 9(4) 301–315

Berecz, John M. The treatment of stuttering through precision punishment and cognitive arousal. Journal of Speech and Hearing Disorders; 1973 May Vol. 38(2) 256–267

Berman, Perry A.; Brady, John P. Miniaturized metronomes in the treatment of stuttering: A survey of clinicians' experience. Journal of Behavior Therapy and Experimental Psychiatry; 1973 Jun Vol. 4(2) 117–119

Burgraff, Roger I. The efficacy of systematic desensitization via imagery as a therapeutic technique with stutterers. British Journal of Disorders of Communication; 1974 Oct Vol 9(2) 134–139

Caron, Chantal; Ladouceur, Robert. Multidimensional behavioral treatment for child stutterers. Behavior Modification; 1989 Apr Vol 13(2) 206–215

Christensen, John E.; Lingwall, James B. The relationship between treatment exposure times and changes in stuttering frequency during contingent stimulation. Journal of Fluency Disorders; 1983 Dec Vol 8(4) 275–281

Costello, Janis. The establishment of fluency with time-out procedures: Three case studies. Journal of Speech and Hearing Disorders; 1975 May Vol 40(2) 216–231

Costello, Janis M.; Hurst, Marilyn R. An analysis of the relationship among stuttering behaviors. Journal of Speech and Hearing Research; 1981 Jan Vol 24(2) 247–256

Craig, Ashley; Andrews, Gavin. The prediction and prevention of relapse in stuttering: The value of self-control techniques and locus of control measures. Behavior Modification; 1985 Oct Vol 9(4) 427–442

Craig, Ashley; Feyer, Anne Marie; Andrews, Gavin. An overview of a behavioural treatment for stuttering. Australian Psychologist; 1987 Mar Vol 22(1) 53–62

Cross, Douglas E.; Cooper, Eugene B. Self- versus investigator-administered presumed fluency reinforcing stimuli. Journal of Speech and Hearing Research; 1976 Jun Vol 19(2) 241–246

Curlee, Richard F. The early history of the behavior modification of stuttering: From laboratory to clinic. Journal of Fluency Disorders; 1993 Mar Vol 18(1) 13–25

Curlee, Richard F.; Perkins, William H. Effectiveness of a DAF conditioning program for adolescent and adult stutterers. Behaviour Research and Therapy; 1973 Nov Vol. 11(4) 395–401

Daly, David A.; Kimbarow, Michael L. Stuttering as operant behavior: Effects of the verbal stimuli wrong, right, and tree on the disfluency rates of school-age stutterers and nonstutterers. Journal of Speech and Hearing Research; 1978 Sep Vol 21(3) 589–600

Devenny, Darlynne A.; Silverman, W.; Balgley, H.; Wall, M. J.; et al. Specific motor abilities associated with speech fluency in Down's syndrome. Journal of Mental Deficiency Research; 1990 Oct Vol 34(5) 437–443

Fukawa, Teruyo; Yoshioka, Hirohide; Ozawa, Emi; Yoshida, Shigeru. Difference of susceptibility to delayed auditory feedback between stutterers and nonstutterers. Journal of Speech and Hearing Research; 1988 Sep Vol 31(3) 475–479

Florin, Irmela. Stuttering: Theoretical approaches, experimental research results, suggestions for therapy. European Journal of Behavioural Analysis and Modification; 1976 Nov Vol 3(1) 189–200

Gagnon, Mireille; Ladouceur, Robert. Behavioral treatment of child stutterers: Replication

and extension. Behavior Therapy; 1992 Win Vol 23(1) 113–129

Gonzalez Valenzuela, M. Jose. Evaluacion y Tratamiento cognitivo-conductual de un caso de tartamudez. / Evaluation and cognitive-behavioral treatment in a severe stuttering case. Analisis y Modificacion de Conducta; 1990 Vol 16(47) 137–148

Greenberg, David; Marks, Isaac. Behavioural psychotherapy of uncommon referrals. British Journal of Psychiatry; 1982 Aug Vol 141 148–153

Gruber, Les. Moses: His speech impediment and behavior therapy. Journal of Psychology and Judaism; 1986 Spr Sum Vol 10(1) 5–13

Grzybowska, Aldona. Behawioraline teorie jakania. / Behavioral theories of stuttering. Przeglad Psychologiczny; 1987 Vol 30(1) 71–80

Halvorson, Jerome A. Punishment of stuttering as a discriminative stimulus for reinforced fluency. Journal of Communication Disorders; 1973 Dec Vol. 6(4) 315–321

Hanson, Bruce R. The effects of a contingent light-flash on stuttering and attention to stuttering. Journal of Communication Disorders; 1978 Sep Vol 11(5) 451–458

Harrington, Jonathan. Stuttering, delayed auditory feedback, and linguistic rhythm. Journal of Speech and Hearing Research; 1988 Mar Vol 31(1) 36–47

Hasbrouck, Jon M. FAMC intensive stuttering treatment program: Ten years of implementation. Military Medicine; 1992 May Vol 157(5) 244–247

Hayden, Paul A.; Adams, Martin R.; Jordahl, Nanette. The effects of pacing and masking on stutterers' and nonstutterers' speech initiation times. Journal of Fluency Disorders; 1982 Mar Vol 7(1–1) 9–19

Hegde, M. N. The effect of shock on stuttering. Journal of the All India Institute of Speech and Hearing; 1971 Jan Vol. 2 104–110

Howie, Pauline M. A response to "On token reinforcement and stuttering therapy: Another view on findings reported by Howie and Woods (1982)." Journal of Applied Behavior Analysis; 1983 Win Vol 16(4) 471–475

Howie, Pauline M.; Tanner, Susan; Andrews, Gavin. Short- and long-term outcome in an intensive treatment program for adult stutterers. Journal of Speech and Hearing Disorders; 1981 Feb Vol 46(1) 104–109

Howie, Pauline M.; Woods, C. Lee. Token reinforcement during the instatement and shaping of fluency in the treatment of stuttering. Journal of Applied Behavior Analysis; 1982 Spr Vol 15(1) 55–64

Hulit, Lloyd M. Influence of suggestion on nonfluencies of normal speakers: A pilot study. Perceptual and Motor Skills; 1987 Aug Vol 65(1) 164

Hurford, David P.; Webster, Ronald L. Decreases in simple reaction time as a function of stutterers' participation in a behavioral therapy. Journal of Fluency Disorders; 1985 Dec Vol 10(4) 301–310

Hutchinson, John M. A review of rhythmic pacing as a treatment strategy for stuttering. Rehabilitation Literature; 1976 Oct Vol 37(10) 297–303

Ingham, Janis C. Current status of stuttering and behavior modification: I. Recent trends in the application of behavior modification in children and adults. Journal of Fluency Disorders; 1993 Mar Vol 18(1) 27–55

Ingham, Roger J. Current status of stuttering and behavior modification: II. Principal issues and practices in stuttering therapy. Journal of Fluency Disorders; 1993 Mar Vol 18(1) 57–79

Ingham, Roger J. On token reinforcement and stuttering therapy: Another view on findings reported by Howie and Woods (1982). Journal of Applied Behavior Analysis; 1983 Win Vol 16(4) 465–470

Ingham, Roger J. The effects of self-evaluation training on maintenance and generalization during stuttering treatment. Journal of Speech and Hearing Disorders; 1982 Aug Vol 47(3) 271–280

Ingham, Roger J.; Adams, Susan; Reynolds, Glenda. The effects on stuttering of self-recording the frequency of stuttering or the word "the." Journal of Speech and Hearing Research; 1978 Sep Vol 21(3) 459–469

Ingham, Roger J.; Andrews, Gavin. An analysis of a token economy in stuttering therapy. Journal of Applied Behavior Analysis; 1973 Sum Vol. 6(2) 219–229

Ingham, Roger J.; Andrews, Gavin. Behavior theory and stuttering: A review. Journal of Speech and Hearing Disorders; 1973 Nov Vol. 38(4) 405–441

Ingham, Roger J.; Packman, Ann. Treatment and generalization effects in an experimental treatment for a stutterer using contingency management and speech rate control. Journal of Speech and Hearing Disorders; 1977 Aug Vol 42(3) 394–407

Jagacinski, Richard J. A qualitative look at feedback control theory as a style of describing behavior. Human Factors; 1977 Aug Vol 19(4) 331–347

James, Jack E. Behavioral self-control of stuttering using time-out from speaking. Journal of Applied Behavior Analysis; 1981 Spr Vol 14(1) 25–37

James, Jack E. Office-based treatment for stuttering: A program of speech retraining and self-management. Scandinavian Journal of Behaviour Therapy; 1982 Vol 11(1) 15–28

James, Jack E. Parameters of the influence of self-initiated time-out from speaking on stuttering. Journal of Communication Disorders; 1983 Mar Vol 16(2) 123–132

James, Jack E. Punishment of stuttering: Contingency and stimulus parameters. Journal of Communication Disorders; 1981 Sep Vol 14(5) 375–386

James, Jack E. The influence of duration on the effects of time-out from speaking. Journal of Speech and Hearing Research; 1976 Jun Vol 19(2) 206–215

James, Jack E.; Ingham, Roger J. The influence of stutterer's expectancies of improvement upon response to time-out. Journal of Speech and Hearing Research; 1974 Mar Vol. 17(1) 86–93

James, Jack E.; Ricciardelli, Lina A.; Rogers, Peter; Hunter, Christine E. A preliminary analysis of the ameliorative effects of time-out from speaking on stuttering. Journal of Speech and Hearing Research; 1989 Sep Vol 32(3) 604–610

Kalveram, Karl T.; Jancke, Lutz. Vowel duration and voice onset time for stressed and nonstressed syllables in stutterers under delayed auditory feedback condition. Folia Phoniatrica; 1989 Jan Feb Vol 41(1) 30–42

Kondas, Ondrej. (The use of a metronome in reeducation of stutterers.) Psychologia a Patopsychologia Dietata; 1974 Vol 9(6) 545–551

Lal, K. K.; Latte, G. A.; Raj, J. Bharath. A case report: Treatment of stuttering with systematic desensitization. Indian Journal of Clinical Psychology; 1976 Sep Vol 3(2) 219–221

Lanyon, Richard I.; Barocas, Victor S. Effects of contingent events on stuttering and fluency. Journal of Consulting and Clinical Psychology; 1975 Dec Vol 43(6) 786–793

Lucke, Herman H. Treatment of language fluency disorders by a procedure combining several techniques. Revista Latinoamericana de Psicologia; 1977 Vol 9(3) 437–441

Madison, Lynda S.; Budd, Karen S.; Itzkowitz, Judy S. Changes in stuttering in relation to children's locus of control. Journal of Genetic Psychology; 1986 Jun Vol 147(2) 233–240

Mallard, A. R. The effects of syllable-timed speech on stuttering behavior: An audiovisual analysis. Behavior Therapy; 1977 Nov Vol 8(5) 947–952

Manning, Walter H.; Trutna, Phyllis A.; Shaw, Candyce K. Verbal versus tangible reward for children who stutter. Journal of Speech and Hearing Disorders; 1976 Feb Vol 41(1) 52–62

Martin, Richard. The future of behavior modification of stuttering: What goes around comes around. JN: Journal of Fluency Disorders; 1993 Mar Vol 18(1) 81–108

Martin, Richard; Haroldson, Samuel. Effect of vicarious punishment on stuttering frequency. Journal of Speech and Hearing Research; 1977 Mar Vol 20(1) 21–26

Martin, Richard; Haroldson, Samuel K. Effects of five experimental treatments on stuttering. Journal of Speech and Hearing Research; 1979 Mar Vol 22(1) 132–146

Martin, Richard R.; Haroldson, Samuel K. Contingent self-stimulation for stuttering. Journal of Speech and Hearing Disorders; 1982 Nov Vol 47(4) 407–413

Martin, Richard; St Louis, Kenneth; Haroldson, Samuel; Hasbrouck, Jon. Punishment and negative reinforcement of stuttering using electric shock. Journal of Speech and Hearing Research; 1975 Sep Vol 18(3) 478–490

McDonough, Alanna N.; Quesal, Robert W. Locus of control orientation of stutterers and nonstutterers. Journal of Fluency Diosrders; 1988 Apr Vol 13(2) 97–106

Mizumachi, Toshiro. (Assessment of the results of stuttering therapy—from the behavior therapeutic point of view.) Japanese Journal of Special Education; 1981 Oct Vol 19(2) 48–55

Moreno, Felipe A. A counterconditioning program (habit-reversal) in treatment of stuttering: A case study. Revista de Psicologia General y Aplicada; 1977 Jul-Aug Vol 32(147) 593–600

Muckenhoff, Elisabeth. Modell zur Genese und Manifestation des Stotterns auf lerntheoretischer Basis. (A learning theory model of the origins of stuttering and stuttering behavior.) Vierteljahresschrift fur Heilpadagogik und ihre Nachbargebiete; 1976 Dec Vol 45(4) 341–346

Newman, Linda L. The effects of punishment of repetitions and the acquisition of "stutter-like" behaviors in normal speakers. Journal of Fluency Disorders; 1987 Feb Vol 12(1) 51–62

Nittrouer, Susan; Cheney, Carl. Operant techniques used in stuttering therapy: A review. Journal of Fluency Disorders; 1984 Sep Vol 9(3) 169–190

Nurnberger, John I.; Hingtgen, Joseph N. Is symptom substitution an important issue in behavior therapy? Biological Psychiatry; 1973 Dec Vol. 7(3) 221–236

Onslow, Mark; Costa, Leanne; Rue, Stephen. Direct early intervention with stuttering: Some preliminary data. Journal of Speech and Hearing Disorders; 1990 Aug Vol 55(3) 405–416

Onslow, Mark; Van Doorn, Janis; Newman, Denis. Variability of acoustic segment durations after prolonged-speech treatment for stuttering. Journal of Speech and Hearing Research; 1992 Jun Vol 35(3) 529–536

Ost, Lars Goran. Experimental studies in behaviour therapy. Scandinavian Journal of Behaviour Therapy; 1976 Vol 5(Suppl 1) 3–36

Petermann, Franz. Aktuelle Trends bei der Verhaltensmodifikation mit Kindern. (Current trends in behavior modification with children.) Psychologische Rundschau; 1981 Oct Vol 32(4) 250–266

Peters, Alice D. The effect of positive reinforcement on fluency: Two case studies. Language,

Speech and Hearing Services in the Schools; 1977 Jan Vol 8(1) 15–22

Peters, M. The view of learning theory. Zeitschrift fur Kinder und Jugendpsychiatrie; 1976 Vol 4(2) 104–112

Prescott, John; Andrews, Gavin. Early and late components of the contingent negative variation prior to manual and speech responses in stutterers and non-stutterers. International Journal of Psychophysiology; 1984 Nov Vol 2(2) 121–130

Prins, David; Hubbard, Carol P. Response contingent stimuli and stuttering: Issues and implications. Journal of Speech and Hearing Research; 1988 Dec Vol 31(4) 696–709

Raj, J. Bharath. Control of stuttering behaviour through response contingent shocks. Journal of the All India Institute of Speech and Hearing; 1974–75 Jan Vol 5–6 10–16

Ramirez, Luis H. (Treatment of stuttering by self-control procedures.) Revista Latinoamericana de Psicologia; 1975 Vol 7(3) 421–434

Reed, Charles G.; Lingwall, James B. Conditioned stimulus effects on stuttering and GSRs. Journal of Speech and Hearing Research; 1980 Jun Vol 23(2) 336–343

Reed, Charles G.; Lingwall, James B. Some relationships between punishment, stuttering, and galvanic skin responses. Journal of Speech and Hearing Research; 1976 Jun Vol 19(2) 197–205

Robb, Michael P.; Lybolt, John T.; Price, Harold A. Acoustic measures of stutterers' speech following an intensive therapy program. Journal of Fluency Disorders; 1985 Dec Vol 10(4) 269–279

Romero, Juan F. Tratamiento multimodal de un caso de tartamudez. / Multimodal treatment in a case of stuttering. First National Symposium: Importance of cognitive and behavioral therapies in child and adolescent psychopathology (1984, Malaga, Spain). Analisis y Modificacion de Conducta; 1985 Vol 11(27) 133–143

Roth U., Erick; Aguilar S., Guido G. Speech therapy: A comparative study of the stutterer. Aprendizaje y Comportamiento; 1979 Vol 2(1–2) 93–108

Runyan, Charles M.; Hames, Patricia E.; Prosek, Robert A. A perceptual comparison between paired stimulus and single stimulus methods of presentation of the fluent utterances of stutterers. Journal of Fluency Disorders; 1982 Mar Vol 7(1–1) 71–77

Rustin, Lena; Kuhr, Armin. The treatment of stammering: A multi-model approach in an in-patient setting. British Journal of Disorders of Communication; 1983 Sep Vol 18(2) 90–97

Ryan, Bruce P.; Van Kirk, Barbara. Programmed stuttering therapy for children: Comparison of four establishment programs. Journal of Fluency Disorders; 1983 Dec Vol 8(4) 291–321

Ryan, Bruce P.; Van Kirk, Barbara. The establishment, transfer, and maintenance of fluent speech in 50 stutterers using delayed auditory feedback and operant procedures. Journal of Speech and Hearing Disorders; 1974 Feb Vol. 39(1) 3–10

Saint Laurent, Lise; Ladouceur, Robert. Analyse des traitements behavioraux du begaiement. (Analyses of behavioral treatments for stuttering.) Canadian Psychology; 1987 Jul Vol 28(3) 239–250

Siegel, Gerald M. Stuttering and behavior modification: Commentary. Journal of Fluency Disorders; Mar Vol 18(1) 109–114

Silverman, Franklin H. Communicative success: A reinforcer of stuttering? Perceptual and Motor Skills; 1976 Oct Vol 43(2) 398

Silverman, Franklin H.; Silverman, Ellen Marie. Effect of threat of shock for being disfluent on fluency of normal speakers. Perceptual and Motor Skills; 1975 Oct Vol 41(2) 353–354

Small, Maurice M. Treatment of stuttering: A case history. Perceptual and Motor Skills; 1975 Dec Vol 41(3) 812

Smit Beek, Eva; Sluijmer Swanenburg, Bep. An experimental group treatment of six stuttering children based on the two-factor theory of Mowrer. Tijdschrift voor Psychotherapie; 1977 Jul Vol 3(4) 175–182

Starkweather, C. W. A behavioral analysis of Van Riperian therapy for stutterers. Journal of Communication Disorders; 1973 Dec Vol 6(4) 273–291

Tyre, Timothy E; Maisto, Stephen A.; Companik, Paul J. The use of systematic desensitation in the treatment of chronic stuttering behavior.

Journal of Spech and Hearing Disorders; 1973 Nov Vol 38(4) 514–519

Viswanath, N. S. Experimental aversion therapy for stuttering: A case study. Journal of the All India Institute of Speech and Hearing; 1971 Jan Vol 2 69–71

Watson, Ben C.; Freeman, Frances J.; Chapman, Sandra B.; Miller, Susan; et al. Linguistic performance deficits in stutterers: Relation to laryngeal reaction time profiles. Journal of Fluency Disorders; 1991 Vol 16(2–3) 85–100

Watts, Fraser. Mechanisms of fluency control in stutterers. British Journal of Disorders of Communication; 1973 Oct Vol 8(2) 131–138

Webster, William G. Sequence reproduction deficits in stutterers tested under nonspeeded response conditions. Journal of Fluency Disorders; 1989 Apr Vol 14(2) 79–86

Webster, William G.; Ryan, C. Lynne. Task complexity and manual reaction times in people who stutter. Journal of Speech and Hearing Research; 1991 Aug Vol 34(4) 708–714

Wendlandt, Wolfgang. (A behavior therapeutic program for adult stutterers.) Praxis der Kinderpsychologie und Kinderpsychiatrie; 1974 Oct Vol 23(7) 255–265

Wendlandt, Wolfgang. (Self-assertive training: A behavioral therapeutic phase in the treatment of adult stutterers.) Zeitschrift fur Klinische Psychologie und Psychotherapie; 1974 Vol 22(3) 236–246

Williams, J. David; Martin, Randall B. Immediate versus delayed consequences of stuttering responses. Journal of Speech and Hearing Research; 1974 Dec Vol 17(4) 569–575

Wolak, Krzysztof. Zastosowanie techniki biofeedback w terapii osab jakajacych sie./Biofeedback technique in stuttering therapy. Psychologia Wychowawcza; 1988 Jan-Feb Vol 31(1) 56– 69

Physiology

Abeleva, I. Yu. Respiration dynamics during speech production in stuttering adults. Defektologiya; 1976 Jan No 1 17–20

Andronova, L. Z. Correction of intonation in stutterers. Defektologiya; 1988 No 6 63–67

Baken, R. J.; McManus, Devin A.; Cavallo, Stephen A. Prephonatory chest wall posturing in stutterers. Journal of Speech and Hearing Research; 1983 Sep Vol 26(3) 444–450

Bakker, Klaas; Brutten, Gene J.; Janssen, Peggy; Van der Meulen, Sjoeke. An eyemarking study of anticipation and dysfluency among elementary school stutterers. Journal of Fluency Disorders; 1991 Feb Vol 16(1) 25–33

Baumgartner, John M.; Brutten, Gene J. Expectancy and heart rate as predictors of the speech performance of stutterers. Journal of Speech and Hearing Research; 1983 Sep Vol 26(3) 383–388

Boudreau, Leonce; Ladouceur, Robert. L'influence de l'aide sociale associee a la respiration regularisee sur le traitement du begaiement. / The influence of social help associated with regularized respiration on the treatment of stuttering. Technologie et Therapie du Comportement; 1985 Fal Vol 8(2) 125–151

Brutten, Gene J.; Bakker, K.; Janssen, P.; Van der Meulen, S. Eye movements of stuttering and nonstuttering children during silent reading. Journal of Speech and Hearing Research; 1984 Dec Vol 27(4) 562–566

Campbell, Michel; Boudreau, Leonce; Ladouceur, Robert. L'influence d'interlocuteurs sur l'evaluation du begaiement. (The influence of speakers on the evaluation of stuttering.) Revue de Modification du Comportement; 1984 Vol 14(3) 112–122

Christensen, John M.; Sacco, Pat R. Association of hair and eye color with handedness and stuttering. Journal of Fluency Disorders; 1989 Feb Vol 14(1) 37–45

Costa, D.; et al. Clinical and paraclinical aspects of tetany in stuttering. Revue Roumaine de Neurologie et Psychiatrie; 1983 Jul Sep Vol 21(3) 277–279

Costa, D.; Pop, A.; Dumitriu, L.; Marinescu, Luzia; et al. Serum immunoreactive parathormone levels correlate with depression and anxiety in hypocalcemic stutterers. Activitas Nervosa Superior; 1986 Vol 28(2) 155–156

Craig, Ashley R.; Cleary, Patrick J. Reduction of stuttering by young male stutterers using EMG feedback. Biofeedback and Self Regulation; 1982 Sep Vol 7(3) 241–255

Cross, Douglas E.; Olson, Patricia. Interaction between jaw kinematics and voice onset for stutterers and nonstutterers in a VRT task. Journal of Fluency Disorders; 1987 Oct Vol 12(5) 367–380

Crowe, Kathryn M.; Kroll, Robert M. Response latency and response class for stutterers and nonstutterers as measured by a word-association task. Journal of Fluency Disorders; 1991 Feb Vol 16(1) 35–54

Dabul, Barbara; Perkins, William H. The effects of stuttering on systolic blood pressure. Journal of Speech and Hearing Research; 1973 Dec Vol 16(4) 586–591

Dellatolas, Georges; Annesi, Isabella; Jallon, Pierre; Chavance, Michel; et al. An epidemiological reconsideration of the Geschwind Galaburda theory of cerebral lateralization. Archives of Neurology; 1990 Jul Vol 47(7) 778–782

Falkowski, Glenn L.; Guilford, Arthur M.; Sandler, Jack. Effectiveness of a modified version of airflow therapy: Case studies. Journal of Speech and Hearing Disorders; 1982 May Vol 47(2) 160–164

Geschwind, Norman. Biological associations of left-handedness. Annals of Dyslexia; 1983 Vol 33 29–40

Guitar, Barry. Reduction of stuttering frequency using analog electromyographic feedback. Journal of Speech and Hearing Research; 1975 Dec Vol 18(4) 672–685

Guitar, Barry; Guitar, Carroll; Neilson, Peter; O'Dwyer, Nicholas; et al. Onset sequencing of selected lip muscles in stutterers and nonstutterers. Journal of Speech and Hearing Research; 1988 Mar Vol 31(1) 28–35

Hanna, Richmond; Wilfling, Franz; McNeill, Brent. A biofeedback treatment for stuttering. Journal of Speech and Hearing Disorders; 1975 May Vol 40(2) 270–273

Harbison, Dan C.; Porter, Robert J.; Tobey, Emily A. Shadowed and simple reaction times in stutterers and nonstutterers. Journal of the Acoustical Society of America; 1989 Oct Vol 86(4) 1277–1284

Harris, Daniel; Fucci, Donald; Petrosino, Linda. Magnitude estimation and cross-modal matching of auditory and lingual vibrotactile sensation by normal speakers and stutterers. Journal of Speech and Hearing Research; 1991 Feb Vol 34(1) 177–182

Hasbrouck, Jon M. FAMC intensive stuttering treatment program: Ten years of implementation. Military Medicine; 1992 May Vol 157(5) 244–247

Hasbrouck, Jon M.; Lowry, Fran. Elimination of stuttering and maintenance of fluency by means of airflow, tension reduction, and discriminative stimulus control procedures. Journal of Fluency Disorders; 1989 Jun Vol 14(3) 165–183

Horovitz, Linda J.; et al. Stapedial reflex and anxiety in fluent and disfluent speakers. Journal of Speech and Hearing Research; 1978 Dec Vol 21(4) 762–767

Hurford, David P.; Webster, Ronald L. Decreases in simple reaction time as a function of stutterers' participation in a behavioral therapy. Journal of Fluency Disorders; 1985 Dec Vol 10(4) 301–310

Hutchinson, John M.; Watkin, Kenneth L. Jaw mechanics during release of the stuttering moment: Some initial observations and interpretations. Journal of Communication Disorders; 1976 Dec Vol 9(4) 269–279

Hutchinson, John M.; Ringel, Robert L. The effect of oral sensory deprivation on stuttering behavior. Journal of Communication Disorders; 1975 Sep Vol 8(3) 249–258

Kalotkin, Madeline; Manschreck, Theo C.; O'Brien, Donna. Electromyographic tension levels in stutterers and normal speakers. Perceptual and Motor Skills; 1979 Aug Vol 49(1) 109–110

Kooman, E. A. Speech disturbance under delayed acoustic feedback and stuttering. Defektologiya; 1975 Jun No 6 27–33

Kraaimaat, Floor; Janssen, Peggy. Are the accessory facial movements of the stutterer learned behaviours? Perceptual and Motor Skills; 1985 Feb Vol 60(1) 11–17

Ladouceur, Robert; Martineau, Guylaine. Evaluation of regulated-breathing method with and without parental assistance in the treatment of child stutterers. Journal of Behavior Therapy and Experimental Psychiatry; 1982 Dec Vol 13(4) 301–306

Lagutina, T. S.; Lovchikova, N. N.; Obukhovskii, N. G. Electrophysiological study of patients with logoneuroses. Soviet Neurology and Psychiatry; 1985 Fal Vol 18(3) 53–61

Lanyon, Richard I. Effect of biofeedback-based relaxation on stuttering during reading and spontaneous speech. Journal of Consulting and Clinical Psychology; 1977 Oct Vol 45(5) 860–866

Lanyon, Richard I.; Barrington, Cecily C.; Newman, Anne C. Modification of stuttering through EMG biofeedback: A preliminary study. Behavior Therapy; 1976 Jan Vol 7(1) 96–103

Lara Cantu, Maria A. Pilot study on electromyographic biofeedback for the treatment of stuttering. Ensenanza e Investigacion en Psicologia; 1978 Jul Dec Vol 4(2) 259–265

Legewie, H.; Cleary, P.; Rackensperger, W. EMG-recording and biofeedback in the diagnosis and therapy of stuttering: A case study. European Journal of Behavioural Analysis and Modification; 1975 Dec Vol 1(2) 137–143

Manschreck, Theo C.; Kalotkin, Madeline; Jacobson, Alan M. Utility of electromyographic biological feedback in chronic stuttering: A clinical study with follow-up. Perceptual and Motor Skills; 1980 Oct Vol 51(2) 535–540

McClean, Michael D. Surface EMG recording of the perioral reflexes: Preliminary observations on stutterers and nonstutterers. Journal of Speech and Hearing Research; 1987 Jun Vol 30(2) 283–287

McClean, Michael D.; Goldsmith, Howard; Cerf, Ann. Lower-lip EMG and displacement during bilabial disfluencies in adult stutterers. Journal of Speech and Hearing Research; 1984 Sep Vol 27(3) 342–349

McClean, Michael D.; Kroll, Robert M.; Loftus, Nirit S. Kinematic analysis of lip closure in stutterers' fluent speech. Journal of Speech and Hearing Research; 1990 Dec Vol 33(4) 755–760

McKnight, Roxanne C.; Cullinan, Walter L. Subgroups of stuttering children: Speech and voice reaction times, segmental durations, and naming latencies. Journal of Fluency Disorders; 1987 Jun Vol 12(3) 217–233

Moore, Walter H. Pathophysiology of stuttering: Cerebral activation differences in stutterers vs. nonstutterers. ASHA-Reports Series

American Speech Language Hearing Association; 1990 Apr No 18 72–80

Muhs, Aribert; Schepank, Heinz. Aspekte des Verlaufs und der geschlectsspezifischen Pravalenz psychogener Erkrankungen bei Kindern und Erwachsenen unter dem Einfluss von Erb und Umweltfaktoren. (Aspects of development of the incidence of psychogenic disorders in children and adults under the influence of hereditary and environmental factors.) Zeitschrift fur Psychosomatische Medizin und Psychoanalyse; 1991 Vol 37(2) 194–206

Murdoch, Bruce E.; Killin, Heather; McCaul, Annette. A kinematic analysis of respiratory function in a group of stutterers pre- and posttreatment. Journal of Fluency Disorders; 1989 Oct Vol 14(5) 323–350

Murray, K. S.; Empson, J. A.; Weaver, S. M. Rehearsal and preparation for speech in stutterers: A psychophysiological study. British Journal of Disorders of Communication; 1987 Aug Vol 22(2) 145–150

Oganesian, Ye. V.; Beliakova, L. I. The rationale for principles of differential application of logopaedic rhythmics in remediation of adult stutterers. Defektologiya; 1982 No 1 3–12

Orta Rodriguez, Martha; Gallegos B., Xochitl. Una evaluacion de tres tecnicas conductuales en el tratamiento de la tartamudez. (An evaluation of 3 behavioral techniques used to treat stuttering.) Revista Mexicana de Psicologia; 1986 Jul-Dec Vol 3(2) 168–173

Pachman, Joseph S.; Oelschlaeger, Mary L.; Hughes, Anita; Hughes, Howard H. Toward identifying effective agents in use of biofeedback to decelerate stuttering behavior. Perceptual and Motor Skills; 1978 Jun Vol 46(3, Pt 1) 1006

Perkins, William; Rudas, Joanna; Johnson, Linda; Bell, Jody. Stuttering: Discoordination of phonation with articulation and respiration. Journal of Speech and Hearing Research; 1976 Sep Vol 19(3) 509–522

Perkins, William H.; Bell, Jody; Johnson, Linda; Stocks, Janice. Phone rate and the effective planning time hypothesis of stuttering. Journal of Speech and Hearing Research; 1979 Dec Vol 22(4) 747–755

Perkins, William H.; et al. Replacement of stuttering with normal speech: III. Clinical effectiveness. Journal of Speech and Hearing Disorders; 1974 Nov Vol 39(4) 416–428

Peters, Herman F.; Boves, Louis. Coordination of aerodynamic and phonatory processes in fluent speech utterances of stutterers. Journal of Speech and Hearing Research; 1988 Sep Vol 31(3) 352–361

Peters, Herman F.; Hulstijn, Wouter; Starkweather, C. Woodruff. Acoustic and physiological reaction times of stutterers and nonstutterers. Journal of Speech and Hearing Research; 1989 Sep Vol 32(3) 668–680

Petrosino, Linda; Fucci, Donald; Gorman, Peter; Harris, Daniel. Midline and off-midline tongue and right- and left-hand vibrotactile thresholds of stutterers and normal-speaking individuals. Perceptual and Motor Skills; 1987 Aug Vol 65(1) 253–254

Platt, L. Jay; Basili, Annamaria. Jaw tremor during stuttering block: An electromyographic study. Journal of Communication Disorders; 1973 Jun Vol. 6(2) 102–109

Prosek, Robert A.; Montgomery, Allen A.; Walden, Brian E. Constancy of relative timing for stutterers and nonstutterers. Journal of Speech and Hearing Research; 1988 Dec Vol 31(4) 654–658

Rastatter, Michael P.; Dell, Carl W. Reaction times of moderate and severe stutterers to monaural verbal stimuli: Some implications for neurolinguistic organization. Journal of Speech and Hearing Research; 1987 Mar Vol 30(1) 21–27

Reed, Charles G.; Lingwall, James B. Some relationships between punishment, stuttering, and galvanic skin responses. Journal of Speech and Hearing Research; 1976 Jun Vol 19(2) 197–205

Sahasi, G.; Pandit, Rama. Indigenous methods of treating stuttering. Journal of Personality and Clinical Studies; 1985 Mar-Sep Vol 1(1–2) 37–40

Saint Laurent, Lise; Ladouceur, Robert. Massed versus distributed application of the regulated-breathing method for stutterers and its long-term effect. Behavior Therapy; 1987 Win Vol 18(1) 38–50

Santacreu Mas, Jose. El condicionamiento ante determinadas palabras en la tartamudez. (Conditioning before some words in stuttering.) Revista de Psicologia General y Aplicada; 1984 Vol 39(6) 1115–1129

Santacreu Mas, Jose. Respuestas psicofisiologicas de sujetos tartamudos durante la pronunciacion de palabras. (Psychophysiological responses of stutterers during pronunciation of words.) Revista de Psicologia General y Aplicada; 1985 Vol 40(2) 221–242

Schultheis, Josef R. Modern theories of stuttering. Praxis der Kinderpsychologie und Kinderpsychiatrie; 1978 Apr Vol 27(3) 83–87

Schultheis, Josef R. Stottern in historischer und "komplexer" Hinsicht. (Stuttering: Historical and complex perpectives.) Vierteljahresschrift fur Heilpadagogik und ihre Nachbargebiete; 1979 Jun Vol 48(2) 125–138

Small, Maurice M. Treatment of stuttering: A case history. Perceptual and Motor Skills; 1975 Dec Vol 41(3) 812

Smith, Anne. Neural drive to muscles in stuttering. Journal of Speech and Hearing Research; 1989 Jun Vol 32(2) 252–264

Smith, Anne; Luschei, Erich S. Assessment of oral-motor reflexes in stutterers and normal speakers: Preliminary observations. Journal of Speech and Hearing Research; 1983 Sep Vol 26(3) 322–328

St. Louis, Kenneth O.; Clausell, Paul L.; Thompson, Jean N.; Rife, Constance C. Preliminary investigation of EMG biofeedback induced relaxation with a preschool aged stutterer. Perceptual and Motor Skills; 1982 Aug Vol 55(1) 195–199

Strub, Richard L.; Black, F. William; Naeser, Margaret A. Anomalous dominance in sibling stutterers: Evidence from CT scan asymmetries, dichotic listening, neuropsychological testing, and handedness. Brain and Language; 1987 Mar Vol 30(2) 338–350

Szelag, Elzbieta; Garwarska Kolek, Danuta; Herman, Anna; Stasiek, Janina. Brain lateralization and severity of stuttering in children. First International Congress of the Polish Neuroscience Society: A congress in the decade of the brain (1992, Warsaw, Poland). Acta Neurobiologiae Experimentalis; 1993 Vol 53(1) 263–267

Till, James A.; Reich, Alan; Dickey, Stanley; Seiber, James. Phonatory and manual reaction times of stuttering and nonstuttering children. Journal of Speech and Hearing Research; 1983 Jun Vol 26(2) 171–180

Timmons, Beverly A. Physiological factors related to delayed auditory feedback and stuttering: A review. Perceptual and Motor Skills; 1982 Dec Vol 55(3, Pt 2) 1179–1189

Van Lieshout, Pascal H.; Peters, Herman F.; Starkweather, C. Woodruff; Hulstijn, Wouter. Physiological differences between stutterers and nonstutterers in perceptually fluent speech: EMG amplitude and duration. Journal of Speech and Hearing Research; 1993 Feb Vol 36(1) 55–63

Walker, Susan T.; Walker, J. M. Differences in heart-rate variability between stutterers and nonstutterers following arousal. Perceptual and Motor Skills; 1973 Jun Vol 36(3, Pt. 1) 926

Ward, David. Voice-onset time and electroglottographic dynamics in stutterers' speech: Implications for a differential diagnosis. British Journal of Disorders of Communication; 1990 Apr Vol 25(1) 93–104

Waterloo, Knut K.; Gotestam, K. Gunnar. The regulated-breathing method for stuttering: An experimental evaluation. Journal of Behavior Therapy and Experimental Psychiatry; 1988 Mar Vol 19(1) 11–19

Watson, Ben C.; Alfonso, Peter J. Physiological bases of acoustic LRT in nonstutterers, mild stutterers, and severe stutterers. Journal of Speech and Hearing Research; 1987 Dec Vol 30(4) 434–447

Watson, Ben C.; Pool, Kenneth D.; Devous, Michael D.; Freeman, Frances J.; et al. Brain blood flow related to acoustic laryngeal reaction time in adult developmental stutterers. Journal of Speech and Hearing Research; 1992 Jun Vol 35(3) 555–561

Watson, Peter; Guitar, Barry. Respiratory stuttering? A case history. Journal of Fluency Disorders; 1986 Jun Vol 11(2) 165–173

Watts, Fraser. Mechanisms of fluency control in stutterers. British Journal of Disorders of Communication; 1973 Oct Vol 8(2) 131–138

Weber, Christine M.; Smith, Anne. Autonomic correlates of stuttering and speech assessed in a range of experimental tasks. Journal of Speech and Hearing Research; 1990 Dec Vol 33(4) 690–706

Wood, Frank; et al. Patterns of regional cerebral blood flow during attempted reading aloud by stutterers both on and off haloperidol medication: Evidence for inadequate left frontal activation during stuttering. Brain and Language; 1980 Jan Vol 9(1) 141–144

Psychological Issues

Abeleva, I. Yu. (Psychology of stuttering in adults during various phases of verbal communication.) Voprosy Psikhologii; 1974 Jul Aug No 4 144–149

Ablon, Steven L. Psychoanalysis of a stuttering boy. Special Issue: Psychoanalysis of children. International Review of Psycho Analysis; 1988 Vol 15(1) 83–91

Adams, Martin R. Learning from negative outcomes in stuttering therapy: I. Getting off on the wrong foot. Journal of Fluency Disorders; 1983 Jun Vol 8(2) 147–153

Angushev, G. I. (An investigation of the interrelationships among mental functions in normal and stuttering adolescents.) Voprosy Psikhologii; 1974 Jul Aug No 4 96–194

Antonucci, Gianfranco; de Rosa, Emilia. La balbuzie: evoluzione dei concetti e prospettive per una comprensione psicodinamica del sintomo. (Stuttering: Evolution of its conceptualizations and prospects for a psychodynamic understanding of this symptom.) Archivio di Psicologia, Neurologia e Psichiatria; 1986 Oct–Dec Vol 47(4) 451–476

Anzieu, Annie. Essai sur le corps fantasmatique du begue. (Essay on the phantasmatic body of the stutterer.) Pratique des Mots; 1982 Sep No 40 14–18

Arkin, Arthur M.; et al. Behavior modification: Present status in psychiatry. New York State Journal of Medicine; 1976 Feb Vol 76(2) 190–196

Asatiani, N. M.; Kazakov, V. G.; Freidin, Yu. L. Some problems of clinical classification of stuttering. Defektologiya; 1988 No 1 28–32

Asatiani, N. M.; Matveeva, E. S.; Sokolova, T. N.; Zhukov, V. F. The neurotic development in the clinical picture of stammering. Zhurnal Nevropatologii i Psikhiatrii imeni S. S. Korsakova; 1985 Vol 85(11) 1684–1688

Atkinson, Leslie. Rational-emotive therapy versus systematic desensitization: A comment on Moleski and Tosi. Journal of Consulting and Clinical Psychology; 1983 Oct Vol 51(5) 776–778

Baker, Lorian; Cantwell, Dennis P. Psychiatric and learning disorders in children with speech and language disorders: A critical review. Advances in Learning and Behavioral Disabilities; 1985 Vol 4 1–28

Ballesteros, Rocio F.; Mas, Jose S.; Carrobles, Jose A. Relaciones entre respuestas psicofisiologicas y autoinformes. / Relationships between psychophysiological responses and self-reports. Analisis y Modificacion de Conducta; 1984 Vol 10(25) 299–311

Banjac Karovic, Milena; Povse Ivkic, Violica; Bojanin, Svetomir. Inhibicija govora i mucanje. (Speech inhibition and stuttering.) Psihijatrija Danas; 1990 Vol 22(1) 99–104

Barblan, Leo. Therapeutique du langage: Science ou intuition? (Therapeutics of language: Science or intuition?) Pratique des Mots; 1983 Sep No 44 23–36

Bloom, Leon. Notes for a history of speech pathology. Psychoanalytic Review; 1978 Fal Vol 65(3) 433–463

Boberg, Einer; Calder, Peter. Stuttering: A review for counsellors and teachers. Canadian Counsellor; 1977 Apr Vol 11(3) 144–148

Bounes, Marika. Test de Rorschach avant et apres traitement de relaxation chez l'enfant. (Rorschach test before and after relaxation treatment of a child.) 11th International Congress on the Rorschach and Projective Methods (1984, Barcelona, Spain). Bulletin de Psychologie; 1986 Jun-Aug Vol 39(11–15) 651–654

Brady, John P. Behavior therapy and American psychiatry. Journal of the National Association of Private Psychiatric Hospitals; 1972 Fal Vol 4(3) 27–35

Bushey, Tahirih; Martin, Richard. Stuttering in children's literature. Language, Speech, and Hearing Services in Schools; 1988 Jul Vol 19(3) 235–250

Butany, V.; Persad, E. Is stuttering a contraindication to psychotherapy? Canadian Journal of Psychiatry; 1982 Jun Vol 27(4) 330–331

Cantwell, Dennis P.; Baker, Lorian. Psychiatric and learning disorders in children with speech and language disorders: A descriptive analysis. Advances in Learning and Behavioral Disabilities; 1985 Vol 4 29–47

Cox, Nancy J.; Seider, Robin A.; Kidd, Kenneth K. Some environmental factors and hypotheses for stuttering in families with several stutterers. Journal of Speech and Hearing Research; 1984 Dec Vol 27(4) 543–548

Craig, Ashley R.; Cleary, Patrick J. Reduction of stuttering by young male stutterers using EMG feedback. Biofeedback and Self Regulation; 1982 Sep Vol 7(3) 241–255

de Rosa, E.; Antonucci, G.; Rinaldi, L. Balbuzie, complesso edipico e angosce primitive: Osservazioni su un caso clinico. / Stuttering, Oedipus complex and earliest anxieties: Some observations on a clinical case. Archivio di Psicologia, Neurologia e Psichiatria; 1987 Vol 48(3) 327–335

Degand, J. (A clinical contribution to the psychodynamic and the pathopsychogenic sources of language problems.) Revue Belge de Psychologie et de Pedagogie; 1972 Vol 34(139) 79–93

Delmonte, Michael M. Meditation as a clinical intervention strategy: A brief review. International Journal of Psychosomatics; 1986 Vol 33(3) 9–12

Devore, Jon E.; Nandur, Mallika S.; Manning, Walter H. Projective drawings and children who stutter. Journal of Fluency Disorders; 1984 Sep Vol 9(3) 217–226

Dharitri, R. Response to therapy by stutterers in relation to their locus of control. Indian Journal of Clinical Psychology; 1985 Sep Vol 12(2) 37–40

Dickson, Stanley. An application of the Blacky Test to a study of the psychosexual development of stutterers. International Journal of Social Psychiatry; 1974 Fal-Win Vol 20(3–4) 269–273

Dolto, Francoise. L'agressivite chez le jeune enfant. (Aggressiveness in the young child.) Pratique des Mots; 1982 Mar No 38 19–25

Ferreiro Diaz, M. D.; Dominguez, M. Dolores; Rodriguez, A. Psicoterapis de grupos infantiles: la madre co-terapeuta. (Group psychotherapy for children: The mother as co-therapist.) Clinica y Analisis Grupal; 1990 May-Aug Vol 12(2) 291–313

Fitzgerald, Hiram E.; Djurdjic, Slavoljub D.; Maguin, Eugene. Assessment of sensitivity to interpersonal stress in stutterers. Journal of Communication Disorders; 1992 Mar Vol 25(1) 31–42

Floyd, Nathaniel M. Billy Budd: A psychological autopsy. American Imago; 1977 Spr Vol 34(1) 28–49

Fogle, Dale O. Learned helplessness and learned restlessness. Psychotherapy Theory, Research and Practice; 1978 Spr Vol 15(1) 39–47

Frankl, Viktor E. The first published cases of paradoxical intention. International Forum for Logotherapy; 1992 15(1) 2–6

Gamelli, Ralph J. Classification of child stuttering: I. Transient developmental, neurogenic acquired, and persistent child stuttering. Child Psychiatry and Human Development; 1982 Sum Vol 12(4) 220–253

Garber, Anath. Psychodramatic treatment of a stutterer. Group Psychotherapy and Psychodrama; 1973 Vol 26(1–2) 34–47

Gerkina, M. I. (The speech of stuttering preschool children under different conditions of communication.) Defektologiya; 1972 Vol 3 29–34

Gottinger, Werner. A concept for the guidance of stutterers. Praxis der Kinderpsychologie und Kinderpsychiatrie; 1980 Feb-Mar Vol 29(2) 55–62

Goraj, Jane T. Stuttering therapy as crisis intervention. British Journal of Disorders of Communication; 1974 Apr Vol. 9(1) 51–57

Greenberg, David; Marks, Isaac. Behavioural psychotherapy of uncommon referrals. British Journal of Psychiatry; 1982 Aug Vol 141 148–153

Greiner, Jay R.; Fitzgerald, Hiram E.; Cooke, Paul A.; Djurdjic, Slavoljub D. Assessment of sensitivity to interpersonal stress in stutterers and nonstutterers. Journal of Communication Disorders; 1985 Jun Vol 18(3) 215–225

Grempel, Franz. Stuttering as a crisis in achieving adult status: Contribution to the etiology and therapy of a stutterer. Praxis der Psychotherapie; 1976 Feb Vol 21(1) 29–41

Guy, Nina. Stuttering as an expression of aggression: Transferential and countertransferential aspects: A case study. Israel Journal of Psychiatry and Related Sciences; 1987 Vol 24(3) 211–221

Halg, Paul. Symbolik und Verlauf in der Therapie eines dreizehnjährigen Stotterers mit dem katathymen Bilderleben. (Symbolism and process in a short term therapy of a male juvenile stutterer using the day dream technique of guided affective imagery (GAI).) Praxis der Kinderpsychologie und Kinderpsychiatrie; 1981 Oct Vol 30(7) 236–243

Halpern, Harvey. Stuttering therapy for nonfluent psychiatric adults. Perceptual and Motor Skills; 1990 Dec Vol 71(3, Pt 1) 914

Halpern, Harvey; McCartin Clark, Marguerite; Wallack, Wendy. The nonfluencies of eight psychiatric adults. Journal of Communication Disorders; 1989 Aug Vol 22(4) 233–241

Harris, Adrienne. Women in relation to power and words. Issues in Ego Psychology; 1987 Vol 10(1) 29–38

Haskell, Rochelle J.; Larr, Alfred L. Psychodramatic role training with stutterers. Group Psychotherapy and Psychodrama; 1974 Vol 27(1–4) 30–36

Hays, Peter; Field, L. Leigh. Postulated genetic linkage between manic-depression and stuttering. Journal of Affective Disorders; 1989 Jan–Feb Vol 16(1) 37–40

Hays, Peter; Field, L. Leigh. Postulated genetic linkage between manic-depression and stuttering. Journal of Affective Disorders; 1989 Jan–Feb Vol 16(1) 37–40

Hays, P. A new sampling strategy for linkage studies in psychoses. Journal of Affective Disorders; 1993 Jun Vol 28(2) 141–142

Horsley, Irmgarde A.; FitzGibbon, Carol T. Stuttering children: Investigation of a stereotype. British Journal of Disorders of Communication; 1987 Apr Vol 22(1) 19–35

Hutchinson, John M.; Ringel, Robert L. The effect of oral sensory deprivation on stuttering behavior. Journal of Communication Disorders; 1975 Sep Vol 8(3) 249–258

Ikezuki, Makoto; Harano, Kotaro; Yamaguchi, Shoji. (Research on the effect of reciprocal inhibition elicited with kinetic response.) Japanese Journal of Behavior Therapy; 1989 Vol 15(1) 56–61

Isshiki, Nobuhiko. Voice and speech disorders requiring surgical treatment. Japanese Psychological Review; 1977 Vol 20(1) 51–60

Itoh, Norihiro; Kamada, Yuko. An analytical study of self-consciousness in stutterers. Japanese Journal of Child and Adolescent Psychiatry; 1981 Vol 22(3) 193–202

Joseph, Anthony B. Transient stuttering in catatonic bipolar patients. Behavioural Neurology; 1991 Win Vol 4(4) 265–269

Kalyagin, V. A. Characteristics of attention in stutterers. Soviet Neurology and Psychiatry; 1985–86 Win Vol 18(4) 85–88

Kaplan, Netta R.; Kaplan, Marvin L. The Gestalt approach to stuttering. Journal of Communication Disorders; 1978 Feb Vol 11(1) 1–9

Kastelova, Darina; Szenteova, Iveta. Socialna interakcia recovo narusenych deti (vo vol'nom case mimo skoly). / Social interaction of speech disordered children (out of school—in their leisure time). Psychologia a Patopsychologia Dietata; 1990 Vol 25(6) 551–557

Kastelova, Darina; Szenteova, Iveta. Sociometricka pozicia recovo naruseneho diet'at'a v triede na ZS. / Sociometric status of speech disordered child in the basic school class. Psychologia a Patopsychologia Dietata; 1991 Vol 26(1) 29–34

Katz-Bernstein, Nitza. Poltern: Therapieansatz fur Kinder. (Tachyphemia: A therapeutic approach for children.) Vierteljahresschrift fur Heilpadagogik und ihre Nachbargebiete; 1986 Dec Vol 55(4) 413–426

Kaubish, V. K.; Linskaia, L. N. Characteristics of neurosislike states and their treatment in children with retarded mental development. Soviet Neurology and Psychiatry; 1991 Fal Vol 24(3) 38–42

Kehrer, H. E. (Behaviour therapy in child and adolescent psychiatry.) Acta Paedopsychiatrica; 1973 Vol 40(2) 58–65

Kerbeshian, Jacob; et al. Gilles de la Tourette disease in multiply disabled children. Special Issue: Children with multiple disabilities. Rehabilitation Literature; 1985 Sep–Oct Vol 46(9–10) 255–258

Khavin, A. B. (Personality reactions to a communication disorder.) Defektologiya; 1974 Vol 1 2 6–29

Khavin, Aleksandr B. Individual psychological factors in prediction of help to stutterers. Voprosy Psikhologii; 1985 Mar–Apr No 2 133–135

Kondas, Ondrej. Emocionalne a situacne premenne pri reci balbutikov. / Emotional and situational variables in the speech of stutterers. Zbornik Univerzity Komenskeho Psychologica; 1982 Vol 26–27 197–208

Kotbi, Naser; Farag, Safwat; Yousif, Mahmoud; Baraka, Mohamed, et al. A comparison between stutterers and non stutterers in intelligence, self-concept, anxiety and depression. Derasat Nafseyah; 1992 2(2) 37–349

Krause, Matthias P. Stottern als Beziehungsstorung—Psychotherapeutische Arbeit mit Eltern stotternder Kinder. / Stuttering as an expression of disturbed parent-child relationship. Praxis der Kinderpsychologie und Kinderpsychiatrie; 1985 Jan Vol 34(1) 15–18

Krause, Rainer. Nonverbal interactive behavior in stutterers and their speaking partners. Psychologie Schweizerische Zeitschrift fur Psychologie und ihre Anwendungen; Vol 37(3) 177–201

Lavkai, I. Yu. On personality deviations in stuttering adolescents. Defektologiya; 1976 Feb No 2 16–18

Leahy, M.; O'Sullivan, B. Psychological change and fluency therapy: A pilot project. British Journal of Disorders of Communication; 1987 Dec Vol 22(3) 245–251

Leith, William R.; Timmons, Jack L. The use of the Psychological Stress Evaluator with stutterers. Journal of Fluency Disorders; 1983 Sep Vol 8(3) 207–213

Levina, R. Ye. On emociogenic factors of stuttering which arise in the course of formation of voluntary speech. Defektologiya; 1981 Jan No 1 7–13

Lomachenkov, A. S.; Martsinkevich, N. E. Maladjustment in children in the form of masked depressions. Trudy Leningradskogo Nauchno Issledovatel'skogo Psikhonevrologicheskogo Instituta i m V M Bekhtereva; 1988 Vol 119 38–42

Lukas, Elisabeth. New ways for dereflection. International Forum for Logotherapy; 1981 Spr–Sum Vol 4(1) 13–28

Lucas, Tina. Communication therapy. Journal of Adolescence; 1982 Sep Vol 5(3) 285–299

Manning, Walter H.; Dailey, Deborah; Wallace, Sue. Attitude and personality characteristics of older stutterers. Journal of Fluency Disorders; 1984 Sep Vol 9(3) 207–215

Matanova-Koleva, Vanja. A conceptual model of stuttering. Psikhologiia Bulgaria; 1985 Vol 13(1) 45–49

McDonough, Alanna N.; Quesal, Robert W. Locus of control orientation of stutterers and nonstutterers. Journal of Fluency Disorders; 1988 Apr Vol 13(2) 97–106

McIntyre, Mary E.; Silverman, Franklin H.; Trotter, William D. Transcendental meditation and stuttering: A preliminary report. Perceptual and Motor Skills; 1974 Aug Vol 39(1) 294

Mempel, Sigurd. Therapiemotivation bei Kindern: Ergebnisse einer empirischen Untersuchung. / Children's motivation for treatment. Praxis der Kinderpsychologie und Kinderpsychiatrie; 1989 May–Jun Vol 38(5) 146–151

Messer, Stanley B. Integrating psychoanalytic and behaviour therapy: Limitations, possibilities and trade-offs. British Journal of Clinical Psychology; 1983 Jun Vol 22(2) 131–132

Miller, Susan; Watson, Ben C. The relationship between communication attitude, anxiety, and depression in stutterers and nonstutterers. Journal of Speech and Hearing Research; 1992 Aug Vol 35(4) 789–798

Moleski, Richard; Tosi, Donald J. Comparative psychotherapy: Rational-emotive therapy versus systematic desensitization in the treatment of stuttering. Journal of Consulting and Clinical Psychology; 1976 Apr Vol 44(2) 309–311

Muhs, Aribert; Schepank, Heinz. Aspekte des Verlaufs und der geschlectsspezifischen Pravalenz psychogener Erkrankungen bei Kindern und Erwachsenen unter dem Einfluss von Erb und Umweltfaktoren. (Aspects of development of the incidence of psychogenic disorders in children and adults under the influence of hereditary and environmental factors.) Zeitschrift fur Psychosoma-

tische Medizin und Psychoanalyse; 1991 Vol 37(2) 194–206

Naidoo, S.; Pillay, Y. G. Personal constructs of fluency: A study comparing stutterers and nonstutterers. Psychological Reports; 1990 Apr Vol 66(2) 375–378

Nammalvar, N.; Rao, A. Venkoba. Identity disturbances among adult stammerers. Indian Journal of Clinical Psychology; 1983 Sep Vol 10(2) 491–496

Nekrasova, Julia B. Wiederherstellung einer gestorten Kommunikation (am Beispiel einer Logoneurose). / Repair of disturbed communication in logoneurosis. Dynamische Psychiatrie; 1989 Vol 22(114–115) 37–50

Nekrasova, Y. B. Psychotherapy sessions and some mental states of stutterers. Voprosy Psikhologii; 1980 Sep–Oct No 5 32–40

Nekrasova, Yu. B. The teacher and the psychological atmosphere in the classroom. Soviet Psychology; 1987–88 Win Vol 26(2) 79–83

Nekrasova, Yuliya B. Dynamics of psychological states in stutterers in the process of logopsychotherapy. Voprosy Psikhologii; 1985 Mar–Apr No 2 127–133

Nekrasova, Yuliya B. (Group emotional and stress psychotherapy to correct mental states of stutterers.) Voprosy Psikhologii; 1984 Mar–Apr No 2 75–82

Nemec, Jiri. Voice-speech fullness of life: Existential analysis in the context of a medical discipline. Zeitschrift fur Klinische Psychologie und Psychotherapie; 1979 Vol 27(3) 196–203

Nemes, Livia. Die klinische Bedeutung der Anklammerungstheorie von Imre Hermann. (The clinical significance of Imre Hermann's theory of clinging.) Zeitschrift fur Psychoanalytische Theorie und Praxis; 1990 Vol 5(2) 112–121

Nicolaidis, Nicos; Papilloud, Janine. Une langue privee pour combler le manque. (A private language to fill a gap.) 47th Congress of Romance Languages Psychoanalysts (1987, Paris, France). Revue Francaise de Psychanalyse; 1988 Mar–Apr Vol 52(2) 523–531

Nurnberger, John I.; Hingtgen, Joseph N. Is symptom substitution an important issue in behavior therapy? Biological Psychiatry; 1973 Dec Vol 7(3) 221–236

Nystul, Michael S.; Muszynska, Eve. Adlerian treatment of a classical case of stuttering. Journal of Individual Psychology; 1976 Nov Vol 32(2) 194–202

Oganesyan, E. V. (Different rhythmic speech therapy exercises for adolescent and adult stutterers.) Defektologiya; 1983 No 1 60–63

Ohashi, Yoshiko; Hagiwara, Sachiko. The onset and development of stuttering problems: Discussion of self-acceptance of stuttering in adolescence. Japanese Journal of Child and Adolescent Psychiatry; 1982 Vol 23(5) 287–299

Ojha, K. N.; Bettagere, R. N. Group psychotherapy with stutterers. Indian Journal of Clinical Psychology; 1982 Sep Vol 9(2) 125–129

Peters, M. The view of learning theory. Zeitschrift fur Kinder und Jugendpsychiatrie; 1976 Vol 4(2) 104–112

Petrunik, Michael; Shearing, Clifford D. Fragile facades: Stuttering and the strategic manipulation of awareness. Social Problems; 1983 Dec Vol 31(2) 125–138

Peutelschmiedova, Alzbeta; Rauerova, Martina. Profesionalni orientace balbutiku. (Vocational orientation of stutterers.) Psychologia a Patopsychologia Dietata; 1990 Vol 25(5) 405–416

Porret, Jean Michel. Psychoanalytic aspects of stammering. IN: SUPEA Faculte de Medecine, Service Acta Paedopsychiatrica International Journal of Child and Adolescent Psychiatry; Apr Vol 56(1) 57–61

Prins, David; Beaudet, Rudolph. Defense preference and stutterers' speech disfluencies: Implications for the nature of the disorder. Journal of Speech and Hearing Research; 1980 Dec Vol 23(4) 757–768

Prins, David; Miller, Michele. Personality, improvement,and regression in stuttering therapy. Journal of Spech and Hearing Research; 1973 Dec Vol 16(4) 685–690

Pukacova, Marianna. (Psychological characteristics of stuttering children.) Psychologia a Patopsychologia Dietata; 1973 Vol 8(3) 233–238

Raou, Ye. Y. Dynamics of some characteristics of stutterer's personality in the process of psychotherapy. Voprosy Psikhologii; 1984 May–Jun Vol 3 67–72

Rodin, Rudolph G.; Roden, Michelle M. Children of Holocaust survisors. Adolescent Pscyhiatry; 1982 Vol 10 66–72

Rudmin, Floyd. Parent's report of stress and articulation oscillation as factors in a preschooler's dysfluencies. Journal of Fluency Disorders; 1984 Feb Vol 9(1) 85–87

Rychkova, N. A. State of voluntary motor activity and speech in preschool children with neurotic and pseudo-neurotic forms of stuttering. Defektologiya; 1981 No 6 73–77

Santacreu Mas, Jose. El condicionamiento ante determinadas palabras en la tartamudez. (Conditioning before some words in stuttering.) Revista de Psicologia General y Aplicada; 1984 Vol 39(6) 1115–1129

Scheiber, Stephen C.; Ziesat, Harold. Clinical and psychological test findings in cerebral dyspraxia associated with hemodialysis. Journal of Nervous and Mental Disease; 1976 Mar Vol 162(3) 212–214

Scopazzo, Maurizio. (Rosenzweig Picture Frustration Study and EEG features in an adolescent stuttering group.) Lavoro Neuropsichiatrico; 1974 Jan–Jun Vol 54(1–3) 49–60

Seidel, Christa; Biesalski, P. (Psychological and clinical experiences with the Frostig Test and the Frostig therapy in speech-impaired chidlren.) Praxis der Kinderpsychologie und Kinderpsychiatrie; 1973 Jan Vol. 22(1) 3–15

Sheehan, Joseph G.; Tanaka, Jeffrey S. Prognostic validity of the Rorschach. Journal of Personality Assessment; 1983 Oct Vol 47(5) 462–465

Sheehan, Joseph G.; Lyon, Martha A. Role perception in stuttering. Journal of Communication Disorders; 1974 Jun Vol 7(2) 113–125

Shklovsky, V. M.; Krol, L. M.; Mikhailova, E. L. Specificity of group psychotherapy in stammering. Trudy Leningradskogo Nauchno Issledovatel'skogo Psikhonevrologicheskogo Instituta i m V M Bekhtereva; 1988 Vol 121 112–117

Shklovsky, Victor M.; Kroll, Leonid M.; Mikhailova, Ekaterina L. Group psychotherapy: Problems of theory and practical application. Psikologicheskii Zhurnal; 1985 May–Jun Vol 6(3) 100–110

Shklovsky, Viktor M.; Krol, Leonid M.; Mikhailova, Ekaterina L. The psychotherapy of stuttering: On the model of stuttering patients' psychotherapy group. Soviet Journal of Psychiatry and Psychology Today; 1988 Vol 1(1) 130–141

Silverman, Lloyd H. An experimental method for the study of unconscious conflict: A progress report. British Journal of Medical Psychology; 1975 Dec Vol 48(4) 291–298

Silverman, Lloyd H. Psychoanalytic theory: "The reports of my death are greatly exaggerated." American Psychologist; 1976 Sep Vol 31(9) 621–637

Silverman, Lloyd H.; Bronstein, Abbot; Mendelsohn, Eric. The further use of the subliminal psychodynamic activation method for the experimental study of the clinical theory of psychoanalysis: On the specificity of the relationship between symptoms and unconscious conflicts. Psychotherapy Theory, Research and Practice; 1976 Spr Vol 13(1) 2–16

Silvestre, Cathie. Corps separe et langage parle. (Body and spoken language.) Topique Revue Freudienne; 1983 Sep Vol 13(31) 105–121

Snyder, Murry A. A psychodynamic approach to the theory and therapy of stuttering. Journal of Communication Disorders; 1977 Mar Vol 10(1–2) 85–88

Srivastava, K. Indira. Socio-psychological factors of stammering and the problem of rehabilitation of stammerers. Indian Psychological Review; 1985 Vol 29(Spec Iss) 24–34

Staffolani, Giuseppe. La balbuzie infantile. / Childhood stuttering. Rivista Internazionale di Psicologia e Ipnosi; 1984 Jan–Mar Vol 25(1) 37–41

Steffen, Hartmut; Seidel, Christa. Perceptive and cognitive school and social behavior of children with language and speech disorders. Zeitschrift fur Kinder und Jugendpsychiatrie; 1976 Vol 4(3) 216–232

Tang, Shenqing; Xu, Jengchen; Luo, Powei. (Preliminary studies on the psychological problems of stuttering children.) Information on Psychological Sciences; 1984 No 6 43–44

Tarkowski, Zbigniew. Psychoterapia osob jakajacych sie. / Psychotherapy of stutterers. Psychologia Wychowawcza; 1987 Mar–Apr Vol 30(2) 184–192

Tkaczenko, Oleh G. Tiefenpsychologische Aspekte des Stotterns. / The depth psychological aspects of stuttering. Zeitschrift fur Individualpsychologie; 1990 Vol 15(4) 298–306

Turnbaugh, Karen; Guitar, Barry; Hoffman, Paul. The attribution of personality traits: The stutterer and nonstutterer. Journal of Speech and Hearing Research; 1981 Jan Vol 24(2) 288–291

Turnbaugh, Karen R.; Guitar, Barry E.; Hoffman, Paul R. Speech clinicians' attribution of personality traits as a function of stuttering severity. Journal of Speech and Hearing Research; 1979 Mar Vol 22(1) 37–45

Van Jaarsveld, Pieter E.; du Plessis, Wynand F. Audio-psycho-phonology at Potchefstroom: A review. South African Journal of Psychology; 1988 Dec Vol 18(4) 136–143

Van Lankveld, Jacques. RET als verlengstuk van stottertherapie. / Rational emotive therapy and stuttering. Gedragstherapie; 1991 Mar Vol 24(1) 29–39

Van Riper, Charles. Henry Freund: 1896–1962. Journal of Fluency Disorders; 1984 May Vol 9(2) 93–102

Vekassy, Laszlo. Idegrendszeri es pszichologiai vizsgalatok dadogoknal. (Psychological and nervous system examination with stutterers.) Magyar Pszichologiai Szemle; 1981 Vol 38(5) 481–494

Virag, Terez. Gyermekkori neurotikus allapotok, magatartaszavarok tortenelmi hattere. / The historical background of neurotic states and conduct disorders in childhood. Magyar Pszichologiai Szemle; 1987–88 Vol 44(3) 227–244

Wagner, Alejandro M. Acera de la tartamudez: Introduccion a la patologia del acto. (Stuttering: An introduction to the pathology of the act.) Revista de Psicoanalisis; 1988 Mar–Apr Vol 45(2) 391–417

Wakabayashi, Shinichiro; Ohtaka, Kazunori; Abe, Tokuichiro; Kaneko, Toshiko. Neuroses in child and adolescent psychiatric clinic. Japanese Journal of Child and Adolescent Psychiatry; 1983 Vol 24(3) 186–195

Wallen, Vincent. A study of the self-concepts of adolescent stutterers. Psychologia An International Journal of Psychology in the Orient; 1973 Dec Vol 16(4) 191–200

Wertheim, Eleanor S. Ego dysfunction in stuttering and its relationship to the subculture of the nuclear family: A predictive study based on the bio-adaptive theory of stuttering: II. British Journal of Medical Psychology; 1973 Jun Vol 46(2) 155–180

Woods, C. Lee; Williams, Dean E. Traits attributed to stuttering and normally fluent males. Journal of Speech and Hearing Research; 1976 Jun Vol 19(2) 267–278

Yamaguchi Wakaba, Yoko. (Neurotic-like behavior in young stuttering children with early onset: The characteristics of the behavior in the male children who began to stutter at the age of two.) RIEEC Report; 1988 Rep 37 39–48

Zelen, Seymour L. Balance and reversal of actor-observer perspectives: An attributional model of pathology. Journal of Social and Clinical Psychology; 1987 Vol 5(4) 435–451

Psychogenic Disfluencies

Bloodstein, Oliver. Verification of stuttering in a suspected malingerer. Journal of Fluency Disorders; 1988 Apr Vol 13(2) 83–88

de Rosa, E.; Antonucci, G.; Rinaldi, L. Balbuzie, complesso edipico e angosce primitive: Osservazioni su un caso clinico. / Stuttering, Oedipus complex and earliest anxieties: Some observations on a clinical case. Archivio di Psicologia, Neurologia e Psichiatria; 1987 Vol 48(3) 327–335

Deal, Jon L. Sudden onset of stuttering: A case report. Journal of Speech and Hearing Disorders; 1982 Aug Vol 47(3) 301–304

Deal, Jon L.; Doro, Joseph M. Episodic hysterical stuttering. Journal of Speech and Hearing Disorders; 1987 Aug Vol 52(3) 299–300

Dempsey, George L.; Granich, Marina. Hypnobehavioral therapy in the case of a traumatic stutterer: A case study. International Journal of Clinical and Experimental Hypnosis; 1978 Jul Vol 26(3) 125–133

Halpern, Harvey. Stuttering therapy for nonfluent psychiatric adults. Perceptual and Motor Skills; 1990 Dec Vol 71(3, Pt 1) 914

Halpern, Harvey; McCartin-Clark, Marguerite; Wallack, Wendy. The nonfluencies of eight psychiatric adults. Journal of Communication Disorders; 1989 Aug Vol 22(4) 233–241

Joseph, Anthony B. Transient stuttering in catatonic bipolar patients. Behavioural Neurology; 1991 Win Vol 4(4) 265–269

Mahr, Greg; Leith, William. Psychogenic stuttering of adult onset. Journal of Speech and Hearing Research; 1992 Apr Vol 35(2) 283–286

Menkes, David B.; Ungvari, Gabor S. Adult-onset stuttering as a presenting feature of schizophrenia: Restoration of fluency with trifluoperazine. Journal of Nervous and Mental Disease; 1993 Jan Vol 181(1) 64–65

Mowrer, Don. Reported use of a Japanese accent to promote fluency. Journal of Fluency Disorders; 1987 Feb Vol 12(1) 19–39

Roth, Carole R.; Aronson, Arnold E.; Davis, Leo J. Clinical studies in psychogenic stuttering of adult onset. Journal of Speech and Hearing Disorders; 1989 Nov Vol 54(4) 634–646

Stewart, Trudy; Grantham, Clare. A case of acquired stammering: The pattern of recovery. European Journal of Communication Disorders; 1993 28(4) 395–403

Watson, Peter; Guitar, Barry. Respiratory stuttering? A case history. Journal of Fluency Disorders; 1986 Jun Vol 11(2) 165–173

Weiner, A. E. A case of adult onset of stuttering. Journal of Fluency Disorders; 1981 Jun Vol 6(2) 181–185

Research and Methodological Issues

Adams, Martin R. Five-year retrospective on stuttering theory, research, and therapy: 1982–1987. Journal of Fluency Disorders; 1988 Dec Vol 13(6) 399–405

Adams, Martin R. Some common problems in the design and conduct of experiments in stuttering. Journal of Speech and Hearing Disorders; 1976 Feb Vol 41(1) 3–9

Adams, Martin R.; Runyan, Charles M. Stuttering and fluency: Exclusive events or points on a continuum? Journal of Fluency Disorders; 1981 Sep Vol 6(3) 197–218

Aguilar, Guido; Berganza, Carlos E. Sesgo en los registros observacionales de la conducta de tartamudeo. (Bias in observational recordings of stuttering behavior.) Revista Intercontinental de Psicologia y Educacion; 1989 Vol 2(1–2) 43–56

Aguilar, Guido; Bohrt, Raul. Interferencia en el diseno de tratamientos alternos. (Interference in the alternating-treatments design.) Ensenanza e Investigacion en Psicologia; 1983 Jan-Jun Vol 9(1) 72–93

Alfonso, Peter J. Subject definition and selection criteria for stuttering research in adult subjects. ASHA Reports Series American Speech Language Hearing Association; 1990 Apr No 18 15–24

Andrews, Gavin; Craig, Ashley. Stuttering: Overt and covert measurement of the speech of treated subjects. Journal of Speech and Hearing Disorders; 1982 Feb Vol 47(1) 96–99

Andrews, Gavin; et al. Stuttering: A review of research findings and theories circa 1982. Journal of Speech and Hearing Disorders; 1983 Aug Vol 48(3) 226–246

Andrews, Gavin; Guitar, Barry; Howie, Pauline M. Meta-analysis of the effects of stuttering treatment. Journal of Speech and Hearing Disorders; 1980 Aug Vol 45(3) 287–307

Andrews, Gavin; Harvey, Robin. Regression to the mean in pretreatment measures of stuttering. Journal of Speech and Hearing Disorders; 1981 May Vol 46(2) 204–207

Andrews, Gavin; Craig, Ashley. Stuttering: Overt and covert measurement of the speech of treated subjects. Journal of Speech and Hearing Disorders; 1982 Feb Vol 47(1) 96–99

Andrews, Moya L.; Smith, Raymond G. Perceptions of auditory components of stuttered speech. Journal of Communication Disorders; 1976 Jun Vol 9(2) 121–128

Armson, Joy; Kalinowski, Joseph. Interpreting results of the fluent speech paradigm in stuttering research: Difficulties in separating cause from effect. Journal of Speech and Hearing Research; 1994 37(1) 69–83

Aron, Myrtle L. Concepts underlying the development of a computer information retrieval programme for research in communication disorders. British Journal of Disorders of Communication; 1981 Sep Vol 16(2) 89–100

Asatiani, N. M.; Kazakov, V. G.; Freidin, Yu. L. Some problems of clinical classification of stuttering. Defektologiya; 1988 No 1 28–32

Attanasio, Joseph S. Research design issues in relationships between anxiety and stuttering: Comments on Craig. Journal of Speech and Hearing Research; 1991 Oct Vol 34(5) 1079–1080

Attanasio, Joseph S. The dodo was Lewis Carroll, you see: Reflections and speculations. Journal of Fluency Disorders; 1987 Apr Vol 12(2) 107–118

Avari, Dinci N.; Bloodstein, Oliver. Adjacency and prediction in school-age stutterers. Journal of Speech and Hearing Research; 1974 Mar Vol 17(1) 33–40

Azrin, Nathan, H. A strategy for applied research: Learning based but outcome oriented. American Psychologist; 1977 Feb Vol 32(2) 140–149

Baker, Lorian; Cantwell, Dennis P. Psychiatric and learning disorders in children with speech and language disorders: A critical review. Advances in Learning and Behavioral Disabilities; 1985 Vol 4 1–28

Barblan, Leo. Therapeutique du langage: Science ou intuition? (Therapeutics of language: Science or intuition?) Pratique des Mots; 1983 Sep No 44 23–36

Boehmler, R. M.; Boehmler, S. I. The cause of stuttering: What's the question? Journal of Fluency Disorders; 1989 Dec Vol 14(6) 447–450

Borden, Gloria J. Initiation versus execution time during manual and oral counting by stutterers. Journal of Speech and Hearing Research; 1983 Sep Vol 26(3) 389–396

Borden, Gloria J. Subtyping adult stutterers for research purposes. ASHA Reports Series American Speech Language Hearing Association; 1990 Apr No 18 58–62

Brown, Shelli L.; Colcord, Roger D. Perceptual comparisons of adolescent stutterers' and nonstutterers' fluent speech. Journal of Fluency Disorders; 1987 Dec Vol 12(6) 419–427

Brundage, Shelley B.; Ratner, Nan B. Measurement of stuttering frequency in children's speech. Journal of Fluency Disorders; 1989 Oct Vol 14(5) 351–358

Brutten, Gene J. A reply to Costello and (Roemer) Hurst. Journal of Speech and Hearing Research; 1983 Mar Vol 26(1) 155–156

Conture, Edward G. Childhood stuttering: What is it and who does it? ASHA Reports Series American Speech Language Hearing Association; 1990 Apr No 18 2–14

Christensen, John M. Did primitive man really talk like an ape? Journal of Speech and Hearing Research; 1992 Aug Vol 35(4) 805

Clutter, Margaret H.; Freeman, Frances J. Stuttering: The six blind men revisited. Journal of Fluency Disorders; 1984 Feb Vol 9(1) 89–92

Colcord, Roger D.; Gregory, Hugo H. Perceptual analyses of stuttering and nonstuttering children's fluent speech productions. Journal of Fluency Disorders; 1987 Jun Vol 12(3) 185–195

Cooper, Eugene B. The chronic perseverative stuttering syndrome: Incurable stuttering. Journal of Fluency Disorders; 1987 Dec Vol 12(6) 381–388

Cooper, Eugene B. Treatment of disfluency: Future trends. Journal of Fluency Disorders; 1986 Dec Vol 11(4) 317–327

Cordes, Anne K.; Ingham, Roger J. The reliability of observational data: II. Issues in the identification and measurement of stuttering events. Journal of Speech and Hearing Research; 1994 37(2) 279–295

Cordes, Anne K.; Ingham, Roger J.; Frank, Peter; Ingham, Janis C. Time-interval analysis of interjudge and intrajudge agreement for stuttering event judgments. Journal of Speech and Hearing Research; 1992 Jun Vol 35(3) 483–494

Craig, Ashley. "Research design issues in relationships between anxiety and stuttering: Comments on Craig": Reply. Journal of Speech and Hearing Research; 1991 Oct Vol 34(5) 1080–1081

Cullinan, Walter L. Consistency measures revisited. Journal of Fluency Disorders; 1988 Feb Vol 13(1) 1–9

Curlee, Richard F. Observer agreement on disfluency and stuttering. Journal of Speech and Hearing Research; 1981 Dec Vol 24(4) 595–600

Cyprus, Shelly; Hezel, Richard T.; Rossi, Debbie; Adams, Martin R. Effects of simulated stuttering on listener recall. Journal of Fluency Disorders; 1984 Sep Vol 9(3) 191–197

Dembowski, James; Watson, Ben C. An instrumented method for assessment and remediation of stuttering: A single-subject case study. Journal of Fluency Disorders; 1991 Vol 16(5–6) 241–273

Evesham, Margaret; Huddleston, Anita. Teaching stutterers the skill of fluent speech as a preliminary to the study of relapse. British Journal of Disorders of Communication; 1983 Apr Vol 18(1) 31–38

Finn, Patrick; Ingham, Roger J. The selection of "fluent" samples in research on stuttering: Conceptual and methodological considerations. Journal of Speech and Hearing Research; 1989 Jun Vol 32(2) 401–418

Gagnon, Mireille; Ladouceur, Robert. Defining clinically significant changes in the treatment of child stutterers. Perceptual and Motor Skills; 1991 Oct Vol 73(2) 375–378

Guitar, Barry. Pretreatment factors associated with the outcome of stuttering therapy. Journal of Speech and Hearing Research; 1976 Sep Vol 19(3) 590–600

Hall, Donald E.; Lynn, James M.; Altieri, Jennifer; Segers, Vicki D.; et al. Inter-intrajudge reliability of the Stuttering Severity Instrument. Journal of Fluency Disorders; 1987 Jun Vol 12(3) 167–173

Ham, Richard E. What are we measuring? Journal of Fluency Disorders; 1989 Aug Vol 14(4) 231–243

Harris, Daniel; Fucci, Donald; Petrosino, Linda. Magnitude estimation and cross-modal matching of auditory and lingual vibrotactile sensation by normal speakers and stutterers. Journal of Speech and Hearing Research; 1991 Feb Vol 34(1) 177–182

Howie, Pauline M.; Woods, C. Lee; Andrews, Gavin J. Relationship between covert and overt speech measures immediately before and immediately after stuttering treatment. Journal of Speech and Hearing Disorders; 1982 Nov Vol 47(4) 419–422

Hulit, Lloyd M. Inter-judge agreement for identifying stuttered words. Perceptual and Motor Skills; 1978 Oct Vol 47(2) 360–362

Ingham, Roger J.; et al. Modification of listener-judged naturalness in the speech of stutterers. Journal of Speech and Hearing Research; 1985 Dec Vol 28(4) 495–504

Ingham, Roger J.; Carroll, Philippa J. Listener judgment of differences in stutterers' nonstuttered speech during chorus- and non-chorus-reading conditions. Journal of Speech and Hearing Research; 1977 Jun Vol 20(2) 293–302

Ingham, Roger J.; Gow, Merrilyn; Costello, Janis M. Stuttering and speech naturalness: Some additional data. Journal of Speech and Hearing Disorders; 1985 May Vol 50(2) 217–219

Ingham, Roger J.; Ingham, Janis C.; Onslow, Mark; Finn, Patrick. Stutterers' self-ratings of speech naturalness: Assessing effects and reliability. Journal of Speech and Hearing Research; 1989 Jun Vol 32(2) 419–431

Ingham, Roger J.; Onslow, Mark. Measurement and modification of speech naturalness during stuttering therapy. Journal of Speech and Hearing Disorders; 1985 Aug Vol 50(3) 261–281

Jagacinski, Richard J. A qualitative look at feedback control theory as a style of describing behavior. Human Factors; 1977 Aug Vol 19(4) 331–347

James, Jack E.; Ingham, Roger J. The influence of stutterer's expectancies of improvement upon response to time-out. Journal of Speech and Hearing Research; 1974 Mar Vol. 17(1) 86–93

James, Jack E. Self-monitoring of stuttering: Reactivity and accuracy. Behaviour Research and Therapy; 1981 Vol 19(4) 291–296

Kooman, E. A. Speech disturbance under delayed acoustic feedback and stuttering. Defektologiya; 1975 Jun No 6 27–33

Krikorian, Carol M.; Runyan, Charles M. A perceptual comparison: Stuttering and nonstuttering children's nonstuttered speech. Journal of Fluency Disorders; 1983 Dec Vol 8(4) 283–290

Kroll, Robert M.; O'Keefe, Bernard M. Molecular self-analyses of stuttered speech via speech time expansion. Journal of Fluency Disorders; 1985 Jun Vol 10(2) 93–105

Kully, Deborah; Boberg, Einer. An investigation of interclinic agreement in the identification of fluent and stuttered syllables. Journal of Fluency Disorders; 1988 Oct Vol 13(5) 309–318

Kurman, Paula. Research: An aerial view. Etc.; 1977 Sep Vol 34(3) 265–276

Ladouceur, Robert; Cote, Christiane; Leblond, Georges; Bouchard, Leandre. Evaluation of regulated-breathing method and awareness training in the treatment of stuttering. Journal of Speech and Hearing Disorders; 1982 Nov Vol 47(4) 422–426

Lankford, Sally D.; Cooper, Eugene B. Recovery from stuttering as viewed by parents of self-diagnosed recovered stutterers. Journal of Communication Disorders; 1974 Jun Vol 7(2) 171–180

Leahy, Margaret M.; Collins, Geraldine. Therapy for stuttering: Experimenting with experimenting. Irish Journal of Psychological Medicine; 1991 Mar Vol 8(1) 37–39

Ludlow, Christy L. Research procedures for measuring stuttering severity. ASHA Reports Series American Speech Language Hearing Association; 1990 Apr No 18 26–31

MacDonald, James D.; Martin, Richard R. Stuttering and disfluency as two reliable and unambiguous response classes. Journal of Speech and Hearing Research; 1973 Dec Vol 16(4) 691–699

Martin, Richard R.; Haroldson, Samuel K. Stuttering and speech naturalness: Audio and audiovisual judgments. Journal of Speech and Hearing Research; 1992 Jun Vol 35(3) 521–528

Martin, Richard R.; Haroldson, Samuel K. Stuttering identification: Standard definition and moment of stuttering. Journal of Speech and Hearing Research; 1981 Mar Vol 24(1) 59–63

Martin, Richard R.; Haroldson, Samuel K.; Woessner, Garry L. Perceptual scaling of stuttering severity. Journal of Fluency Disorders; 1988 Feb Vol 13(1) 27–47

Metz, Dale E.; Schiavetti, Nicholas; Sacco, Pat R. Acoustic and psychophysical dimensions of the perceived speech naturalness of nonstutterers and posttreatment stutterers. Journal of Speech and Hearing Disorders; 1990 Aug Vol 55(3) 516–525

Moore, Walter H. Pathophysiology of stuttering: Cerebral activation differences in stutterers vs. nonstutterers. ASHA Reports Series American Speech Language Hearing Association; 1990 Apr No 18 72–80

Moscicki, Eve K. Fundamental methodological considerations in controlled clinical trials.

Journal of Fluency Disorders 1993 18(2–3) 183–196

Motsch, Hans Joachim. Idiographische Logopadie. (Idiographic speech science.) Vierteljahresschrift fur Heilpadagogik und ihre Nachbargebiete; 1990 Mar Vol 59(1) 2–13

Nippold, Marilyn A. Concomitant speech and language disorders in stuttering children: A critique of the literature. Journal of Speech and Hearing Disorders; 1990 Feb Vol 55(1) 51–60

Onslow, Mark; Gardner, Kate; Bryant, Kathryn M.; Stuckings, Cathi L.; et al. Stuttered and normal speech events in early childhood: The validity of a behavioral data language. Journal of Speech and Hearing Research; 1992 Feb Vol 35(1) 79–87

Perkins, William H.; Bell, Jody; Johnson, Linda; Stocks, Janice. Phone rate and the effective planning time hypothesis of stuttering. Journal of Speech and Hearing Research; 1979 Dec Vol 22(4) 747–755

Perkins, William H. Implications of scientific research for treatment of stuttering: A lecture. Journal of Fluency Disorders; 1981 Jun Vol 6(2) 155–162

Peters, Herman F.; Boves, Louis; Van Dielen, Ineke C. Perceptual judgment of abruptness of voice onset in vowels as a function of the amplitude envelope. Journal of Speech and Hearing Disorders; 1986 Nov Vol 51(4) 299–308

Prosek, Robert A.; Runyan, Charles M. Effects of segment and pause manipulations on the identification of treated stutterers. Journal of Speech and Hearing Research; 1983 Dec Vol 26(4) 510–516

Prosek, Robert A.; Runyan, Charles M. Temporal characteristics related to the discrimination of stutterers' and nonstutterers' speech samples. Journal of Speech and Hearing Research; 1982 Mar Vol 25(1) 29–33

Quesal, Robert W. Stuttering research: Have we forgotten the stutterer? Journal of Fluency Disorders; 1989 Jun Vol 14(3) 153–164

Ramig, Peter R. The impact of self-help groups on persons who stutter: A call for research. Journal of Fluency Disorders; 1993 18(2–3) 351–361

Rentschler, Gary J. Effects of subgrouping in stuttering research. Journal of Fluency Disorders; 1984 Dec Vol 9(4) 307–311

Resnick, Sylvia; Tureen, Phyllis. Evaluation of fluent and disfluent speech segments by stutterers and nonstutterers. Journal of Fluency Disorders; 1990 Feb Vol 15(1) 1–8

Riley, Glyndon D. "Inter-intrajudge reliability of the Stuttering Severity Instrument": Comment. Journal of Fluency Disorders; 1988 Apr Vol 13(2) 153–155

Robey, Randall R. The analysis of one-way between effects in fluency research. Journal of Fluency Disorders; 1990 Oct–Dec Vol 15(5–6) 275–289

Ryan, Bruce P.; Ryan, Barbara V. Additions to Andrews, Craig, Feyer, Hoddinott, Howie, and Neilson (1983) and to Andrews, Guitar, and Howie (1980). Journal of Speech and Hearing Disorders; 1984 Nov Vol 49(4) 429

Schiavetti, Nicholas; Martin, Richard M.; Haroldson, Samuel K.; Metz, Dale Evan. Psychophysical analysis of audiovisual judgements of speech naturalness on nonstutterers and stutterers. Journal of Speech and Hearing Research; 1994 37(1) 46–53

Schiavetti, Nicholas; Sacco, Pat R.; Metz, Dale E.; Sitler, Ronald W. Direct magnitude estimation and interval scaling of stuttering severity. Journal of Speech and Hearing Research; 1983 Dec Vol 26(4) 568–573

Schliesser, Herbert F. Psychological scaling of speech by students in training compared to that by experienced speech-language pathologists. Perceptual and Motor Skills; 1985 Dec Vol 61(3, Pt 2) 1299–1302

Schliesser, Herbert F. Psychological scaling of speech by students in training compared to that by experienced speech-language pathologists. Perceptual and Motor Skills; 1985 Dec Vol 61(3, Pt 2) 1299–1302

Schwartz, Howard D. Adolescents who stutter. Journal of Fluency Disorders; 1993 18(2–3) 289–302

Shames, George H. Stuttering: An RFP for a cultural perspective. Journal of Fluency Disorders; 1989 Feb Vol 14(1) 67–77

Starkweather, C. Woodruff. Current trends in therapy for stuttering children and suggestions for future research. ASHA Reports Series American Speech Language Hearing Association; 1990 Apr No 18 82–90

Still, A. W.; Griggs, S. Changes in the probability of stuttering following a stutter: A test of some recent models. Journal of Speech and Hearing Research; 1979 Sep Vol 22(3) 565–571

Still, A. W.; Sherrard, Carol A. Formalizing theories of stuttering. British Journal of Mathematical and Statistical Psychology; 1976 Nov Vol 29(2) 129–138

Tarkowski, Zbigniew; Jaworska, Malgorzata. Gielkot: Stan i perspektywy badan. / Disorderly speech: State and perspectives of research. Psychologia Wychowawcza; 1987 Sep–Oct Vol 30(4) 440–447

Webster, Ronald L. Concept and theory in stuttering: An insufficiency of empiricism. Journal of Communication Disorders; 1977 Mar Vol 10(1–2) 65–71

Wingate, M. E. Expectancy as basically a short-term process. Journal of Speech and Hearing Research; 1975 Mar Vol 18(1) 31–42

Wingate, Marcel E. The immediate source of stuttering: An integration of evidence. Journal of Communication Disorders; 1977 Mar Vol 10(1–2) 45–51

Wingate, Marcel E. The relationship of theory to therapy in stuttering. Journal of Communication Disorders; 1977 Mar Vol 10(1–2) 37–44

Yairi, Ehud. Item analysis for parental behavior rated by stutterers and nonstutterers. Perceptual and Motor Skills; 1973 Apr Vol 36(2) 451–452

Yairi, Ehud. Subtyping child stutterers for research purposes. ASHA Reports Series American Speech Language Hearing Association; 1990 Apr No18 50–57

Young, Martin A. Evaluating differences between stuttering and nonstuttering speakers: The group difference design. Journal of Speech and Hearing Research; 1994 37(3) 522–535

Young, Martin A. Increasing the frequency of stuttering. Journal of Speech and Hearing Research; 1985 Jun Vol 28(2) 282–293

Young, Martin A. Observer agreement for marking moments of stuttering. Journal of Speech

and Hearing Research; 1975 Sep Vol 18(3) 530–540

Zimmermann, Gerald N.; Smith, Anne; Hanley, John M. Stuttering: In need of a unifying conceptual framework. Journal of Speech and Hearing Research; 1981 Mar Vol 24(1) 25–31

Self-Evaluation

Acosta, Miryam; Rodriguez, Pedro R. Tartamudez y si mismo. (Stuttering and the self.) Revista Intercontinental de Psicologia y Educacion; 1991 Vol 4(2) 105–119

Bar, Asher. Increasing fluency in young stutterers vs decreasing stuttering: A clinical approach. Journal of Communication Disorders; 1973 Dec Vol 6(4) 247–258

Ballesteros, Rocio F.; Mas, Jose S.; Carrobles, Jose A. Relaciones entre respuestas psicofisiologicas y autoinformes. / Relationships between psychophysiological responses and self-reports. Analisis y Modificacion de Conducta; 1984 Vol 10(25) 299–311

Brown, C. J.; Zimmermann, G. N.; Linville, R. N.; Hegmann, J. P. Variations in self-paced behaviors in stutterers and nonstutterers. Journal of Speech and Hearing Research; 1990 Jun Vol 33(2) 317–323

Burley, Peter M.; Morley, Ruth. Self-monitoring processes in stutterers. Journal of Fluency Disorders; 1987 Feb Vol 12(1) 71–78

Collins, Constance R.; Blood, Gordon W. Acknowledgment and severity of stuttering as factors influencing nonstutterers' perceptions of stutterers. Journal of Speech and Hearing Disorders; 1990 Feb Vol 55(1) 75–81

Craig, Ashley; Feyer, Anne Marie; Andrews, Gavin. An overview of a behavioural treatment for stuttering. Australian Psychologist; 1987 Mar Vol 22(1) 53–62

Craig, Ashley R.; Cleary, Patrick J. Reduction of stuttering by young male stutterers using EMG feedback. Biofeedback and Self Regulation; 1982 Sep Vol 7(3) 241–255

Cross, Douglas E.; Cooper, Eugene B. Self- versus investigator-administered presumed fluency reinforcing stimuli. Journal of Speech and Hearing Research; 1976 Jun Vol 19(2) 241–246

Finn, Patrick; Ingham, Roger J. Stutterers' self-ratings of how natural speech sounds and feels. Journal of Speech and Hearing Research; 1994 37(2) 326–341

Gonzalez-Valenzuela, M. Jose. Evaluacion y Tratamiento cognitivo-conductual de un caso de tartamudez. / Evaluation and cognitive-behavioral treatment in a severe stuttering case. Analisis y Modificacion de Conducta; 1990 Vol 16(47) 137–148

Guitar, Barry. Reduction of stuttering frequency using analog electromyographic feedback. Journal of Speech and Hearing Research; 1975 Dec Vol 18(4) 672–685

Hanna, Richmond; Wilfling, Franz; McNeill, Brent. A biofeedback treatment for stuttering. Journal of Speech and Hearing Disorders; 1975 May Vol 40(2) 270–273

Hasbrouck, Jon M. FAMC intensive stuttering treatment program: Ten years of implementation. Military Medicine; 1992 May Vol 157(5) 244–247

Ingham, Roger J. The effects of self-evaluation training on maintenance and generalization during stuttering treatment. Journal of Speech and Hearing Disorders; 1982 Aug Vol 47(3) 271–280

Ingham, Roger, J. The effects on stuttering of self-recording the frequency of stuttering or the word "the". Journal of Speech and Hearing reserach; 1978 Sep Vol 21(3) 459–469 1978.

Ingham, Roger J.; Ingham, Janis C.; Onslow, Mark; Finn, Patrick. Stutterers' self-ratings of speech naturalness: Assessing effects and reliability. Journal of Speech and Hearing Research; 1989 Jun Vol 32(2) 419–431

Itoh, Norihiro; Kamada, Yuko. An analytical study of self-consciousness in stutterers. Japanese Journal of Child and Adolescent Psychiatry; 1981 Vol 22(3) 193–202

James, Jack E. Behavioral self-control of stuttering using time-out from speaking. Journal of Applied Behavior Analysis; 1981 Spr Vol 14(1) 25–37

James, Jack E. Self-monitoring of stuttering: Reactivity and accuracy. Behaviour Research and Therapy; 1981 Vol 19(4) 291–296

James, Jack E.; Ingham, Roger J. The influence of stutterer's expectancies of improvement upon response to time-out. Journal of Speech and Hearing Research; 1974 Mar Vol. 17(1) 86–93

Johnson, Gerald F. Ten commandments for long-term maintenance of acceptable self-help skills for persons who are hard-core stutterers. Journal of Fluency Disorders; 1987 Feb Vol 12(1) 9–18

Kalinowski, Joseph S.; Lerman, Jay W.; Watt, James. A preliminary examination of the perceptions of self and others in stutterers and nonstutterers. Journal of Fluency Disorders; 1987 Oct Vol 12(5) 317–331

Klinger, Herbert. Effects of pseudostuttering on normal speakers' self-ratings of beauty. Journal of Communication Disorders; 1987 Aug Vol 20(4) 353–358

Kotbi, Naser; Farag, Safwat; Yousif, Mahmoud; Baraka, Mohamed, et al. A comparison between stutterers and nonstutterers in intelligence, self-concept, anxiety and depression. Derasat Nafseyah; 1992 2(2) 37–349

Kroll, Robert M.; O'Keefe, Bernard M. Molecular self-analyses of stuttered speech via speech time expansion. Journal of Fluency Disorders; 1985 Jun Vol 10(2) 93–105

La Croix, Zane E. Management of disfluent speech through self-recording procedures. Journal of Speech and Hearing Disorders; 1973 May Vol 38(2) 272–274

Lankford, Sally D.; Cooper, Eugene B. Recovery from stuttering as viewed by parents of self-diagnosed recovered stutterers. Journal of Communication Disorders; 1974 Jun Vol 7(2) 171–180

Lanyon, Richard I. Effect of biofeedback-based relaxation on stuttering during reading and spontaneous speech. Journal of Consulting and Clinical Psychology; 1977 Oct Vol 45(5) 860–866

Lanyon, Richard I.; Barrington, Cecily C.; Newman, Anne C. Modification of stuttering through EMG biofeedback: A preliminary study. Behavior Therapy; 1976 Jan Vol 7(1) 96–103

Lara-Cantu, Maria A. Pilot study on electromyographic biofeedback for the treatment of stuttering. Ensenanza e Investigacion en Psicologia; 1978 Jul–Dec Vol 4(2) 259–265

Legewie, H.; Cleary, P.; Rackensperger, W. EMG-recording and biofeedback in the diagnosis and therapy of stuttering: A case study. European Journal of Behavioural Analysis and Modification; 1975 Dec Vol 1(2) 137–143

Manschreck, Theo C.; Kalotkin, Madeline; Jacobson, Alan M. Utility of electromyographic biological feedback in chronic stuttering: A clinical study with follow-up. Perceptual and Motor Skills; 1980 Oct Vol 51(2) 535–540

Martin, Richard R.; Haroldson, Samuel K.; Woessner, Garry L. Perceptual scaling of stuttering severity. Journal of Fluency Disorders; 1988 Feb Vol 13(1) 27–47

Martin, Richard R.; Haroldson, Samuel K. Contingent self-stimulation for stuttering. Journal of Speech and Hearing Disorders; 1982 Nov Vol 47(4) 407–413

McCabe, Robert B.; McCollum, Judith D. The personal reactions of a stuttering adult to delayed auditory feedback. Journal of Speech and Hearing Disorders; 1972 Nov Vol. 37(4) 536–541

Moore, Walter H. Hemispheric alpha asymmetries during an electromyographic biofeedback procedure for stuttering: A single-subject experimental design. Journal of Fluency Disorders; 1984 May Vol 9(2) 143–162

Mullen, Brian. Stuttering, audience size, and the Other Total Ratio: A self-attention perspective. Journal of Applied Social Psychology; 1986 Vol 16(2) 139–149

Nigam, J. C. Stuttering and its self treatment. Hearing Aid Journal; 1985 Jul Vol 4(3) 78–79

Ohashi, Yoshiko; Hagiwara, Sachiko. The onset and development of stuttering problems: Discussion of self-acceptance of stuttering in adolescence. Japanese Hournal of Child and Adolescent Psychiatry; 1982 Vol 23(5) 287–299

Ornstein, Amy F.; Manning, Walter H. Self-efficacy scaling by adult stutterers. Journal of Communication Disorders; 1985 Aug Vol 18(4) 313–320

Orta-Rodriguez, Martha; Gallegos, B. Xochitl. Una evaluacion de tres tecnicas conductuales en el tratamiento de la tartamudez. (An evaluation of 3 behavioral techniques used to treat stuttering.) Revista Mexicana de Psicologia; 1986 Jul–Dec Vol 3(2) 168–173

Pachman, Joseph S.; Oelschlaeger, Mary L.; Hughes, Anita; Hughes, Howard H. Toward identifying effective agents in use of biofeedback to decelerate stuttering behavior. Perceptual and Motor Skills; 1978 Jun Vol 46(3, Pt 1) 1006

Prins, David. Stutterers' perceptions of therapy improvement and of posttherapy regression: Effects of certain program modifications. Journal of Speech and Hearing Disorders; 1976 Nov Vol 41(4) 452–463

Prins, David; Nichols, Anne. Client impressions of the effectiveness of stuttering therapy: A comparison of two programs. British Journal of Disorders of Communication; 1974 Oct Vol 9(2) 123–133

Ramirez, Luis H. (Treatment of stuttering by self-control procedures.) Revista Latinoamericana de Psicologia; 1975 Vol 7(3) 421–434

Resnick, Sylvia; Tureen, Phyllis. Evaluation of fluent and disfluent speech segments by stutterers and nonstutterers. Journal of Fluency Disorders; 1990 Feb Vol 15(1) 1–8

Rudolf, Sharon R.; Manning, Walter H.; Sewell, William R. The use of self-efficacy scaling in training student clinicians: Implications for working with stutterers. Journal of Fluency Disorders; 1983 Mar Vol 8(1) 55–75

Sherrard, Carol A. Stuttering as "false alarm" responding. British Journal of Disorders of Communication; 1975 Oct Vol 10(2) 83–91

St. Louis, Kenneth O.; Clausell, Paul L.; Thompson, Jean N.; Rife, Constance C. Preliminary investigation of EMG biofeedback induced relaxation with a preschool aged stutterer. Perceptual and Motor Skills; 1982 Aug Vol 55(1) 195–199

Watson, Jennifer B. A comparison of stutterers' and nonstutterers' affective, cognitive, and behavioral self-reports. Journal of Speech and Hearing Research; 1988 Sep Vol 31(3) 377–385

Wendlandt, Wolfgang. (Self-assertive training: A behavioral therapeutic phase in the treatment of adult stutterers.) Zwitschrift fur Klinische Psychologie und Psychotherapie; 1974 Vol 22(3) 236–246.

Wolak, Krzysztof. Zasstosowanie techniki biofeedback w terapii osab jakajacych sie./Biofeedback technique in stuttering therapy.

Psychologia Wychowawcza; 1988 Jan–Feb Vol 31(1) 56–69

Therapeutic Strategies and Stuttering

Ablon, Steven L. Psychoanalysis of a stuttering boy. Special Issue: Psychoanalysis of children. International Review of Psycho-Analysis; 1988 Vol 15(1) 83–91

Adams, Martin R. Five-year retrospective on stuttering theory, research, and therapy: 1982–1987. Journal of Fluency Disorders; 1988 Dec Vol 13(6) 399–405

Adams, Martin R. Learning from negative outcomes in stuttering therapy: I. Getting off on the wrong foot. Journal of Fluency Disorders; 1983 Jun Vol 8(2) 147–153

Adams, Martin R.; Hotchkiss, John. Some reactions and responses of stutterers to a miniaturized metronome and metronome-conditioning therapy: Three case reports. Behavior Therapy; 1973 Jul Vol 4(4) 565–569

Adams, Martin R.; Hutchinson, John. The effects of three levels of auditory masking on selected vocal characteristics and the frequency of disfluency of adult stutterers. Journal of Speech and Hearing Research; 1974 Dec Vol 17(4) 682–688

Adams, Martin R.; Runyan, Charles M. A response to Roger Ingham. Journal of Fluency Disorders; 1983 Jun Vol 8(2) 175–179

Adams, Martin R.; Webster, L. Michael. Case selection strategies with children "at risk" for stuttering. Journal of Fluency Disorders; 1989 Feb Vol 14(1) 11–16

Aguilar, Guido; de Aguilar, Maria T.; de Berganza, Maria R. El tartamudeo y su deteccion temprana. / Stuttering and its early detection. 5th Latin-American Congress of Behavior Analysis and Behavior Modification: Applied behavior analysis (1986, Caracas, Venezuela). Avances en Psicologia Clinica Latinoamericana; 1988 Vol 6 41–51

Ainsworth, Stanley. The relationships of theory and clinician characteristics to therapy for stutterers: A discussion of the Murphy and Wingate papers. Journal of Communication Disorders; 1977 Mar Vol 10(1–2) 53–59

Alarcia, J.; Pinard, Gilbert; Serrano, M.; Tetreault, L. Etude comparative de trois traitements du begaiement: relaxation, desensibilisation, reeducation. (A comparative study of three treatments for stuttering: Relaxation, desensitization, reeducation.) Revue de Psychologie Appliquee; 1982 Vol 32(1) 1–25

Ananthamurthy, H. S.; Parameswaran, T. M. Management of speech problems. Child Psychiatry Quarterly; 1978 Jan Vol 11(1) 10–13

Andrews, Gavin. Stuttering: A tutorial. Australian and New Zealand Journal of Psychiatry; 1981 Jun Vol 15(2) 105–109

Andrews, Gavin J.; Howie, Pauline M.; Dozsa, Melinda; Guitar, Barry E. Stuttering: Speech pattern characteristics under fluency-inducing conditions. Journal of Speech and Hearing Research; 1982 Jun Vol 25(2) 208–216

Andrews, Gavin; et al. Stuttering: A review of research findings and theories circa 1982. Journal of Speech and Hearing Disorders; 1983 Aug Vol 48(3) 226–246

Andrews, Gavin; Craig, Ashley. Stuttering: Overt and covert measurement of the speech of treated subjects. Journal of Speech and Hearing Disorders; 1982 Feb Vol 47(1) 96–99

Andrews, Gavin; Cutler, Jeffrey. Stuttering therapy: The relation between changes in symptom level and attitudes. Journal of Speech and Hearing Disorders; 1974 Aug Vol 39(3) 312–319

Andrews, Gavin; Guitar, Barry; Howie, Pauline M. Meta-analysis of the effects of stuttering treatment. Journal of Speech and Hearing Disorders; 1980 Aug Vol 45(3) 287–307

Andrews, Gavin; Tanner, Susan. Stuttering treatment: An attempt to replicate the regulated-breathing method. Journal of Speech and Hearing Disorders; 1982 May Vol 47(2) 138–140

Andrews, Gavin J.; Tanner, Susan. Stuttering: The results of 5 days treatment with an airflow technique. Journal of Speech and Hearing Disorders; 1982 Nov Vol 47(4) 427–429

Andronova, L. Z. Correction of intonation in stutterers. Defektologiya; 1988 No 6 63–67

Arkin, Arthur M.; et al. Behavior modification: Present status in psychiatry. New York State

Journal of Medicine; 1976 Feb Vol 76(2) 190–196

Atkinson, Leslie. Rational-emotive therapy versus systematic desensitization: A comment on Moleski and Tosi. Journal of Consulting and Clinical Psychology; 1983 Oct Vol 51(5) 776–778

Azrin, Nathan H.; Nunn, Robert G.; Frantz, Sharmon E. Comparison of regulated-breathing versus abbreviated desensitization on reported stuttering episodes. Journal of Speech and Hearing Disorders; 1979 Aug Vol 44(3) 331–339

Bar, Asher. Increasing fluency in young stutterers vs decreasing stuttering: A clinical approach. Journal of Communication Disorders; 1973 Dec Vol. 6(4) 247–258

Beattie, Michael S. A behaviour therapy programme for stuttering. British Journal of Disorders of Communication; 1973 Oct Vol. 8(2) 120–130

Beaty, David T. A multimodal approach to elimination of stuttering. Perceptual and Motor Skills; 1980 Feb Vol 50(1) 51–55

Becker, Peter; Kessler, Bernd; Fuchsgruber, Konrad. (A comparative therapeutic experiment on the theory and the efficiency of operant methods of treatment of stutterers.) Archiv fur Psychologie; 1975 Vol 127(1–2) 78–92

Berecz, John. Treatment of smoking with cognitive conditioning therapy: A self-administered aversion technique. Behavior Therapy; 1976 Oct Vol 7(5) 641–648

Berecz, John M. Cognitive conditioning therapy in the treatment of stuttering. Journal of Communication Disorders; 1976 Dec Vol 9(4) 301–315

Berecz, John M. The treatment of stuttering through precision punishment and cognitive arousal. Journal of Speech and Hearing Disorders; 1973 May Vol 38(2) 256–267

Berkowitz, Mozelle; Cook, Harriet; Haughey, Mary Jo. A non-traditional fluency program developed for the public school setting. Language, Speech and Hearing Services in the Schools; 1994 25(2) 94–100

Berman, Perry A.; Brady, John P. Miniaturized metronomes in the treatment of stuttering: A survey of clinicians' experience. Journal of Behavior Therapy and Experimental Psychiatry; 1973 Jun Vol. 4(2) 117–119

Bhargava, S. C. Participant modelling: An effective treatment strategy for stammering. Indian Journal of Psychiatry; 1981 Jul Vol 23(3) 259–262

Boberg, Einer; Yeudall, Lorne T.; Schopflocher, Donald; Bo Lassen, Peter. The effect of an intensive behavioral program on the distribution of EEG alpha power in stutterers during the processing of verbal and visuospatial information. Journal of Fluency Disorders; 1983 Sep Vol 8(3) 245–263

Boberg, Julia M.; Boberg, Einer. The other side of the block: The stutterer's spouse. Journal of Fluency Disorders; 1990 Feb Vol 15(1) 61–75

Boudreau, Leonce; Ladouceur, Robert. L'influence de l'aide sociale associee a la respiration regularisee sur le traitement du begaiement. / The influence of social help associated with regularized respiration on the treatment of stuttering. Technologie et Therapie du Comportement; 1985 Fal Vol 8(2) 125–151

Boudreau, Leonce A.; Jeffrey, Clarence J. Stuttering treated by desensitization. Journal of Behavior Therapy and Experimental Psychiatry; 1973 Sep Vol. 4(3) 209–212

Bounes, Marika. Test de Rorschach avant et apres traitement de relaxation chez l'enfant. (Rorschach test before and after relaxation treatment of a child.) 11th International Congress on the Rorschach and Projective Methods (1984, Barcelona, Spain). Bulletin de Psychologie; 1986 Jun Aug Vol 39(11–15) 651–654

Brady, John P. Behavior therapy and American psychiatry. Journal of the National Association of Private Psychiatric Hospitals; 1972 Fal Vol 4(3) 27–35

Brady, John P. The pharmacology of stuttering: A critical review. American Journal of Psychiatry; 1991 Oct Vol 148(10) 1309–1316

Brady, John P.; Price, Trevor R.; McAllister, Thomas W.; Dietrich, Kimberly. A trial of verapamil in the treatment of stuttering in adults. Biological Psychiatry; 1989 Mar Vol 25(5) 630–633

Burgraff, Roger I. The efficacy of systematic desensitization via imagery as a therapeutic technique with stutterers. British Hournal of Disorders of Communication; 1974 Oct Vol 9(2) 134–139

Caron, Chantal; Dugas, Michel; Ladouceur, Robert. Le traitement individuel et en groupe de begues adultes. (Individual and group treatment of adult stutterers.) Science et Comportement; 1990 Vol 20(3–4) 185–193

Caron, Chantal; Ladouceur, Robert. Multidimensional behavioral treatment for child stutterers. Behavior Modification; 1989 Apr Vol 13(2) 206–215

Code, Chris. Dichotic listening with the communicatively impaired: Results from trials of a short. British English dichotic word test. Journal of Phonetics; 1981 Oct Vol 9(4) 375–383

Code, Christopher; Muller, David. Comments on paper: The long-term use of an automatically triggered masking device in the treatment of stammering. British Journal of Disorders of Communication; 1980 Sep Vol 15(2) 141–142

Conture, Edward G. Youngsters who stutter: Diagnosis, parent counseling, and referral. Journal of Developmental and Behavioral Pediatrics; 1982 Sep Vol 3(3) 163–169

Cooper, Eugene B. The chronic perseverative stuttering syndrome: Incurable stuttering. Journal of Fluency Disorders; 1987 Dec Vol 12(6) 381–388

Cooper, Eugene B. Treatment of disfluency: Future trends. Journal of Fluency Disorders; 1986 Dec Vol 11(4) 317–327

Cote, Christiane; Ladouceur, Robert. Effects of social aids and the regulated breathing method in the treatment of stutterers. Journal of Consulting and Clinical Psychology; 1982 Jun Vol 50(3) 450

Cox, Nancy J.; Kidd, Kenneth K. Can recovery from stuttering be considered a genetically milder subtype of stuttering? Behavior Genetics; 1983 Mar Vol 13(2) 129–139

Craig, A. R.; Calver, P. Following up on treated stutterers: Studies of perceptions of fluency and job status. Journal of Speech and Hearing Research; 1991 Apr Vol 34(2) 279–284

Craig, Ashley; Andrews, Gavin. The prediction and prevention of relapse in stuttering: The value of self-control techniques and locus of control measures. Behavior Modification; 1985 Oct Vol 9(4) 427–442

Craig, Ashley; Feyer, Anne Marie; Andrews, Gavin. An overview of a behavioural treatment for stuttering. Australian Psychologist; 1987 Mar Vol 22(1) 53–62

Craig, Ashley R.; Cleary, Patrick J. Reduction of stuttering by young male stutterers using EMG feedback. Biofeedback and Self Regulation; 1982 Sep Vol 7(3) 241–255

Craven, Duane C.; Ryan, Bruce P. The use of a portable delayed auditory feedback unit in stuttering therapy. Journal of Fluency Disorders; 1984 Sep Vol 9(3) 237–243

Curlee, Richard F.; Perkins, William H. Effectiveness of a DAF conditioning program for adolescent and adult stutterers. Behaviour Research and Therapy; 1973 Nov Vol 11(4) 395–401

Daly, David A. Use of the home VCR to facilitate transfer of fluency. Journal of Fluency Disorders; 1987 Apr Vol 12(2) 103–106

de Vries, Ursula. "Laut—langsam—deutlich"—eine Phase aus der Therapie stotternder Schuler. / "Loudly—slowly—intelligibly": One phase of the therapy for children who stutter. Vierteljahresschrift fur Heilpadagogik und ihre Nachbargebiete; 1990 Mar Vol 59(1) 60–72

Degand, J. (A clinical contribution to the psychodynamic and the pathopsychogenic sources of language problems.) Revue Belge de Psychologie et de Pedagogie; 1972 Vol 34(139) 79–93

Delmonte, Michael M. Meditation as a clinical intervention strategy: A brief review. International Journal of Psychosomatics; 1986 Vol 33(3) 9–12

Dembowski, James; Watson, Ben C. An instrumented method for assessment and remediation of stuttering: A single-subject case study. Journal of Fluency Disorders; 1991 Vol 16(5–6) 241–273

Dempsey, George L.; Granich, Marina. Hypnobehavioral therapy in the case of a traumatic stutterer: A case study. International Journal of Clinical and Experimental Hypnosis; 1978 Jul Vol 26(3) 125–133

Dewar, A. D. Influence of auditory feedback masking on stammering and its use in treatment. International Journal of Rehabilitation Research; 1984 Vol 7(3) 341–342

Dharitri, R. Response to therapy by stutterers in relation to their locus of control. Indian Journal of Clinical Psychology; 1985 Sep Vol 12(2) 37–40

DiGiuseppe, Ray; Wilner, R. Stefanie. An eclectic view of family therapy: When is family therapy the treatment of choice? When is it not? Journal of Clinical Child Psychology; 1980 Spr Vol 9(1) 70–72

Dopheide, Bill. Competencies expected of beginning clinicians working with children who stutter. Journal of Fluency Disorders; 1987 Jun Vol 12(3) 157–166

Dorgan, Barbara J.; Dorgan, Richard E. A theoretical rationale for total family therapy with stutterers. British Journal of Social Psychiatry and Community Health; 1972–1973 Vol 6(3) 214–222

Doughty, Patricia. Case study: The use of hypnosis with a stammerer. British Journal of Experimental and Clinical Hypnosis; 1990 Feb Vol 7(1) 65–67

Dugas, Michel; Ladouceur, Robert. Traitement multidimensionnel et progressif des begues severes. (Multidimensional and progressive treatment of severe stuttering.) Science et Comportement; 1988 Win Vol 18(4) 221–232

Ecker, Willi; Meyer, Victor. Individualized behavioural treatment of severe stuttering. Behavioural Psychotherapy; 1991 Vol 19(4) 347–357

Falkowski, Glenn L.; Guilford, Arthur M.; Sandler, Jack. Effectiveness of a modified version of airflow therapy: Case studies. Journal of Speech and Hearing Disorders; 1982 May Vol 47(2) 160–164

Ferreiro-Diaz, M. D.; Dominguez, M. Dolores; Rodriguez, A. Psicoterapis de grupos infantiles: la madre co-terapeuta. (Group psychotherapy for children: The mother as co-therapist.) Clinica y Analisis Grupal; 1990 May–Aug Vol 12(2) 291–313

Finn, Patrick; Gow, Merrilyn. Prediction of outcome after treatment for stuttering. British Journal of Psychiatry; 1989 Feb Vol 154 273–274

Florin, Irmela. Stuttering: Theoretical approaches, experimental research results, suggestions for therapy. European Journal of Behavioural Analysis and Modification; 1976 Nov Vol 3(1) 189–200

Gagnon, Mireille; Ladouceur, Robert. Behavioral treatment of child stutterers: Replication and extension. Behavior Therapy; 1992 Win Vol 23(1) 113–129

Garber, Anath. Psychodramatic treatment of a stutterer. Group Psychotherapy and Psychodrama; 1973 Vol 26(1–2) 34–47

Garcia-Moreno, Juan. Eficacia clinica de dos alternativas terapeuticas en el tratamiento de la tartamudez. (Clinical efficacy of two therapeutic alternatives to the treatment of stuttering.) Revista de Psicologia General y Aplicada; 1984 Vol 39(6) 1093–1113

Garcia-Moreno, Juan. Tratamiento de la tartamudez por el metodo de la regulacion de la respiracion. (Treatment of stuttering by the regulated-breathing method.) Informes de Psicologia; 1985 Vol 4(1–2) 67–72

Gemelli, Ralph J. Classification of child stuttering: II. Persistent late onset male stuttering, and treatment issues for persistent stutterers—psychotherapy or speech therapy, or both? Child Psychiatry and Human Development; 1982 Fal Vol 13(1) 3–34

Gendelman, Evelyn G. Confrontation in the treatment of stuttering. Journal of Speech and Hearing Disorders; 1977 Feb Vol 42(1) 85–89

Goldberg, S. A. The development of fluency through behavioral cognitive stuttering therapy, Journal of Communication Disorders; 1983 8(7) 89–107

Gonzalez-Valenzuela, M. Jose. Evaluacion y Tratamiento cognitivo-conductual de un caso de tartamudez. / Evaluation and cognitive-behavioral treatment in a severe stuttering case. Analisis y Modificacion de Conducta; 1990 Vol 16(47) 137–148

Goraj, Jane T. Stuttering therapy as crisis intervention. British Journal of Disorders of Communication; 1974 Apr Vol 9(1) 51–57

Gottinger, Werner. A concept for the guidance of stutterers. Praxis der Kinderpsychologie und Kinderpsychiatrie; 1980 Feb Mar Vol 29(2) 55–62

Gottwald, Sheryl R.; Goldbach, Peggy; Isack, Audrey H. Stuttering: Prevention and detection. Young Children; 1985 Nov Vol 41(1) 9–14

Greenberg, David; Marks, Isaac. Behavioural psychotherapy of uncommon referrals. British Journal of Psychiatry; 1982 Aug Vol 141 148–153

Grube, M. Marshall; Smith, Debra S. Paralinguistic intonation rhythm intervention with a developmental stutterer. Journal of Fluency Disorders; 1989 Jun Vol 14(3) 185–208

Guy, Nina. Stuttering as an expression of aggression: Transferential and countertransferential aspects: A case study. Israel Journal of Psychiatry and Related Sciences; 1987 Vol 24(3) 211–221

Halg, Paul. Symbolik und Verlauf in der Therapie eines dreizehnjahrigen Stotterers mit dem katathymen Bilderleben. (Symbolism and process in a short term therapy of a male juvenile stutterer using the day dream technique of guided affective imagery (GAI).) Praxis der Kinderpsychologie und Kinderpsychiatrie; 1981 Oct Vol 30(7) 236–243

Halpern, Harvey. Stuttering therapy for nonfluent psychiatric adults. Perceptual and Motor Skills; 1990 Dec Vol 71(3, Pt 1) 914

Ham, Richard E. Clinician preparation: Experiences with pseudostuttering: "It was the longest day of my life" Journal of Fluency Diosrders; 1990 Oct–Dec Vol 15(5–6) 305–315

Ham, Richard E. Unison speech and rate control therapy. Journal of Fluency Disorders; 1988 Apr Vol 13(2) 115–126

Ham, Richard E. Unison speech and rate control therapy. Journal of Fluency Disorders; 1988 Apr Vol 13(2) 115–126

Hamre, Curt. Another perspective on Silverman's "dimensions of improvement in stuttering." Journal of Speech and Hearing Research; 1981 Sep Vol 24(3) 470–471

Haney, R. R.; Gill, Kinloch. Modification of oral reading disfluency by paced oral reading with subsequent fading of the pacing stimulus: A case report. American Corrective Therapy Journal; 1975 Mar–Apr Vol 29(2) 51–55

Hanna, Richmond; Wilfling, Franz; McNeill, Brent. A biofeedback treatment for stuttering. Journal of Speech and Hearing Disorders; 1975 May Vol 40(2) 270–273

Hasbrouck, Jon M. FAMC intensive stuttering treatment program: Ten years of implementation. Military Medicine; 1992 May Vol 157(5) 244–247

Hasbrouck, Jon M.; Lowry, Fran. Elimination of stuttering and maintenance of fluency by means of airflow, tension reduction, and discriminative stimulus control procedures. Journal of Fluency Disorders; 1989 Jun Vol 14(3) 165–183

Hayden, Paul A.; Adams, Martin R.; Jordahl, Nanette. The effects of pacing and masking on stutterers' and nonstutterers' speech initiation times. Journal of Fluency Disorders; 1982 Mar Vol 7(1–1) 9–19

Healey, E. Charles; Ramig, Peter R. The relationship of stuttering severity and treatment length to temporal measures of stutterers' perceptually fluent speech. Journal of Speech and Hearing Disorders; 1989 Aug Vol 54(3) 313–319

Hegde, M. N. The short and long term effects of contingent aversive noise on stuttering. Journal of the All India Institute of Speech and Hearing; 1971 Jan Vol 2 7–14

Heinzel, Joachim. The problem of stuttering and the therapy methods of the behaviour therapy. Praxis der Kinderpsychologie und Kinderpsychiatrie; 1976 Aug–Sep Vol 25(6) 197–205

Herscovitch, A.; LeBow, M. D. Imaginal pacing in the treatment of stuttering. Journal of Behavior Therapy and Experimental Psychiatry; 1973 Dec Vol 4(4) 357–360

Howie, Pauline M. A response to "On token reinforcement and stuttering therapy: Another view on findings reported by Howie and Woods (1982)." Journal of Applied Behavior Analysis; 1983 Win Vol 16(4) 471–475

Howie, Pauline M.; Tanner, Susan; Andrews, Gavin. Short- and long-term outcome in an intensive treatment program for adult stutterers. Journal of Speech and Hearing Disorders; 1981 Feb Vol 46(1) 104–109

Howie, Pauline M.; Woods, C. Lee. Token reinforcement during the instatement and shaping of fluency in the treatment of stuttering. Journal of Applied Behavior Analysis; 1982 Spr Vol 15(1) 55–64

Hurford, David P.; Webster, Ronald L. Decreases in simple reaction time as a function of stutterers' participation in a behavioral therapy. Journal of Fluency Disorders; 1985 Dec Vol 10(4) 301–310

Hutchinson, John M. A review of rhythmic pacing as a treatment strategy for stuttering. Rehabilitation Literature; 1976 Oct Vol 37(10) 297–303

Hutchinson, John M.; Burk, Kenneth W. An investigation of the effects of temporal alterations in auditory feedback upon stutterers and clutterers. Journal of Communication Disorders; 1973 Sep Vol. 6(3) 193–205

Ibanez-Ramirez, Manuel. Tratamiento de un caso de tartamudez. / Treatment of a stuttering case. Analisis y Modificacion de Conducta; 1985 Vol 11(30) 605–611

Ignatieva, S. A. Active regulated games in the system of correctional education of stuttering preschoolers. Defektologiya; 1986 No 3 67–71

Ikezuki, Makoto; Harano, Kotaro; Yamaguchi, Shoji. (Research on the effect of reciprocal inhibition elicited with kinetic response.) Japanese Journal of Behavior Therapy; 1989 Vol 15(1) 56–61

Ingham, Roger J. Current status of stuttering and behavior modification: II. Principal issues and practices in stuttering therapy. Journal of Fluency Disorders; 1993 Mar Vol 18(1) 57–79

Ingham, Roger J. Modification of maintenance and generalization during stuttering treatment. Journal of Speech and Hearing Research; 1980 Dec Vol 23(4) 732–745

Ingham, Roger J. On token reinforcement and stuttering therapy: Another view on findings reported by Howie and Woods (1982). Journal of Applied Behavior Analysis; 1983 Win Vol 16(4) 465–470

Ingham, Roger J. Research on stuttering treatment for adults and adolescents: A perspective on how to overcome a malaise. ASHA Reports Series American Speech Language Hearing Association; 1990 Apr No 18 91–95

Ingham, Roger J. The effects of self-evaluation training on maintenance and generalization during stuttering treatment. Journal of Speech and Hearing Disorders; 1982 Aug Vol 47(3) 271–280

Ingham, Roger J.; Andrews, Gavin. An analysis of a token economy in stuttering therapy. Journal of Applied Behavior Analysis; 1973 Sum Vol. 6(2) 219–229

Ingham, Roger J.; Packman, Ann. Treatment and generalization effects in an experimental treatment for a stutterer using contingency management and speech rate control. Journal of Speech and Hearing Disorders; 1977 Aug Vol 42(3) 394–407

Ingham, Roger J.; Southwood, Helen; Horsburgh, Gay. Some effects of the Edinburgh Masker on stuttering during oral reading and spontaneous speech. Journal of Fluency Disorders; 1981 Jun Vol 6(2) 135–154

James, Jack E. Office-based treatment for stuttering: A program of speech retraining and self-management. Scandinavian Journal of Behaviour Therapy; 1982 Vol 11(1) 15–28

James, Jack E. Self-monitoring of stuttering: Reactivity and accuracy. Behaviour Research and Therapy; 1981 Vol 19(4) 291–296

James, Jack E.; Ricciardelli, Lina A.; Hunter, Christine E.; Rogers, Peter. Relative efficacy of intensive and spaced behavioral treatment of stuttering. Behavior Modification; 1989 Jul Vol 13(3) 376–395

Jehle, Peter; Boberg, Einer. Intensivbehandlung fur jugendliche und erwachsene Stotternde von Boberg und Kully. / Intensive treatment for adolescent and adult stutterers by Boberg and Kully. Folia Phoniatrica; 1987 Sep–Oct Vol 39(5) 256–268

Johannesson, Goran. (Two behavior therapy techniques in the treatment of stuttering.) Scandinavian Journal of Behaviour Therapy; 1975 Vol 4(1) 11–22

Johnson, Gerald F. Ten commandments for long-term maintenance of acceptable self-help skills for persons who are hard-core stutterers. Journal of Fluency Disorders; 1987 Feb Vol 12(1) 9–18

Jones, R. Barrie. Modified regulated-breathing in treatment of a single case of stuttering. Perceptual and Motor Skills; 1981 Feb Vol 52(1) 130

Kaplan, Netta R.; Kaplan, Marvin L. The Gestalt approach to stuttering. Journal of Communication Disorders; 1978 Feb Vol 11(1) 1–9

Katz-Bernstein, Nitza. Poltern: Therapieansatz fur Kinder. (Tachyphemia: A therapeutic approach for children.) Vierteljahresschrift fur Heilpadagogik und ihre Nachbargebiete; 1986 Dec Vol 55(4) 413–426

Kehrer, H. E. (Behaviour therapy in child and adolescent psychiatry.) Acta Paedopsychiatrica; 1973 Vol 40(2) 58–65

Kern, Horst J.; Kern, Marijke. Verhaltenstherapie beim Stottern: Videoruckmeldung und willentliches Stottern. (Behavioral stuttering therapy: Video feedback and intentional stuttering.) Zeitschrift fur Klinische Psychologie. Forschung und Praxis; 1991 Vol 20(4) 389–401

Kharatinov, A. V. (Methodological principles of art therapy in a system of social rehabilitation for adult stutterers.) Novye Issledovaniya v Psikhologii; 1981 No 1(24) 94–97

Khavin, A. B.; Diakova, E. A. (Characteristics of communication impairments in adult stutterers and effectiveness of medical-rehabilitation work.) Defektologiya; 1988 No 3 20–24

Kondas, Ondrej. (The use of a metronome in reeducation of stutterers.) Psychologia a Patopsychologia Dietata; 1974 Vol 9(6) 545–551

Kraaimaat, Floor W.; Janssen, Peggy. Een werkmodel voor een differentiele diagnostiek en behandeling van stotteren. (A working model for the differential diagnosis and treatment of stuttering.) Gedragstherapie; 1983 Dec Vol 16(4) 299–309

Krause, Rainer. Problems of psychological research and treatment of stuttering. Zeitschrift fur Klinische Psychologie und Psychotherapie; 1976 Vol 24(2) 128–143

Kuhr, Armin; Rustin, Lena. The maintenance of fluency after intensive in-patient therapy: Long-term follow-up. Journal of Fluency Disorders; 1985 Sep Vol 10(3) 229–236

Kully, Deborah; Boberg, Einer. An investigation of interclinic agreement in the identification of fluent and stuttered syllables. Journal of Fluency Disorders; 1988 Oct Vol 13(5) 309–318

La Croix, Zane E. Management of disfluent speech through self-recording procedures. Journal of Speech and Hearing Disorders; 1973 May Vol 38(2) 272–274

Ladouceur, Robert; Saint Laurent, Lise. Stuttering: A multidimensional treatment and evaluation package. Journal of Fluency Disorders; 1986 Jun Vol 11(2) 93–103

Ladouceur, Robert; Boudreau, Leonce; Theberge, Sylvie. Awareness training and regulated-breathing method in modification of stuttering. Perceptual and Motor Skills; 1981 Aug Vol 53(1) 187–194

Ladouceur, Robert; Cote, Christiane; Leblond, Georges; Bouchard, Leandre. Evaluation of regulated-breathing method and awareness training in the treatment of stuttering. Journal of Speech and Hearing Disorders; 1982 Nov Vol 47(4) 422–426

Lal, K. K.; Latte, G. A.; Raj, J. Bharath. A case report: Treatment of stuttering with systematic desensitization. Indian Journal of Clinical Psychology; 1976 Sep Vol 3(2) 219–221

Langlois, Aimee; Long, Steven H. A model for teaching parents to facilitate fluent speech. Journal of Fluency Disorders; 1988 Jun Vol 13(3) 163–172

Lankford, Sally D.; Cooper, Eugene B. Recovery from stuttering as viewed by parents of self-diagnosed recovered stutterers. Journal of Communication Disorders; 1974 Jun Vol 7(2) 171–180

Lanyon, Richard I. Effect of biofeedback-based relaxation on stuttering during reading and spontaneous speech. Journal of Consulting and Clinical Psychology; 1977 Oct Vol 45(5) 860–866

Lanyon, Richard I.; Barrington, Cecily C.; Newman, Anne C. Modification of stuttering through EMG biofeedback: A preliminary study. Behavior Therapy; 1976 Jan Vol 7(1) 96–103

Lara-Cantu, Maria A. Pilot study on electromyographic biofeedback for the treatment of stuttering. Ensenanza e Investigacion en Psicologia; 1978 Jul–Dec Vol 4(2) 259–265

Lasogga, Frank; Kondring, Irmgard. Stotterer in Selbsthilfegruppen und in Einzeltherapie. (Stutterers in self-help groups and in individual therapy.) Zeitschrift fur Klinische Psychologie. Forschung und Praxis; 1982 Vol 11(3) 201–214

Lay, Thomas. Stuttering: Training the therapist. Journal of Fluency Disorders; 1982 Mar Vol 7(1-1) 63–69

Leahy, M.; O'Sullivan, B. Psychological change and fluency therapy: A pilot project. British

Journal of Disorders of Communication; 1987 Dec Vol 22(3) 245–251

Leahy, Margaret M.; Collins, Geraldine. Therapy for stuttering: Experimenting with experimenting. Irish Journal of Psychological Medicine; 1991 Mar Vol 8(1) 37–39

Lee, Bernard S.; McGough, W. Edward; Peins, Maryann. Automated desensitization of stutterers to use of the telephone. Behavior Therapy; 1976 Jan Vol 7(1) 110–112

Lees, Roberta M. The effect of foreperiod length on the acoustic voice reaction times of stutterers. Journal of Fluency Disorders; 1988 Jun Vol 13(3) 157–162

Legewie, H.; Cleary, P.; Rackensperger, W. EMG-recording and biofeedback in the diagnosis and therapy of stuttering: A case study. European Journal of Behavioural Analysis and Modification; 1975 Dec Vol 1(2) 137–143

Leith, William R.; Mims, Howard A. Cultural influences in the development and treatment of stuttering: A preliminary report on the Black stutterer. Journal of Speech and Hearing Disorders; 1975 Nov Vol 40(4) 459–466

Leith, William R.; Timmons, Jack L. The stutterer's reaction to the telephone as a speaking situation. Journal of Fluency Disorders; 1983 Sep Vol 8(3) 233–243

Lockhart, Myra S.; Robertson, Alan W. Hypnosis and speech therapy as a combined therapeutic approach to the problem of stammering: A study of thirty patients. British Journal of Disorders of Communication; 1977 Oct Vol 12(2) 97–108

Lokhov, M. I. Interhemispheric asymmetry in mechanisms of nonaphasic speech disturbances. Human Physiology; 1988 Jan–Feb Vol 14(1) 27–31

Lokhov, M. I.; Vartanyan, G. A. Stammering: New therapeutic approaches. Zhurnal Nevropatologii i Psikhiatrii imeni S.S. Korsakova; 1989 Vol 89(3) 68–73

Lucas, Tina. Communication therapy. Journal of Adolescence; 1982 Sep Vol 5(3) 285–299

Lucke, Herman H. Treatment of language fluency disorders by a procedure combining several techniques. Revista Latinoamericana de Psicologia; 1977 Vol 9(3) 437–441

Lukas, Elisabeth. New ways for dereflection. International Forum for Logotherapy; 1981 Spr–Sum Vol 4(1) 13–28

Mallard, A. R.; Westbrook, J. B. Variables affecting stuttering therapy in school settings. Language, Speech, and Hearing Services in Schools; 1988 Oct Vol 19(4) 362–370

Manders, Eric; Bastijns, Paul. The regulated-breathing method for stuttering: An experimental evaluation. Journal of Behavior Therapy and Experimental Psychiatry; 1988 Mar Vol 19(1) 11–19

Manohar, P. D.; Jayaram, M.; Rangasayee; Narendiran. Correspondence therapy for stuttering. Journal of the All India Institute of Speech and Hearing; 1973 Jan Vol 4 113–122

Manschreck, Theo C.; Kalotkin, Madeline; Jacobson, Alan M. Utility of electromyographic biological feedback in chronic stuttering: A clinical study with follow-up. Perceptual and Motor Skills; 1980 Oct Vol 51(2) 535–540

Market, Karen E.; Montague, James C.; Buffalo, M. D.; Drummond, Sakina S. Acquired stuttering: Descriptive data and treatment outcome. Journal of Fluency Disorders; 1990 Feb Vol 15(1) 21–33

Martin, Richard; Haroldson, Samuel K. Effects of five experimental treatments on stuttering. Journal of Speech and Hearing Research; 1979 Mar Vol 22(1) 132–146

Martin, Richard R.; Haroldson, Samuel K. Some comments on "Effects of five experimental treatments on stuttering": A reply. Journal of Speech and Hearing Research; 1980 Mar Vol 23(1) 214–216

Martin, Richard R.; Lindamood, Linda P. Stuttering and spontaneous recovery: Implications for the speech-language pathologist. Language, Speech, and Hearing Services in Schools; 1986 Jul Vol 17(3) 207–218

Martin, Richard; St Louis, Kenneth; Haroldson, Samuel; Hasbrouck, Jon. Punishment and negative reinforcement of stuttering using electric shock. Journal of Speech and Hearing Research; 1975 Sep Vol 18(3) 478–490

Mehta, M. Comparison of abbreviated and full relaxation therapy in systematic desensitization of stutterers. Journal of Personality and

Clinical Studies; 1985 Mar–Sep Vol 1(1–2) 7–10

Mempel, Sigurd. Therapiemotivation bei Kindern: Ergebnisse einer empirischen Untersuchung. / Children's motivation for treatment. Praxis der Kinderpsychologie und Kinderpsychiatrie; 1989 May–Jun Vol 38(5) 146–151

Messer, Stanley B. Integrating psychoanalytic and behaviour therapy: Limitations, possibilities and trade-offs. British Journal of Clinical Psychology; 1983 Jun Vol 22(2) 131–132

Meyers, Susan C.; Strang, Harold R.; Hall, Emily L. Impact of microcomputer simulation training on student-clinicians' ability to effectively intervene with preschool stutterers. Journal of Fluency Disorders; 1989 Apr Vol 14(2) 135–151

Mironova, S. (On the work of a speech therapist in a preschool children's home.) Defektologiya; 1985 No 1 89–90

Mokrovskaya, A. A. Therapeutic and corrective work with stammering preschool children in conditions of a day-time semi-hospital institution. Zhurnal Nevropatologii i Psikhiatrii imeni S.S. Korsakova; 1986 Vol 86(10) 1565–1569

Mokrovskaya, A. A. Therapeutic and remedial work with stuttering preschoolers in a day hospital. Soviet Neurology and Psychiatry; 1988 Spr Vol 21(1) 53–61

Moleski, Richard; Tosi, Donald J. Comparative psychotherapy: Rational-emotive therapy versus systematic desensitization in the treatment of stuttering. Journal of Consulting and Clinical Psychology; 1976 Apr Vol 44(2) 309–311

Moore, James C.; Rigo, Thomas G. An awareness approach to the covert symptoms of stuttering. Journal of Fluency Disorders; 1983 Jun Vol 8(2) 133–145

Moore, James C.; Rigo, Thomas G. An awareness approach to the covert symptoms of stuttering. Journal of Fluency Disorders; 1983 Jun Vol 8(2) 133–145

Moore, Mary S.; Adams, Martin R. The Edinburgh Masker: A clinical analog study. Journal of Fluency Disorders; 1985 Dec Vol 10(4) 281–290

Moreno, Felipe A. A counterconditioning program (habit-reversal) in treatment of stuttering: A case study. Revista de Psicologia General y Aplicada; 1977 Jul–Aug Vol 32(147) 593–600

Motsch, Hans Joachim. Idiographische Logopadie. (Idiographic speech science.) Vierteljahresschrift fur Heilpadagogik und ihre Nachbargebiete; 1990 Mar Vol 59(1) 2–13

Murphy, Albert T. Authenticity and creativity in stuttering theory and therapy. Journal of Communication Disorders; 1977 Mar Vol 10(1–2) 25–36

Murray, K. S.; Empson, J. A.; Weaver, S. M. Rehearsal and preparation for speech in stutterers: A psychophysiological study. British Journal of Disorders of Communication; 1987 Aug Vol 22(2) 145–150

Nekrasova, Julia B. Wiederherstellung einer gestorten Kommunikation (am Beispiel einer Logoneurose). / Repair of disturbed communication in logoneurosis. Dynamische Psychiatrie; 1989 Vol 22(114–115) 37–50

Nekrasova, Y. B. Psychotherapy sessions and some mental states of stutterers. Voprosy Psikhologii; 1980 Sep–Oct No 5 32–40

Nekrasova, Yuliya B. Dynamics of psychological states in stutterers in the process of logopsychotherapy. Voprosy Psikhologii; 1985 Mar–Apr No 2 127–133

Nekrasova, Yuliya B. (Group emotional and stress psychotherapy to correct mental states of stutterers.) Voprosy Psikhologii; 1984 Mar–Apr No 2 75–82

Newman, Linda L. The effects of punishment of repetitions and the acquisition of "stutter-like" behaviors in normal speakers. Journal of Fluency Disorders; 1987 Feb Vol 12(1) 51–62

Nigam, J. C. Stuttering and its self treatment. Hearing Aid Journal; 1985 Jul Vol 4(3) 78–79

Nowack, William J.; Stone, R. Edward. Acquired stuttering and bilateral cerebral disease. Journal of Fluency Disorders; 1987 Apr Vol 12(2) 141–146

Nurnberger, John I.; Hingtgen, Joseph N. Is symptom substitution an important issue in behavior therapy? Biological Psychiatry; 1973 Dec Vol. 7(3) 221–236

Nystul, Michael S.; Muszynska, Eve. Adlerian treatment of a classical case of stuttering. Journal of Individual Psychology; 1976 Nov Vol 32(2) 194–202

Oganesian, E. V. On unification of registration and assessment of rehabilitation effects in adult stutterers. Defektologiya; 1986 No 4 75–78

Oganesian, E. V. (Study of the effectiveness of speech correction within the context of a complex approach to the treatment of stuttering in adults in specialized hospital departments.) Defektologiya; 1985 No 4 23–28

Oganesian, Ye. V.; Beliakova, L. I. The rationale for principles of differential application of logopaedic rhythmics in remediation of adult stutterers. Defektologiya; 1982 No 1 3–12

Oganesyan, E. V. (Different rhythmic speech therapy exercises for adolescent and adult stutterers.) Defektologiya; 1983 No 1 60–63

Ojha, K. N.; Bettagere, R. N. Group psychotherapy with stutterers. Indian Journal of Clinical Psychology; 1982 Sep Vol 9(2) 125–129

Onslow, Mark; Costa, Leanne; Rue, Stephen. Direct early intervention with stuttering: Some preliminary data. Journal of Speech and Hearing Disorders; 1990 Aug Vol 55(3) 405–416

Onslow, Mark; Ingham, Roger J. Speech quality measurement and the management of stuttering. Journal of Speech and Hearing Disorders; 1987 Feb Vol 52(1) 2–17

Orta-Rodriguez, Martha; Gallegos B., Xochitl. Una evaluacion de tres tecnicas conductuales en el tratamiento de la tartamudez. (An evaluation of 3 behavioral techniques used to treat stuttering.) Revista Mexicana de Psicologia; 1986 Jul–Dec Vol 3(2) 168–173

Ost, Lars Goran. Experimental studies in behaviour therapy. Scandinavian Journal of Behaviour Therapy; 1976 Vol 5(Suppl 1) 3–36

Ost, Lars Goran; Gotestam, K. Gunnar; Melin, Lennart. A controlled study of two behavioral methods in the treatment of stuttering. Behavior Therapy; 1976 Oct Vol 7(5) 587–592

Ottoni, Thais M. (The use of the technique of speech modeling in modification of verbal behavior.) Revista Interamericana de Psicologia; 1974 Vol 8(3–4) 197–203

Palenzuela-Sanchez, Angeles. Intervencion sobre contingencias externas como tratamiento psicologico en un caso de tartamudez de desarrollo. (Intervention based on external contingencies as psychological treatment in a case of stuttering in a young child.) Analisis y Modificacion de Conducta; 1993 Vol 19(64) 287–298

Pauls, David L.; Kidd, Kenneth K. Genetic strategies for the analysis of childhood behavioral traits. Schizophrenia Bulletin; 1982 Vol 8(2) 253–266

Perkins, William H. Replacement of stuttering with normal speech: I. Rationale. Journal of Speech and Hearing Disorders; 1973 Aug Vol. 38(3) 283–294

Perkins, William H. Replacement of stuttering with normal speech: II. Clinical procedures. Journal of Speech and Hearing Disorders; 1973 Aug Vol. 38(3) 295–303

Perkins, William H.; et al. Replacement of stuttering with normal speech: III. Clinical effectiveness. Journal of Speech and Hearing Disorders; 1974 Nov Vol 39(4) 416–428

Perkins, William H. Implications of scientific research for treatment of stuttering: A lecture. Journal of Fluency Disorders; 1981 Jun Vol 6(2) 155–162

Petermann, Franz. Aktuelle Trends bei der Verhaltensmodifikation mit Kindern. (Current trends in behavior modification with children.) Psychologische Rundschau; 1981 Oct Vol 32(4) 250–266

Peters, M. The view of learning theory. Zeitschrift fur Kinder und Jugendpsychiatrie; 1976 Vol 4(2) 104–112

Petrunik, Michael; Shearing, Clifford D. Fragile facades: Stuttering and the strategic manipulation of awareness. Social Problems; 1983 Dec Vol 31(2) 125–138

Pill, Jaan. A comparison between two treatment programs for stuttering: A personal account. Journal of Fluency Disorders; 1988 Dec Vol 13(6) 385–398

Polaino Lorente, Aquilino M. Experiences in the treatment of childhood stuttering. Revista de Psicologia General y Aplicada; 1976 Mar–Apr Vol 31(139) 171–183

Porter, Jeannie F. Homosexuality treated adventitiously in a stuttering therapy program: A case report presenting a heterophobic orientation. Australian and New Zealand Journal of Psychiatry; 1976 Jun Vol 10(2) 185–189

Preus, Alf. Treatment of mentally retarded stutterers. Journal of Fluency Disorders; 1990 Aug Vol 15(4) 223–233

Prins, David; Miller, Michele. Personality, improvement, and regression in stuttering therapy. Journal of Speech and Hearing Research; 1973 Dec Vol 16(4) 685–690

Prins, David. Stutterers' perceptions of therapy improvement and of posttherapy regression: Effects of certain program modifications. Journal of Speech and Hearing Disorders; 1976 Nov Vol 41(4) 452–463

Prins, David; Nichols, Anne. Client impressions of the effectiveness of stuttering therapy: A comparison of two programs. British Journal of Disorders of Communication; 1974 Oct Vol 9(2) 123–133

Quarrington, Bruce. How do the various theories of stuttering facilitate our therapeutic approach? Journal of Communication Disorders; 1977 Mar Vol 10(1–2) 77–83

Raj, J. Bharath. Control of stuttering behaviour through response contingent shocks. Journal of the All India Institute of Speech and Hearing; 1974–75 Jan Vol 5–6 10–16

Raj, J. Bharath. Treatment of stuttering. Indian Journal of Clinical Psychology; 1976 Sep Vol 3(2) 157–163

Raj, J. Bharath; Latte, G. A. Recoveries from stuttering. Indian Journal of Clinical Psychology; 1977 Sep Vol 4(2) 185–187

Ramig, Peter R. Rate changes in the speech of stutterers after therapy. Journal of Fluency Disorders; 1984 Dec Vol 9(4) 285–294

Ramirez, Luis H. (Treatment of stuttering by self-control procedures.) Revista Latinoamericana de Psicologia; 1975 Vol 7(3) 421–434

Ratner, Nan B. Measurable outcomes of instructions to modify normal parent-child verbal interactions: Implications for indirect stuttering therapy. Journal of Speech and Hearing Research; 1992 Feb Vol 35(1) 14–20

Resick, Patricia A.; Wendiggensen, Paul; Ames, Sean; Meyer, Victor. Systematic slowed speech: A new treatment for stuttering. Behaviour Research and Therapy; 1978 Vol 16(3) 161–167

Resnick, Sylvia; Tureen, Phyllis. Evaluation of fluent and disfluent speech segments by stutterers and nonstutterers. Journal of Fluency Disorders; 1990 Feb Vol 15(1) 1–8

Rochford, E. Burke. Stutterers' practices: Folk remedies and therapeutic intervention. Journal of Communication Disorders; 1983 Sep Vol 16(5) 373–384

Rojahn, Johannes; Pesta, Thekla. Stuttering behaviors incompatible with speech interruption: Therapeutic limitations and usefulness with stutterers. Zeitschrift fur Klinische Psychologie; 1977 Vol 6(4) 281–302

Romero, Juan F. Tratamiento multimodal de un caso de tartamudez. / Multimodal treatment in a case of stuttering. First National Symposium: Importance of cognitive and behavioral therapies in child and adolescent psychopathology (1984, Malaga, Spain). Analisis y Modificacion de Conducta; 1985 Vol 11(27) 133–143

Rosenberger, Peter B.; Wheelden, Julie A.; Kalotkin, Madeline. The effect of haloperidol on stuttering. American Journal of Psychiatry; 1976 Mar Vol 133(3) 331–334

Roth U., Erick; Aguilar S., Guido G. Speech therapy: A comparative study of the stutterer. Aprendizaje y Comportamiento; 1979 Vol 2(1–2) 93–108

Rousey, Carol G.; Arjunan, K. N.; Rousey, Clyde L. Successful treatment of stuttering following closed head injury. Journal of Fluency Disorders; 1986 Sep Vol 11(3) 257–261

Runyan, Charles M.; Runyan, Sara E. A fluency rules therapy program for young children in the public schools. Language, Speech, and Hearing Services in Schools; 1986 Oct Vol 17(4) 276–284

Rustin, Lena; Kuhr, Armin. The treatment of stammering: A multi-model approach in an in-patient setting. British Journal of Disorders of Communication; 1983 Sep Vol 18(2) 90–97

Rustin, Lena; Ryan, Bruce P.; Ryan, Barbara V. Use of the Monterey programmed stuttering therapy in Great Britain. British Journal of Disorders of Communication; 1987 Aug Vol 22(2) 151–162

Ryan, Bruce P.; Van Kirk, Barbara. Programmed stuttering therapy for children: Comparison of four establishment programs. Journal of Fluency Disorders; 1983 Dec Vol 8(4) 291–321

Ryan, Bruce P.; Van Kirk, Barbara. Speech therapy rhythmics in the correctional system for preschool stutterers. Defektologiya; 1987 No 3 60–64

Ryan, Bruce P.; Van Kirk, Barbara. The establishment, transfer, and maintenance of fluent speech in 50 stutterers using delayed auditory feedback and operant procedures. Journal of Speech and Hearing Disorders; 1974 Feb Vol. 39(1) 3–10

Rychkova, N. A. Speech therapy rhythmics in the correctional system for preschool stutterers. Defektologiya; 1987 No 3 60–64

Sacco, Pat R.; Metz, Dale E. Changes in stutterers' fundamental frequency contours following therapy. Journal of Fluency Disorders; 1987 Feb Vol 12(1) 1–8

Sahasi, G.; Pandit, Rama. Indigenous methods of treating stuttering. Journal of Personality and Clinical Studies; 1985 Mar–Sep Vol 1(1–2) 37–40

Saint-Laurent, Lise; Ladouceur, Robert. Analyse des traitements behavioraux du begaiement. (Analyses of behavioral treatments for stuttering.) Canadian Psychology; 1987 Jul Vol 28(3) 239–250

Saint-Laurent, Lise; Ladouceur, Robert. Massed versus distributed application of the regulated-breathing method for stutterers and its long-term effect. Behavior Therapy; 1987 Win Vol 18(1) 38–50

Salend, Spencer J.; Andress, Marilyn J. Decreasing stuttering in an elementary-level student. Language, Speech, and Hearing Services in Schools; 1984 Jan Vol 15(1) 16–21

Scheidegger, Ursula. Spieltherapie mit stotternden Kindern: Ein Erfahrungsbericht. / Play therapy with stuttering children: Practical experiences. Vierteljahresschrift fur Heilpadagogik und ihre Nachbargebiete; 1987 Dec Vol 56(4) 619–629

Schultheis, Josef R. Modern theories of stuttering. Praxis der Kinderpsychologie und Kinderpsychiatrie; 1978 Apr Vol 27(3) 83–87

Schulze, Christa C. Kontrolle von Stottervorlaufern durch GSR-Biofeedback. (Control of stuttering precursors through GSR biofeedback.) Zeitschrift fur Klinische Psychologie. Forschung und Praxis; 1982 Vol 11(2) 116–143

Schwartz, Arthur H.; Daly, David A. Elicited imitation in language assessment: A tool for formulating and evaluating treatment programs. Journal of Communication Disorders; 1978 Feb Vol 11(1) 25–35

Seidel, Christa; Biesalski, P. (Psychological and clinical experiences with the Frostig Test and the Frostig therapy in speech-impaired chidlren.) Praxis der Kinderpsychologie und Kinderpsychiatrie; 1973 Jan Vol 22(1) 3–15

Seider, Robin A.; Gladstien, Keith L.; Kidd, Kenneth K. Recovery and persistence of stuttering among relatives of stutterers. Journal of Speech and Hearing Disorders; 1983 Nov Vol 48(4) 402–409

Shelton, John L. The elimination of persistent stuttering by the use of homework assignments involving speech shadowing: A case report. Behavior Therapy; 1975 May Vol 6(3) 392–393

Shenker, Rosalee C.; Finn, Patrick. An evaluation of the effects of supplemental "fluency" training during maintenance. Journal of Fluency Disorders; 1985 Dec Vol 10(4) 257–267

Shklovskii, Viktor M.; Krol, Leonid M.; Mikhailova, Ekaterina L. The psychotherapy of stuttering: On the model of stuttering patients' psychotherapy group. Soviet Journal of Psychiatry and Psychology Today; 1988 Vol 1(1) 130–141

Shklovsky, V. M.; Krol, L. M.; Mikhailova, E. L. Specificity of group psychotherapy in stammering. Trudy Leningradskogo Nauchno Issledovatel'skogo Psikhonevrologicheskogo Instituta i m V M Bekhtereva; 1988 Vol 121 112–117

Shklovsky, Victor M.; Kroll, Leonid M.; Mikhailova, Ekaterina L. Group psychotherapy: Problems of theory and practical application. Psikologicheskii Zhurnal; 1985 May–Jun Vol 6(3) 100–110

Silverman, Franklin H. Communicative success: A reinforcer of stuttering? Perceptual and Motor Skills; 1976 Oct Vol 43(2) 398

Silverman, Franklin H. Dimensions of improvement in stuttering. Journal of Speech and Hearing Research; 1980 Mar Vol 23(1) 137–151

Silverman, Franklin H. Long-term impact of a miniature metronome on stuttering: An interim report. Perceptual and Motor Skills; 1976 Jun Vol 42(3, Pt 2) 1322

Silverman, Franklin H.; Umberger, Forrest G. Effect of pacing speech with a miniature electronic metronome on the frequency and duration of selected disfluency behaviors in the spontaneous speech of adult stutterers. Behavior Therapy; 1974 May Vol 5(3) 410–414

Small, Maurice M. Treatment of stuttering: A case history. Perceptual and Motor Skills; 1975 Dec Vol 41(3) 812

Smit-Beek, Eva; Sluijmer-Swanenburg, Bep. An experimental group treatment of six stuttering children based on the two-factor theory of Mowrer. Tijdschrift voor Psychotherapie; 1977 Jul Vol 3(4) 175–182

Snyder, Murry A. A psychodynamic approach to the theory and therapy of stuttering. Journal of Communication Dis Vol 10(1–2) 85–88

Srivastava, K. Indira. Soc fac- tors of stammering and eha- bilitation of stammerers. ical Review; 1985 Vol 29(Spe

St. Louis, Kenneth O.; L.; Thompson, Jean N.; Rif Pre- liminary investigation ack induced relaxation wit ged stutterer. Perceptual an 982 Aug Vol 55(1) 195–199

Staffolani, Giuseppe. La . / Childhood stuttering. R ale di Psicologia e Ipnosi; 19 5(1) 37–41

Starkweather, C. Woodruf in therapy for stuttering c es- tions for future research Se- ries American Speech ing Association; 1990 Apr No 18 82–90

Starkweather, C. Woodruff; Gottwald, Sheryl R. The demands and capacities model: II. Clinical applications. Journal of Fluency Disorders; 1990 Jun Vol 15(3) 143–157

Stewart, Trudy; Wright, Louise. An overview of services in Britain for people who stutter. American Journal of Speech-Language Pathology; 1994 3(1) 5–8

Stigora, Joseph A.; DiSimoni, Frank G. Resolution of opposing forces: An approach to the understanding and clinical management of stuttering. Journal of Fluency Disorders; 1989 Aug Vol 14(4) 293–302

Stocker, Beatrice; Gerstman, Louis J. A comparison of the Probe technique and conventional therapy for young stutterers. Journal of Fluency Disorders; 1983 Dec Vol 8(4) 331–339

Strang, Harold R.; Meyers, Susan C. A microcomputer simulation to evaluate and train effective intervention techniques in listening partners of preschool stutterers. Journal of Fluency Disorders; 1987 Jun Vol 12(3) 205–215

Stromer, Jeffrey M. Some comments on "Biofeedback in the treatment of psychophysiologic disorders: Stuttering." Biofeedback and Self Regulation; 1979 Dec Vol 4(4) 383–385

Swan, Ann M. Helping children who stutter: What teachers need to know. Childhood Education; 1993 Spr Vol 69(3) 138–141

Tang, Shenqing; Xu, Jengchen; Luo, Powei. (Preliminary studies on the psychological problems of stuttering children.) Information on Psychological Sciences; 1984 No 6 43–44

Tarkowski, Zbigniew. Psychoterapia osob jakajacych sie. / Psychotherapy of stutterers. Psychologia Wychowawcza; 1987 Mar–Apr Vol 30(2) 184–192

Trotter, William D.; Silverman, Franklin H. Does the effect of pacing speech with a miniature metronome on stuttering wear off? Perceptual and Motor Skills; 1974 Aug Vol 39(1, Pt 2) 429–430

Trotter, William D.; Silverman, Franklin H. Experiments with the Stutter Aid. Perceptual and Motor Skills; 1973 Jun Vol 36(3, Pt. 2) 1129–1130

Turkat, Ira D.; Pomeranz, Jane F.; Bruch, Michael H. Rapid treatment of a twenty-two-year stammering problem by slow speech training. Scandinavian Journal of Behaviour Therapy; 1981 Vol 10(1) 49–53

Tyre, Timothy E.; Maisto, Stephen A.; Companik, Paul J. The use of systematic desensitization in the treatment of chronic stuttering behavior. Journal of Speech and Hearing Disorders; 1973 Nov Vol 38(4) 514–519

Van Jaarsveld, Pieter E.; du Plessis, Wynand F. Audio-psycho-phonology at Potchefstroom: A review. South African Journal of Psychology; 1988 Dec Vol 18(4) 136–143

Vekassy, Laszlo. Gyogyult dadogok utanvizsgalata. / The catamnestic study of cured stutterers. Magyar Pszichologiai Szemle; 1989 Vol 45(1) 37–57

Vekassy, Laszlo. Az autogen trening a dadogo komplex kezeleseben. (Autogenic training in the complex treatment of the stutterer.) Magyar Pszichologiai Szemle; 1981 Vol 38(1) 43–56

Viswanath, N. S. Experimental aversion therapy for stuttering: A case study. Journal of the All India Institute of Speech and Hearing; 1971 Jan Vol 2 69–71

Vlasenko, I. T. Study of and principles of analysis of verbal and non-verbal processes in children with developmental language impairments. Defektologiya; 1988 No 4 3–11

Waterloo, Knut K.; Gotestam, K. Gunnar. The regulated-breathing method for stuttering: An experimental evaluation. Journal of Behavior Therapy and Experimental Psychiatry; 1988 Mar Vol 19(1) 11–19

Watts, Fraser. Mechanisms of fluency control in stutterers. British Journal of Disorders of Communication; 1973 Oct Vol 8(2) 131–138

Webster, Ronald L. A few observations on the manipulation of speech response characteristics in stutterers. Journal of Communication Disorders; 1977 Mar Vol 10(1–2) 73–76

Wendlandt, Wolfgang. (A behavior therapeutic program for adult stutterers.) Praxis der Kinderpsychologie und Kinderpsychiatrie; 1974 Oct Vol 23(7) 255–265

Wendlandt, Wolfgang. (Self-assertive training: A behavioral therapeutic phase in the treatment of adult stutterers.) Zeitschrift fur Klinische Psychologie und Psychotherapie; 1974 Vol 22(3) 236–246

Williams, J. David; Martin, Randall B. Immediate versus delayed consequences of stuttering responses. Journal of Speech and Hearing Research; 1974 Dec Vol 17(4) 569–575

Wingate, Marcel E. The relationship of theory to therapy in stuttering. Journal of Communication Disorders; 1977 Mar Vol 10(1–2) 37–44

Wolak, Krzysztof. Zastosowanie techniki biofeedback w terapii osob jakajacych sie. / Biofeedback technique in stuttering therapy. Psychologia Wychowawcza; 1988 Jan–Feb Vol 31(1) 56–69

Wolff, Tore. En teori om hur stamning uppkommer. (A theory about the cause of stuttering.) Psykisk Halsa; 1989 Vol 30(1) 45–49

Yovetich, William S. Message therapy: Language approach to stuttering therapy with children. Journal of Fluency Disorders; 1984 Feb Vol 9(1) 11–20

Zibelman, Robert. Avoidance-reduction therapy for stuttering. American Journal of Psychotherapy; 1982 Oct Vol 36(4) 489–496

Voice and Laryngeal Behaviors

Abeleva, I. Yu. Respiration dynamics during speech production in stuttering adults. Defektologiya; 1976 Jan No 1 17–20

Adams, Martin R. Voice onsets and segment durations of normal speakers and beginning stutterers. Journal of Fluency Disorders; 1987 Apr Vol 12(2) 133–139

Adams, Martin R.; Hutchinson, John. The effects of three levels of auditory masking on selected vocal characteristics and the frequency of disfluency of adult stutterers. Journal of Speech and Hearing Research; 1974 Dec Vol 17(4) 682–688

Adams, Martin R.; Ramig, Peter. Vocal characteristics of normal speakers and stutterers during choral reading. Journal of Speech and Hearing Research; 1980 Jun Vol 23(2) 457–469

Adams, Martin R.; Sears, Rosa L.; Ramig, Peter R. Vocal changes in stutterers and nonstutterers during monotoned speech. Journal of Fluency Disorders; 1982 Mar Vol 7(1–1) 21–35

Andronova, L. Z.; Arutiunyan, M. A.; Aleksandrovskaya, A. S. On the influence of singing on stuttering. Defektologiya; 1987 No 4 58–60

Anitha, H. P. Phonation and stuttering. Journal of the All India Institute of Speech and Hearing; 1982 Vol 13 105–111

Bakker, Klaas; Brutten, Gene J. A comparative investigation of the laryngeal premotor, adjustment, and reaction times of stutterers and nonstutterers. Journal of Speech and Hearing Research; 1989 Jun Vol 32(2) 239–244

Bakker, Klaas; Brutten, Gene J. Speech-related reaction times of stutterers and nonstutterers: Diagnostic implications. Journal of Speech and Hearing Disorders; 1990 May Vol 55(2) 295–299

Bakker, Klaas; Brutten, Gene J. A comparative investigation of the laryngeal premotor, adjustment, and reaction times of stutterers and nonstutterers. Journal of Speech and Hearing Research; 1989 Jun Vol 32(2) 239–244

Bergmann, Gunther. Studies in stuttering as a prosodic disturbance. Journal of Speech and Hearing Research; 1986 Sep Vol 29(3) 290–300

Bishop, Judith H.; Williams, Harriet G.; Cooper, William A. Age and task complexity variables in motor performance of children with articulation-disordered, stuttering, and normal speech. Journal of Fluency Disorders; 1991 Vol 16(4) 219–228

Borden, Gloria J.; Baer, Thomas; Kenney, Mary K. Onset of voicing in stuttered and fluent utterances. Journal of Speech and Hearing Research; 1985 Sep Vol 28(3) 363–372

Borden, Gloria J.; Kim, Daniel H.; Spiegler, Karin. Acoustics of stop consonant-vowel relationships during fluent and stuttered utterances. Journal of Fluency Disorders; 1987 Jun Vol 12(3) 175–184

Bosshardt, Hans Georg. Subvocalization and reading rate differences between stuttering and nonstuttering children and adults. Journal of Speech and Hearing Research; 1990 Dec Vol 33(4) 776–785

Caruso, Anthony J.; Conture, Edward G.; Colton, Raymond H. Selected temporal parameters of coordination associated with stuttering in children. Journal of Fluency Disorders; 1988 Feb Vol 13(1) 57–82

Ciambrone, Sarah W.; Adams, Martin R.; Berkowitz, Michael. A correlational study of stutterers' adaptation and voice initiation times. Journal of Fluency Disorders; 1983 Mar Vol 8(1) 29–37

Colcord, Roger D.; Adams, Martin R. Voicing duration and vocal SPL changes associated with stuttering reduction during singing. Journal of Speech and Hearing Research; 1979 Sep Vol 22(3) 468–479

Conture, Edward G. Some effects of noise on the speaking behavior of stutterers. Journal of Speech and Hearing Research; 1974 Dec Vol 17(4) 714–723

Conture, Edward G.; McCall, Gerald N.; Brewer, David W. Laryngeal behavior during stuttering. Journal of Speech and Hearing Research; 1977 Dec Vol 20(4) 661–668

Conture, Edward G.; Rothenberg, Martin; Molitor, Richard D. Electroglottographic observations of young stutterers' fluency. Journal of Speech and Hearing Research; 1986 Sep Vol 29(3) 384–393

Conture, Edward G.; Schwartz, Howard D.; Brewer, David W. Laryngeal behavior during stuttering: A further study. Journal of Speech and Hearing Research; 1985 Jun Vol 28(2) 233–240

Cross, Douglas E.; Luper, Harold L. Relation between finger reaction time and voice reaction time in stuttering and nonstuttering children and adults. Journal of Speech and Hearing Research; 1983 Sep Vol 26(3) 356–361

Cross, Douglas E.; Olson, Patricia. Interaction between jaw kinematics and voice onset for stutterers and nonstutterers in a VRT task. Journal of Fluency Disorders; 1987 Oct Vol 12(5) 367–380

Cross, Douglas E.; Olson, Patricia L. Articulatory-laryngeal interaction in stutterers and normal speakers: Effects of a bite-block on rapid voice initiation. Journal of Fluency Disorders; 1987 Dec Vol 12(6) 407–418

Cullinan, Walter L.; Springer, Mark T. Voice initiation and termination times in stuttering and nonstuttering children. Journal of Speech and Hearing Research; 1980 Jun Vol 23(2) 344–360

de Nil, Luc F.; Brutten, Gene J. Speech-associated attitudes: Stuttering, voice disordered, articulation disordered, and normal speaking children. Journal of Fluency Disorders; 1990 Apr Vol 15(2) 127–134

de Nil, Luc F.; Brutten, G. J. Voice onset times of stuttering and nonstuttering children: The influence of externally and linguistically imposed time pressure. Journal of Fluency Disorders; 1991 Vol 16(2–3) 143–158

Dembowski, James; Watson, Ben C. Preparation time and response complexity effects on stutterers' and nonstutterers' acoustic LRT. Journal of Speech and Hearing Research; 1991 Feb Vol 34(1) 49–59

Ferrand, Carole T.; Gilbert, Harvey R.; Blood, Gordon W. Selected aspects of central processing and vocal motor function in stutterers and nonstutterers. Journal of Fluency Disorders; 1991 Vol 16(2–3) 101–115

Garber, Sharon F.; Martin, Richard R. Effects of noise and increased vocal intensity on stuttering. Journal of Speech and Hearing Research; 1977 Jun Vol 20(2) 233–240

Hayden, Paul A.; Jordahl, Nanette; Adams, Martin R. Stutterers' voice initiation times during conditions of novel stimulation. Journal of Fluency Disorders; 1982 Mar Vol 7(1–1) 1–7

Healey, E. Charles; Mallard, A. R.; Adams, Martin R. Factors contributing to the reduction of stuttering during singing. Journal of Speech and Hearing Research; 1976 Sep Vol 19(3) 475–480

Healey, E. Charles. Speaking fundamental frequency characteristics of stutterers and nonstutterers. Journal of Communication Disorders; 1982 Jan Vol 15(1) 21–29

Healey, E. Charles; Gutkin, Barbara. Analysis of stutterers' voice onset times and fundamental frequency contours during fluency. Journal of Speech and Hearing Research; 1984 Jun Vol 27(2) 219–225

Healey, E. Charles. Fundamental frequency contours of stutterers' vowels following fluent stop consonant productions. Folia Phoniatrica; 1984 May–Jun Vol 36(3) 145–151

Healey, E. Charles; Ramig, Peter R. Acoustic measures of stutterers' and nonstutterers' fluency in two speech contexts. Journal of Speech and Hearing Research; 1986 Sep Vol 29(3) 325–331

Healey, E. Charles; Ramig, Peter R. The relationship of stuttering severity and treatment length to temporal measures of stutterers' perceptually fluent speech. Journal of Speech and Hearing Disorders; 1989 Aug Vol 54(3) 313–319

Horii, Yoshiyuki. Phonatory initiation, termination, and vocal frequency change reaction times of stutterers. Journal of Fluency Disorders; 1984 May Vol 9(2) 115–124

Horii, Yoshiyuki; Ramig, Peter R. Pause and utterance durations and fundamental frequency characteristics of repeated oral readings by stutterers and nonstutterers. Journal of Fluency Disorders; 1987 Aug Vol 12(4) 257–270

Howell, Peter. Changes in voice level caused by several forms of altered feedback in fluent speakers and stutterers. Language and Speech; 1990 Oct–Dec Vol 33(4) 325–338

Howell, Peter; Powell, David J. Hearing your voice through bone and air: Implications for explanations of stuttering behavior from studies of normal speakers. Journal of Fluency Disorders; 1984 Dec Vol 9(4) 247–263

Howell, Peter; Williams, Mark. Acoustic analysis and perception of vowels in children's and teenagers' stuttered speech. Journal of the Acoustical Society of America; 1992 Mar Vol 91(3) 1697–1706

Howell, Peter; Wingfield, Trudie. Perceptual and acoustic evidence for reduced fluency in the vicinity of stuttering episodes. Language and Speech; 1990 Jan–Mar Vol 33(1) 31–46

Hutchinson, John M.; Watkin, Kenneth L. Jaw mechanics during release of the stuttering moment: Some initial observations and interpretations. Journal of Communication Disorders; 1976 Dec Vol 9(4) 269–279

Jancke, Lutz. Variability and duration of voice onset time and phonation in stuttering and nonstuttering adults. Journal of Fluency Disorders; 1994 19(1) 21–39

Jancke, Lutz; Kalveram, Karl T. Kontrolle von on-time (Phonationsdauer) und voice-onset-time bei rechts- bzw. linksohrig dargebotener auditiver Ruckmeldungen: Unterschiedliche Lateralisierung bei stotternden und nichtstotternden Personen? (Control of on-time (phonation duration) and voice-onset time with right- or left-ear auditory feedback: Different lateralization in stutterers and nonstutterers?) Zeitschrift fur Experimentelle und Angewandte Psychologie; 1987 Vol 34(1) 54–63

Kalveram, Karl T.; Jancke, Lutz. Vowel duration and voice onset time for stressed and nonstressed syllables in stutterers under delayed auditory feedback condition. Folia Phoniatrica; 1989 Jan–Feb Vol 41(1) 30–42

Kelly, Ellen M.; Conture, Edward G. Acoustic and perceptual correlates of adult stutterers' typical and imitated stutterings. Journal of Fluency Disorders; 1988 Aug Vol 13(4) 233–252

Klich, Richard J.; May, Gaylene M. Spectrographic study of vowels in stutterers' fluent speech. Journal of Speech and Hearing Research; 1982 Sep Vol 25(3) 364–370

Klouda, Gayle V.; Cooper, William E. Contrastive stress, intonation, and stuttering frequency. Language and Speech; 1988 Jan–Mar Vol 31(1) 3–20

Klouda, Gayle V.; Cooper, William E. Contrastive stress, intonation, and stuttering frequency. Language and Speech; 1988 Jan–Mar Vol 31(1) 3–20

Lee, Bernard S.; McGough, W. Edward; Peins, Maryann. Automated desensitization of stutterers to use of the telephone. Behavior Therapy; 1976 Jan Vol 7(1) 110–112

Lees, Roberta M. The effect of foreperiod length on the acoustic voice reaction times of stutterers. Journal of Fluency Disorders; 1988 Jun Vol 13(3) 157–162

Mallard, A. R.; Hicks, Douglas M.; Riggs, Donald E. A comparison of stutterers and nonstutterers in a task of controlled voice onset. Journal of Speech and Hearing Research; 1982 Jun Vol 25(2) 287–290

Manning, Walter H.; Coufal, Kathy J. The frequency of disfluencies during phonatory transitions in stuttered and nonstuttered speech. Journal of Communication Disorders; 1976 Mar Vol 9(1) 75–81

McFarlane, Stephen C.; Shipley, Kenneth G. Latency of vocalization onset for stutterers and nonstutterers under conditions of auditory and visual cueing. Journal of Speech and Hearing Disorders; 1981 Aug Vol 46(3) 307–312

McGee, Sandra R.; Hutchinson, John M.; Deputy, Paul N. The influence of the onset of phonation on the frequency of disfluency among children who stutter. Journal of Speech and Hearing Research; 1981 Jan Vol 24(2) 269–272

McKnight, Roxanne C.; Cullinan, Walter L. Subgroups of stuttering children: Speech and voice reaction times, segmental durations, and naming latencies. Journal of Fluency Disorders; 1987 Jun Vol 12(3) 217–233

McLean-Muse, Ann; Larson, Charles R.; Gregory, Hugo H. Stutterers' and nonstutterers' voice fundamental frequency changes in response to auditory stimuli. Journal of Speech and Hearing Research; 1988 Dec Vol 31(4) 549–555

Metz, Dale E.; Conture, Edward G.; Caruso, Anthony. Voice onset time, frication, and aspiration during stutterers' fluent speech. Journal of Speech and Hearing Research; 1979 Sep Vol 22(3) 649–656

Metz, Dale E.; Schiavetti, Nicholas; Sacco, Pat R. Acoustic and psychophysical dimensions of the perceived speech naturalness of nonstutterers and posttreatment stutterers. Journal of Speech and Hearing Disorders; 1990 Aug Vol 55(3) 516–525

Montgomery, Allen A.; Cooke, Paul A. Perceptual and acoustic analysis of repetitions in stuttered speech. Journal of Communication Disorders; 1976 Dec Vol 9(4) 317–330

Murphy, Marianne; Baumgartner, John M. Voice initiation and termination time in stuttering and nonstuttering children. Journal of Fluency Disorders; 1981 Sep Vol 6(3) 257–264

Nemec, Jiri. Voice-speech fullness of life: Existential analysis in the context of a medical discipline. Zeitschrift fur Klinische Psychologie und Psychotherapie; 1979 Vol 27(3) 196–203

Newman, Parley W.; Harris, Richard W.; Hilton, Laurence M. Vocal jitter and shimmer in stuttering. Journal of Fluency Disorders; 1989 Apr Vol 14(2) 87–95

Onslow, Mark; Van Doorn, Janis; Newman, Denis. Variability of acoustic segment durations after prolonged-speech treatment for stuttering. Journal of Speech and Hearing Research; 1992 Jun Vol 35(3) 529–536

Perkins, William H. Implications of scientific research for treatment of stuttering: A lecture. Journal of Fluency Disorders; 1981 Jun Vol 6(2) 155–162

Perkins, William H.; Kent, Raymond D.; Curlee, Richard F. A theory of neuropsycholinguistic function in stuttering. Journal of Speech and Hearing Research; 1991 Aug Vol 34(4) 734–752

Peters, Herman F.; Hulstijn, Wouter; Starkweather, C. Woodruff. Acoustic and physiological reaction times of stutterers and nonstutterers. Journal of Speech and Hearing Research; 1989 Sep Vol 32(3) 668–680

Peters, Herman F.; Boves, Louis. Coordination of aerodynamic and phonatory processes in fluent speech utterances of stutterers. Journal of Speech and Hearing Research; 1988 Sep Vol 31(3) 352–361

Reich, Alan; Till, James A.; Goldsmith, Howard. Laryngeal and manual reaction times of stuttering and nonstuttering adults. Journal of

Speech and Hearing Research; 1981 Jan Vol 24(2) 192–196

Peters, Herman F.; Boves, Louis; Van Dielen, Ineke C. Perceptual judgment of abruptness of voice onset in vowels as a function of the amplitude envelope. Journal of Speech and Hearing Disorders; 1986 Nov Vol 51(4) 299–308

Prosek, Robert A.; Montgomery, Allen A.; Walden, Brian E. Constancy of relative timing for stutterers and nonstutterers. Journal of Speech and Hearing Research; 1988 Dec Vol 31(4) 654–658

Prosek, Robert A.; Montgomery, Allen A.; Walden, Brian E.; Hawkins, David B. Formant frequencies of stuttered and fluent vowels. Journal of Speech and Hearing Research; 1987 Sep Vol 30(3) 301–305

Rastatter, Michael P.; Dell, Carl W. Simple visual versus lexical decision vocal reaction times of stuttering and normal subjects. Journal of Fluency Disorders; 1987 Feb Vol 12(1) 63–69

Rastatter, Michael P.; Dell, Carl. Vocal reaction times of stuttering subjects to tachistoscopically presented concrete and abstract words: A closer look at cerebral dominance and language processing. Journal of Speech and Hearing Research; 1987 Sep Vol 30(3) 306–310

Reich, Alan; Till, James A.; Goldsmith, Howard. Laryngeal and manual reaction times of stuttering and nonstuttering adults. Journal of Speech and Hearing Research; 1981 Jan Vol 24(2) 192–196

Robb, Michael P.; Lybolt, John T.; Price, Harold A. Acoustic measures of stutterers' speech following an intensive therapy program. Journal of Fluency Disorders; 1985 Dec Vol 10(4) 269–279

Rosenfield, David B.; Freeman, Frances J. Stuttering onset after laryngectomy. Journal of Fluency Disorders; 1983 Sep Vol 8(3) 265–268

Runyan, Charles M.; Bonifant, Debra C. A perceptual comparison: All-voiced versus typical reading passage read by children. Journal of Fluency Disorders; 1981 Sep Vol 6(3) 247–255

Sacco, Pat R.; Metz, Dale E. Changes in stutterers' fundamental frequency contours following therapy. Journal of Fluency Disorders; 1987 Feb Vol 12(1) 1–8

Schmitt, Lane S.; Cooper, Eugene B. Fundamental frequencies in the oral reading behavior of stuttering and nonstuttering male children. Journal of Communication Disorders; 1978 Feb Vol 11(1) 17–23

Shenker, Rosalee C.; Finn, Patrick. An evaluation of the effects of supplemental "fluency" training during maintenance. Journal of Fluency Disorders; 1985 Dec Vol 10(4) 257–267

St. Louis, Kenneth O.; Hinzman, Audrey R. A descriptive study of speech, language, and hearing characteristics of school-aged stutterers. Journal of Fluency Disorders; 1988 Oct Vol 13(5) 331–355

St. Louis, Kenneth O.; Murray, Cheryl D.; Ashworth, Melanie S. Coexisting communication disorders in a random sample of school-aged stutterers. Journal of Fluency Disorders; 1991 Feb Vol 16(1) 13–23

Stager, Sheila V. Heterogeneity in stuttering: Results from auditory brainstem response testing. American Speech Language Hearing Association Convention (1982, Toronto, Canada). Journal of Fluency Disorders; 1990 Feb Vol 15(1) 9–19

Starkweather, C. Woodruff; Franklin, Sharon; Smigo, Therese M. Vocal and finger reaction times in stutterers and nonstutterers: Differences and correlations. Journal of Speech and Hearing Research; 1984 Jun Vol 27(2) 193–196

Starkweather, C. Woodruff; Hirschman, Paula; Tannenbaum, Robert S. Latency of vocalization onset: Stutterers versus nonstutterers. Journal of Speech and Hearing Research; 1976 Sep Vol 19(3) 481–492

Stephen, Simon C.; Haggard, Mark P. Acoustic properties of masking/delayed feedback in the fluency of stutterers and controls. Journal of Speech and Hearing Research; 1980 Sep Vol 23(3) 527–538

Venkatagiri, Horabail S. Reaction time for /s/ and /z/ in stutterers and nonstutterers: A test of discoordination hypothesis. Journal of Communication Disorders; 1982 Jan Vol 15(1) 55–62

Venkatagiri, Horabail S. Reaction time for voiced and whispered /a/ in stutterers and nonstutterers. Journal of Fluency Disorders; 1981 Sep Vol 6(3) 265–271

Ward, David. Voice-onset time and electroglottographic dynamics in stutterers' speech: Implications for a differential diagnosis. British Journal of Disorders of Communication; 1990 Apr Vol 25(1) 93–104

Watson, Ben C.; Pool, Kenneth D.; Devous, Michael D.; Freeman, Frances J.; et al. Brain blood flow related to acoustic laryngeal reaction time in adult developmental stutterers. Journal of Speech and Hearing Research; 1992 Jun Vol 35(3) 555–561

Watson, Ben C.; Alfonso, Peter J. Foreperiod and stuttering severity effects on acoustic laryngeal reaction time. Journal of Fluency Disorders; 1983 Sep Vol 8(3) 183–205

Watson, Ben C.; Alfonso, Peter J. Physiological bases of acoustic LRT in nonstutterers, mild stutterers, and severe stutterers. Journal of Speech and Hearing Research; 1987 Dec Vol 30(4) 434–447

Watson, Ben C.; Freeman, Frances J.; Chapman, Sandra B.; Miller, Susan; et al. Linguistic performance deficits in stutterers: Relation to laryngeal reaction time profiles. Journal of Fluency Disorders; 1991 Vol 16(2–3) 85–100

Weiner, A. E. Patterns of vocal fold movement during stuttering. Journal of Fluency Disorders; 1984 Feb Vol 9(1) 31–49

Wells, G. B. A feature analysis of stuttered phonemes. Journal of Fluency Disorders; 1983 Jun Vol 8(2) 119–124

Wingate, Marcel E. Questionnaire study of laryngectomee stutterers. Journal of Fluency Disorders; 1981 Sep Vol 6(3) 273–281

Wingate, Marcel E. Sound and pattern in artificial fluency: Spectrographic evidence. Journal of Fluency Disorders; 1981 Jun Vol 6(2) 95–118

Zebrowski, Patricia M.; Conture, Edward G.; Cudahy, Edward A. Acoustic analysis of young stutterers' fluency: Preliminary observations. Journal of Fluency Disorders; 1985 Sep Vol 10(3) 173–192

Australia/New Zealand

Andrews, Gavin. Stuttering: A tutorial. Australian and New Zealand Journal of Psychiatry; 1981 Jun Vol 15(2) 105–109

Cassar, Mary C. Hypnosis and stuttering intervention. Australian Journal of Clinical Hypnotherapy and Hypnosis; 1987 Mar Vol 8(1) 37–49

Cassar, Mary C. Stuttering and hypnosis: Processes of cortical control. Australian Journal of Clinical Hypnotherapy and Hypnosis; 1988 Sep Vol 9(2) 49–65

Craig, Ashley; Feyer, Anne Marie; Andrews, Gavin. An overview of a behavioural treatment for stuttering. Australian Psychologist; 1987 Mar Vol 22(1) 53–62

Francis, J. G. Stopping stuttering starting with hypnosis. Australian Journal of Clinical and Experimental Hypnosis; 1984 May Vol 12(1) 9–21

Kelemen, Z. Hypno-behavioural therapy for the treatment of stuttering. Australian Journal of Clinical Hypnotherapy; 1980 Mar Vol 1(1) 17–23

London, Ray W. International perspectives on pediatric hypnosis. Australian Journal of Clinical Hypnotherapy and Hypnosis; 1983 Sep Vol 4(2) 83–91

Porter, Jeannie F. Homosexuality treated adventitiously in a stuttering therapy program: A case report presenting a heterophobic orientation. Australian and New Zealand Journal of Psychiatry; 1976 Jun Vol 10(2) 185–189

British Isles

Andrews, Gavin; Craig, Ashley. Prediction of outcome after treatment for stuttering. British Journal of Psychiatry; 1988 Aug Vol 153 236–240

Aron, Myrtle L. Concepts underlying the development of a computer information retrieval programme for research in communication disorders. British Journal of Disorders of Communication; 1981 Sep Vol 16(2) 89–100

Beattie, Michael S. A behaviour therapy programme for stuttering. British Journal of Disorders of Communication; 1973 Oct Vol. 8(2) 120–130

Burgraff, Roger I. The efficacy of systematic desensitization via imagery as a therapeutic technique with stutterers. British Journal of Disorders of Communication; 1974 Oct Vol 9(2) 134–139

Code, Chris. Dichotic listening with the communicatively impaired: Results from trials of a short British-English dichotic word test. Journal of Phonetics; 1981 Oct Vol 9(4) 375–383

Code, Christopher; Muller, David. Comments on paper: The long-term use of an automatically triggered masking device in the treatment of stammering. British Journal of Disorders of Communication; 1980 Sep Vol 15(2) 141–142

Dewar, A. D. Influence of auditory feedback masking on stammering and its use in treatment. International Journal of Rehabilitation Research; 1984 Vol 7(3) 341–342

Dorgan, Barbara J.; Dorgan, Richard E. A theoretical rationale for total family therapy with stutterers. British Journal of Social Psychiatry and Community Health; 1972–1973 Vol 6(3) 214–222

Doughty, Patricia. Case study: The use of hypnosis with a stammerer. British Journal of Experimental and Clinical Hypnosis; 1990 Feb Vol 7(1) 65–67

Evesham, Margaret; Fransella, Fay. Stuttering relapse: The effect of a combined speech and psychological reconstruction programme. British Journal of Disorders of Communication; 1985 Dec Vol 20(3) 237–248

Evesham, Margaret; Huddleston, Anita. Teaching stutterers the skill of fluent speech as a preliminary to the study of relapse. British Journal of Disorders of Communication; 1983 Apr Vol 18(1) 31–38

Fransella, Fay. The development of attitudes to prejudice: A personal construct psychology view. Educational and Child Psychology; 1985 Vol 2(3) 150–156

Gibney, Noel J. Delayed auditory feedback: Changes in the volume intensity and the delay interval as variables affecting the fluency of stutterers' speech. British Journal of Psychology; 1973 Feb Vol. 64(1) 55–63

Goraj, Jane T. Stuttering therapy as crisis intervention. British Journal of Disorders of Communication; 1974 Apr Vol. 9(1) 51–57

Greenberg, David; Marks, Isaac. Behavioural psychotherapy of uncommon referrals. British Journal of Psychiatry; 1982 Aug Vol 141 148–153

Horsley, Irmgarde A.; FitzGibbon, Carol T. Stuttering children: Investigation of a stereotype. British Journal of Disorders of Communication; 1987 Apr Vol 22(1) 19–35

Leahy, M.; O'Sullivan, B. Psychological change and fluency therapy: A pilot project. British Journal of Disorders of Communication; 1987 Dec Vol 22(3) 245–251

Leahy, Margaret M.; Collins, Geraldine. Therapy for stuttering: Experimenting with experimenting. Irish Journal of Psychological Medicine; 1991 Mar Vol 8(1) 37–39

Lees, Roberta M. Some thoughts on the use of hypnosis in the treatment of stuttering. British Journal of Experimental and Clinical Hypnosis; 1990 Jun Vol 7(2) 109–114

Lockhart, Myra S.; Robertson, Alan W. Hypnosis and speech therapy as a combined therapeutic approach to the problem of stammering: A study of thirty patients. British Journal of Disorders of Communication; 1977 Oct Vol 12(2) 97–108

MacKenzie, Catherine. Aphasic articulatory defect and aphasic phonological defect. British Journal of Disorders of Communication; 1982 Apr Vol 17(1) 27–46

McCormick, Barry. Therapeutic and diagnostic applications of delayed auditory feedback. British Journal of Disorders of Communication; 1975 Oct Vol 10(2) 98–110

Messer, Stanley B. Integrating psychoanalytic and behaviour therapy: Limitations, possibilities and trade-offs. British Journal of Clinical Psychology; 1983 Jun Vol 22(2) 131–132

Moore, Margaret; Nystul, Michael S. Parent-child attitudes and communication processes in families with stutterers and families with non-stutterers. British Journal of Disorders of Communication; 1979 Dec Vol 14(3) 173–180

Moore, W. H.; Craven, Duane C.; Faber, Michele M. Hemispheric alpha asymmetries of words with positive, negative, and neutral arousal values preceding tasks of recall and recognition: Electrophysiological and behavioral results from stuttering males and nonstuttering males and females. Brain and Language; 1982 Nov Vol 17(2) 211–224

Moore, W. H. Bilateral tachistoscopic word perception of stutterers and normal subjects. Brain and Language; 1976 Jul Vol 3(3) 434–442

Murray, K. S.; Empson, J. A.; Weaver, S. M. Rehearsal and preparation for speech in stutterers: A psychophysiological study. British Journal of Disorders of Communication; 1987 Aug Vol 22(2) 145–150

Murray, T. J.; Kelly, Patrick; Campbell, Lynda; Stefanik, Kathy. Haloperidol in the treatment of stuttering. British Journal of Psychiatry; 1977 Apr Vol 130 370–373

Pinsky, Seth D.; McAdam, Dale W. Electroencephalographic and dichotic indices of cerebral laterality in stutterers. Brain and Language; 1980 Nov Vol 11(2) 374–397

Prins, David; Nichols, Anne. Client impressions of the effectiveness of stuttering therapy: A comparison of two programs. British Journal of Disorders of Communication; 1974 Oct Vol 9(2) 123–133

Rosenbek, John; Messert, Bernard; Collins, Michael; Wertz, Robert T. Stuttering following brain damage. Brain and Language; 1978 Jul Vol 6(1) 82–96

Rosenfield, David B.; Goodglass, Harold. Dichotic testing of cerebral dominance in stutterers. Brain and Language; 1980 Sep Vol 11(1) 170–180

Rustin, Lena; Kuhr, Armin. The treatment of stammering: A multi-model approach in an in-patient setting. British Journal of Disorders of Communication; 1983 Sep Vol 18(2) 90–97

Rustin, Lena; Ryan, Bruce P.; Ryan, Barbara V. Use of the Monterey programmed stuttering therapy in Great Britain. British Journal of Disorders of Communication; 1987 Aug Vol 22(2) 151–162

Sherrard, Carol A. Stuttering as "false alarm" responding. British Journal of Disorders of Communication; 1975 Oct Vol 10(2) 83–91

Silverman, Lloyd H. An experimental method for the study of unconscious conflict: A progress report. British Journal of Medical Psychology; 1975 Dec Vol 48(4) 291–298

Silverman, Lloyd H.; Bronstein, Abbot; Mendelsohn, Eric. The further use of the subliminal psychodynamic activation method for the experimental study of the clinical theory of psychoanalysis: On the specificity of the relationship between symptoms and unconscious conflicts. Psychotherapy Theory, Research and Practice; 1976 Spr Vol 13(1) 2–16

Stansfield, Jois. Stuttering and cluttering in the mentally handicapped population: A review of the literature. British Journal of Mental Subnormality; 1988 Jan Vol 34(1)(66) 54–61

Stewart, Trudy M. The relationship of attitudes and intentions to behave to the acquisition of fluent speech behaviour by stammerers. British Journal of Disorders of Communication; 1982 Sep Vol 17(2) 3–13

Stewart, Trudy; Grantham, Clare. A case of acquired stammering: The pattern of recovery. European Journal of Communication Disorders; 1993 28(4) 395–403

Still, A. W.; Griggs, S. Changes in the probability of stuttering following a stutter: A test of some recent models. Journal of Speech and Hearing Research; 1979 Sep Vol 22(3) 565–571

Still, A. W.; Sherrard, Carol A. Formalizing theories of stuttering. British Journal of Mathematical and Statistical Psychology; 1976 Nov Vol 29(2) 129–138

Strub, Richard L.; Black, F. William; Naeser, Margaret A. Anomalous dominance in sibling stutterers: Evidence from CT scan asymmetries, dichotic listening, neuropsychological testing, and handedness. Brain and Language; 1987 Mar Vol 30(2) 338–350

Sussman, Harvey M.; MacNeilage, Peter F. Studies of hemispheric specialization for speech production. Brain and Language; 1975 Apr Vol 2(2) 131–151

Tozman, Seymour; Kramer, Steven S. A speech deficit syndrome associated with addictive drug use. British Journal of Addiction; 1977 Mar Vol 72(1) 37–40

Ward, David. Voice-onset time and electroglottographic dynamics in stutterers' speech: Implications for a differential diagnosis. British Journal of Disorders of Communication; 1990 Apr Vol 25(1) 93–104

Watts, Fraser. Mechanisms of fluency control in stutterers. British Journal of Disorders of Communication; 1973 Oct Vol. 8(2) 131–138

Wells, Betsy G.; Moore, W. H. EEG alpha asymmetries in stutterers and non-stutterers: Effects of linguistic variables on hemispheric processing and fluency. Neuropsychologia; 1990 Vol 28(12) 1295–1305

Wood, Frank; et al. Patterns of regional cerebral blood flow during attempted reading aloud by stutterers both on and off haloperidol medication: Evidence for inadequate left frontal activation during stuttering. Brain and Language; 1980 Jan Vol 9(1) 141–144

Canada

Boberg, Einer; Calder, Peter. Stuttering: A review for counsellors and teachers. Canadian Counsellor; 1977 Apr Vol 11(3) 144–148

Boudreau, Leonce; Ladouceur, Robert. L'influence de l'aide sociale associee a la respiration regularisee sur le traitement du begaiement. / The influence of social help associated with regularized respiration on the treatment of stuttering. Technologie et Therapie du Comportement; 1985 Fal Vol 8(2) 125–151

Butany, V.; Persad, E. Is stuttering a contraindication to psychotherapy? Canadian Journal of Psychiatry; 1982 Jun Vol 27(4) 330–331

Byrne, Alan; Byrne, Mary K.; Zibin, Terry O. Transient neurogenic stuttering. International Journal of Eating Disorders; 1993 14(4) 511–514

Campbell, Michel; Boudreau, Leonce; Ladouceur, Robert. L'influence d'interlocuteurs sur l'evaluation du begaiement. (The influence of speakers on the evaluation of stuttering.) Revue de Modification du Comportement; 1984 Vol 14(3) 112–122

Caron, Chantal; Dugas, Michel; Ladouceur, Robert. Le traitement individuel et en groupe de begues adultes. (Individual and group treatment of adult stutterers.) Science et Comportement; 1990 Vol 20(3–4) 185–193

Dugas, Michel; Ladouceur, Robert. Traitement multidimensionnel et progressif des begues severes. (Multidimensional and progressive treatment of severe stuttering.) Science et Comportement; 1988 Win Vol 18(4) 221–232

Forster, David C.; Webster, William G. Concurrent task interference in stutterers: Dissociating hemispheric specialization and activation. Canadian Journal of Psychology; 1991 Sep Vol 45(3) 321–335

Quarrington, Bruce. The parents of stuttering children: The literature re-examined. Canadian Psychiatric Association Journal; 1974 Feb Vol 19(1) 103–110

Saint-Laurent, Lise; Ladouceur, Robert. Analyse des traitements behavioraux du begaiement. (Analyses of behavioral treatments for stuttering.) Canadian Psychology; 1987 Jul Vol 28(3) 239–250

China

Tang, Shenqing; Xu, Jengchen; Luo, Powei. (Preliminary studies on the psychological problems of stuttering children.) Information on Psychological Sciences; 1984 No 6 43–44

Europe (Eastern)

Abeleva, I. Yu. (Psychology of stuttering in adults during various phases of verbal communication.) Voprosy Psikhologii; 1974 Jul Aug No 4 144–149

Abeleva, I. Yu. Respiration dynamics during speech production in stuttering adults. Defektologiya; 1976 Jan No 1 17–20

Andronova, L. Z. Correction of intonation in stutterers. Defektologiya; 1988 No 6 63–67

Andronova, L. Z.; Arutiunyan, M. A.; Aleksandrovskaya, A. S. On the influence of singing on stuttering. Defektologiya; 1987 No 4 58–60

Asatiani, N. M.; Kazakov, V. G.; Freidin, Yu. L. Some problems of clinical classification of stuttering. Defektologiya; 1988 No 1 28–32

Asatiani, N. M.; Matveeva, E. S.; Sokolova, T. N.; Zhukov, V. F. The neurotic development in the clinical picture of stammering. Zhurnal Nevropatologii i Psikhiatrii imeni S.S. Korsakova; 1985 Vol 85(11) 1684–1688

Banjac Karovic, Milena; Povse Ivkic, Violica; Bojanin, Svetomir. Inhibicija govora i mucanje. (Speech inhibition and stuttering.) Psihijatrija Danas; 1990 Vol 22(1) 99–104

Beliakova, L. I; Kumalia, I. (Comparative analysis of motor and speech-motor functions in preschool stutterers.) Defektologiya; 1985 No 1 69–74

Belyakova, Lidiya I.; Matanova, Vanya. Psycholinguistic characteristics of stammering preschoolers' speech. Voprosy Psikhologii; 1990 Jul–Aug No 4 61–67

Berezhkovskaya, E. L.; Golod, V. I.; Turovskaya, Z. G. Sensory asymmetry in stutterers and normal individuals. Voprosy Psikhologii; 1980 No 1 57–63

Bojanin, Svetomir; Vuletic-Peco, Aleksandra; Radojkovic, Dejan. Porodica dece sa razvojnim hiperkinetskim sindromom, tikovima i mucanjem. (Families of children with developing hyperkinetic syndrome, tics, and stuttering.) Psihijatrija Danas; 1991 Vol 23(1–2) 37–48

Buyanov, M. I.; Bogdanova, E. V.; Subbotina, R. A.; Trebuleva, V. N. On heredity in stuttering. Defektologiya; 1987 No 3 20–22

Buyanov, M. I.; et al. Follow-up data on quasi-neurotic stuttering. Defektologiya; 1981 No 5 10–13

Cheveliova, N. A. Toward the problem of stuttering in children. Defektologiya; 1977 Jan No 1 20–23

Costa, D.; et al. Clinical and paraclinical aspects of tetany in stuttering. Revue Roumaine de Neurologie et Psychiatrie; 1983 Jul–Sep Vol 21(3) 277–279

Costa, D.; Antoniac, Maria; Berghianu, S.; Marinescu, Rodica; et al. Clinical and paraclinical aspects of tetany in stuttering. Activitas Nervosa Superior; 1986 Vol 28(2) 156–158

Costa, D.; Pop, A.; Dumitriu, L.; Marinescu, Luzia; et al. Serum immunoreactive parathormone levels correlate with depression and anxiety in hypocalcemic stutterers. Activitas Nervosa Superior; 1986 Vol 28(2) 155–156

Degand, J. (A clinical contribution to the psychodynamic and the pathopsychogenic sources of language problems.) Revue Belge de Psychologie et de Pedagogie; 1972 Vol 34(139) 79–93

Filimoshkina, N. M.; Timchenko, V. A. (Counsel for parents of a stuttering child.) Defektologiya; 1982 Vol 5 69–72

Gerkina, M. I. (The speech of stuttering preschool children under different conditions of communication.) Defektologiya; 1972 Vol 3 29–34

Grzybowska, Aldona. Behawioraline teorie jakania. / Behavioral theories of stuttering. Przeglad Psychologiczny; 1987 Vol 30(1) 71–80

Grzybowska, Aldona; Lapinska, Irena; Michalska, Roza. Postawy nauczycieli wobec jakania. / Teachers' attitudes to stuttering. Psychologia Wychowawcza; 1991 Mar–Apr Vol 34(2) 139–150

Ignatieva, S. A. Active regulated games in the system of correctional education of stuttering preschoolers. Defektologiya; 1986 No 3 67–71

Ivanova, G. A.; Lapa, A. Z.; Lokhov, M. I.; Movsisyants, S. A. EEG features in stammering pre-school children. Zhurnal Nevropatologii i Psikhiatrii imeni S.S. Korsakova; 1990 Vol 90(3) 78–81

Ivanova, G. A.; Lapa, A. Z.; Lokhov, M. I.; Movsisyants, S. A. Features of stuttering pre-school children. Neuroscience and Behavioral Physiology; 1991 May–Jun Vol 21(3) 284–287

Kalyagin, V. A. Characteristics of attention in stutterers. Soviet Neurology and Psychiatry; 1985–86 Win Vol 18(4) 85–88

Kastelova, Darina; Szenteova, Iveta. Sociometricka pozicia recovo naruseneho diet'at'a v triede na ZS. / Sociometric status of speech disordered child in the basic school class. Psychologia a Patopsychologia Dietata; 1991 Vol 26(1) 29–34

Kaubish, V. K.; Linskaia, L. N. Characteristics of neurosislike states and their treatment in children with retarded mental development. Soviet Neurology and Psychiatry; 1991 Fal Vol 24(3) 38–42

Kharatinov, A. V. (Methodological principles of art therapy in a system of social rehabilitation for adult stutterers.) Novye Issledovaniya v Psikhologii; 1981 No 1(24) 94–97

Khavin, A. B. (Personality reactions to a communication disorder.) Defektologiya; 1974 Vol 12 6–29

Khavin, A. B.; Diakova, E. A. (Characteristics of communication impairments in adult stutterers and effectiveness of medical-rehabilitation work.) Defektologiya; 1988 No 3 20–24

Khavin, Aleksandr B. Individual-psychological factors in prediction of help to stutterers. Voprosy Psikhologii; 1985 Mar–Apr No 2 133–135

Kondas, Ondrej. Emocionalne a situacne premenne pri reci balbutikov. / Emotional and situational variables in the speech of stutterers. Zbornik Univerzity Komenskeho Psychologica; 1982 Vol 26–27 197–208

Kooman, E. A. Speech disturbance under delayed acoustic feedback and stuttering. Defektologiya; 1975 Jun No 6 27–33

Kulas, Henryk. Sytuacja szkolna dzieci jakajacych sie. / The school situation of stuttering children. Psychologia Wychowawcza; 1990 Nov–Dec Vol 33(5) 331–344

Kuz'min, Yu. I.; Dmitrieva, E. S.; Zaitseva, K. A. Functional asymmetry of the brain in stuttering children during perception of emotions. Human Physiology; 1989 Mar–Apr Vol 15(2) 129–131

Lagutina, T. S.; Lovchikova, N. N.; Obukhovskii, N. G. Electrophysiological study of patients with logoneuroses. Soviet Neurology and Psychiatry; 1985 Fal Vol 18(3) 53–61

Lavkai, I. Yu. On personality deviations in stuttering adolescents. Defektologiya; 1976 Feb No 2 16–18

Lechta, Viktor; Vanhara, Ladislav. Analyza postojov uciteliek a matiek k zajakavemu diet'at'u. / Analysis of attitudes of teachers and mothers towards a stammering child. Jednotna Skola; 1985 Apr Vol 37(4) 357–362

Levina, R. Ye. On emociogenic factors of stuttering which arise in the course of formation of voluntary speech. Defektologiya; 1981 Jan No 1 7–13

Lokhov, M. I.; Vartanyan, G. A. Stammering: New therapeutic approaches. Zhurnal Nevropatologii i Psikhiatrii imeni S.S. Korsakova; 1989 Vol 89(3) 68–73

Lomachenkov, A. S.; Martsinkevich, N. E. Maladjustment in children in the form of masked depressions. Trudy Leningradskogo Nauchno Issledovatel'skogo Psikhonevrologicheskogo Instituta i m V M Bekhtereva; 1988 Vol 119 38–42

Matanova Koleva, Vanja. A conceptual model of stuttering. Psikhologiia Bulgaria; 1985 Vol 13(1) 45–49

Meshcherskaya, L. N. Use of external acoustic influence for correction of stuttering. Defektologiya; 1985 No 3 14–19

Mironova, S. (On the work of a speech therapist in a preschool children's home.) Defektologiya; 1985 No 1 89–90

Mokrovskaya, A. A. Therapeutic and corrective work with stammering preschool children in conditions of a day-time semi-hospital institution. Zhurnal Nevropatologii i Psikhiatrii imeni S.S. Korsakova; 1986 Vol 86(10) 1565–1569

Mokrovskaya, A. A. Therapeutic and remedial work with stuttering preschoolers in a day hospital. Soviet Neurology and Psychiatry; 1988 Spr Vol 21(1) 53–61

Morozov, V. P.; Kuz'min, Yu. I.; Zaitseva, K. A.; Dmitrieva, E. S. Hemispheric functional asymmetry in stuttering. Human Physiology; 1988 May–Jun Vol 14(3) 188–194

Nekrasov, Y. B. (Diagnosis and prognosis of stutterers: II. A differentiated approach to stutterers based on the use of a set of methods.) Novye Issledovaniya v Psikhologii; 1981 No 1(24) 90–93

Nekrasova, Y. B. Psychotherapy sessions and some mental states of stutterers. Voprosy Psikhologii; 1980 Sep–Oct No 5 32–40

Nekrasova, Yuliya B. Dynamics of psychological states in stutterers in the process of logopsychotherapy. Voprosy Psikhologii; 1985 Mar–Apr No 2 127–133

Nekrasova, Yuliya B. (Group emotional and stress psychotherapy to correct mental states of stutterers.) Voprosy Psikhologii; 1984 Mar–Apr No 2 75–82

Nekrasova, Yu. B. The teacher and the psychological atmosphere in the classroom. Soviet Psychology; 1987–88 Win Vol 26(2) 79–83

Oganesyan, E. V. (Analysis of interrelations among some aspects of the motor sphere and speech in adult stutterers.) Defektologiya; 1983 No 3 16–20

Oganesyan, E. V. (Different rhythmic speech therapy exercises for adolescent and adult stutterers.) Defektologiya; 1983 No 1 60–63

Oganesian, E. V. On unification of registration and assessment of rehabilitation effects in adult stutterers. Defektologiya; 1986 No 4 75–78

Oganesian, E. V. (Study of the effectiveness of speech correction within the context of a complex approach to the treatment of stuttering in adults in specialized hospital departments.) Defektologiya; 1985 No 4 23–28

Oganesian, Ye. V.; Beliakova, L. I. The rationale for principles of differential application of logopaedic rhythmics in remediation of adult stutterers. Defektologiya; 1982 No 1 3–12

Peutelschmiedova, Alzbeta; Rauerova, Martina. Profesionalni orientace balbutiku. (Vocational orientation of stutterers.) Psychologia a Patopsychologia Dietata; 1990 Vol 25(5) 405–416

Pukacova, Marianna. (Psychological characteristics of stuttering children.) Psychologia a Patopsychologia Dietata; 1973 Vol 8(3) 233–238

Raou, Ye. Y. Dynamics of some characteristics of stutterer's personality in the process of psychotherapy. Voprosy Psikhologii; 1984 May–Jun Vol 3 67–72

Rychkova, N. A. Speech therapy rhythmics in the correctional system for preschool stutterers. Defektologiya; 1987 No 3 60–64

Rychkova, N. A. State of voluntary motor activity and speech in preschool children with neurotic and pseudo-neurotic forms of stuttering. Defektologiya; 1981 No 6 73–77

Shklovskii, Viktor M.; Krol, Leonid M.; Mikhailova, Ekaterina L. The psychotherapy of stuttering: On the model of stuttering patients' psychotherapy group. Soviet Journal of Psychiatry and Psychology Today; 1988 Vol 1(1) 130–141

Shklovsky, V. M.; Krol, L. M.; Mikhailova, E. L. Specificity of group psychotherapy in stammering. Trudy Leningradskogo Nauchno Issledovatel'skogo Psikhonevrologicheskogo Instituta i m V M Bekhtereva; 1988 Vol 121 112–117

Shklovsky, Victor M.; Kroll, Leonid M.; Mikhailova, Ekaterina L. Group psychotherapy: Problems of theory and practical application. Psikologicheskii Zhurnal; 1985 May–Jun Vol 6(3) 100–110

Shurgaya, German G.; Korolyova, Inna V.; Kuzmin, Urii I.; Sakhnovskaya, Oksana S. Interhemispheric asymmetry at the perception of speech signals in stutterers. Psikologicheskii Zhurnal; 1987 Jul–Aug Vol 8(4) 80–91

Souvorova, V. V.; Matova, M. A.; Tourovskaya, Z. G. Binocular reproductive images under conditions of atypical interhemispheric rela-

tions (in stutterers). Voprosy Psikhologii; 1984 Jan–Feb No 1 105–110

Szelag, Elzbieta; Garwarska-Kolek, Dantua; Heerman, Anna; Stasiek, Janina. Brain lateralization and severity of stuttering in children. Acta Neurobiologiae Experimentalis; 1993 Vol 53(1) 263–267

Tarkowski, Zbigniew. Psychoterapia osob jakajacych sie. / Psychotherapy of stutterers. Psychologia Wychowawcza; 1987 Mar–Apr Vol 30(2) 184–192

Tarkowski, Zbigniew; Jaworska, Malgorzata. Gielkot: Stan i perspektywy badan. / Disorderly speech: State and perspectives of research. Psychologia Wychowawcza; 1987 Sep–Oct Vol 30(4) 440–447

Traugott, N. N.; Onopriychuk, E. I. EEG peculiarities of different clinical types of stuttering in preschoolers. Defektologiya; 1985 No 4 79–83

Vekassy, Laszlo. Idegrendszeri es pszichologiai vizsgalatok dadogoknal. (Psychological and nervous system examination with stutterers.) Magyar Pszichologiai Szemle; 1981 Vol 38(5) 481–494

Vekassy, Laszlo. Az autogen-trening a dadogo komplex kezeleseben. (Autogenic training in the complex treatment of the stutterer.) Magyar Pszichologiai Szemle; 1981 Vol 38(1) 43–56

Vekassy, Laszlo. Dadogok oral-praxia es oral stereognosis vizsgalata. / Oral praxia and oral stereognosis examinations in stutterers. Magyar Pszichologiai Szemle; 1987–88 Vol 44(4) 291–304

Vekassy, Laszlo. Gyogyult dadogok utanvizsgalata. / The catamnestic study of cured stutterers. Magyar Pszichologiai Szemle; 1989 Vol 45(1) 37–57

Virag, Terez. Gyermekkori neurotikus allapotok, magatartaszavarok tortenelmi hattere. / The historical background of neurotic states and conduct disorders in childhood. Magyar Pszichologiai Szemle; 1987–88 Vol 44(3) 227–244

Vlasenko, I. T. Study of and principles of analysis of verbal and non-verbal processes in children with developmental language impairments. Defektologiya; 1988 No 4 3–11

Wallen, Vincent. A study of the self-concepts of adolescent stutterers. Psychologia: An International Journal of Psychology in the Orient; 1973 Dec Vol. 16(4) 191–200

Wolak, Krzysztof. Zastosowanie techniki biofeedback w terapii osob jakajacych sie. / Biofeedback technique in stuttering therapy. Psychologia Wychowawcza; 1988 Jan–Feb Vol 31(1) 56–69

Yastrebova, A. V.; Voronova, G. G. Examination of stuttering students. Defektologiya; 1980 No 5 51–57

Europe (Western)

Ablon, Steven L. Psychoanalysis of a stuttering boy. Special Issue: Psychoanalysis of children. International Review of Psycho-Analysis; 1988 Vol 15(1) 83–91

Adamczyk, Bogdan; Kuniszyk Jozkowiak, Wieslawa. Effect of echo and reverberation of a restricted information capacity on the speech process. Folia Phoniatrica; 1987 Jan–Feb Vol 39(1) 9–17

Aguilar, Guido; Berganza, Carlos E. Sesgo en los registros observacionales de la conducta de tartamudeo. (Bias in observational recordings of stuttering behavior.) Revista Intercontinental de Psicologia y Educacion; 1989 Vol 2(1–2) 43–56

Aguilar, Guido; Bohrt, Raul. Interferencia en el diseno de tratamientos alternos. (Interference in the alternating-treatments design.) Ensenanza e Investigacion en Psicologia; 1983 Jan–Jun Vol 9(1) 72–93

Alarcia, J.; Pinard, Gilbert; Serrano, M.; Tetreault, L. Etude comparative de trois traitements du begaiement: relaxation, desensibilisation, reeducation. (A comparative study of three treatments for stuttering: Relaxation, desensitization, reeducation.) Revue de Psychologie Appliquee; 1982 Vol 32(1) 1–25

Antonucci, Gianfranco; de Rosa, Emilia. La balbuzie: evoluzione dei concetti e prospettive per una comprensione psicodinamica del sintomo. (Stuttering: Evolution of its conceptualizations and prospects for a psychodynamic understanding of this symptom.) Archivio di Psicologia, Neurologia e Psichiatria; 1986 Oct–Dec Vol 47(4) 451–476

Anzieu, Annie. Essai sur le corps fantasmatique du begue. (Essay on the phantasmatic body of the stutterer.) Pratique des Mots; 1982 Sep No 40 14–18

Azorin, Jean-Michel; Pringuey, Dominique; Samuelian, Jean-Claude; Benychou, Michele. Les Nouvelles benzodiazepines. / The new benzodiazepines. XXth Psychiatric Meeting (1986, Marseille, France). Psychologie Medicale; 1987 Mar Vol 19(3) 363–365

Ballesteros, Rocio F.; Mas, Jose S.; Carrobles, Jose A. Relaciones entre respuestas psicofisiologicas y autoinformes. / Relationships between psychophysiological responses and self-reports. Analisis y Modificacion de Conducta; 1984 Vol 10(25) 299–311

Banjac-Karovic, Milena; Povse-Ivkic, Violica; Bojanin, Svetomir. Inhibicija govora i mucanje. (Speech inhibition and stuttering.) Psihijatrija Danas; 1990 Vol 22(1) 99–104

Barblan, Leo. Therapeutique du langage: Science ou intuition? (Therapeutics of language: Science or intuition?) Pratique des Mots; 1983 Sep No 44 23–36

Becker, H. Ungewohnliche Sprechstorungen bei der endogenen Depression. / Unusual speech disorders in endogenous depression. Nervenarzt; 1989 Dec Vol 60(12) 757–758

Becker, Peter; Kessler, Bernd; Fuchsgruber, Konrad. (A comparative therapeutic experiment on the theory and the efficiency of operant methods of treatment of stutterers.) Archiv fur Psychologie; 1975 Vol 127(1–2) 78–92

Bojanin, Svetomir; Vuletic-Peco, Aleksandra; Radojkovic, Dejan. Porodica dece sa razvojnim hiperkinetskim sindromom, tikovima i mucanjem. (Families of children with developing hyperkinetic syndrome, tics, and tuttering.) Psihijatrija Danas; 1991 Vol 23(1–2) 37–48

Boudreau, Leonce; Ladouceur, Robert. L'influence de l'aide sociale associee a la respiration regularisee sur le traitement du begaiement. / The influence of social help associated with regularized respiration on the treatment of stuttering. Technologie et Therapie du Comportement; 1985 Fal Vol 8(2) 125–151

Bounes, Marika. Test de Rorschach avant et apres traitement de relaxation chez l'enfant. (Rorschach test before and after relaxation treatment of a child.) 11th International Congress on the Rorschach and Projective Methods (1984, Barcelona, Spain). Bulletin de Psychologie; 1986 Jun–Aug Vol 39(11–15) 651–654

D'Onofrio, Angelo. Occhio per occhio, dente per dente. / An eye for an eye, a tooth for a tooth. Centro Ricerche Biopsichiche, Padova; 1987–88 Vol 30–31 17–23

de Rosa, E.; Antonucci, G.; Rinaldi, L. Balbuzie, complesso edipico e angosce primitive: Osservazioni su un caso clinico. / Stuttering, Oedipus complex and earliest anxieties: Some observations on a clinical case. Archivio di Psicologia, Neurologia e Psichiatria; 1987 Vol 48(3) 327–335

de Vries, Ursula. "Laut—langsam—deutlich"—eine Phase aus der Therapie stotternder Schuler. / "Loudly—slowly—intelligibly": One phase of the therapy for children who stutter. Vierteljahresschrift fur Heilpadagogik und ihre Nachbargebiete; 1990 Mar Vol 59(1) 60–72

Degand, J. (A clinical contribution to the psychodynamic and the pathopsychogenic sources of language problems.) Revue Belge de Psychologie et de Pedagogie; 1972 Vol 34(139) 79–93

Dolto, Francoise. L'agressivite chez le jeune enfant. (Aggressiveness in the young child.) Pratique des Mots; 1982 Mar No 38 19–25

Elbers, L. Ontwikkelingsstotteren: Wat ontwikkelt? / The development of stuttering in young children. Gedrag Tijdschrift voor Psychologie; 1983 Vol 11(1) 28–43

Emrich, H. M.; Eilert, P. Evaluation of speech and language in neuropsychiatric disorders. Archiv fur Psychiatrie und Nervenkrankheiten; 1978 Vol 225(3) 209–221

Ferreiro-Diaz, M. D.; Dominguez, M. Dolores; Rodriguez, A. Psicoterapis de grupos infantiles: la madre co-terapeuta. (Group psychotherapy for children: The mother as co-therapist.) Clinica y Analisis Grupal; 1990 May–Aug Vol 12(2) 291–313

Fink, Hans; Niebergall, Gerhard. An attempt to measure anxieties in children who stutter. Heilpadagogik; 1975 Sep Vol 44(3) 220–227

Florin, Irmela. Stuttering: Theoretical approaches, experimental research results, suggestions for therapy. European Journal of Behavioural Analysis and Modification; 1976 Nov Vol 3(1) 189–200

Franke, Ulrike. Zur Frage de mannlichen Disposition fur Kommunikationsstorungen. / Predisposition of males for communication disorders. Folia Phoniatrica; 1985 Jan–Feb Vol 37(1) 36–43

Garcia-Moreno, Juan. Tratamiento de la tartamudez por el metodo de la regulacion de la respiracion. (Treatment of stuttering by the regulated-breathing method.) Informes de Psicologia; 1985 Vol 4(1–2) 67–72

Gonzalez-Valenzuela, M. Jose. Evaluacion y Tratamiento cognitivo-conductual de un caso de tartamudez. / Evaluation and cognitive-behavioral treatment in a severe stuttering case. Analisis y Modificacion de Conducta; 1990 Vol 16(47) 137–148

Gottinger, Werner. A concept for the guidance of stutterers. Praxis der Kinderpsychologie und Kinderpsychiatrie; 1980 Feb–Mar Vol 29(2) 55–62

Grempel, Franz. Stuttering as a crisis in achieving adult status: Contribution to the etiology and therapy of a stutterer. Praxis der Psychotherapie; 1976 Feb Vol 21(1) 29–41

Halg, Paul. Symbolik und Verlauf in der Therapie eines dreizehnjahrigen Stotterers mit dem katathymen Bilderleben. (Symbolism and process in a short term therapy of a male juvenile stutterer using the day dream technique of guided affective imagery (GAI).) Praxis der Kinderpsychologie und Kinderpsychiatrie; 1981 Oct Vol 30(7) 236–243

Healey, E. Charles. Fundamental frequency contours of stutterers' vowels following fluent stop consonant productions. Folia Phoniatrica; 1984 May–Jun Vol 36(3) 145–151

Heinzel, Joachim. The problem of stuttering and the therapy methods of the behaviour therapy. Praxis der Kinderpsychologie und Kinderpsychiatrie; 1976 Aug–Sep Vol 25(6) 197–205

Ibanez-Ramirez, Manuel. Tratamiento de un caso de tartamudez. / Treatment of a stuttering case. Analisis y Modificacion de Conducta; 1985 Vol 11(30) 605–611

James, Jack E. Office-based treatment for stuttering: A program of speech retraining and self-management. Scandinavian Journal of Behaviour Therapy; 1982 Vol 11(1) 15–28

Jancke, Lutz; Kalveram, Karl T. Kontrolle von on-time (Phonationsdauer) und voice-onset-time bei rechts- bzw. linksohrig dargebotener auditiver Ruckmeldungen: Unterschiedliche Lateralisierung bei stotternden und nichtstotternden Personen? (Control of on-time (phonation duration) and voice-onset time with right- or left-ear auditory feedback: Different lateralization in stutterers and nonstutterers?) Zeitschrift fur Experimentelle und Angewandte Psychologie; 1987 Vol 34(1) 54–63

Janssen, Peggy; Kraaimaat, Floor. Angst als predictor van het behandelingsresultaat bij stotteren. / Anxiety as a predictor in the outcome of stuttering therapy. Gedragstherapie; 1986 Sep Vol 19(3) 161–170

Jehle, Peter; Boberg, Einer. Intensivbehandlung fur jugendliche und erwachsene Stotternde von Boberg und Kully. / Intensive treatment for adolescent and adult stutterers by Boberg and Kully. Folia Phoniatrica; 1987 Sep–Oct Vol 39(5) 256–268

Johannesson, Goran. (Two behavior therapy techniques in the treatment of stuttering.) Scandinavian Journal of Behaviour Therapy; 1975 Vol 4(1) 11–22

Johannsen, H. S.; Schulze, H. Zur Situation der Stottertherapie bei Vorschul- und Grundschulkindern in der Bundesrepublik: Ergebnisse einer Befragung von Stottertherapeuten und einer Analyse von Fachzeitschriften. / Current status of stuttering therapy in preschool and school-age children in FRG: Results of a questionnaire study among therapists and analysis of the literature. Folia Phoniatrica; 1989 Jan–Feb Vol 41(1) 10–22

Kalveram, K. A neural-network model enabling sensorimotor learning: Application to the control of arm movements and some implications for speech motor control and stuttering. Psychological Research/Psychologische Forschung; 1993 55(4) 299–314

Kalveram, Karl T.; Jancke, Lutz. Vowel duration and voice onset time for stressed and nonstressed syllables in stutterers under delayed auditory feedback condition. Folia Phoniatrica; 1989 Jan–Feb Vol 41(1) 30–42

Katz-Bernstein, Nitza. Poltern: Therapieansatz fur Kinder. (Tachyphemia: A therapeutic approach for children.) Vierteljahresschrift fur Heilpadagogik und ihre Nachbargebiete; 1986 Dec Vol 55(4) 413–426

Kehrer, H. E. (Behaviour therapy in child and adolescent psychiatry.) Acta Paedopsychiatrica; 1973 Vol 40(2) 58–65

Kern, Horst J.; Kern, Marijke. Verhaltenstherapie beim Stottern: Videoruckmeldung und willentliches Stottern. (Behavioral stuttering therapy: Video feedback and intentional stuttering.) Zeitschrift fur Klinische Psychologie. Forschung und Praxis; 1991 Vol 20(4) 389–401

Klepel, Helene; Kuhne, Gert Eberhard; Mackerodt, Gerd. Untersuchungen zur Haufigkeit elektroenzephalographischer Befunde bei Kindern mit Stottern im Vergleich zu gesunden Gleichaltrigen. / Studies on the frequency of encephalographic findings in stuttering children in comparison to healthy children of the same age group. Psychiatrie, Neurologie und medizinische Psychologie; 1982 Aug Vol 34(8) 488–492

Kondas, Ondrej. (The use of a metronome in reeducation of stutterers.) Psychologia a Patopsychologia Dietata; 1974 Vol 9(6) 545–551

Kraaimaat, Floor W.; Janssen, Peggy. Een werkmodel voor een differentiele diagnostiek en behandeling van stotteren. (A working model for the differential diagnosis and treatment of stuttering.) Gedragstherapie; 1983 Dec Vol 16(4) 299–309

Kramer, Josefine. Wesen, Haufigkeit, Ursachen und Erscheinungsformen der geistigen Behinderung: II. (Nature, frequency, causes, and forms of mental retardation: II.) Vierteljahresschrift fur Heilpadagogik und ihre Nachbargebiete; 1976 Sep Vol 45(3) 270–283

Krause, Matthias P. Stottern als Beziehungsstorung—Psychotherapeutische Arbeit mit Eltern stotternder Kinder. / Stuttering as an expression of disturbed parent-child relationship. Praxis der Kinderpsychologie und Kinderpsychiatrie; 1985 Jan Vol 34(1) 15–18

Krause, Rainer. Nonverbal interactive behavior in stutterers and their speaking partners. Psychologie Schweizerische Zeitschrift fur Psychologie und ihre Anwendungen; 1978 Vol 37(3) 177–201

Krause, Rainer. Problems of psychological research and treatment of stuttering. Zeitschrift fur Klinische Psychologie und Psychotherapie; 1976 Vol 24(2) 128–143

Lara-Cantu, Maria A. Pilot study on electromyographic biofeedback for the treatment of stuttering. Ensenanza e Investigacion en Psicologia; 1978 Jul–Dec Vol 4(2) 259–265

Lasogga, Frank; Kondring, Irmgard. Stotterer in Selbsthilfegruppen und in Einzeltherapie. (Stutterers in self-help groups and in individual therapy.) Zeitschrift fur Klinische Psychologie. Forschung und Praxis; 1982 Vol 11(3) 201–214

Lasogga, Frank; Wedemeyer, Marina. The child-rearing practices of parents of stuttering children. Zeitschrift fur Klinische Psychologie. Forschung und Praxis; 1979 Vol 8(4) 270–282

Lasogga, Frank; Wedemeyer, Marina. The child-rearing practices of parents of stuttering children. Zeitschrift fur Klinische Psychologie. Forschung und Praxis; 1979 Vol 8(4) 270–282

Lawson, R.; Pring, T.; Fawcus, M. The effects of short courses in modifying the attitudes of adult and adolescent stutterers to communication. European Journal of Disorders of Communication; 1993 Vol 28(3) 299–308

Legewie, H.; Cleary, P.; Rackensperger, W. EMG-recording and biofeedback in the diagnosis and therapy of stuttering: A case study. European Journal of Behavioural Analysis and Modification; 1975 Dec Vol 1(2) 137–143

Lukas, Elisabeth. New ways for dereflection. International Forum for Logotherapy; 1981 Spr–Sum Vol 4(1) 13–28

Macioszek, Gisela. (On delayed auditory feedback in stutterers with various levels of stuttering severity.) Zeitschrift fur Klinische Psychologie; 1973 Vol 2(4) 278–299

Mempel, Sigurd. Therapiemotivation bei Kindern: Ergebnisse einer empirischen Untersuchung. / Children's motivation for treatment. Praxis der Kinderpsychologie und Kinderpsychiatrie; 1989 May-Jun Vol 38(5) 146–151

Minderaa, R. B.; Van Gemert, T. M.; Van de Wetering, B. J. Onverwachte presentatiewijzen van het syndroom van Gilles de la Tourette. / Unexpected types of presentation of Gilles de la Tourette's syndrome. Tijdschrift voor Psychiatrie; 1988 Vol 30(4) 246–254

Motsch, Hans Joachim. Idiographische Logopadie. (Idiographic speech science.) Vierteljahresschrift fur Heilpadagogik und ihre Nachbargebiete; 1990 Mar Vol 59(1) 2–13

Mouren-Simeoni, M. C.; Bouvard, M. P. Les indications des neuroleptiques chez l'enfant. / Neuroleptic indications in children. Encephale; 1990 Mar–Apr Vol 16(2) 133–141

Muckenhoff, Elisabeth. Modell zur Genese und Manifestation des Stotterns auf lerntheoretischer Basis. (A learning theory model of the origins of stuttering and stuttering behavior.) Vierteljahresschrift fur Heilpadagogik und ihre Nachbargebiete; 1976 Dec Vol 45(4) 341–346

Muhs, Aribert; Schepank, Heinz. Aspekte des Verlaufs und der geschlectsspezifischen Pravalenz psychogener. Erkrankungen bei Kindern und Erwachsenen unter dem Einfluss von Erb- und Umweltfaktoren. (Aspects of development of the incidence of psychogenic disorders in children and adults under the influence of hereditary and environmental factors.) Zeitschrift fur Psychosomatische Medizin und Psychoanalyse; 1991 Vol 37(2) 194–206

Nekrasova, Julia B. Wiederherstellung einer gestorten Kommunikation (am Beispiel einer Logoneurose). / Repair of disturbed communication in logoneurosis. Dynamische Psychiatrie; 1989 Vol 22(114–115) 37–50

Nemec, Jiri. Voice-speech fullness of life: Existential analysis in the context of a medical discipline. Zeitschrift fur Klinische Psychologie und Psychotherapie; 1979 Vol 27(3) 196–203

Nemes, Livia. Die klinische Bedeutung der Anklammerungstheorie von Imre Hermann. (The clinical significance of Imre Hermann's theory of clinging.) Zeitschrift fur Psychoanalytische Theorie und Praxis; 1990 Vol 5(2) 112–121

Nicolaidis, Nicos; Papilloud, Janine. Une langue privee pour combler le manque. (A private language to fill a gap.) 47th Congress of Romance Languages Psychoanalysts (1987, Paris, France). Revue Francaise de Psychanalyse; 1988 Mar–Apr Vol 52(2) 523–531

Ost, Lars Goran. Experimental studies in behaviour therapy. Scandinavian Journal of Behaviour Therapy; 1976 Vol 5(Suppl 1) 3–36

Palenzuela-Sanchez, Angeles. Intervencion sobre contingencias externas como tratamiento psicologico en un caso de tartamudez de desarrollo. (Intervention based on external contingencies as psychological treatment in a case of stuttering in a young child.) Analisis y Modificacion de Conducta; 1993 Vol 19(64) 287–298

Pesci, Guido. Nuove modalita diagnostiche e ipnoterapeutiche per ridurre o annullare la balbuzie. / New diagnostic methods and hypnotherapy in the reduction or cure of stammering. 2nd National Hypnotherapy and Handwriting Psychology Convention (1985, Milan, Italy). Rivista Internazionale di Psicologia e Ipnosi; 1985 Apr–Sep Vol 26(2–3) 181–188

Petermann, Franz. Aktuelle Trends bei der Verhaltensmodifikation mit Kindern. (Current trends in behavior modification with children.) Psychologische Rundschau; 1981 Oct Vol 32(4) 250–266

Peters, M. The view of learning theory. Zeitschrift fur Kinder und Jugendpsychiatrie; 1976 Vol 4(2) 104–112

Pimental, Patricia A.; Gorelick, Philip B. Aphasia, apraxia and neurogenic stuttering as complications of metrizamide myelography: Speech deficits following myelography. Acta Neurologica Scandinavica; 1985 Nov Vol 72(5) 481–488

Porret, Jean-Michel. Psychoanalytic aspects of stammering. IN: SUPEA Faculte de Medecine, Service. Acta Paedopsychiatrica International Journal of Child and Adolescent Psychiatry; Apr Vol 56(1) 57–61

Raisova, Vera; Hyanek, J. Speech disorders associated with histidinemia and other hereditary disorders of amino acid metabolism. Folia Phoniatrica; 1986 Jan–Feb Vol 38(1) 43–48

Raou, Ye. Y. Dynamics of some characteristics of stutterer's personality in the process of psychotherapy. Voprosy Psikhologii; 1984 May–Jun Vol 3 67–72

Reich, Gunter. Stotternde Kinder und ihre Familien. / Stuttering children and their families. Praxis der Kinderpsychologie und Kinderpsychiatrie; 1987 Jan Vol 36(1) 16–22

Rojahn, Johannes; Pesta, Thekla. Stuttering behaviors incompatible with speech interruption: Therapeutic limitations and usefulness with stutterers. Zeitschrift fur Klinische Psychologie; 1977 Vol 6(4) 281–302

Romero, Juan F. Tratamiento multimodal de un caso de tartamudez. / Multimodal treatment in a case of stuttering. First National Symposium: Importance of cognitive and behavioral therapies in child and adolescent psychopathology (1984, Malaga, Spain). Analisis y Modificacion de Conducta; 1985 Vol 11(27) 133–143

Roth U., Erick; Aguilar S., Guido G. Speech therapy: A comparative study of the stutterer. Aprendizaje y Comportamiento; 1979 Vol 2(1–2) 93–108

Samuel-Lajeunesse, B.; Degleris, N.; Brouri, R.; Agathon, M. Appreciation des effets des techniques assertives en groupe en milieu psychiatrie. (Group training in assertive techniques in a psychiatric milieu.) Annales Medico-Psychologiques; 1985 May Vol 143(5) 458–464

Santacreu-Mas, Jose. El condicionamiento ante determinadas palabras en la tartamudez. (Conditioning before some words in stuttering.) Revista de Psicologia General y Aplicada; 1984 Vol 39(6) 1115–1129

Scheidegger, Ursula. Spieltherapie mit stotternden Kindern: Ein Erfahrungsbericht. / Play therapy with stuttering children: Practical experiences. Vierteljahresschrift fur Heilpadagogik und ihre Nachbargebiete; 1987 Dec Vol 56(4) 619–629

Schultheis, Josef R. Modern theories of stuttering. Praxis der Kinderpsychologie und Kinderpsychiatrie; 1978 Apr Vol 27(3) 83–87

Schultheis, Josef R. Stottern in historischer und "komplexer" Hinsicht. (Stuttering: Historical and complex perpectives.) Vierteljahresschrift fur Heilpadagogik und ihre Nachbargebiete; 1979 Jun Vol 48(2) 125–138

Schulze, Christa C. Kontrolle von Stottervor-laufern durch GSR-Biofeedback. (Control of stuttering precursors through GSR bio-feedback.) Zeitschrift fur Klinische Psychologie. Forschung und Praxis; 1982 Vol 11(2) 116–143

Schulze, Hartmut; Johannsen, H. S. Importance of parent-child interaction in the genesis of stuttering. Folia Phoniatrica; 1991 May–Jun Vol 43(3) 133–143

Scopazzo, Maurizio. (Rosenzweig Picture Frus-tration Study and EEG features in an ado-lescent stuttering group.) Lavoro Neuropsi-chiatrico; 1974 Jan–Jun Vol 54(1–3) 49–60

Seidel, Christa; Biesalski, P. (Psychological and clinical experiences with the Frostig Test and the Frostig therapy in speech-impaired chidl-ren.) Praxis der Kinderpsychologie und Kin-derpsychiatrie; 1973 Jan Vol 22(1) 3–15

Silvestre, Cathie. Corps separe et langage parle. (Body and spoken language.) Topique Revue Freudienne; 1983 Sep Vol 13(31) 105–121

Smit-Beek, Eva; Sluijmer Swanenburg, Bep. An experimental group treatment of six stutter-ing children based on the two-factor theory of Mowrer. Tijdschrift voor Psychotherapie; 1977 Jul Vol 3(4) 175–182

Soroker, N.; Bar-Israel, Y.; Schechter, I.; Solzi, P. Stuttering as a manifestation of right-hemi-spheric subcortical stroke. European Neurol-ogy; 1990 Sep–Oct Vol 30(5) 268–270

Staffolani, Giuseppe. La balbuzie infantile. / Childhood stuttering. Rivista Internazionale di Psicologia e Ipnosi; 1984 Jan–Mar Vol 25(1) 37–41

Steffen, Hartmut; Seidel, Christa. Perceptive and cognitive school and social behavior of children with language and speech disorders. Zeitschrift fur Kinder und Jugendpsychiatrie; 1976 Vol 4(3) 216–232

Steidl, Ladislav; Pesak, Josef; Chytilova, Hana. Stuttering and tetanic syndrome. Folia Phoni-atrica; 1991 Jan–Feb Vol 43(1) 7–12

Sussman, Harvey M. Contrastive patterns of in-trahemispheric interference to verbal and spatial concurrent tasks in right-handed, left-handed and stuttering populations. Neurop-sychologia; 1982 Vol 20(6) 675–684

Tkaczenko, Oleh G. Tiefenpsychologische Aspekte des Stotterns. / The depth psycho-

logical aspects of stuttering. Zeitschrift fur Individualpsychologie; 1990 Vol 15(4) 298–306

Turkat, Ira D.; Pomeranz, Jane F.; Bruch, Michael H. Rapid treatment of a twenty-two-year stammering problem by slow speech training. Scandinavian Journal of Behaviour Therapy; 1981 Vol 10(1) 49–53

Turkat, Ira D.; Pomeranz, Jane F.; Bruch, Michael H. Rapid treatment of a twenty-two-year stammering problem by slow speech training. Scandinavian Journal of Behaviour Therapy; 1981 Vol 10(1) 49–53

Van Lankveld, Jacques. RET als verlengstuk van stottertherapie. / Rational emotive therapy and stuttering. Gedragstherapie; 1991 Mar Vol 24(1) 29–39

von Deuster, C. Untersuchungen zur Hemi-spharendominanz und Handigkeit bei stam-melnden Kindern mit normaler und gestorter auditiver Wahrnehmung. / Studies of hemi-sphere dominance and handedness of stam-mering children with normal and disturbed auditory perception. Folia Phoniatrica; 1983 Nov–Dec Vol 35(6) 265–272

Wagner, Alejandro M. Acera de la tartamudez: Introduccion a la patologia del acto. (Stutter-ing: An introduction to the pathology of the act.) Revista de Psicoanalisis; 1988 Mar–Apr Vol 45(2) 391–417

Wendlandt, Wolfgang. (A behavior therapeutic program for adult stutterers.) Praxis der Kin-derpsychologie und Kinderpsychiatrie; 1974 Oct Vol 23(7) 255–265

Wendlandt, Wolfgang. (Self-assertive training: A behavioral therapeutic phase in the treatment of adult stutterers.) Zeitschrift fur Klinische Psychologie und Psychotherapie; 1974 Vol 22(3) 236–246

Wolff, Tore. En teori om hur stamning uppkom-mer. (A theory about the cause of stuttering.) Psykisk Halsa; 1989 Vol 30(1) 45–49

India

Anitha, H. P. Phonation and stuttering. Journal of the All India Institute of Speech and Hear-ing; 1982 Vol 13 105–111

Bhargava, S. C. Participant modeling in stuttering. Indian Journal of Psychiatry; 1988 Jan Vol 30(1) 91–93

Dharitri, R. Response to therapy by stutterers in relation to their locus of control. Indian Journal of Clinical Psychology; 1985 Sep Vol 12(2) 37–40

Hegde, M. N. The effect of shock on stuttering. Journal of the All India Institute of Speech and Hearing; 1971 Jan Vol. 2 104–110

Jayaram, M. Relationship of stuttering to word information value in a phonemic clause. Journal of the All India Institute of Speech and Hearing; 1982 Vol 13 1–6

Lal, K. K.; Latte, G. A.; Raj, J. Bharath. A case report: Treatment of stuttering with systematic desensitization. Indian Journal of Clinical Psychology; 1976 Sep Vol 3(2) 219–221

Manohar, P. D.; Jayaram, M.; Rangasayee; Narendiran. Correspondence therapy for stuttering. Journal of the All India Institute of Speech and Hearing; 1973 Jan Vol 4 113–122

Mehta, M. Comparison of abbreviated and full relaxation therapy in systematic desensitization of stutterers. Journal of Personality and Clinical Studies; 1985 Mar–Sep Vol 1(1–2) 7–10

Nammalvar, N.; Rao, A. Venkoba. Identity disturbances among adult stammerers. Indian Journal of Clinical Psychology; 1983 Sep Vol 10(2) 491–496

Nandur, V. U. Effect of binaural masking noise on stuttering: A spectographic analysis. Journal of the All India Institute of Speech and Hearing; 1982 Vol 13 164–169

Nataraja, N. P.; Rajkumar, P.; Ramesh, M. V. Disfluencies in normals under DAF—in reading combined and voiced passages. Hearing Aid Journal; 1983 Jul–Dec Vol 4(1) 23–26

Nigam, J. C. Stuttering and its self treatment. Hearing Aid Journal; 1985 Jul Vol 4(3) 78–79

Ojha, K. N.; Bettagere, R. N. Group psychotherapy with stutterers. Indian Journal of Clinical Psychology; 1982 Sep Vol 9(2) 125–129

Raj, J. Bharath. A case report: Treatment of stuttering with systematic desensitization. Lal, K. K.; Latte, G. A.; Raj, J. Bharath. Indian Journal of Clinical Psychology; 1976 Sep Vol 3(2) 219–221

Raj, J. Bharath. Control of stuttering behaviour through response contingent shocks. Journal of the All India Institute of Speech and Hearing; 1974–75 Jan Vol 5–6 10–16

Raj, J. Bharath; Latte, G. A. Recoveries from stuttering. Indian Journal of Clinical Psychology; 1977 Sep Vol 4(2) 185–187

Raj, J. Bharath. Treatment of stuttering. Indian Journal of Clinical Psychology; 1976 Sep Vol 3(2) 157–163

Raj, J. Bharath; Latte, G. A. Recoveries from stuttering. Indian Journal of Clinical Psychology; 1977 Sep Vol 4(2) 185–187

Sahasi, G.; Pandit, Rama. Indigenous methods of treating stuttering. Journal of Personality and Clinical Studies; 1985 Mar–Sep Vol 1(1–2) 37–40

Srivastava, K. Indira. Socio-psychological factors of stammering and the problem of rehabilitation of stammerers. Indian Psychological Review; 1985 Vol 29(Spec Iss) 24–34

Stewart, Joseph L. Cross-cultural studies and linguistic aspects of stuttering. Journal of the All India Institute of Speech and Hearing; 1971 Jan Vol 2 1–6

Viswanath, N. S. Experimental aversion therapy for stuttering: A case study. Journal of the All India Institute of Speech and Hearing; 1971 Jan Vol 2 69–71

Japan

Aoki, Tsuyoshi. (Delayed auditory feedback and stuttering.) Japanese Journal of Educational Psychology; 1974 Sep Vol 22(3) 186–191

Hirasawa, Hajima; Ohashi, Yoshiko; Hagiwara, Sachiko. (Listeners' attitudes toward stuttering—a study on some illustrative cases in literary works.) Japanese Journal of Special Education; 1982 Feb Vol 19(3) 39–46

Ikezuki, Makoto; Harano, Kotaro; Yamaguchi, Shoji. (Research on the effect of reciprocal inhibition elicited with kinetic response.) Japanese Journal of Behavior Therapy; 1989 Vol 15(1) 56–61

Isshiki, Nobuhiko. Voice and speech disorders requiring surgical treatment. Japanese Psychological Review; 1977 Vol 20(1) 51–60

Itoh, Norihiro; Kamada, Yuko. An analytical study of self-consciousness in stutterers. Japanese Journal of Child and Adolescent Psychiatry; 1981 Vol 22(3) 193–202

Mizumachi, Toshiro. An experimental study of listeners' attitudes toward stuttering children: I. The influence different encounter modes in the stuttering situation exercise on listeners' attitude changes. Japanese Journal of Special Education; 1983 Jun Vol 21(1) 21–26

Mizumachi, Toshiro. Assertiveness in stutterers—with reference to within-group differences. Japanese Journal of Special Education; 1985 Mar Vol 22(4) 1–9

Mizumachi, Toshiro. (Assessment of the results of stuttering therapy—from the behavior therapeutic point of view.) Japanese Journal of Special Education; 1981 Oct Vol 19(2) 48–55

Mizumachi, Toshiro. Study on the assertiveness in stutterers. Japanese Journal of Behavior Therapy; 1987 Mar Vol 12(2) 50–58

Mizumachi, Toshiro. (The factor analytic study on listeners' attitudes toward stuttering children.) Japanese Journal of Special Education; 1982 Jul Vol 20(1) 27–33

Ohashi, Yoshiko. The development of stuttering in children: A cross-sectional study. Japanese Journal of Child Psychiatry; 1976 Dec–Feb Vol 17(1) 57–68

Ohashi, Yoshiko; Hagiwara, Sachiko. The onset and development of stuttering problems: Discussion of self-acceptance of stuttering in adolescence. Japanese Journal of Child and Adolescent Psychiatry; 1982 Vol 23(5) 287–299

Tsunoda, Tadanobu; Moriyama, Haruyuki. Specific patterns of cerebral dominance for various sounds in adult stutterers. Journal of Auditory Research; 1972 Jul Vol 12(3) 216–227

Wakaba, Yoko. The process of onset of stuttering: A survey of male children who started to stutter in the first six months of the third year. RIEEC-Report; 1990 Feb Vol 39 35–41

Wakabayashi, Shinichiro; Ohtaka, Kazunori; Abe, Tokuichiro; Kaneko, Toshiko. Neuroses in child and adolescent psychiatric clinic. Japanese Journal of Child and Adolescent Psychiatry; 1983 Vol 24(3) 186–195

Yamaguchi Wakaba, Yoko. (Neurotic-like behavior in young stuttering children with early onset: The characteristics of the behavior in the male children who began to stutter

at the age of two.) RIEEC-Report; 1988 Rep 37 39–48

Yanagawa, Mitsuaki. On the etiology of stuttering and personality tendencies in mothers and children. Japanese Journal of Child Psychiatry; 1973–74 Dec–Feb Vol 15(1) 22–28

Latin America

Acosta, Miryam; Rodriguez, Pedro R. Tartamudez y si mismo. (Stuttering and the self.) Revista Intercontinental de Psicologia y Educacion; 1991 Vol 4(2) 105–119

Aguilar, Guido. Ansiedad y comportamiento de tartamudeo. / Anxiety and stuttering behavior. Avances en Psicologia Clinica Latinoamericana; 1982 Vol 1 33–60

Aguilar, Guido; de Aguilar, Maria T.; de Berganza, Maria R. El tartamudeo y su deteccion temprana. / Stuttering and its early detection. 5th Latin American Congress of Behavior Analysis and Behavior Modification: Applied behavior analysis (1986, Caracas, Venezuela). Avances en Psicologia Clinica Latinoamericana; 1988 Vol 6 41–51

Friedman, Silvia. Fluencia, disfluencia, gagueira. / Fluency, disfluency, stuttering. Revista Interamericana de Psicologia; 1991 Vol 25(1) 83–92

Garcia-Moreno, Juan. Eficacia clinica de dos alternativas terapeuticas en el tratamiento de la tartamudez. (Clinical efficacy of two therapeutic alternatives to the treatment of stuttering.) Revista de Psicologia General y Aplicada; 1984 Vol 39(6) 1093–1113

Gonzalez-Ochoa, A. M.; Parra-Parra, M. L.; Rodriguez-Carillo, P. R. Actitudes y tartamudez II. (Attitudes and stuttering: II.) Revista de Psicologia General y Aplicada; 1990 Jul 43(3) 393–400

Lucke, Herman H. Treatment of language fluency disorders by a procedure combining several techniques. Revista Latinoamericana de Psicologia; 1977 Vol 9(3) 437–441

Moreno, Felipe A. A counterconditioning program (habit-reversal) in treatment of stuttering: A case study. Revista de Psicologia General y Aplicada; 1977 Jul–Aug Vol 32(147) 593–600

Orta-Rodriguez, Martha; Gallegos B., Xochitl. Una evaluacion de tres tecnicas conductuales en el tratamiento de la tartamudez. (An evaluation of 3 behavioral techniques used to treat stuttering.) Revista Mexicana de Psicologia; 1986 Jul–Dec Vol 3(2) 168–173

Ottoni, Thais M. (The use of the technique of speech modeling in modification of verbal behavior.) Revista Interamericana de Psicologia; 1974 Vol 8(3–4) 197–203

Polaino-Lorente, Aquilino M. Experiences in the treatment of childhood stuttering. Revista de Psicologia General y Aplicada; 1976 Mar–Apr Vol 31(139) 171–183

Ramirez, Luis H. (Treatment of stuttering by self-control procedures.) Revista Latinoamericana de Psicologia; 1975 Vol 7(3) 421–434

Rodriguez, Pedro R. Actitudes y conductas de los maestros de educacion primaria hacia la tartamudez. (Attitudes and behaviors of primary school teachers toward stuttering.) Revista Intercontinental de Psicologia y Educacion; 1988 Dec Vol 1(2) 165–183

Rodriguez, Pedro R. Actitudes y tartamudez. (Attitudes and stuttering.) Revista de Psicologia General y Aplicada; 1986 Vol 41(6) 1229–1252

Rodriguez, Pedro R.; Silva, Celia. Perfil de la tartamudez y del tartamudo. (Profile of stuttering and the stutterer.) Revista Latinoamericana de Psicologia; 1985 Vol 17(1) 87–112

Santacreu-Mas, Jose. El condicionamiento ante determinadas palabras en la tartamudez. (Conditioning before some words in stuttering.) Revista de Psicologia General y Aplicada; 1984 Vol 39(6) 1115–1129

Santacreu-Mas, Jose. Respuestas psicofisiologicas de sujetos tartamudos durante la pronunciacion de palabras. (Psychophysiological responses of stutterers during pronunciation of words.) Revista de Psicologia General y Aplicada; 1985 Vol 40(2) 221–242

Middle East/Africa

Guy, Nina. Stuttering as an expression of aggression: Transferential and countertransferential aspects: A case study. Israel Journal of Psychiatry and Related Sciences; 1987 Vol 24(3) 211–221

Kotbi, Naser; Farag, Safwat; Yousif, Mahmoud; Baraka, Mohamed, et al. A comparison between stutterers and non stutterers in intelligence, self-concept, anxiety and depression. Derasat Nafseyah; 1992 2(2) 37–349

Van Jaarsveld, Pieter E.; du Plessis, Wynand F. Audio-psycho-phonology at Potchefstroom: A review. South African Journal of Psychology; 1988 Dec Vol 18(4) 136–143

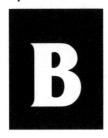

Self Help and Professional Interest Groups

Self Help Groups

National Stuttering Project
2151 Irving Street
Suite 208
San Francisco, California 94122
Phone: (415) 566-5324

National Council on Stuttering
558 Russell Road
DeKalb, Illinois 60115
Phone: (815) 756-6986

Speak Easy International
233 Concord Drive
Paramus, New Jersey 07652
Phone: (201) 262-0895

Professional Interest Groups

American Speech-Language and Hearing
    Association
Special Interest Division 4: Fluency and
    Fluency Disorders
10801 Rockville Pike
Rockville, Maryland 20852
Phone: (310) 897-5700

Stuttering Foundation of America
P.O. Box 11749
Memphis, Tennessee 38111
Phone: (800) 992-9329

Stuttering Resource Foundation
123 Oxford Road
New Rochelle, New York 10804
Phone: (914) 632-3925
            (800) 232-4773

International Fluency Association
C. Woodruff Starkweather, Secretary
457 Old Farm Road
Wyncote, Pennsylvania 19095

Bibliography

Adams, M.R. (1976). Some common problems in the design and conduct of experiments in Stuttering. *Journal of Speech and Hearing Disorders, 41,* 3–9.

Adams, M.R (1981). The speech production abilities of stutterers: Recent, ongoing, and future research. *Journal of Fluency Disorders, 6,* 311–326.

Adams, M.R. (1982). Fluency, nonfluency and stuttering in children. *Journal of Fluency Disorders, 7,* 171–185.

Adams, M.R. (1987). Personal Communication.

Adams, M.R. & Hutchinson (1974). The effects of three levels of auditory masking on selected vocal characteristics and the frequency of disfluency of adult stutterers. *Journal of Speech and Hearing Research, 17,* 682–688.

Adams, M.R. & Popelka, G. (1971). The influence of "time-out" on stutterers and their dysfluency. *Behavior Therapy, 2,* 334–339.

Adams, M.R. & Ramig, P. (1980). Vocal characteristics of normal speakers and stutterers during choral reading. *Journal of Speech and Hearing Research, 23,* 457–469.

Adams, M.R. & Runyan, C.M. (1981) Stuttering and fluency: Exclusive events or points on a continuum? *Journal of Fluency Disorders, 6*(3) 197–218.

Ager, A. (1987). Minimal intervention: A strategy for generalized behavior change with mentallyhandicapped individuals, *Behavioral Psychotherapy, 15,* 1, 16–30.

Allen, C.P. & Daly, D.A. (1978). Effects of transcendental meditation and EMG biofeedback relaxation on stuttering. *ASHA, 20,* 730.

American Speech-Language-Hearing Association (1988). Position statement: Prevention of communication disorders. *ASHA, 30,* 90.

American Speech-Language-Hearing Association (1992). Code of ethics. *ASHA, 34:3,* 1–2.

American Speech-Language-Hearing Association (1993). *Demographic Data.* Rockville, MD.

Ammons, L.J. (1993). Followup study of direct fluency training with the young stutterer. Master Thesis, East Carolina University, Greenville, North Carolina.

Anderson, G.R. & Anderson, S.K (1983). The exceptional native American. In D.R. Omark & J.G. Erickson (Eds.), *The Bilingual Exceptional Child.* San Diego: College-Hill Press, 163–180.

Andrews, G. (1984). Epidemiology of stuttering. In R. Curlee & W. Perkins (Eds.), *Nature & Treatment of Stuttering.* San Diego: College Hill Press.

Andrews, G. & Craig, A. (1988). Prediction of outcome after treatment for stuttering. *British Journal of Psychiatry, 154,* 273–274.

Andrews, G., Craig, A., Feyer, A.M., Hoddinott, S., Howie, P. & Neilson, M. (1983). Stuttering: A review of research findings and theories: Circa 1982. *Journal of Speech and Hearing Disorders, 48,* 226–264.

Andrews, G., Guitar, B. & Howie, P. (1980). Meta-analysis of the effects of stuttering treatment. *Journal of Speech Hearing Disorders, 45,* 287–307.

Andrews, G. & Harris, M. (1964). *The Syndrome of Stuttering. Clinics in Developmental Med.,* 17, London: Spastics Society Medical Education and Information Unit in association with Wm. Heinemann Medical Books.

Andrews, G. & Harvey, R. (1981). Regression to the mean in pretreatment measuresof stuttering. *Journal of Speech and Hearing Disorders, 46,* 204–207.

Andrews, G., Howie, P.M., Doza, M. & Guitar, B.F. (1982). Stuttering: Speech pattern characteristics under fluency-inducing conditions. *Journal of Speech and Hearing Research, 25,* 208–216.

Andrews, G. & Ingham, R. (1971). Stuttering: Considerations in the evaluation of treatment. *British Journal of Communication Disorders, 6,* 129–138.

Arnold, M. (1984). *Memory and the Brain.* Hillsdale, NJ.: Lawrence Erlbaum Associates.

Aron, M.L. (1962). Nature and incidence of stuttering among a Bantu group of school-going children. *Journal of Speech and Hearing Disorders, 27,* 116–128.

Avari & Bloodstein (1974). Adjacency and prediction in school-age stutterers. *Journal of Speech and Hearing Research, 17,* 32–40.

Azrin, N.H. & Nunn, R.G. (1974). A rapid method of eliminating stuttering by a regulated breathing approach. *Behavioral Research Therapy, 12,* 279–286.

Baer, D.M. (1990). The critical issue in treatment efficacy is knowing why treatment was applied: A student's response to Roger Ingham. *In Treatment Efficacy Research in Communication Disorders.* Rockville, MD: American Speech-Hearing-Language Association.

Baker, L. & Cantwell, D.P. (1985). Psychiatric and learning disorders in children with speech and language disorders: A critical review. *Advances in Learning and Behavioral Disabilities, 41,* 28.

Bandura, A. (1969). *Principles of Behavior Modification.* N.Y.: Holt Rinehart & Winston.

Bar, A. Singer, J. & Feldman, R.G. (1969). Subvocal muscle activity during stuttering and fluent speech: A comparison. *Journal of South African Logopedic Society, 16,* 9–14.

Barbara, D.A. (1954). *Stuttering: A Psychodynamic Approach to its Understanding and Treatment.* New York: Julian Press.

Barber, V. (1939). Studies in the psychology of stuttering: XV. Chorus reading as a distraction in stuttering. *Journal of Speech Disorders, 4,* 371–383.

Barber, V. (1940). Studies in the psychology of stuttering: XVI. Rhythm as distraction in stuttering. *Journal of Speech and Hearing Disorders, 5,* 29–42.

Barfield, A. (1976). Biological influences on sex differences in behavior. In M.S. Teitelbaum (Ed.), *Sex Differences; Social and Biological Perspectives.* Garden City, NY: Anchor Press.

Bebout, L. & Arthur, B. (1992). Cross-cultural attitudes toward speech disorders. *Journal of Speech and Hearing Research, 35*(1) 45–52.

Beilin, H. (1975). *Studies in The Cognitive Basis of Language Development.* New York: Academic Press.

Benjamin, A. (1974). *The Helping Interview, 2nd. Ed.* Boston, Mass: Houghton Mifflin Co.

Berecz, J.M. (1973). The treatment of stuttering through precision punishment and cognitive arousal. *Journal of Speech and Hearing Disorders, 38,* 256–267.

Berlo, D.K. (1960). *The Process of Communication.* New York: Holt, Rinehart & Winston.

Bernthal, J. & Bankson, N. (1981). *Articulation Disorders.* Englewood Cliffs, NJ: Prentice Hall.

Berry, M.F. (1938). A study of the medical history of stuttering children. *Speech Monographs, 5,* 97–114.

Blood, G.W.& Seider, R.(1981). The concomitant problems of young stutterers. *Journal of Speech and Hearing Disorders, 46,* 31–33.

Bloodstein, O. (1944). Studies in the psychology of stuttering:IXI. The relationship between oral reading rate and severity of stuttering. *Journal of Speech Disorders, 9,* 161–173.

Bloodstein, O. (1958). Stuttering as an anticipatory struggle reaction. In J. Eisenson (Ed.), *Stuttering: A Symposium.* New York: Harper & Row.

Bloodstein, O. (1960). The development of stuttering: Part II developmental phases. *Journal of Speech and Hearing Disorders, 25,* 366–376.

Bloodstein, O. (1981). *Handbook on Stuttering.* Chicago: National Easter Seals Society.

Bloodstein, O. (1984). Stuttering as an anticipatory struggle disorder. In R. Curlee & W. Perkins (Eds.), *Nature and Treatment of Stuttering*. San Diego, CA: College-Hill Press.

Bloodstein, O. (1987). *Handbook on Stuttering*. Chicago: National Easter Seals Society.

Boberg, E. (1981). Maintenance of fluency: An experimental program. In E. Boberg, (Ed.), *Maintenance of Fluency*. New York: Elsevier, 71–112.

Boberg, E., Howie, P., Woods, L. (1979). Maintenance of fluency: A review. *Journal of Fluency Disorders, 4*, 93–116.

Boberg, E. & Kully, D. (1984). Techniques for transferring fluency. In W.H. Perkins (Ed.), *Current Therapy of Communication Disorders*. New York: N.Y.: Thieme-Stratton.

Boberg, E., Yeudall, L.T., Schopflocher, D. & Bo-Lassen, P. (1983). The effect of an intensive behavioral program on the distribution of EEG alpha power in stutterers during the processing of verbal and visuaospatial information. *Journal of Fluency Disorders, 8*, 245–263.

Boorstein, D.J. (1985). *The Discoverers*. New York: Vintage Books, 625.

Borden, G.J., Kim, Daniel H. & Spiegler, K. (1991). Acoustics of stop consonant-vowel relationships during fluent and stuttered utterances. *Journal of Fluency Disorders, 12*, 3, 175–184.

Brady, J.P. (1969). Studies of the metronome effect on stuttering. *Behavior Research and Therapy, 7*, 197–205.

Brady, J.P. (1991) The pharmacology of stuttering: A critical review. *American Journal of Psychiatry, 148*(10) 1309–1316.

Brady, W.A. & Hall, D.E. (1976). The prevalence of stuttering among school-age children. *Language Speech Hearing Services in Schools, 7*, 75–81.

Brayton, E.R. & Conture, E.G. (1978). Effects of noise and rhythmic stimulation on the speech of stutterers. *Journal of Speech and Hearing Research, 21*, 285–294.

Briggs, K.A. (1977). Charismatic Christians. In H.L. Marx, Jr. (Ed.), *Religions in America*. New York: Wilson.

Browder, D., Schoen, S. & Francis, E. (1986). Learning to learn through observation. *Journal of Special Education, 20*, 4, 447–461.

Bruce, M.C. & Adams, M.R. (1978). Effects of two types of motor practice on stuttering adaptation. *Journal of Speech and Hearing Disorders, 21*, 421–428.

Bruder, M. (1986). Acquisition and generalization of teaching techniques: A study with parents of toddlers. *Behavior Modification, 10,4*, 391–414.

Brutten, E.J. (1963). Palmar sweat investigation of disfluency and expectancy adaptation. *Journal of Speech and Hearing Research, 6*, 40–48.

Brutten, E.J. (1980). The effect of punishment on a Factor I stuttering behavior. *Journal of Fluency Disorders, 5*, 77–85.

Brutten, E.J. (1986). The Two-Factor Theory. In G. H. Shames & H. Rubin (Eds.), *Stuttering Then and Now*. Columbus,OH: Charles Merrill Pub, 155–183.

Brutten, E.J. & Miller, R. (1988). The disfluencies of normally fluent black first graders. *Journal of Fluency Disorders, 13*, 291–299.

Brutten, E.J., & Shoemaker, D.J. (1967). *The Modification of Stuttering*. Englewood Cliffs, NJ: Prentice-Hall,Inc.

Brutten, E.J. & Shoemaker, D.J. (1969). Stuttering: The disintegration of speech due to conditioned negative emotion. In B.B. Gray and G. England (Eds.), *Stuttering and the Conditioning Therapies*. Monterey, CA: Monterey Institute of Speech and Hearing.

Bubeickova, M. (1977). The stuttering child's relation to school. *Psychologia a Patopsychologia Dietata, 12*(6) 535–545.

Buckingham, H. Jr.(1982). Neuropsychological models of language. In N. Lass, L. McReynolds, J. Northern & D. Yoder (Eds.), *Speech, Language and Hearing, Vol. I.,* Philadelphia: W.B. Saunders.

Bull, P.E. (1987). *Posture and Gesture*. New York: Pergamon Press.

Bullen, A.K. (1945). A cross cultural approach to the problem of stuttering, *Child Development, 16*, 1–88.

Butterworth, B. & Goldman-Eisler, F. (1979). Recent studies in cognitive rhythm. In A.W. Siegman & S. Feldstein (Eds.), *Of Speech and Time*. Hillsdale, NJ: Erlbaum.

California Department of Education. (1991). *Special education enrollment data: State total, ages 0–22, enrollment and annual growth by dis-*

ability. Sacramento, CA: California Department of Education.

Campbell, J. (1988). *The Power of Myth*. New York: Doubleday

Canter, G.J. (1971). Observations on neurogenic stuttering: A contribution to differential diagnosis. *British Journal of Disorders of Communication, 6*, 139–143.

Cantwell, D.P. & Baker, L. (1985). Psychiatric and learning disorders in children with speech and language disorders: A descriptive analysis. *Advances in Learning and Behavioral Disabilities, 4*, 29–47.

Caplan, L. (1972). An investigation of some aspects of stuttering-like speech in adult dysphasic subjects. *Journal of South Africa Speech and Hearing Association, 19*, 52–66.

Casey, E. (1987). *Remembering*. Bloomington, Ind.: Indiana University Press.

Cheng, L.R.I. (1987). Cross cultural and linguistic considerations in working with Asian populations. *ASHA, 29*, 33–37.

Cherry, C. & Sayers, B. (1956). Experiments upon the total inhibition of stammering by external control and some clinical results. *Journal of Psychosomatic Research, 1*, 233–246.

Cherry, C., Sayers, B.M. & Marland, P.M. (1955). Experiments on the complete suppression of stammering. *Nature, 176*, 874–875.

Christensen, J.E. & Lingwall, J.B. (1982). Verbal contingent stimulation of stuttering in laboratory and home settings. *Journal of Fluency Disorders, 7*, 359–368.

Clifford, S., et.al. (1965). Stuttering in South Dakota Indians. *Central States Speech Journal, 16*, 59–60.

Coelho, C. & Duffy, R. (1987). The relationship of the acquisition of manual signs to severity of aphasia: A training study. *Brain & Language, 31*, 328–345.

Colburn, N. & Mysak, E.D. (1982a). Developmental disfluency and emerging grammar I. Disfluency characteristics in early syntactic utterances, *Journal of Speech and Hearing Research, 25*, 414–421.

Colburn, N. & Mysak, E.D. (1982b). Developmental disfluency and emerging grammar II. Co-occurrence of disfluency with specified semantic-syntactic structures. *Journal of Speech and Hearing Research, 25*, 421–427.

Cole, L. (1989). E pluribus pluribus: Multicultural imperatives for the 1990's and beyond. *ASHA, 31*, 65–70.

Cole, L. Deal, V.R. (Eds.), (In Press). *Communication Disorders in Multicultural Populations*. Rockville, MD: American Speech-Language-Hearing Association.

Commodore, R.W. (1980). Communicative stress and stuttering during normal, whispered and articulation-without-phonation speech modes: A further study. *Human Communication, 5*, 143–150.

Commodore, R.W. & Cooper, E.B. (1978). Communicative stress and stuttering frequency during normal whispered and articulation-without-phonation speech modes. *Journal of Fluency Disorders, 3*, 1–12.

Connell, P. (1987). An effect of modeling and imitation teaching procedures on children with and without specific language impairment. *Journal of Speech and Hearing Research, 30*, 105–113.

Conrad, C. (1980). *An Incidence Study of Stuttering Among Black Adults*. Unpublished research project. Northwestern University, Evanston, Illinois.

Conture, E.G. (1990). *Stuttering*, 2nd Ed. Englewood Cliffs, NJ: Prentice-Hall.

Conture, E.G. & Brayton, E.R. (1975). The influence of noise on stutterer's different disfluency types. *Journal of Speech and Hearing Research, 18*, 381–384.

Conture, E.G., McCall, G.N. & Brewer, D.W. (1977). Laryngeal behavior during stuttering Journal of Speech and Hearing Research, *20*, 661–668.

Conture, E.G., Rothenberg, M. & Molitar, R.D. (1986). Electroglottographic observations of young stutterers' fluency. *Journal of Speech Hearing and Research, 29*, 384–393.

Cooper, E.B. (1975). Clinician attitudes toward stutterers: A study in bigotry? Paper presented at the convention of the American Speech-Language-Hearing Association, Washington, D.C.

Cooper, E.B. (1979). Intervention procedures for the young stutterer. In H.H. Gregory (Ed.),

Controversies About Stuttering Therapy. Baltimore: University Park Press.

Cooper, E.B., Cady, B.B. & Robbins, C.J. (1970). The effect of the verbal stimulus words wrong, right, and tree on the disfluency rates of stutterers and nonstutterers. *Journal of Speech and Hearing Research, 13,* 239–244.

Cooper, E.B. & Cooper, C.S. (1985), *Cooper Personalized Fluency Control Therapy, Revised.* Allen, IX: DLM Teaching Resources.

Cooper, E.B. & Cooper, C.S. (1991), Multicultural considerations in the assessment and treatment of fluency disorders. American Speech-Language-Hearing Association Annual Convention, Atlanta.

Cooper, E. B. & Cooper, C.S. (1993). Fluency Disorders. In D. Battle (Ed.), *Communication Disorders in Multicultural Populations.* Boston: Andover Medical Pub, 189–211.

Costello, J. (1975). The establishment of fluency with time-out procedures: Three case studies. *Journal of Speech Hearing Disorders, 40,* 216–31.

Costello, J. (1983a). Current behavioral treatments for children. In D. Prins & R.J. Ingham (Eds.), *Treatment of Stuttering in Early Childhood: Methods and Issues.* San Diego: College-Hill Press.

Costello, J.M. (1980). Operant conditioning and the treatment of stuttering. *Seminars in Speech, Language and Hearing, 1,* 311–325.

Costello, J. (1983b). Generalization across settings. In J. Miller, D. Yoder & R. Schiefelbush (Eds.), *Contemporary Issues in Language Intervention (ASHA Reports, No. 12).* Rockville, MD: American Speech and Hearing Association, 275–297.

Costello, J.C. (1989). Generalization in the treatment of stuttering. In L.V. McReynolds & J.E. Spradlin. *Generalization Strategies in the Treatment of Communication Disorders.* Philadelphia: B.C. Decker, Inc., 63–81.

Costello, J.M. (1984a). Operant conditioning and the treatment of stuttering. In W.H. Perkins (Ed.), *Stuttering Disorders.* New York: Thieme-Stratton, Inc.

Costello, J.M. (1984b). Treatment of the young chronic stutterer: Managing fluency. In R.F. Curlee & W. H. Perkins (Eds.), *Nature and Treatment of Stuttering: New Directions.* San Diego: College-Hill Press.

Costello, J.M. (1984c). Current behavioral treatments for children. In D. Prins & R.J. Ingham (Eds.), *Treatment of Stuttering in Early Childhood: Methods and Issues.* San Diego: College-Hill Press.

Costello, J. & Ingham, R.J. (1984a). Assessment strategies for stuttering. In R. Curlee & W. Perkins (Eds.), *Nature and Treatment of Stuttering.* San Diego. CA: College-Hill Press.

Costello, J. & Ingham, R.J. (1984b). Stuttering as an operant disorder. In R. Curlee & W. Perkins (Eds.), *Nature and Treatment of Stuttering.* San Diego. CA: College-Hill Press.

Costello-Ingham, J. (1993). Behavioral treatment of stuttering children. In R.F. Curlee (Ed.), *Stuttering and Related Disorders of Fluency.* New York: Thieme Medical Publishers, Inc.

Craig, A., Feyer, A.M. & Andrews, G. (1987). An overview of a behavioural treatment for stuttering. *Australian Psychologist, 22,* 1, 53–62.

Craig, A., Franklin, J. & Andrews, G. (1981). A scale to measure the locus of control of behavior. *British Journal of Medical Psychology, 57,* 2, 173–180.

Craig, A.R. & Cleary, P.J. (1982). Reduction of stuttering by young male stutterers using EMG feedback. *Biofeedback and Self-Regulation, 7,* 241–55.

Craven, D.C. & Ryan, B.P. (1984) The use of a portable delayed auditory feedback unit in stuttering therapy. *Journal of Fluency Disorders, 9(3),* 237–243.

Cronbach, L. & Snow, R. (1977). *Aptitudes and Instructional Methods.* New York: Irvington Publishers.

Crowder, R. (1976). *Principles of Learning and Memory.* Hillsdale, NJ.: Lawrence Erlbaum Associates.

Crowe, T. & Walton, J.H. (1981). Teacher attitudes toward stuttering. *Journal of Fluency Disorders, 6,* 2, 163–174.

Culatta, B. & Page, J. (1982). Strategies for achieving generalization of grammatical structures. *Communicative Disorders, 7,* 31–44.

Culatta, R. (1970). The conscious and direct control of fluent and disfluent speech by stutterers. Dissertation, University of Pittsburgh.

Culatta, R. (1976). Fluency: The other side of the coin. *ASHA, 18* (11)795–799.

Culatta, R. (1990). China is not an island in the Pacific Ocean. *ASHA, 22, 2, 51–53.*

Culatta, R. & Goldberg, S.A. (In Press). *A Test for the Screening, Diagnosis and Treatment of Stuttering (TSDTS).* San Francisco, CA: Intelli-Group Publishers.

Culatta, R. & Leeper, L. (1987). Disfluency in childhood: It's not always stuttering. *Journal of Childhood Communication Disorders, 10,* 96–106.

Culatta, R. & Leeper, L. (1988). Dysfluency isn't always stuttering. *Journal of Speech and Hearing Disorders, 53,* 483–488.

Culatta, R. & Leeper, L. (1989). The differential diagnosis of disfluency. *National Student Speech Language Hearing Association Journal, 17,* 50–59.

Culatta, R. & Leeper, L. (1989b). Speech rates of elderly speakers. American Speech-Language and Hearing Association Annual Convention, St. Louis, MO.

Culatta, R. Page, J.L. & Wilson, L. (1987). Speech rates of normally communicative children. American Speech-Language and Hearing Association's Annual Convention, New Orleans, LA.

Culatta, R. & Rubin, H. (1973). A program for the initial stages of fluency therapy. *Journal of Speech and Hearing Research, 16,* 556–567.

Culp, D.M. (1984). The preschool fluency development program: Assessment and treatment. In M. Peins (Ed.), *Contemporary Approaches to Stuttering Therapy.* Boston: Little Brown & Company, 39–71.

Curlee, R.F. & Perkins, W.H. (1969). Conversational rate control therapy for stuttering. *Journal of Speech and Hearing Disorders, 34,* 245–250.

Daley, F.L. (1955). The relationship of parental attitudes and adjustments to the development of stuttering. In W. Johnson & R.R. Leutenegger (Eds.), *Stuttering in Children and Adults.* Minneapolis: University of Minnesota Press.

Daly, D.A. (1988a). *The Freedom of Fluency: A Therapy Program for the Chronic Stutterer.* Moline, Ill.: LinguiSystems, Inc.

Daly, D.A. (1984). Treatment of the young chronic stutterer: Managing stuttering. In R.F. Curlee & W.H. Perkins (Eds.), *Nature and Treatment of Stuttering: New Directions.* San Diego: College-Hill Press.

Daly, D.A. (1988a). A practitioner's view of stuttering. *ASHA, 30,* 34–35.

Daly D.A. (1988b). *The Freedom of Fluency: A therapy Program for the Chronic Stutterer.* Moline IL: LinguiSystems, Inc.

Daly, D.A. (1992). Management of stuttering and cluttering in adolescence. North Carolina Speech Language Hearing Association Annual Meeting, Wilminton, N.C.

Darley, F.L, Aronson, A.E. & Brown, J.R. (1969). Differential diagnostic patterns of dysarthria. *Journal of Speech and Hearing Research, 12,* 246–269.

Darley, F.L, Aronson, A.E. & Brown, J.R. (1975). *Motor Speech Disorders.* Philadelphia: W.B. Saunders Co.

Deal, J.L. (1982). Sudden onset of stuttering: A case report. *Journal of Speech and Hearing Research, 47,* 301–304.

DeBlassie, R.R. & Franco, J.N. (1983). Psychological and educational assessment of bilingual children. In D.R. Omark & J.G. Erickson (Eds.), *The Bilingual Exceptional Child.* San Diego: College-Hill Press, 55–68

Dell, C. (1979). *Treating the school age stutterer: A guide for clinicians.* Memphis, TN: Speech Foundation of America.

Dempsey, G.L & Granich, M. (1978). Hypno-behavioral therapy in the case of a traumatic stutterer: A case study. *International Journal of Clinical and Experimental Hypnosis, 26,* 125–133.

Dewar, A., Dewar, A.D., Austin, W.T.S. & Brash, H.M. (1979). The longterm use of an automatically triggered auditory feedback masking device in the treatment of stammering. *British Journal of Disorders of Communication, 14,* 219–229.

Diaz-Duque, O.F. (1989). Communication barriers in medical settings: Hispanics in the United States. *International Journal of the Sociology of Language, 79,* 93–102.

Dickson, S. (1971). Incipient stuttering and spontaneous remission of stuttered speech. *Journal of Communication Disorders, 4,* 99–110.

Donahue-Kilburg, G. (1992). *Family-Centered Early Intervention for Communication Disorders.* Gaithersburg, MD: Aspen Publishers.

Douglas, E. & Quarrington, B. (1952). The differentiation of internalized and externalized secondary stuttering. *Journal of Speech and Hearing Disorders, 17,* 377–385.

Doyle, P. Goldstein. H. & Bourgeois, M. (1987). "Experimental analysis of syntax training in Broca's aphasia: A generalization and social validation study," *Journal of Speech and Hearing Disorders, 52,* 143–155.

Dunlap, K. (1932). *Habits: Their Making and Unmaking.* New York: Liveright.

Dunn, R., Gemake, J., Jalali, F., Zenhausern, R., et. al. (1990). Cross-cultural differences in learning styles of elementary-age students from four ethnic backgrounds. *Journal of Multicultural Counseling and Development, 18,* 68–93.

Eccles, J. (1973). *The Understanding of the Brain.* New York: McGraw-Hill.

Edgren, B., Leanderson, R. & Levi, L (1970). A research program on stuttering and stress. *Acta Otolaryngology,* Supplement No. 263, 113–118.

Egolf, D.B., Shames, G.H., Johnson, P. & Kaspirison-Burelli, A. (1972). The use of parent-child interaction patterns in therapy for young stutterers. *Journal of Speech and Hearing Disorders, 37,* 22–232.

Egolf, D.B., Shames, G.H. & Seltzer, H.N. (1971). The effects of time-out on the fluency of stutterers in group therapy. *Journal of Communication Disorders, 4,* 111–118.

Eisenberg, A.M. & Smith, R.R., Jr. (1971). *Nonverbal Communication.* New York: Bobbs-Merrill.

Eisenson, J. (1958). A perseverative theory of stuttering. In J. Eisenson (Ed.), *Stuttering: A Symposium.* New York: Harper & Row.

Eisenson, J. & Horowitz, E. (1945) The influence of propositionality on stuttering. *Journal of Speech Disorders, 10,* 193–197.

Ekman, P. & Friesen, W. (1971). *Emotion in the Human Face.* New York: Bobbs-Merrill.

Elbert, M. & McReynolds, L. (1985), The generalization hypothesis: Final consonant deletion, *Language and Speech, 28,* 281–294.

Ellis, A. (1962). *Reason and Emotion in Psychotherapy.* New York: Lyle Stuart.

Ellis, E., Lenz, B. & Sabornie, E. (1987). Generalization and adaptation of learning strategies to natural environments: II. Research into practice. *RASE: Remedial & Special Education, 8,* 20–23.

Ellis, E., Lenz, B. & Sabornie, E.(1987). Generalization and adaptation of learning strategies to natural environments: I. Critical agents, *RASE: Remedial & Special Education, 8,* 6–20.

Erickson, J.G. (1981). Suggestions for interviewing children. In J.G. Erickson & D.R. Omark (Eds.), *Communication Assessment of the Bilingual Bicultural Child.* Baltimore: University Park Press, 285–289.

Erickson, J.G. & Walker, C.L (1983), Bilingual exceptional children: What are the issues? In D.R. Omark & J.G. Erickson (Eds.), *The Bilingual Exceptional Child.* San Diego: College-Hill Press, 3–22.

Erickson, R.L. (1969). Assessing communication attitudes among stutterers. *Journal of Speech and Hearing Research, 12,* 711–724.

Esch, J. (1987), Toward a technology of generalization. *Behavior Analyst 10,* 303–305.

Eversham, M. & Fransella, F. (1985). Stuttering relapse: The effect of a combined speech and psychological reconstruction programme. *British Journal of Disorders of Communication, 20* (3), 237–248

Falconer, D.S. (1965). The inheritance of liability to certain diseases estimated from the incidence among relatives. *Annals of Human Genetics, 29,* 51–76.

Farr, M. (1986). *The Long-Term Retention of Knowledge and Skills.* New York: Springer-Verlag.

Farver, J.A. & Howes, C. (1988). Cross-cultural differences in social interaction: A comparison of American and Indonesian children. *Journal of Cross-Cultural Psychology, 19*(2), 203–215.

Fetz, D.L. & Landers, D.M. (1983). The effects of mental practice on motor skill learning and performance: A meta-analysis. *Journal of Sport Psychology, 5,* 25–27.

Fink, H. & Niebergall, G. (1975). An attempt to measure anxieties in children who stutter. *Heilpadagogik, 44,* 3, 220–227.

Finn, P. & Ingham, R. (1989). The selection of "fluent" samples in research on stuttering: Conceptual and methodological considerations. *Journal of Speech and Hearing Research, 33,* 401–408.

Flanagan, B., Goldiamond, I. & Azrin, N.H. (1958). Operant stuttering: The control of stuttering behavior through response-contingent consequences. *Journal of Experimental Behavior 1,* 173–177.

Flanagan, B. (1986). Operant update. In G. Shames & H. Rubin (Eds.), *Stuttering Then and Now.* Columbus, OH: Charles Merrill.

Flanagan, J.C. (1954). The critical incident technique. *Psychological Bulletin, 51,* 327–358.

Frankel, S.A. & Frankel, E.B. (1970). Nonverbal behavior in a selected group of negro and white males. *Psychosomatics, 11, 2,* 127–132.

Frazier, N. & Sadker, M. (1973). *Sexism in School and Society.* New York: Harper & Row.

Freeman, F. & Ushijimma, T. (1975). Laryngeal activity accompanying the moment of stuttering: A preliminary report of EMG investigations. *Journal of Fluency Disorders, 1,* 36–45.

Freeman, F. & Ushijimma, T. (1978). Laryngeal muscle activity during stuttering. *Journal of Speech and Hearing Research, 21,* 538–562.

Freestone, N.W. (1942) An electroencephalographic study on the moment of stuttering. *Speech Monographs, 9,* 28–60.

Gagne', R. (1970). *The Conditions of Learning.* New York: Holt, Rinehart & Winston.

Gagne', R. & Briggs, L. (1974). *Principles of Instructional Design.* New York: Holt, Rinehart & Winston.

Garber, S.F. & Martin, R.R. (1974). The effects of white noise on the frequency of stuttering, *Journal of Speech and Hearing Research, 17,* 73–79.

Garber, S.F. & Martin, R.R. (1977). Effects of noise on increased vocal intensity on stuttering, *Journal of Speech and Hearing Research, 20,* 233–240.

Garrett, A. (1972). *Interviewing: Its Principles and Methods,* 2nd. Ed. E. Zaki & M. Mangold (Eds.). New York: Family Service Association of America.

Gautheron, B., Liorzou, A., Even, C. & Vallancien, B. (1973). The role of the larynx in stuttering. In Y. Lebrun & R. Hoops (Eds.), *Neurolinguistic Approaches to Stuttering.* The Hague: Mouton.

Gerber, S.E. (1990). *Prevention.* Englewood Cliffs, NJ: Prentice-Hall.

Gierut, J., Elbert, M. & Dinnsen, D. (1987). A functional analysis of phonological knowledge and generalization learning in misarticulating children. *Journal of Speech and Hearing Research, 30, 4,* 462–479.

Gillespie, S.K. & Cooper, E.B. (1973). Prevalence of speech problems in junior and senior high schools. *Journal of Speech and Hearing Research, 16,* 739–743.

Gillis-Olion, M., et. al. (1986). Strategies for interacting with black parents of handicapped children. *Negro Educational Review, 37,* 8–16.

Gladstein, K.L., Seider, R.A. & Kidd, K. K. (1981). Analysis of sibship patterns of stutterers. *Journal of Speech and Hearing Research, 24,* 460–462.

Glasner, P.J. (1949). Personality characteristics and emotional problems in stutterer under age five. *Journal of Speech and Hearing Disorders, 14,* 135–138.

Glogowski, K. (1976). Ist dos Stottern erbbedingt? *Folia Phoniat, 28,* 235–36. Abstract.

Goebal, M.D. (1994) *CAFT Program.* Annandale, Virginia: Annandale Fluency Clinic.

Goldberg, S.A. (1981). *Behavioral Cognitive Stuttering Therapy (BCST): The Rapid Development of Fluent Speech.* San Francisco: IntelliGroup Publishers.

Goldberg, S.A. (1983). The development of fluency through behavioral cognitive stuttering therapy. *Journal of Communication Disorders, 8,* 7, 89–107.

Goldberg, S.A. (1990a). Identification of technical and interpersonal clinical skills. American Speech-Language-Hearing Association Annual Convention, Seattle.

Goldberg, S.A. (1990b). Evaluation of clinical skills based on experience and education. California Speech-Language-Hearing Association Annual Convention, Seattle.

Goldberg, S.A. (1992). Genetics in stuttering treatment: Its use and limitations. American Speech-Language-Hearing Association Audioteleconference on an Overview of genetic considerations in speech and language disorders.

Goldberg, S.A. (1993) *Introduction to Clinic Practice: A Methodology and Philosophy*. Columbus, OH: Merrill/MacMillin Publishing

Goldberg, S.A., Brutten, E., Cooper, E. & Culatta, R. (1992). Criteria for the selection of stuttering intervention techniques and programs. American Speech-Language-Hearing Association Annual Convention, San Antonio, Tx.

Goldberg, S.A., & Culatta, R.A. (1991). The demise of stuttering therapy: An indictment. American Speech-Language-Hearing Association Annual Convention, Atlanta.

Goldiamond, I. (1965). Stuttering and fluency as manipulative operant response classes. In L. Kraner & L.P. Ullmann (Eds.), *Research in Behavior Modification*. New York: Holt, Rinehart, & Winston.

Goldman, R. (1967). Cultural influences in the sex ratio in the incidence of stuttering. *American Anthropologist, 69,* 78–81.

Goldman - Eisner, F. (1961) A comparative study of two hesitation phenomena. *Language and Speech 4,* 18–26.

Gollnick, D. & Chinn, P. (1990). *Multicultural Education in a Pluralistic Society*. Columbus, OH: Merrill Publishers.

Goodenough, W. (1987). Multi-culturalism as the normal human experience. In E. M. Eddy & W.L. Partridge (Eds.), *Applied Anthropology in America* (2nd. Ed.). New York: Columbia University Press.

Gorman, W.F. (1982). Defining malingering. *Journal of Forensic Science, 2,* 401–407.

Gow, L, Ward, J. & Balla, J. (1986), The use of verbal self-instruction training to promote indirect generalization, *Australia & New Zealand Journal of Developmental Disabilities, 12,*123–132.

Gottwald, S. & Halfond, B. (1985). Parent counseling in stuttering prevention. Miniseminar, American Speech-Language-Hearing Association Annual Convention, Washington, DC.

Gregory, H.H. (1968). Application of learning theory concepts in the management of stuttering. In H.H. Gregory (Ed.), *Learning Theory and Stuttering Therapy*. Evanston, IL: Northwestern University Press.

Gregory, H.H. & Hill, D. (1980). Stuttering therapy for child. In W. Perkins (Ed.), *Strategies in Stuttering Therapy*. New York: Thieme-Stratton.

Gregory, H.H. (1984). Prevention of stuttering: Management of early stages. In R.F. Curlee & W.H. Perkins (Eds.), *Nature and Treatment of Stuttering: New Directions*. San Diego, CA: College-Hill Press.

Gregory, H.H. (1986a). Environmental manipulation and family counseling. In G.H. Shames & H. Rubin (Eds.), *Stuttering Then and Now*. Columbus OH:Charles Merrill, 273–291.

Gregory, H.H. (1986b). *Stuttering: Differential Evaluation and Therapy*. Austin, TX:Pro-Ed.

Guitar, B.E. (1975). Reduction of stuttering frequency using analog electromyographic feedback. *Journal of Speech and Hearing Research, 18,* 672–685.

Guitar, B.E. (1976). Pretreatment factors associated with the outcome of stuttering therapy. *Journal of Speech and Hearing Research, 19,* 590–600.

Guitar, B.E. (1992), Parent verbal interactions and speech rate: A case study in stuttering. *Journal of Speech and Hearing Research, 35,* 742.

Guitar, B.E. & Bass, C. (1978). Stuttering therapy: The relation between attitude change and long-term outcome. *Journal of Speech and Hearing Disorders, 43,* 392–400

Guitar, B., Schaefer, H.K., Donahue-Kilburg, G., & Bond, L. (1992). Parent verbal interactions and speech rate: A case study in stuttering. *Journal of Speech and Hearing Research, 35(4)* 742–754.

Hall, D.E., Wray, D.F. & Conti, D.M. (1986). The language-disfluency relationship: A case study. *Hearsay, Fall,* 110–113.

Hall, E.T. (1959). *The Silent Language*. Garden City, NY: Doubleday and Co.

Hall, J.W. & Jerger, J. (1978). Central auditory function in stutterers. *Journal of Speech and Hearing Research, 21, 2,* 324–337.

Hall, P.K. (1977). The occurrence of disfluencies in language-disordered school-age children. *Journal of Speech and Hearing Disorders, 42,* 364–369.

Halvorson, J.A. (1971). The effects on stuttering frequency of pairing punishment (response cost) with reinforcement. *Journal of Speech and Hearing Research, 14,* 356–364.

Ham, R.E. (1986). *Techniques of stuttering therapy.* Englewood Cliffs, NJ: Prentice Hall.

Ham, R.E. (1990). *Therapy of Stuttering.* Englewood Cliffs, NJ: Prentice-Hall.

Hanna, E.P. & Owen, N. (1977). Facilitating transfer and maintenance of fluency in stuttering therapy. *Journal of Speech and Hearing Disorders, 42,* 65–76.

Hannley, M. & Dorman, M.F. (1982). Some observations on auditory function and stuttering. *Journal of Fluency Disorders, 7,* 93–108.

Haroldson, S.K., Martin, R.R. & Starr, C.D. (1968). Time-out as a punishment for stuttering. *Journal of Speech and Hearing Research, 11,* 560–566.

Harris, C.M., Martin, R.R. & Haroldson, S.K. (1971). Punishment of expectancy responses by stutterers. *Journal of Speech and Hearing Research, 14,* 710–717.

Healey, E.C. & Adams, M.R. (1981). Speech timing skills of normally fluent and stuttering children and adults. *Journal of Fluency Disorders, 6,* 3, 233–246.

Hedge, M.N. & Brutten, G.J. (1977). Reinforcing fluency in stutterers: An experimental study. *Journal of Fluency Disorders, 2,* 315–328.

Helm, N.A., Butler, R.B. & Canter, G.J. (1980). Neurogenic acquired stuttering. *Journal of Fluency Disorders, 5,* 269–279.

Helm-Estabrooks, N. (1987). Diagnosis and management of neurogenic stuttering in adults. In K.O. St. Louis (Ed.), *Atypical Stutterer: Principals and Practices of Rehabilitation.* San Diego: Academic Press, 193–217.

Helmreich, H.G. & Bloodstein, O. (1973). The grammatical factor in childhood disfluency in relation to the continuity hypothesis. *Journal of Speech and Hearing Research, 16,* 731–738.

Hendler, M., Weisberg, P. & O'Dell, N. (1987). Developing the receptive and productive use of pronouns in an autistic child: Use of modeling and programming for generalization. *Child and Family Behavior Therapy, 9,* 3–34.

Henja, R. (1960). *Speech Disorders and Non-Directive Therapy.* New York: Ronald Press.

Henry, J. (1940). Speech disturbances in Pilaga Indian children. *American Journal of Orthopsychiatry, 10,* 362, 369.

Hewes, G.W. (1957). World distribution of certain postural habits. *American Anthropologist, 57,* 213–244.

Hill, H. (1944). Stuttering: I. A critical review and evaluation of biochemical investigations. *Journal of Speech Disorders, 9,* 245–61.

Hillis, J.W. (1993). Ongoing assessment in the management of stuttering: A clinical perspective. *American Journal of Speech-Language Pathology, 2,* 24–37.

Hird, J.S., Landers, D.M., Thomas, J.R. & Horan, J.J. (1991). Physical practice is superior to mental practice in enhancing cognitive and motor task performance. *Journal of Sports Exercise Psychology, 13,* 281–293.

Hoffman, L.W. (1988). Cross-cultural differences in childrearing goals. Special Issue: Parental behavior in diverse societies. *New Directions for Child Development, 40,* 99–122.

Holland, A.L. (1967). Communicative ability in daily living: Its measurement and observation. Paper presented at *Academy of Aphasia,* Montreal, Canada.

Homzie, M.J., Lindsay, J.S., Simpson, J. & Hasenstab, S. (1988). Concomitant speech, language, and learning problems in adult stutterers and in members of their families. *Journal of Fluency Disorders, 13*(4) 39–48.

Howie, P.M. (1981). Concordance for stuttering in monozygotic and dizygotic twin pairs. *Journal of Speech and Hearing Research, 24,* 317–321.

Howie, P.M., Tanner, S. & Andrews, G. (1981). Short- and long-term outcome in an intensive treatment program for adult stutterers. *Journal of Speech and Hearing Disorders. 46,* 104–109.

Howie, P. & Andrews, G. (1984). Treatment of adult stutterers: Managing fluency. In R.F. Curlee & W.H. Perkins (Eds.), *Nature and Treatment of Stuttering: New Directions.* San Diego: College-Hill Press.

Hughes, D. (1985). *Language Treatment and Generalization.* San Diego: College-Hill Press.

Hunt, P., Goetz, L, Alwell, M. & Sailor, W. (1986). Using an interrupted behavior chain strategy to teach generalized communication responses. *Journal of the Association for Persons With Severe Handicaps, 11,* 3, 196–204.

Hutchinson, J.M. & Norris, G.M. (1977). The differential effect of three auditory stimuli on the frequency of stuttering behaviors. *Journal of Fluency Disorders, 2,* 283–293.

Hymes, D. (1984). Linguistic problems in defining the concept of "tribe." In J. Baugh & J. Sherzer (Eds.), in *Language in Use.* Englewood Cliffs, NJ: Prentice-Hall, 7–25.

Ickes, W.K. & Pierce, S. (1973). The stuttering moment: A plethysmographic study. *Journal of Communication Disorders, 6,* 155–64

Ihrig, K. & Wolchik, S. (1988). Peer versus adult models and autistic children's learning: Acquisition, generalization, and maintenance. *Journal of Autism & Developmental Disorders, 18,* 67–79.

Ingham, R.J. & Packman, A. (1979). A further evaluation of the speech of stutterers during chorus- and nonchorus-reading. *Journal of Speech and Hearing Research, 22,* 784–793.

Ingham, R.J. (1990) Theoretical, methodological, and ethical issues in treatment efficacy research: Stuttering therapy as a case study. In *Treatment Efficacy Research in Communicative Disorders.* Rockville, MD: ASHA Foundation, 15–29.

Ingham, R. (1980). Modification of maintenance and generalization during stuttering treatment. *Journal of Speech and Hearing Research, 23,* 732–745.

Ingham, R. (1984a). Generalization and maintenance of treatment. In R. Curlee and W. Perkins (Eds.), *Nature and Treatment of Stuttering: New Directions.* San Diego: College-Hill Press.

Ingham, R. (1984b). Techniques for maintaining fluency. In W.H. Perkins (Ed.), *Stuttering Disorders.* pp. 209–221. New York: Thieme-Stratton.

Ingham, R. (1993). Transfer and maintenance of treatment gains of chronic stutterers. In R. Curlee (Ed.) *Stuttering and Related Disorders of Fluency.* New York: Thieme Medical Publishers.

Ingham, R.J. (1975). Operant methodology in stuttering therapy. In J. Eisenson (Ed.), *Stuttering: A Second Symposium.* New York: Harper & Row.

Ingham, R.J. (1984a). *Stuttering and Behavior Therapy: Current Status and Experimental Foundations.* San Diego, CA: College-Hill Press.

Ingham, R.J. (1990). Commentary on Perkins (1990) and Moore and Perkins (1990): On the valid role of reliability in identifying "What is stuttering?" *Journal of Speech and Hearing Disorders, 55,* 394–397.

Ingham, R.J., Andrews, G. & Winkler, R. (1972). Stuttering: A comparative evaluation of the short-term effectiveness of four treatment techniques, *Journal of Communication Disorders, 5,* 91–117.

Ingham, R.J. & Carroll, P.J. (1977). Listener judgement differences in stutterers' nonstuttered speech during chorus-and nonchorus-reading. *Journal of Speech and Hearing Research, 20,* 293–302.

Ingham, R.J. & Ingham, J. (1992). Personal communication.

Ingham, R.J., Martin, R.R. & Kuhl, P. (1974). Modification and control of rate of speaking by stutterers. *Journal of Speech and Hearing Research, 17,* 489–496.

Ingham, R.J. & Packman, A.C. (1978). Perceptual assessment of normalcy of speech following stuttering therapy. *Journal of Speech and Hearing Research, 21,* 63–73.

Irwin, O.C. (1948). Infant speech: The effects of occupational status and age on the use of sound types. *Journal of Speech and Hearing Disorders, 13,* 224–226.

Jacobson, E. (1938). *Progressive Relaxation.* Chicago: University of Chicago Press.

James, J.E. & Ingham, R.J. (1974). The influence of stutterers' expectancies of improvement upon response to time-out. *Journal of Speech and Hearing Research, 17,* 83–96.

James, J.E., Ricciandelli, L.A., Hunter, C.E. & Rogers, P. (1989). Relative efficacy of intensive and spaced behaviorial treatment of stuttering. *Behavior Modification, 13, 3,* 376–395.

Janssen, P. & Brutten, G.J. (1973). The differential effects of punishment of oral prolongations. In Y. Lebrun & R. Hoops, (Eds.), *Neurolinguistic Approaches to Stuttering.* The Hague: Mouton.

Janssen, P., Wieneke, G. & Vaane, E.(1983). Variability in the initiation of articulatory movements in the speech of stutterers and normal speakers. *Journal of Fluency Disorders, 8,* 341–358.

Jasper, H.H. & Murray, E. (1932). A study of the eye-movements of stutterers during oral reading. *Journal of Experimental Psychology, 15,* 528–538.

Jayaram, M. (1983). Phonetic influences on stuttering in monolingual and bilingual stutterers. *Journal of Communication Disorders, 16,* 287–297.

Johns, D.F. & Darley, F.L. (1970). Phonemic variability in apraxia of speech. *Journal of Speech and Hearing Research, 13,* 556–583.

Johnson, G.F., Coleman, K. & Rasmussen, K. (1978). Multidays: Multidimensional approach for the young stutterer. *Language Speech and Hearing Services in the School, 9,* 2, 129–132.

Johnson, L.J. (1980). Facilitating parental involvement in therapy of the disfluent child. In W.H. Perkins (Ed.), *Strategies in Stuttering Therapy. Seminars in Speech, Language and Hearing I.* New York: Thieme-Stratton, 301–310.

Johnson, W. (1944). The Indians have no word for it. I. Stuttering in children. *Quarterly Journal of Speech, 30,* 330–337.

Johnson, W. (1955). A study of the onset and development of stuttering. In W. Johnson (Ed.), *Stuttering in Children and Adults.* Minneapolis: University of Minnesota Press.

Johnson, W. & Associates (1959). *The Onset of Stuttering.* Minneapolis: University of Minnesota Press.

Johnson, W. & Inness, M. (1939). Studies in the psychology of stuttering: XIII. A statistical analysis of the adaptation and consistency effects in relation to stuttering. *Journal of Speech Disorder, 4,* 79–86.

Johnson, W. & Knott, J.R. (1937). Studies in the psychology of stuttering: I. The distribution of moments of stuttering in successive readings of the same passage. *Journal of Speech and Hearing Disorders, 2,* 17–19.

Johnson, W. & Rosen, L. (1937). Studies in the psychology of stuttering: VII. Effect of certain changes in speech pattern upon frequency of stuttering. *Journal of Speech Disorders, 2,* 105–109.

Jung, C.G. (1968). *Analytical Psychology: Its Theory and Practice* (The Taistock Lectures). New York: Pantheon.

Kamhi, A.G. & McOsker, T.G. (1982), Attention and stuttering: Do stutterers think too much about speech? *Journal of Fluency Disorders, 7,* 309–321.

Karr, G.M. (1977). The performance of stutterers on central auditory tests. *South African Journal of Communication Disorders, 24,* 100–109.

Kayser, H. (1985). A Study of Speech and Language Pathologists and their Mexican-American Language Disordered Caseloads. Unpublished doctoral dissertation. New Mexico State University, Las Cruces, New Mexico.

Kelly, E. & Conture, E. (1991). Intervention with school aged stutterers: A parent-child fluency group approach. *Seminars in Speech and Language, 12,* 310–322.

Kennett, R.J. (1976). *Zen is Eternal Life.* Emeryville, CA: Dharma Publishing

Kent, R.G. (1983). Facts about stuttering: Neuropsychologic perspectives. *Journal of Speech and Hearing Disorders, 48,* 249–255.

Kenyon, E. (1943). The etiology of stammering: The psychophysiological facts which concern the production of speech sounds and stammering. *Journal of Speech and Hearing Disorders, 8,* 347–348.

Kidd, K.K. (1977). A genetic perspective on stuttering. *Journal of Fluency Disorders, 2,* 259–269.

Kidd, K.K. (1983). Recent progress on the genetics of stuttering. In C.L. Ludlow and J.A. Cooper (Eds.), *Genetic Aspects of Speech and Language Disorders,* 197–231, New York: Academic Press.

Kidd, K.K., Heimbuch, R.C. & Records, M.A. (1981). Vertical transmission of susceptibility to stuttering with sex-modified expression. *Proceedings of the National Academy of Science, 78,* 606–610.

Kidd, K.K., Heinbuch, R.C., Records, Oehlert, G., & Webster, R.L. (1980). Familial stuttering patterns are not related to one measure of severity. *Journal of Speech and Hearing Research, 23,* 539–545.

Kidd, K.K., Kidd, J.R., & Records, M.A. (1978). The possible causes of the sex ratio in stuttering and its implications. *Journal of Fluency Disorders, 3,* 13–23.

Kidd, K.K. & Records, M.A. (1978). Genetic methodologies for the study of speech. In E.O. Breakefield (Ed.), *Neurogenetics: Genetic Approaches to the Nervous System*. New York: Elsevier, 311–344.

Kidd, R.D. (1980). Genetic model of stuttering. *Journal of Fluency Disorders, 5,* 187–201.

Kluckhohn, C. (1954). Culture and behavior. In G. Lindsey, (Ed.), *Handbook of Social Psychology*. Reading, MA: Addison-Wesley.

Kohler, R. & Greenwood, C. (1986). Toward a technology of generalization: The identification of natural contingencies of reinforcement, *Behavior Analyst, 9,* 19–26.

Kondras, O. (1967). The treatment of stammering in children by the shadow method. *Behavior Research & Therapy, 5,* 325–329.

Kopp, H.G. (1963). Eye movements in reading as related to speech dysfunction in male stutterers. *Speech Monographs, 30,* 248.

Korn, E. R. & Johnson, K. (1987). *Visualization: The Uses of Imagery in the Health Professions*. Homewood, IL: Dow Jones-Irwin.

Kraaimaat, F.W., Janssen, P., Van Dam Baggen, R. (1991). *Perceptual and Motor Skills, 72*(3, Pt 1) 766.

Krumboltz, J.D. & Thorensen, C.E. (1969). The effect of behavioral counseling in group and individual settings on information seeking behavior. *Journal of Counseling, Psychology, 11,* 324–333.

Kully, D. & Boberg, E. (1988). An investigation of interclinic agreement in the identification of fluent and stuttered syllables. *Journal of Fluency Disorders, 13,* 309–318.

Kyrios, M., Prio, M., Oberklaid, F. & Demetriou, A. (1989). Cross-cultural studies of temperament: Temperament in Greek infants. *International Journal of Psychology, 24,* 585–603.

La Croix, Z. (1973). Management of disfluent speech through self-recording procedures. *Journal of Speech and Hearing Disorders, 39,* 272–274.

Lahey, M. (1988). *Language Disorders and Language Development*. New York: MacMillan Publishers.

Lambert, M.C., Weisz, J.R. & Knight, F. (1989). Over- and undercontrolled clinic referral problems of Jamaican and American children and adolescents: The culture general and the culture specific. *Journal of Consulting and Clinical Psychology, 57,* 467–472.

Lanyon, R.I. (1967). The measurement of stuttering severity. *Journal of Speech and Hearing Research, 10,* 836–843.

Lawson, M. (1986). A framework for describing strategy use. *Mental Retardation and Learning Disability Bulletin, 14,* 2–19.

Leeper, L. H. & Culatta, R. (1989). Stuttering and dysfluency: Differences and treatment implications. Unpublished manuscript.

Leith, W.R. & Mims, H.A. (1975). Cultural influences in the development and treatment of stuttering: A preliminary report on the black stutterer. *Journal of Speech and Hearing Disorders, 40,* 459–466.

Lemert, E.M. (1952). Stuttering among the North Pacific Coastal Indians. *Southwestern Journal of Anthropology, 8,* 429–441.

Lemert, E.M. (1953). Some Indians who stutter. *Journal of Speech and Hearing Disorders, 18,* 168–174.

Lemert, E.M. (1962). Stuttering and social structure in two Pacific societies. *Journal of Speech and Hearing Disorders, 27,* 3–10.

Lemert, E.M. (1979). A sociological perspective. In J.G. Sheehan (Ed.), *Stuttering: Research and Therapy*. New York: Harper & Row, 172–187.

Leonard, L. (1981). Facilitating linguistic skills in children with specific language impairment. *Applied Psycholinguistics, 2,* 89–118.

Linares, N. (1983). Management of communicatively handicapped Hispanic American children. In D.R. Omark & J.G. Erickson (Eds.), *The Bilingual Exceptional Child*. San Diego: College-Hill Press, 145–162

Luper, H.I. & Mulder, R.I. (1966). *Stuttering Therapy for Children*. Englewood Cliffs, NJ: Prentice-Hall.

Marion, R.L (1981). Strategies for communicating with parents of black exceptional children. *Momentum, 12,* 20–22.

Martin, R.R. (1981). Introduction and perspective: Review of published research. In E. Boberg (Ed.), *Maintenance of Fluency*. Proceeding of the Banff Conference, New York: Elsevier North-Holland, 1–30.

Martin, R.R. & Berndt, L.A. (1970). The effects of time-out on stuttering in a 12 year old boy. *Exceptional Children, 36,* 303–304.

Martin, R.R. & Haroldson, S.K. (1971). Time-out as a punishment for stuttering during conversation. *Journal of Communication Disorders, 4,* 15–19.

Martin, R.R. & Haroldson, S.K. (1979). Effects of five experimental treatments on stuttering. *Journal of Speech and Hearing Research, 22,* 132–146.

Martin, R.R., Haroldson, S.K. & Trident, K.A. (1984). Stuttering and speech naturalness. *Journal of Speech and Hearing Research, 49,* 53–58.

Martin, R.R., Johnson, L.J., Siegel, G.M. & Haroldson, S.K. (1985). Auditory stimulation, rhythm and stuttering. *Journal of Speech and Hearing Research, 28,* 487–495.

Martin, R.R. & Siegel, G.M. (1966a). The effects of response contingent shock on stuttering. *Journal of Speech and Hearing Research, 9,* 340–352.

Martin, R.R. & Siegel, G.M. (1966b). The effects of simultaneously punishing stuttering and rewarding fluency. *Journal of Speech and Hearing Research, 9,* 466–475.

Maslow, A.H. (1968). *Toward a Psychology of Being.* New York: Van Nostrand Reinhold.

Mason, D. & Shine, R. (1981). A follow-up study of fluency training with the young stutterer (Ages 2–9 to 8–0 years). Masters Thesis, East Carolina University, North Carolina.

Matthews, J. (1986). Historical prologue. In G.H. Shames & H. Rubin (Eds.), *Stuttering Then and Now.* Columbus: Charles Merrill.

McCarthy, M.M. (1981). Speech effect of theophylline. *Pediatrics, 6,* 5.

McDonald, E.T. (1964). *A Deep Test of Articulation.* Tucson, AZ: Communication Skill Builders, Inc.

McReynolds, L V. & Elbert, M. (1981). Generalization of correct articulation in clusters. *Applied Psycholinguistics, 2,* 119–132.

McReynolds, L.V. & Kearns, K.P. (1983). *Single-Subject Experimental Designs in Communicative Disorders.* Baltimore: University Park Press.

Meltzer, H. (1935). Talkativeness in stuttering and non-stuttering children. *Journal of Genetic Psychology, 46,* 371–390.

Merits-Patterson, R. & Reed, C.G. (1981). Disfluencies in the speech of language-delayed children. *Journal of Speech and Hearing Research, 24,* 55–58.

Merton, R.K (1957). *Social Theory and Social Structure.* New York: Free Press.

Metz, D.E., Conture, E.G. & Colton, R.H. (1976). Temporal relations between the respiratory and laryngeal systems prior to stuttered disfluencies. *ASHA, 18,* 664.

Meyers, S.C. & Freeman, F.J. (1985). Mother and child speech rate as a variable in stuttering and disfluency. *Journal of Speech and Hearing Research, 28,* 436–444.

Milisen, R. & Johnson, W. (1936). A comparative study of stutterers, former stutterers, and normal speakers whose handedness has been changed. *Archives of Speech, 1,* 61–86.

Miller, S. & Watson, B.C. (1992). The relationship between communication attitude, anxiety, and depression in stutterers and nonstutterers. *Journal of Speech and Hearing Research,* 35(4) 789–798.

Molyneaux, D. & Lane, V.W. (1982). *Effective Interviewing.* New York: Allyn & Bacon.

Moncur, J.P. (1951). Parental domination in stuttering. *Journal of Speech and Hearing Disorders, 17,* 155–165.

Montagu, A. (1972). *Statement on Race: An Annotated Elaboration and Exposition of the Four Statements on Race Issues by the United Nations Educational, Scientific, and Cultural Organization.* New York: Oxford University Press.

Montes, J. & Erickson, J.G. (1990), Bilingual stuttering: Exploring a diagnostic dilemma. *Ethnotes, 1,* 14–15.

Moore, M.S. & Adams, M.R. (1985). The Edinburgh masker: A clinical analog study. *Journal of Fluency Disorders, Vol 10 (4),* 281–290.

Moore, S.E. & Perkins, W.H. (1990). Validity and reliability of judgments of authentic and simulated stuttering. *Journal of Speech and Hearing Disorders, 55,* 383–391.

Moore, W.E. (1959). A study of the blood chemistry of stutterers under two hypnotic conditions. *Speech Monographs, 26,* 64–68.

Morgenstern, J. (1953). Psychological and Social Factors in Children's Stammering. Doctoral Dissertation, University of Edinburgh.

Morgenstern, J. (1956). Socioeconomic factors in stuttering. *Journal of Speech and Hearing Disorders, 21,* 25–33.

Moser, H.M. (1938). A qualitative analysis of eye-movements during stuttering. *Journal of Speech Disorders, 3,* 131–39.

Mowrer, D.E. (1975). An instructional program to increase fluent speech of stutterers. *Journal of Fluency Disorders, 1,* 25–35.

Mowrer, D.E. (1979). *A Program to Establish Fluent Speech.* Columbus: Merrill Publishing Co.

Murphy, A.T. (1982). The clinical process and the speech-language pathologist. In G.H. Shames and E.H. Wiig, *Human Communication Disorders.* Columbus, OH: Merrill, 453–474.

Murray, H.A. (1943). *Thematic Apperception Test.* Cambridge, MA: Harvard University Press.

Murray, F.P. (1958). Observations of therapy for stuttering in Japan. *Journal of Speech and Hearing Disorders, 23,* 243–249.

Nekrasova, Y.B. (1985). Dynamics of psychological states in stutterers in the process of logopsychotherapy. *Voprosy Psikhologii, Mar-Apr, 2,* 127–133.

Nelson, S.E. (1939). The role of heredity in stuttering. *Journal of Pediatrics, 14,* 642–654.

Newsweek (1991). Was he really Bruno Borrowheim?, Feb 18, p.75.

Nicolosi, L., Harryman, E. & Kresheck, J. (1978). *Terminology of Communication Disorders.* Baltimore: The Williams & Wilkins Company.

Nurnberg, H.G. & Greenwald, B. (1981). Stuttering: An unusual side effect of phenothiazines. *American Journal of Psychiatry, 138,* 386–387.

Nurnberger, J.I. & Hingtgen, J.N. (1973). Is symptom substitution an important issue in behavior therapy? *Biological Psychiatry 7, 3,* 221–236.

Nwokah, E.E. (1988). The imbalance of stuttering behavior in bilingual speakers. *Journal of Fluency Disorders, 13, 5* 357–373.

Ojemann, G. & Mateer, C. (1979). Human language cortex: Localization of memory, syntax, and sequential motor-phoneme identification systems. *Science, 205,* 1401–1403.

Okasha, A., Bishry, Z., Kamel, M. & Hassan, A.H. (1974). Psychosocial study of stammering in Egyptian children. *British Journal of Psychiatry, 124,* 531–533.

Orton, S. & Travis, L. (1929). Studies in stuttering: IV. Studies of action currents in stutterers. *Archives of Neurological Psychiatry, 21,* 61–68.

Pancsofar, E. & Bates, P. (1985). The impact of the acquisition of successive training exemplars on generalization. *Journal of the Association for Persons with Severe Handicaps, 10, 2,* 95–104.

Paivio, A. (1971). *Imagery and Verbal Processes.* New York: Holt, Rinehart and Winston.

Pearl, S. & Berenthal, J. (1980). The effect of grammatical complexity on disfluency behavior of nonstuttering preschool children. *Journal of Fluency Disorders, 5,* 55–58.

Peins, M., McGough, W.E. & Lee, Bernard (1984). Double tape recorder therapy. In M. Peins (Ed.), *Contemporary Approaches to Stuttering Therapy.* Boston: Little Brown.

Perigoe, C. & Ling, D. (1986). Generalization of speech skills in hearing-impaired children." *Volta Review, 8, 7,* 351–366.

Perkins, W.H. (1971). *Speech Pathology: An Applied Behavioral Science.* St. Louis, MO: C.V. Mosby.

Perkins, W.H. (1973a). Replacement of stuttering with normal speech: I. Rational. *Journal of Speech Hearing Disorders, 38,* 283–294.

Perkins, W.H. (1973b). Replacement of stuttering with normal speech: II Clinical procedures. *Journal of Speech and Hearing Disorders, 38,* 295–303.

Perkins, W.H. (1975). Articulatory rate in the evaluation of stuttering treatments. *Journal of Speech and Hearing Disorders, 40,* 277–278.

Perkins, W.H. (1979). From psychoanalysis to discoordination. In H.H. Gregory (Ed.), *Controversies About Stuttering Therapy.* Baltimore: University Park Press.

Perkins, W.H. (1981). An alternative to automatic fluency. In *Stuttering Therapy: Transfer and Maintenance.* Memphis: Speech Foundation of America.

Perkins, W.H. (1983). Learning from negative outcomes in stuttering therapy: II An epiphany of failure. *Journal of Fluency Disorders, 8,* 155–160.

Perkins, W.H. (1984). Techniques for establishing fluency. In W.H. Perkins (Ed.), *Stuttering Disorders.* New York: Thieme-Straton.

Perkins, W.H. (1990a). What is stuttering? *Journal of Speech and Hearing Disorders, 55,* 370–382.

Perkins, W.H. (1990b). Gratitude, good intentions, and red herrings: A response to commentaries. *Journal of Speech and Hearing Disorders, 55,* 402–404.

Perkins, W.H. (1991). Preface. In W.H. Perkins (Guest Ed.), Stuttering: Challenges of therapy. *Seminars in Speech and Language 12,* 4, 263–264.

Perkins, W.H., Bell, J., Johnson, L. & Stocks, J. (1979). Phone rate and the effective planning time hypothesis of stuttering. *Journal of Speech and Hearing Research, 22,* 247–255.

Perkins, W.H., Kent, R.D. & Curlee, R.F. (1991). A theory of neuropsycholinguistic function. *Journal of Speech and Hearing Research, 34,* 734–752.

Perkins, W.H., Rudas, J., Johnson, L. & Bell, J. (1976). Stuttering: Discoordination of phonation with articulation and respiration. *Journal of Speech and Hearing Research, 19,* 509–522.

Perls, F.S., Hefferline, R.E. & Goodman, P. (1951). *Gestalt Therapy.* New York: Dell Publishing.

Peters, A.D. (1977). The effect of positive reinforcement of fluency: Two case studies. *Language, Speech and Hearing Services in the Schools, 8,* 15–22.

Peters, T.J. & Guitar, B. (1991). *Stuttering: An Integrated Approach to its Nature and Treatment.* Baltimore, MD: Williams & Wilkins.

Pindzola, R., Jenkins, M. & Loken, K. (1989). Speaking rates of young children. *Language, Speech and Hearing Services in the Schools, 20,* 133–138.

Pindzola, R. & White, D.T. (1986). A protocol for differentiating the incipient stutterer. *Speech and Hearing Services in the Schools, 17,* 2–15.

Pindzola, R.H. (1986). A description of some selected stuttering instruments. *Journal of Childhood Communicative Disorders, 9,* 183–200.

Pinzola, R. H. (1987). *Stuttering Intervention Program.* Tulsa, OK: Modern Education Corporation.

Poulos, M.G. & Webster, W.G. (1991). Family history as a basis for subgrouping people who stutter. *Journal of Speech and Hearing Research, 34,* 5–10.

Powell, S. (1987). Improving critical thinking: A review. *Educational Psychology, 7,* 169–185.

Prins, D. (1970). Improvement and regression in stutterers following short-term intensive ther-

apy. *Journal of Speech Hearing Disorders, 35,* 123–135.

Prins, D. (1984). Treatment of adults: Managing stuttering. In R.F. Curlee & W.H. Perkins (Eds.), *Nature and Treatment of Stuttering.* San Diego: College-Hill Press.

Prins, D. & Miller, M. (1973). Personality, improvement, and regression in stuttering therapy. *Journal of Speech and Hearing Research, 16,* 685–690.

Prins, D. & Nichols, A. (1974). Client impressions of the effectiveness of stuttering therapy. A comparison of two programs. *British Journal of Disorders of Communication, 9,* 123–133.

Pryor, R. (1985). *Live on Sunset Strip.* RCA/Columbia Pictures Home Video.

Purcell, R. & Runyan, C. (1980). Normative study of speech rates of children. *Journal of Speech and Hearing Association of Virginia, 21,* 6–14.

Quader, S.E. (1977). Dysarthria: An unusual side effect of tricyclic antidepressants. *British Medical Journal, 9,* 97.

Quist, R.W. & Martin, R.R. (1967). The effect of response contingent verbal punishment on stuttering. *Journal of Speech and Hearing Research, 10,* 795–800.

Ramig, P.R., Krieger, S.M. & Adams, M.R. (1982). Vocal changes in stutterers and nonstutterers when speaking to children. *Journal of Fluency Disorders, 7,* 369–384.

Ramirez, M. & Castaneda, A. (1974). *Cultural Democracy, Bicognitive Development, and Education.* New York: Academic Press.

Reed, C.G. & Lingwall, J.B. (1976). Some relationships between punishment, stuttering, and galvanic skin responses. *JSHR, 23(2),* 336–343.

Reed, C.G. & Godden, A.L. (1977). An experimental treatment using verbal punishment with two preschool stutterers. *Journal of Fluency Disorders, 2,* 225–233.

Resendiz, R.S. & Fox, R.A. (1985). Reflection-impulsivity in Mexican children: Cross-cultural relationships. *Journal of General Psychology, 112,* 285–290.

Richard, H.C. & Mundy, M.B. (1965). Direct manipulation of stuttering behavior: An experimental-clinical approach. In L.P. Ullmann and L. Krasner (Eds.) *Case Studies in Behavior Modi-*

fication. New York: Holt, Rinehart and Winston.

Richardson, A. (1969). *Mental Imagery*. New York: Springer Pub. Co.

Riley, G. & Riley, J. (1980). Motoric and linguistic variables among children who stutter: A factor analysis. *Journal of Speech and Hearing Disorders, 45*, 4, 504–514.

Riley, G. & Riley, J. (1986). Oral motor discoordination among children who stutter. *Journal of Fluency Disorders, 11*, 4, 335–344.

Riley, G. (1972). A stuttering severity instrument for children and adults. *Journal of Speech and Hearing Disorders, 37*, 314–322.

Riley G.D. & Riley J. (1984). A component model for treating stuttering in children. In M. Peins (Ed.), *Contemporary Approaches in Stuttering Therapy*. Boston, MA: Little Brown.

Robinson, T.L. Jr. & Crowe, T.A. (1987). A comparative study of speech disfluencies in nonstuttering black and white college athletes. *Journal of Fluency Disorders, 12*, 147–156.

Rogers, C.R. (1942). *Counseling and Psychotherapy*. New York: Houghton-Mifflin.

Rogers, C.R. (1951). *Client-Centered Therapy*. New York: Houghton-Mifflin.

Rollin, W.J. (1987). *The Psychology of Communication Disorders in Individuals and Their Families*. Englewood Cliffs, NJ: Prentice-Hall.

Roschach, H. (1937). *Psychodiagnostik. Methodik und Ergebnisse eines wahrnehmungdiagnostischen Experiments*, 3rd. Ed., Berlin: Huber.

Rosenbek, J.C. (1980). Apraxia of speech-relationship to stuttering. *Journal of Fluency Disorders, 5*, 233–253.

Rosenbek, J.C. (1984). Stuttering secondary to nervous system damage. In R. Curlee & W. Perkins (Eds.), *Nature and Treatment of Stuttering: New Directions*. San Diego: College Hill Press.

Rosenbek, J.C., McNeil, M.R., Lemme, M.L., Prescott, T.E. & Alfre, AC. (1975). Speech and language findings in a chronic hemodialysis patient: A case report. *Journal of Speech and Hearing Disorders, 40*, 245–252.

Rosenbek, J.C., Messert, B., Collins, M. & Wertz, R. (1978). Stuttering following brain damage. *Brain and Language, 6*, 82–96.

Rotenberg, K.J. & Cranwell, F.R. (1989). Self-concept in American Indian and white children. *Journal of Cross-Cultural Psychology, 20*, 39–53.

Rubin, H. (1986). Cognitive therapy. In G.H. Shames & H. Rubin (Eds.), *Stuttering: Then and Now*. Columbus: Merrill Publishing Company.

Rubin, H. & Culatta, R. (1971). A point of view about fluency. *ASHA, 13*, 380–384.

Runyan, C.M. & Adams, M.R. (1978). Perceptual study of the speech of "successfully therapeutized" stutterers. *Journal of Fluency Disorders, 3*, 25–39.

Russell, B. (1961). *The Basic Writings of Bertrand Russell*, R.E. Egner and L. E. Denonn (Eds.), New York: Simon & Schuster.

Rustin, L., Ryan, B. & Ryan, B. (1987). Use of the Monterey programmed stuttering therapy in Great Britain. *British Journal of Disorders of Communication, 22*, 151–162.

Ryan, B. (1985). Training the professional. In E. Boberg (Ed.), *Stuttering. Part One. Seminars in Speech and Language*. New York: Thieme-Stratten, Inc.

Ryan, B.P. (1974). *Programmed Therapy for Stuttering in Children and Adults*. Springfield, IL :C.C. Thomas.

Ryan, B.P. & Van Kirk, B. (1983). Programmed stuttering therapy for children; comparison of four establishment programs. *Journal of Fluency Disorders, 8*(4), 291–321.

Ryan, B. (1981). Maintenance programs. In E. Boberg (Ed.), *Maintenance of Fluency*. New York: Elsevier.

Ryan, B. (1992). Articulation, language, rate, and fluency characteristics of stuttering and nonstuttering preschool children. *Journal of Speech and Hearing Research, 35*(2) 333–342.

Ryan, B.P. (1971). Operant procedures applied to stuttering therapy in children. *Journal of Speech and Hearing Disorders, 36*, 264–280.

Ryan, B.P. (1974a). Maintenance programs in progress. In Boberg, E. (Ed.), *Maintenance of Fluency*. New York: Elsevier, 113–146.

Ryan, B.P. (1974b). *Programmed Therapy for Stuttering in Children and Adults*. Springfield, IL: Charles C. Thomas.

Ryan, B.P. (1979). Stuttering therapy in a framework of operant conditioning and programmed learning. In H.H. Gregory (Ed.), *Controversies About Stuttering Therapy*. Baltimore: University Park Press.

Ryan, B.P. (1984). Treatment of stuttering in school children. In W.H. Perkins (Ed.), *Stuttering Disorders*. New York: Thieme-Stratton.

Ryan, B.P. (1986). Operant therapy for children. In G. Shames and H. Rubin (Eds.), *Stuttering Therapy Then and Now*. Columbus, OH: Charles E. Merrill.

Ryan, B.P. & Ryan, B. (1983). Programmed stuttering therapy for children: Comparison of four establishment programs. *Journal of Fluency Disorders 8*, 4, 291–321.

Ryan, B.P. & Van Kirk, B. (1971). *Monterey Fluency Program*. Palo Alto, CA: Monterey Learning Systems.

Ryan, B.P. & Van Kirk, B. (1974). *Programmed Stuttering Therapy for Children. (Final Report, Office of Education Project 0–72–4222)* Washington, DC: U.S. Department of Health, Education and Welfare.

Sabin, E.J., Clemmer, E.J., O'Connell, D.C. & Kowal, A.A. (1979). Pausological approach to speech development. In A.W. Siegman & S. Feldstein (Eds.), *Of Speech and Time*. Hillsdale, NJ: Erlbaum.

Sadker, M., Sadker, & Steindam, S. (1989). Gender equity and educational reform. *Educational Leadership, 46*, 44–47.

Sagen, C. (1977). *The Dragons of Eden*. New York: Ballantine Books.

Saleh, M.A. (1986). Cultural perspectives: Implications for counselling in the Arab world. *School Psychology International, 7*, 71–76.

Samuels, M. & Samuels, N. (1975). *Seeing Through the Mind's Eye*. New York: Random House.

Saskia, K., Janssen, P., Kraaimaat, F. & Brutten, G.J. (1992). Communicative Style of mothers of incipient stutterers prior to onset. American Speech-Language-Hearing Association Annual Convention, San Antonio.

Satir, V. (1967). *Conjoint Family Therapy (Rev. Ed.)* Palo Alto, CA:Science and Behavior Books.

Scheflen, A.E. (1967). On the structuring of human communication. *American Behavioral Scientist, 10*, 8, 8–12.

Scheuerle, J. (1992). *Counseling in Speech-Language Pathology and Audiology*. New York: MacMillian Publishers.

Schnidler, M.D. (1955). A study of educational adjustments of stuttering and non-stuttering children. In W. Johnson & R.R. Lentenberger, (Eds.), *Stuttering in Children and Adults*. Minneapolis: University of Minnesota Press.

Schuell, H. (1946). Sex differences in relation to stuttering. *Journal of Speech and Hearing Disorders, 11*, 277–298.

Schwartz, M. (1977). *Stuttering Solved*. New York: Lippencott.

Seeman, J. (1986). Client-Centered Therapy. In G.H. Shames & H. Rubin (Eds.), *Stuttering Then and Now*. Columbus: Charles Merrill.

Seeman, M. (1937). The significance of twin pathology for the investigation of speech disorders. *Archive Gesamte Phonetik, Part II, 1*, 88–92.

Seltzer, H. & Culatta, R. (1979). A modeling approach to stuttering therapy for young children. *Journal of Childhood Communication Disorders, 3*, 103–110.

Shames, G.H. (1986). A current view of stutter-free speech. In G.H. Shames & H. Rubin (Eds.), *Stuttering Then and Now*. Columbus, OH: Charles Merrill.

Shames, G.H. (1989). Stuttering: An RFP for a cultural perspective. *Journal of Fluency Disorders, 14*, 67–77.

Shames, G.H. (1990). Disorders of fluency. In G.H. Shames & E.H. Wiig (Eds.), *Human Communication Disorders* (3rd ed.). Columbus: Merrill Publishing Co, 311.

Shames, G.H. & Beams, H.L. (1956). Incidence of stuttering in older age groups. *Journal of Speech and Hearing Disorders, 21*, 313–316.

Shames, G.H. & Egolf, D.B. (1976). *Operant Conditioning and the Management of Stuttering. A Book for Clinicians*. Englewood Cliffs, NJ: Prentice-Hall.

Shames, G.H. & Florence, C.L. (1980). *Stutter-free Speech: A Goal for Therapy*. Columbus, OH: Charles Merrill.

Shames, G.H. & Rubin, H. (1986). *Stuttering Then and Now*. Columbus, OH: Charles Merrill.

Shames, G.H. & Sherrick, C.E., Jr. (1963). A discussion of nonfluency and stuttering as operant behavior. *Journal of Speech and Hearing Research, 28*, 3–18.

Shane, M.L.S. (1955). Effect on stuttering of alteration in auditory feedback. In W. Johnson

& R.R. Leutenegger (Eds.), *Stuttering in Children and Adults*. Minneapolis: University of Minnesota Press.

Shapiro, A.I. (1980). An electromyographic analysis of the fluent and dysfluent utterances of several types of stutterers. *Journal of Fluency Disorders, 5*, 203–231.

Shaw, C.K. and Strum, W.F. (1972). The effects of response-contingent reward on the connected speech of children who stutter. *Journal of Speech and Hearing Disorders 7*, 75–88.

Shearer, W.M. (1966). Behavior of middle ear muscle during stuttering. *Science, 152*, 1280.

Sheehan, J. & Martyn, M.M. (1966). Spontaneous recovery from stuttering. *Journal of Speech and Hearing Research, 9*, 121–135.

Sheehan, J.C. (1975). Conflict theory and avoidance-reduction therapy. In J. Eisenson (Ed.), *Stuttering: A Second Symposium*. New York: Harper & Row.

Sheehan, J.G. (1953). Theory and treatment of stuttering as an approach-avoidance conflict. *Journal of Psychology, 36*, 27–49.

Sheehan, J.G. (1958). Conflict theory of stuttering. In J. Eisenson (Ed.), *Stuttering: A Symposium*. New York: Harper & Row.

Sheehan, J.G. (1970). *Stuttering: Research and Therapy*. New York: Harper & Row.

Sheehan, J.G. (1980). Problems in the evaluation of progress and outcome. In W.H. Perkins (Guest Ed.), Strategies in Stuttering Therapy, Vol. 14 of Northern, J.L (Ed.), *Seminars in Speech, Language and Hearing*, 389–401.

Sheehan, J.G. (1984). Problems in the evaluation of progress and outcome. In W.H. Perkins (Ed.), *Stuttering Disorders*. New York: Thieme-Stratton.

Sheehan, J.G., Hadley, R. & Gould, E. (1967). Impact of authority on stuttering. *Journal Abnormal Psychology, 72*, 290–293.

Sheehan, J.G. & Voas, R.B. (1954). Tension patterns during stuttering in relation to conflict, anxiety-binding, and reinforcement. *Speech Monograph, 21*, 272–279.

Shine, R.E. (1980a). *Systematic Fluency Training for Children : A Fluency Training Kit*. Tigard, OR: C.C. Publications.

Shine, R. (1980b). Direct management of the beginning stutterer. In W. Perkins (Ed.), *Strategies in Stuttering Therapy: Seminars in Speech,*

Language and Hearing. New York: Thieme-Stratton.

Shine, R. (1983). Helping the stuttering child. *North Carolina Medical Journal, 44*, 12, 795–799.

Shine, R. (1984). Assessment and fluency training with the young stutterer. In M. Peins (Ed.), *Contemporary Approaches in Stuttering Therapy*. Boston: Little Brown & Company.

Shine, R. (1988). *Systematic Fluency Training for Young Children: Third Edition*. Austin, Texas: Pro-Ed.

Shipley, K.G. (1992). *Interviewing and Counseling in Communicative Disorders*. New York:MacMillan Publishers.

Shriberg, L. & Kwiatkowski, J. (1987). A retrospective study of spontaneous generalization in speech-delayed children. *Language, Speech and Hearing Services in Schools, 18*, 172–178.

Shumak, I.C. (1955). A speech situation rating sheet for stutterers. In W. Johnson (Ed.), *Stuttering in Children and Adults: Thirty Years of Research at the University of Iowa*. Minneapolis: University of Minneapolis Press, 341–347.

Siegel, G.M. (1970). Punishment, stuttering, and disfluency. *Journal of Speech and Hearing Research, 13*, 677–714.

Siegle, G.M. & Hauagen, D. (1964). Audience size and variations in stuttering behavior. *Journal of Speech and Hearing Research, 7*, 381–388.

Silverman, E.M. & Zimmer, C.H. (1982). Demographic characteristics and treatment experiences of women and men who stutter. *Journal of Fluency Disorders, 7*, 273–285.

Silverman, F.H. (1980). The stuttering problem profile: A task that assists both client and clinician in defining therapy goals. *Journal of Speech and Hearing Disorders, 45*, 119–123.

Silverman, F.H. (1983). *Legal Aspects of Speech-Language Pathology and Audiology*. Englewood Cliffs, NJ: Prentice-Hall.

Silverman, F.H. (1992). *Stuttering and Other Fluency Disorders*. Englewood Cliffs, NJ: Prentice-Hall.

Silverman, F.H. (1970). A note on the degree of adaptation by stutterers and nonstutterers' during oral reading.

Silverman, F.H. & Goodban, M.T. (1972). The effect of auditory masking on the fluency of normal speakers. *Journal of Speech and Hearing Research, 14,* 525–530.

Snidecor, J C. (1947). Why the Indian does not stutter. *Quarterly Journal of Speech, 38,* 493–495.

Snidecor, J.C. (1955). Tension and facial appearance in stuttering. In W. Johnson & R.R. Leutenegger (Eds.), *Stuttering in Children and Adults.* Minneapolis: University of Minnesota Press.

Sommer, R. (1978). *The Mind's Eye: Imagery in Everyday Life.* New York: Delacorte Press.

Sperber, D. (1986). Salvaging parts of the "classical theory" of categorization. *Behavioral and Brain Sciences, 9.*

St. Louis, K.O. & Hinzman, A.R. (1988). A descriptive study of speech, language, and hearing characteristics of school-aged stutterers. *Journal of Fluency Disorders, 13*(5) 331–355.

Stager, S., Ludlow, C., Gordon, C., Cotelingham, M. & Rapoport, J. (1994). Maintenance of fluency following long-term clomipramine treatment. First World Congress on Fluency Disorders, Munich, Germany, August, 1994.

Starkweather, C.W. (1980). A multiprocess behavioral approach to stuttering therapy. *Seminars in Speech, Language and Hearing, 1,* 327–337.

Starkweather, C.W. (1987). *Fluency and Stuttering.* Englewood Cliffs, NJ: Prentice Hall.

Starkweather, C.W. (1990) Current trends in therapy for stuttering children and suggestions for future research. *ASA Reports, ASHA.*

Starkweather, C.W. (1992). Response and reaction to Hamre, "Stuttering Prevention I." *Journal of Fluency Disorders, 17,* 43–55.

Starkweather, C.W., Gottwald, S.R. & Halfond, M.M. (1990). *Stuttering Prevention: A Clinical Method.* Englewood Cliffs, NJ: Prentice-Hall.

Stefankiewicz & Bloodstein (1974). The effect of a 4 week interval on the consistency of stuttering. *Journal of Speech and Hearing Research, 17,* 141–145.

Stevens, H. (1986). Is it organic or is it functional: Is it hysteria or malingering. *Psychiatric Clinics of North America, 60.*

Stewart, J.L. (1971). Cross-cultural studies and linguistic aspects of stuttering. *Journal of the All India Institute of Speech and Hearing, 2,* 1–6.

Stewart, J.L. (1983). Communication disorders in the American Indian population. In D.R. Omark & J.G. Erickson (Eds.), *The Bilingual Exceptional Child.* San Diego: College-Hill Press, 181–195

Stockard, J. & Johnson, M.M. (1980). *Sex Roles: Sex Inequality and Sex Role Development.* Englewood Cliffs, NJ: Prentice-Hall.

Stocker, B., & Gerstman, L.J. (1983). A comparison of the probe technique and conventional therapy for young stutterers. *Journal of Fluency Disorders, 8,* 331–339.

Stokes, T. & Baer, D. (1978). An implicit technology of generalization. *Journal of Applied Behavior Analyst, 11,* 285–303.

Stromsta, C. (1965). A spectrographic study of dysfluencies labeled as stuttering by parents. *De Therapia Vocis et Loguela, 1,* XIII. Congress of the International Society of Logopedics and Phoniatrics.

Taylor, O.L. (1989). Old wine and new bottles: Some things change yet remain the same. ASHA, 31, 9, 72–73.

Taylor, O.L. (In Press). In L. Cole & V.R. Deal, *Communication Disorders in Multicultural Populations.* Rockville, MD: American Speech-Language-Hearing Association.

Thagard, P. (1986). The pragmatics of induction. *Behavioral and Brain Sciences, 9,* 668–669.

Tint, D. (1984). Rate Assessment and Dysfluent Behaviors in Normal Spanish-Speaking Children. Unpublished manuscript. Temple University, Philadelphia.

Toliver-Weddington, G. & Meyerson, M.D. (1983). Training paraprofessionals for identification and intervention with communicatively disordered bilinguals. In D.R. Omark & J.G. Erickson (Eds.), *The Bilingual Exceptional Child.* San Diego: College-Hill Press, 379–396.

Toronto, A.S. & Merrill, S.M. (1983). Developing local normed assessment instruments. In D.R. Omark & J.G. Erickson (Eds.), *The Bilingual Exceptional Child.* San Diego: College-Hill Press, 105–121.

Toscher, M.M. & Rupp, R.R. (1978). A study of the central auditory processes in stutterers using the Synthetic Sentence Identification (SSI) Test battery. *Journal of Speech and Hearing Research, 21*(4) 779–792.

Travis, L.E. (1957). The unspeakable feelings of people with special reference to stuttering. In

L.E. Travis (Ed.), *Handbook of Speech Pathology*. New York: Appleton-Century-Crofts.

Travis, L.E. (1978). The cerebral dominance theory of stuttering. *Journal of Speech and Hearing Disorders, 43,* 278–281.

Travis, L.E. & Knott, J.R. (1936). Brain potentials from normal speakers and stutterers. *Journal of Speech Disorders, 2* 239–41.

Travis, L.E. & Malamud, W. (1937). Brain potentials from normal subjects, stutterers, and schizophrenic patients. *American Journal of Psychiatry, 93,* 929–936.

Ulliana & Ingham (1984). Behavioral and nonbehavioral variables in the measurement of stutterers' communication attitudes. *Journal of Speech and Hearing Research, 49,* 83–93.

Van Riper, C. (1939). *Speech Correction: Principles and Methods.* New York: Prentice-Hall.

Van Riper, C. (1958). Experiments in stuttering therapy. In J. Eisenson (Ed.), *Stuttering: A Symposium.* New York: Harper & Row.

Van Riper, C. (1968). *Stuttering Successes and Failures. Publication #6.* Memphis, TN: Speech Foundation of America.

Van Riper, C. (1971). *The Nature of Stuttering.* Englewood Cliffs, NJ: Prentice-Hall.

Van Riper, C. (1973). *The Treatment of Stuttering.* Englewood Cliffs, NJ: Prentice-Hall.

Van Riper, C. (1978). *Speech Correction* (6th Ed.) Englewood Cliffs, NJ: Prentice-Hall.

Van Riper, C. (1982). *The Nature of Stuttering.* Englewood Cliffs, NJ: Prentice-Hall.

Vealey, R.S. (1986). Imagery training for performance enhancement. In J.M. William (Ed.), *Applied Sport Psychology,* pp 209–234, California: Mayfield Pub.

Waddle, P. (1934). *A Comparison of Speech Defectives Among Colored and White Children.* Thesis. University of Iowa, Iowa City, Iowa.

Wakefield, L. (1985). Non-fluent Behaviors in Normal Spanish-Speaking Adults. Unpublished manuscript. Temple University, Philadelphia.

Wall, M.J. & Meyers, F.L. (1982). A review of linguistic factors associated with early childhood stuttering. *Journal of Communication Disorders, 15,* 441–449.

Wall, M.J. & Meyers, F.L. (1984). *Clinical Management of Childhood Stuttering.* Austin, TX: Pro-Ed.

Webster, R. (1979). Empirical considerations regarding stuttering therapy. In H.H. Gregory (Ed.), *Controversies About Stuttering Therapy.* Baltimore: University Park Press.

Webster, R.L. (1974). A behavioral analysis of stuttering: Treatment and theory. In Calhoun, K.S., Adams, H.E. & Mitchell, H.E. (Eds.), *Innovative Treatment Methods in Psychopathology.* New York: Wiley, 17–61.

Webster, R.L. (1980). Evolution of a target based behavioral therapy for stuttering. *Journal of Fluency Disorders, 5,* 303–320.

Webster, R.L. & Dorman, M.F. (1970). Decreases in stuttering frequency as a function of continuous and contingent forms of auditory masking. *Journal of Speech and Hearing Research, 14,* 307–311.

Webster, R.L., Stigora, J.A., Monkhouse, K.A. & Goebel, M.A. (1991). Technology and fluency building with various patient populations. American Speech, Language, Hearing Association, Annual Meeting, Atlanta, GA.

Webster, W.G. (1990). Motor performance of stutterers: A search for mechanisms. *Journal of Motor Behavior, 22,* 4 553–571.

Wei, T.T.D. (1983). The Vietnamese refugee child: Understanding cultural differences.In D.R. Omark & J.G. Erickson (Eds.), *The Bilingual Exceptional Child.* San Diego: College-Hill Press, 197–212

Weiner, A.E. (1978). Vocal control therapy for stutterers: A trial program. *Journal of Fluency Disorders, 3,* 115–126.

Weiner, A.E. (1984). Vocal control therapy for stutterers. In M. Peins (Ed.), *Contemporary Approaches in Stuttering Therapy.* Boston: Little Brown & Company.

Weiss, A.L. & Zebrowski, P.M. (1991). Patterns of assertiveness and responsiveness in parental interactions with stuttering and fluent children. *Journal of Fluency Disorders, 16*(2–3) 125–141.

Wepman, J.M. (1935). Is stuttering inherited? *Proceedings of the American Speech Correction Association, 5,* 39–52.

Wepman, J.M. (1939). Familial incidence in stammering. *Journal of Speech Disorders, 4,* 199–204.

Wertz, R.T., Collins, M.J., Weiss, D., Kurtske, J.K., Friden, T., Brookshsire, R.H., Pierce, J.,

Holtzapple, P., Hubbard, D.J., Porch, B.E., West, J.A., Davis, L., Matovick, V., Morle, G.K., Resurrection, E. (1981). Veterans Administration cooperative study on aphasia: A comparison of individual and group treatment. *Journal of Speech and Hearing Research, 24,* 580–594.

Wertz, R.T., Weiss, D.G., Arew, J.A., Brookshire, R.A., Garcia-Bunvel, L., Holland, A.L., Kurtzke, J.F., LaPointe, L.L., Miliatti, F.J., Brannegan, R., Greenbaum, H., Marchall, R.C., Vogul, D., Carter, J., Barnes, W.S., Goodman, R. (1986). Comparison of clinic, home and defined language treated for aphasia. *Archives of Neurology, 43,* 653–658.

West, R., Nelson, S., Berry, M.F. (1939). The heredity of stuttering. *Quarterly Journal of Speech, 25,* 23–30.

Wexler, K.B. (1982). Developmental disfluency in 2-, 4- and 6-year old boys in neutral and stress situations. *Journal of Speech and Hearing Research, 25,* 229–234.

Wilfling & McNeill (1975). Biofeedback treatment for stuttering. *Journal of Speech and Hearing Disorders, 40,* 270–273.

Williams, D.E. (1957). A point of view about "stuttering." *Journal of Hearing Disorders, 22,* 390–397.

Williams, D.E. (1971). Stuttering therapy for children. In L.E. Travis (Ed.), *Handbook of Speech Pathology.* New York: Appleton-Century-Crofts.

Williams, D.E. (1978). The problem of stuttering. In F.L. Darley & D.C. Spriestersbach, (Eds.), *Diagnostic Methods in Speech Pathology.* New York: Harper & Row.

Williams, D.E. (1979). A perspective on approaches to stuttering therapy. In H.H. Gregory (Ed.), *Controversies About Stuttering Therapy.* Baltimore: University Park Press.

Williams, D.E., Darley, F.L. & Spriestersbach, D.C. (1978) In F.L. Darley & D.C. Spriestersbach, (Eds.), *Diagnostic Methods in Speech Pathology.* New York: Harper & Row.

Williams, R.L. (1973). *Black Intelligence Test of Cultural Homogeneity (BITCH).* St. Louis: Williams & Associates.

Wingate, M.E. (1962). Evaluation and stuttering. Part I: Speech characteristics of young children. *Journal of Speech and Hearing Disorders, 27,* 106–115.

Wingate, M.E. (1964). A standard definition of stuttering. *Journal of Speech and Hearing Disorders, 29,* 484–489.

Wingate, M.E. (1975). Expectancy as basically a short-term process. *Journal of Speech and Hearing Research, 18,* 31–42.

Winner, M. & Elbert, M. (1988). Evaluating the treatment effect of repeated probes. *Journal of Speech and Hearing Disorders, 53,* 211–218.

Wischner, G.J. (1950). Stuttering behavior and learning: A preliminary theoretical formulation. *Journal of Speech and Hearing Disorders, 15,* 329–335.

Wolpe, J. (1958). *Psychotherapy by Reciprocal Inhibition.* Stanford, CA: Stanford University Press.

Wood, F., Stump, D., McKeehan, A., Sheldon, S. & Proctor, J. (1980). Patterns of regional cerebral blood flow during attempted reading aloud by stutterers both on and off haloperidol medication: Evidence for inadequate left frontal activation during stuttering. *Brain Language, 9,* 141–144.

Woods, T. (1987), Programming common antecedents: A practical strategy for enhancing the generality of learning. *Behavioral Psychotherapy, 15,* 158–180.

Woolf, G. (1967). The assessment of stuttering as struggle, avoidance and expectancy. *British Journal of Disorders of Communication, 2,* 158–177.

Yairi, E. (1981). Disfluencies of normally speaking 2 year old children. *Journal of Speech and Hearing Research, 24,* 490–495.

Yairi, E. (1983). The onset of stuttering in two- and three-year old children: A preliminary report. *Journal of Speech and Hearing Research, 48,* 171–178.

Yairi, E. & Ambrose, N. (1992). A longitudinal study of stuttering in children: A preliminary report. *JSHR, 35,* 755–788.

Yairi, E. & Clifton, N.F., Jr. (1972). Disfluent speech behavior of preschool children, high school seniors and geriatric persons. *Journal of Speech and Hearing Research, 15,* 714–719.

Yairi, E., & Lewis, E. (1984). Disfluencies at the onset of stuttering. *Journal of Speech and Hearing Research, 27,* 155–159.

Yairi, E., & Williams, D.E. (1971). Reports of parental attitudes by stuttering & by nonstuttering children. *Journal of Speech and Hearing Research, 14*, 596–604.

Yeakle, M.K. & Cooper E.B. (1986). Teacher perceptions of stuttering. *Journal of Fluency Disorders, 11*(4) 345–359.

Yetman, N.R. (Ed.), (1985). *Majority and Minority: The Dynamics of Racial and Ethnic Relations* (4th Ed.). Boston: Allyn and Bacon.

Young, M.A. (1984). Identification of stuttering and stutterers. In R.F. Curlee & W.H. Perkins (Eds.), *Nature and Treatment of Stuttering: New Directions.* San Diego:College-Hill Press.

Zebrowski, P.E. & Schum, R. (1993). Counsel parents of children who stutter. *American Journal of Speech-Language Pathology, 2*, 265–74.

Zeskind, P.S. (1983). Cross-cultural differences in maternal perceptions of cries of low- and high-risk infants. *Child Development, 54*, 1119–1128.

Zimmerman, G. (1980). Stuttering: A disorder of movement. *Journal of Speech and Hearing Research, 23*, 122–36.

Zimmerman, G., Liljeblad, S., Frank, A. & Cleeland, C.(1983). The Indians have many terms for it: Stuttering among the Bannock-Shosoni. *Journal of Speech and Hearing Research, 26*, 315–318.

Author Index

Adams, M.R., 10, 42–43, 75, 98, 103, 106, 134, 202, 205, 228
Ager, A., 196
Alfre, A.C., 36
Allen, C.P., 202
Alwell, M., 197
Ambrose, N., 96, 134
Ammons, L.J., 248
Andrews, G., 10, 16, 58, 75, 78, 104, 117, 119, 133, 141, 160, 161, 190, 191, 196, 202, 203, 205, 206
Arew, J.A., 160
Aron, M.L., 114, 117, 119
Aronson, A.E., 35, 36, 44
Arthur, B., 133
Austin, W.T.S., 172, 228
Azrin, N.H., 19, 167, 178, 180, 184, 250

Baer, D.M., 159, 195
Baker, L., 134
Bandura, A., 242
Barbara, D.A., 12
Barber, V., 32, 97, 106
Barnes, W.S., 160
Bass, C., 104–5
Beams, H.L., 6
Bebout, L., 133
Bell, J., 11, 103, 173
Benjamin, A., 53, 54
Berndt, L.A., 106
Berry, M.F., 10
Bishry, Z., 119
Blood, G.W., 134
Bloodstein, O., 6, 9, 10, 12, 13, 14, 15, 17, 19, 20, 26, 28, 31, 32, 42, 56, 70,

74, 96, 98, 115, 117, 119, 120, 133, 173, 190, 202, 204
Boberg, E., 21, 159, 203, 204, 211, 212
Bond, L., 155
Borden, G.J., 167
Brady, J.P., 106
Brady, W.A., 119, 133, 134
Brannegan, R., 160
Brash, H.M., 172, 228
Brayton, E.R., 106
Briggs, K.A., 118
Brookshire, R., 160
Brown, J.R., 35, 36, 44
Bruce, M.C., 103
Brutten, E.J., 14, 15, 16, 104, 120, 161, 163, 170, 178, 181, 183, 213–15
Bubenickova, M., 134
Bulatta, R., 133
Bullen, A.K., 114
Burlee, R.F., 4–5
Butler, R.B., 35
Butterworth, B., 42

Cady, B.B., 103
Campbell, J., 123
Canter, G.J., 35, 36
Cantwell, D.P., 134
Caplan, L., 35
Carroll, P.J., 97, 106
Carter, J., 160
Castaneda, A., 123
Cheng, L.R.I., 123, 126
Cherry, C., 32, 106
Chinn, P., 111, 112, 124
Christensen, J.E., 103

Cleary, P.J., 105
Clemmer, E.J., 42
Clifford, S., 117
Clifton, N.F., Jr., 41
Colburn, N., 42
Cole, L., 111, 124, 126
Coleman, K., 186–87
Collins, M., 35, 160
Colton, R.J., 167
Commodore, R.W., 103
Conti, D.M., 41, 42, 43
Conture, E.G., 106, 144, 154, 155, 167
Cooper, C.S., 66, 79, 80–81, 84, 86, 92,
       117, 144, 154, 180, 215, 216, 269
Cooper, E., 13–14, 66, 79, 80–81, 84, 86,
       92, 103, 117, 121, 134, 144, 154,
       161, 163, 180, 190–91, 215, 216,
       269
Costello, J., 74, 75, 78, 98, 101, 104, 121,
       144, 178, 183, 184, 205, 218
Costello, J.C., 195
Costello, J.M., 105, 134, 149, 158, 187,
       190, 191
Cotelingham, M., 173
Craig, A., 16, 58, 104, 105, 133, 160, 161,
       196
Craven, D.C., 195
Cronbach, L., 122
Crowe, T.A., 134
Culatta, R.A., 4, 21, 23, 34, 36, 39, 40, 41,
       42, 75, 76, 80–81, 105, 119, 120,
       122, 133, 137, 144, 161, 162, 163,
       174–75, 182, 194, 205, 218–19,
       242–43, 266, 270
Culp, D.M., 79, 80–81, 220–21
Curlee, R.F., 221–22, 240, 270

Daly, D.A., 102, 168, 202, 203, 222–23,
       264, 266, 270
Darley, F.L., 35, 36, 44, 69, 70, 72, 73, 77,
       81, 86, 89
Davis, L., 160
Deal, J.L., 38, 39
Deal, V.R., 124, 126
Dell, C., 155, 223–25
Dempsey, G.L., 39
Dewar, A.D., 172, 228
Dinnsen, D., 197
Donahue-Kilburg, G., 151, 155
Dorman, M.F., 171

Douglas, E., 7
Doza, M., 133
Dunlap, K., 17
Dunn, R., 123

Edgren, B., 173
Egolf, D.B., 21, 52, 106, 121, 122, 154,
       163, 182
Eisenson, J., 14, 97
Elbert, M., 197
Ellis, A., 153
Erickson, J.G., 120, 124
Erickson, R.L., 66
Eversham, M., 195

Falconer, D.S., 11
Farver, J.A., 123
Fetz, D.L., 171
Feyer, A.M., 16, 58, 133, 160, 161,
       196
Fink, H., 133
Finn, P., 24
Flanagan, B., 19, 178, 184
Florance, C.L., 14, 53, 103, 104, 105, 141,
       142, 174, 180, 190, 194, 196, 201,
       244–45, 264, 266
Fox, R.A., 123
Fransella, F., 195
Frazier, N., 124
Freeman, F.J., 75, 134, 155
Friden, T., 160

Garcia-Bunvel, L., 160
Gemake, J., 123
Gerber, S.E., 158
Gerstman, L.J., 188
Gierut, J., 197
Gillespie, S.K., 117
Gladstein, K.L., 134
Glasner, P.H., 116
Glogowski, K., 119
Godden, A.L., 103
Goebel, M.A., 225–26, 270
Goetz, L., 197
Goldberg, S.A., 4, 11, 21, 66, 78, 80–81,
       82, 86, 89, 98, 103, 119, 120, 124,
       126, 133, 144, 151, 154, 155, 156,
       161, 162, 163, 173, 174, 180, 183,
       184, 190, 194, 204, 226, 228, 260,
       267, 270

Goldiamond, I., 19, 20, 103, 174, 178, 184, 240
Goldman, R., 117, 119
Goldman-Eisler, F., 42
Gollnick, D., 111, 112, 124
Goodenough, W., 111
Goodman, P., 154
Goodman, R., 160
Gordon, C., 173
Gorman, W.F., 40
Gottwald, S.R., 158, 204
Gould, E., 201
Granich, M., 39
Greenbaum, H., 160
Greenwald, B., 37
Gregory, H.H., 158, 190, 229–30
Guitar, B.E., 104–5, 133, 144, 154, 155, 190, 192, 202, 204, 205, 206, 234–36

Hadley, R., 201
Halfond, M.M., 158, 204
Hall, D.E., 41, 42, 43, 119, 134
Hall, E.T., 121
Hall, J.W., 171
Halvorson, J.A., 133, 178, 179
Ham, R.E., 144
Hanna, E.P., 205
Hannley, M., 171
Haroldson, S., 76, 103, 105, 106
Harris, M., 117, 119
Harryman, E., 4
Harvey, R., 78
Hassan, A.H., 119
Haugen, D., 133
Healey, E.C., 134
Hedge, M.N., 104
Hefferline, R.E., 154
Hejna, R., 147
Helm, N.A., 35
Helm-Estabrooks, N., 34, 36
Helmreich, H.G., 42
Hill, D., 229–30
Hill, H., 172, 173
Hillis, J.W., 193
Hingtgen, J.N., 133
Hinzman, A.R., 134
Hird, J.S., 171
Hoddinott, S., 16, 58, 160, 161, 196
Hoffman, L.W., 121

Holland, A.L., 160
Holtzapple, P., 160
Homzie, M.J., 134
Horowitz, E., 97
Howes, C., 123
Howie, P., 10–11, 16, 21, 58, 133, 160, 161, 190, 191, 196, 202, 203, 204, 206
Hubbard, D.J., 160
Hunt, P., 197
Hunter, C.E., 133, 195
Hutchinson, J.M., 106

Ingham, R.J., 6, 9, 10, 11, 14, 15, 20, 24, 74, 75, 78, 84, 97, 98, 101, 103, 104, 106, 121, 133, 141, 144, 155, 159, 173, 196, 203, 205, 217–18, 230–31
Inness, M., 97

Jacobson, E., 15, 168
Jalali, F., 123
James, J.E., 106, 133, 195
Janssen, P., 15, 16, 133, 167, 178
Jenkins, M., 75
Jerger, J., 171
Johns, D.F., 35
Johnson, G.F., 186–87
Johnson, L.J., 11, 103, 104, 106, 171, 173, 186–87
Johnson, M.M., 124
Johnson, P., 52, 121, 182
Johnson, W., 14, 16, 17, 32, 58, 97, 103, 106, 114, 116, 120
Jung, C.G., 153

Kamel, M., 119
Kamhi, A.G., 204
Karr, G.M., 171
Kaspirison-Burelli, A., 52, 121, 182
Kearns, K.P., 3, 102
Kelly, E., 155
Kent, R.D., 4–5
Kent, R.G., 34, 133
Kenyon, E., 10
Kidd, J.R., 10
Kidd, K.K., 10, 134
Kidd, R.D., 32, 118, 133, 204
Kluckhohn, C., 113
Knight, F., 118, 124
Knott, J.R., 32

Kondras, O., 106
Korn, E.R., 171
Kowal, A.A., 42
Kraaimaat, F.W., 15, 16, 133
Kresheck, J., 4
Krieger, S.M., 202
Krumboltz, J.D., 154
Kuhl, P., 103
Kully, D., 159, 211, 212
Kurtske, J., 160

La Croix, Z., 105
Lambert, M.C., 118, 124
Landers, D.M., 171
Lanyon, R.I., 86, 89
LaPointe, L.L., 160
Leanderson, R., 173
Lee, B., 193, 194
Leeper, L., 23, 34, 36, 39, 40, 41, 42, 75,
        76, 119, 133
Leith, W.R., 120
Lemert, E.M., 113, 114, 115, 117
Lemme, M.L., 36
Levi, L., 173
Lewis, E., 15, 25, 26
Ling, D., 197
Lingwall, J.B., 103, 133
Loken, K., 75
Ludlow, C., 173
Luper, J.I., 80–81, 82, 102, 189, 232–33

McCarthy, M.M., 37
McDonald, E.T., 104
McGough, W.E., 193, 194
McNeil, M.R., 36
McOsker, T.G., 204
McReynolds, L.V., 3, 102
Marchall, R.C., 160
Marland, P.M., 32
Martin, N., 133
Martin, R.R., 20, 76, 103, 105, 106, 204
Martyn, M.M., 161, 163
Mason, D., 248
Matovick, V., 160
Matthews, J., 9
Merits-Patterson, R., 41
Messert, B., 35
Metz, D.E., 167
Meyers, F.L., 41, 253–54
Meyers, S.C., 75, 134, 155

Miliatti, F.J., 160
Miller, M., 238
Miller, S., 133
Mims, H.A., 120
Montes, J., 120, 124
Moore, M.S., 228
Moore, W.E., 173
Morgenstern, J., 114, 116, 133
Morle, G.K., 160
Mowrer, D.E., 186, 233–34, 270
Mulder, R.I., 80–81, 82, 102, 189, 232–33
Mundy, M.B., 186
Murray, H.A., 13
Mysak, E.D., 42

Neilson, M., 16, 58, 160, 161, 196
Nekrasova, Y.B., 134
Nelson, S.E., 10
Nichols, A., 238
Nicolosi, L., 4
Niebergall, G., 133
Norris, G.M., 106
Nunn, R.G., 167, 180, 250
Nurnberg, H.G., 37
Nurnberger, J.I., 133
Nwokah, E.E., 133

O'Connell, D.C., 42
Okasha, A., 119
Orton, S., 9–10
Owen, N., 205

Packman, A.C., 75, 98, 106
Page, J.L., 75, 76
Paivio, A., 171
Peins, M., 193, 194
Perigoe, C., 197
Perkins, W., 4–5, 11, 21, 25, 75, 84, 103,
        133, 173, 182, 191, 204, 205,
        221–22, 240, 259, 267, 270
Perls, F.S., 154
Peters, A.D., 104
Peters, T.J., 144, 154, 155, 190, 192, 205,
        234–36
Pierce, J., 160
Pindzola, R.H., 26, 75, 82, 236–37
Popelka, G., 106
Porch, B.E., 160
Poulos, M.G., 10
Prescott, T.E., 36

Prins, D., 237–38
Purcell, R., 75

Quader, S.E., 37
Quarrington, B., 7
Quist, R.W., 103

Ramig, P.R., 98, 106, 202
Ramirez, M., 123
Rapoport, J., 173
Rasmussen, K., 186–87
Records, M.A., 10
Reed, C.G., 41, 103, 133
Resendiz, R.S., 123
Resurrection, E., 160
Ricciandelli, L.A., 133, 195
Richardson, A., 171
Riley, G.D., 80–81, 82, 83, 134, 152, 154,
    236, 239–40
Riley, J., 134, 152, 154, 239–40
Robbins, C.J., 103
Rogers, C.R., 13, 145, 153
Rogers, P., 133, 195
Rollin, W.J., 153, 182, 201
Rorschach, J., 13
Rosen, L., 97, 103, 106
Rosenbek, J.C., 34, 35, 36
Rubin, H., 105, 144, 190, 191, 194, 205,
    218–19, 230, 266, 270
Rubin, J., 21, 122, 174–75, 182, 193, 194,
    218–19
Rudas, J., 11, 103, 173
Runyan, C.M., 75, 205
Rupp, R.R., 171
Rustin, L., 241, 242
Ryan, B., 134, 240, 241, 242, 267
Ryan, B.P., 26, 104, 134, 154, 186, 187,
    188, 190, 195, 196, 202, 203, 205,
    240–42, 267

Sabin, E.J., 42
Sadker, M., 124
Sailor, W., 197
St. Louis, K.O., 134
Saleh, M.A., 122
Samuels, M., 171
Samuels, N., 171
Saskia, K., 15, 16
Sayers, B.M., 32, 106
Schaefer, H.K., 155

Scheuerle, J., 152
Schnidler, M.D., 116
Schuell, H., 118
Schum, R., 155
Schwartz, M.F., 167, 249–50
Seeman, J., 13
Seeman, M., 10
Seider, R.A., 134
Seltzer, H.N., 106, 243
Seltzer, J., 242–43
Shames, G.H., 3, 6, 13, 14, 19, 21, 39, 53,
    103–6, 111, 121, 122, 133, 141,
    142, 154, 163, 174, 178, 179, 180,
    182, 189, 190, 191, 194, 196, 201,
    230, 243–45, 264, 266
Shane, M.L.S., 32
Shaw, C.K., 104
Sheehan, J.G., 15, 97, 151, 155, 161, 163,
    189, 193, 196, 201, 245–47
Sherrick, C.E., Jr., 14, 19, 39, 178, 179
Shine, R.E., 81, 82, 126, 247–49, 260, 264
Shipley, K.G., 153
Shoemaker, D.J., 14, 15, 120, 170, 181,
    183, 213–15
Shumak, I.C., 85
Siegel, G.M., 20, 103, 105, 106, 133, 178,
    183, 184, 186
Silverman, E.M., 190
Silverman, F.H., 86, 89, 95, 156, 204
Snidecor, J.C., 114
Snow, R., 122
Sommer, R., 171
Spriestersbach, D.C., 69, 70, 72, 73, 77,
    81, 86, 89
Stager, S., 173
Starkweather, C.W., 28, 158, 159, 189,
    190, 204, 250–51
Starr, D.C., 106
Stevens, H., 39
Stewart, J.L., 133
Stockard, J., 124
Stocker, B., 188
Stocks, J., 103
Stokes, T., 195
Stromsta, C., 30
Strum, W.F., 104

Tanner, S., 203
Taylor, O.L., 123, 129
Thomas, C.C., 241

Thorensen, C.E., 154
Toscher, M.M., 171
Travis, L.E., 9–10, 12
Trident, K.A., 76

Ulliana, 133

Vaane, E., 167
Van Dam Baggen, R., 133
Van Kirk, B., 154, 188, 195, 203, 205, 240–42
Van Riper, C., 4, 18, 30, 39, 102, 114, 120, 122, 144, 151, 155, 173, 189, 193, 196, 240, 251–52, 269
Vealey, R.S., 171
Vogul, D., 160

Waddle, P., 117
Wall, M.J., 41, 253–54
Walton, J.H., 134
Watson, B.C., 133
Webster, R.L., 167, 180, 190, 203, 247, 254–55
Webster, W.G., 10, 133
Weiner, A.E., 255–57
Weiss, A.L., 134
Weiss, D.G., 160
Weisz, J.R., 118, 124

Wepman, J.M., 10
Wertz, R.T., 35, 160
West, J.A., 160
West, R., 10
White, D.T., 26, 236
Wieneke, G., 167
Williams, D.E., 19, 69, 70, 72, 73, 77, 79, 81, 85, 86, 89, 102, 134, 192
Wilson, L., 75, 76
Wingate, M.E., 4, 168
Winkler, R., 141, 205
Wischner, G.J., 14, 15
Wolpe, J., 14, 15, 168, 189, 256
Woods, L., 21, 203, 204
Woods, T., 201
Woolf, G., 66, 86, 92, 98, 126
Wray, D.F., 41, 42, 43

Yairi, E., 6, 15, 25, 26, 41, 96, 133, 134
Yates, M., 133
Yeakle, M.K., 134
Yetman, N.R., 121
Young, M.A., 159

Zebrowski, P., 134, 155
Zenhausern, R., 123
Zeskind, P.S., 122
Zimmer, C.H., 190

Subject Index

Abnormal overt (or covert)
    communication behavior,
    stuttering as, 6–7
Aboriginal cultures, stuttering in, 114–15
Adaptation, 97
Adolescents, question outline for
    diagnostic interview with, 61, 66
Adults
    effective therapy for, 150–51
    question outline for diagnostic
        interview with, 62
African Americans, occurrence of
    stuttering by gender in, 119
Age
    effective therapy and, 148–51
        mature adults, 150–51
        preschool-aged children, 148–49
        primary school-aged children, 149
        young adults, 150
    fluency and, 201
    occurrence of stuttering and, 119
    speech behaviors and, 120
    test instruments appropriate by, 126
Air Flow Therapy, 249–50
American Speech-Language-Hearing
    Association (ASHA), 136, 137,
    157, 163
Anticipatory-struggle reaction,
    stuttering as, 15–16
Anxiety response, stuttering as learned,
    15–16
Assessment techniques, 69–107
    comprehensive testing procedure,
        95–106

Differential Screening for
    Stuttering, 96–98
Stuttering Assessment Protocol,
    80, 82, 96, 98–106, 127, 260
for covert characteristics of
    stuttering, 82–95
    covert assessment protocols, 85–95
    covert stuttering behaviors, 84–85
    measurement procedures, 85
cultural differences and, effect of,
    125–29
    data gathering procedures,
        126–28
    instruments and protocols, 126
    procedures for conveying
        information, 128–29
for overt characteristics of stuttering,
    69–82
    measurement procedures, 77–79
    overt assessment protocols, 79–82
    overt stuttering behaviors, 69–77
Associations, enhancing generalization
    through, 201
Attitude(s), 165, 189–93
    to be changed, 191–93, 205
        responsibility for change, 192
    clinician's decision to modify, 189–91
Attitude probes in Stuttering
    Assessment Protocol, 100, 104–5
Auditory feedback, 171–72
    delayed (DAF), 19–20, 221, 240, 241
Automatic speech, 97
Avoidance, 84
Avoidance-reduction therapy, 246

Bantu culture, occurrence of stuttering in, 117
  by gender, 119
Baseline data
  analysis of, 260, 263–64, 265–66, 268, 271
  collection of, 98–101
Behavioral changeability, probes of, 101–6
  case study illustrations of, 260–62, 264, 266, 268–69, 271–72
Behavioral Cognitive Stuttering Therapy, 80, 82, 98, 226–28, 264, 267, 270
Behavioral expectations of sexes, ethnic cultural values and, 124
Belief system of parents, 57–58
Bounce (speech modification technique), 18

Cancellation (speech modification technique), 18
Case history
  cultural differences and obtaining, 127
  data from parents, 57
Case history models, 262–72
  of disfluency pattern that is not stuttering, 271–72
  for selecting published protocols, 263–65
  for selecting technique from various protocols, 265–67
  using all PROLAM strategies, 267–70
Cause of stuttering
  information from client on, 63
  as unknown, 6
Cerebral dominance, theory of, 9–10
Changeability, probes of behavioral, 99–106
  case study illustrations of, 260–62, 264, 266, 268–69, 271–72
Checklist of Stuttering Behavior, 73, 79, 80
Chemical reaction disfluencies, 36–37
Childhood developmental disorder, stuttering as, 6, 7
Child rearing, ethnic cultural values and, 121–22

Children, question outline for diagnostic interview with, 60, 66
Choral reading, 97, 106
Circumlocutions, 71
Class, stuttering by, 116–17
Client. See also Informed client
  information from. See under Diagnostic interview
  resistive, 64–66
Client-centered therapy. See Nondirective (client-centered) therapy
Client-initiated interviews, guidelines for, 53–54
Client observations, 51–53
  outside clinic, 51–52
  informal clinic observation, 52–53
Clinical contacts, scheduling of, 203
Clinical efficacy, 159–61
  general efficacy of therapy, 160–61
  of specific intervention programs, 161
Clinical failures, explanations of, 162–63
  clinician incompetence, 163
  lack of motivation, 162–63
  nature of the disorder, 162
  use of inappropriate treatment protocols, 163
Clinical Management of Childhood Stuttering, 253–54
Clinics
  hospital, 138–39
  private practice, 138–39
  university training, 140–41
Cognitive fluency program, 218–19
Communication, stutterers' different view of, 6, 7
Communication behavior, stuttering as abnormal overt (or covert), 6–7
Communication styles, 112. See also Culture
Complexity of utterance
  controlling, in PROLAM-GM, 165, 186, 187–89
  in Stuttering Assessment Protocol, 100, 104
Component Model for Treating Stuttering in Children, 239–40
Comprehensive Alberta Stuttering Program, 211–12

Computer-Aided Fluency Establishment Trainer (CAFET), 225–26, 270
Concomitant Stuttering Behavior Checklist, 79, 80
Concrete speech probe, 104
Content, fluency and, 201
Continuous phonation, combining rate reduction with, 174, 176
Conversational Rate Control Therapy, 221–22, 270
Cooper Personalized Fluency Control Therapy Revised, 215–17, 269
Counselling, parental, 151–57
    on changes in environment, 154
    discussing feelings and emotions, 153–54
    general counselling principles, 152–53
    genetic counselling, 155–57
    on helping with intervention strategies, 154–55
    providing information, 133, 134, 153
Counterconditioning, 213
Covert characteristics of stuttering, 82–95
    covert assessment protocols, 85–95
    covert stuttering behaviors, 84–85
    measurement procedures for, 85
Covert communication behavior, stuttering as abnormal, 6–7
Culture, 111–30
    evaluation and intervention and, 125–29
        data gathering procedures, 126–28
        instruments and protocols, 126
        procedures for conveying information, 128–29
    incidence and occurrence of stuttering and, 113–19
        macroculture, 113–15
        microcultures, 115–19
    speech behaviors and, 119–20
        age, 120
        ethnic and language groups, 120
    therapy and, effect on, 120–25
        ethnic or national origin, 121–24
        gender/sex, 124–25
        religion, 124

Daily self-monitoring activities, 203
Data gathering procedures, cultural differences and, 126–28

Decision-making process, steps in, 260–62
Deconditioning, 213
Definitions of stuttering, 3–8
    comparison of definitions, 4
    four-factor definition, 5–8
    from historical perspective, 3–5
Delayed auditory feedback (DAF), 19–20, 221, 240, 241
Demographic data, 132
Desensitization, 250, 252
    systematic, 169–70, 255
Developmental disfluencies, normal, 25–26
Developmental disorder of childhood, stuttering as, 6, 7
Developmental phases of stuttering, 28, 31
Diagnosogenic Theory, 16
Diagnostic evaluation, impact of culture on, 125–29
    data gathering procedures, 127–28
    instruments and protocols, 126
    procedures for conveying information, 128–29
Diagnostic interview, 54–64
    guidelines for constructing, 53–54
    information from clients, 59–64
        behaviors during stuttering, 62
        cause of stuttering, 63
        control over changes, 64
        description of behavior, 61
        efforts to speak fluently, 64
        feelings during stuttering, 63
        happenings during fluent speech, 64
        occurrences when speech changes, 64
        previous speech therapy, 64
        reasons for coming, 59–60
        speech changes during last 6 months, 63
        thoughts during stuttering, 62–63
    information from parents, 55–59
        belief system, 57–58
        case history data, 57
        description of the behavior, 56–57
        parental guilt and defensiveness, 58–59
        previous treatment, 57

reasons for seeking professional
help, 55–56
Differential Screening for Stuttering
(DSS), 96–98
behavioral information, 96–98
case history information, 96
speech sample analysis, 98
Directive therapy, 143–45
advantages and disadvantages of,
143–45
diagnosis, 143
treatment plans, 143
Direct questioning, cultural differences
and, 126
Disclosure laws, 156–57
Discriminative stimulus, 177
Disfluency, 23–46
language disorders, 41–44
illustrative case history, 43–44
measures of, 72
mixed disfluencies, 44–45
neurogenic, 34–38
chemical reaction disfluencies,
36–37
motor speech disfluencies, 36,
37–38
neurolinguistic disfluencies, 36
normal developmental, 25–26
psychogenic disfluency, 38–41
emotionally-based disfluencies,
38–39, 40–41
malingering, 39–40
manipulative disfluency, 39
stuttering, 26–34
developmental phases, 28, 31
illustrative case history, 33–34
schemata for development of,
26–30
that is not stuttering, case history of,
271–72
Drug therapies, 172–73
Duration of moments of stuttering, 101
measurements of, 71–74

Edinburgh Masker Device, 228
Effective therapy, variables in, 131–64
age-related characteristics and,
148–51
mature adults, 150–51
preschool-aged children, 148–49

primary school-aged children, 149
young adults, 150
clinical efficacy, 159–61
general efficacy of therapy, 160–61
of specific intervention programs,
161
clinical failures, explanations for,
162–63
clinical incompetence, 163
lack of motivation, 162–63
nature of the disorder, 162
use of inappropriate treatment
protocols, 163
genetic counselling, 155–57
information to be conveyed,
156–57
informed client and, 131–32
cultural differences and
procedures for conveying
information, 128–29
information to share with clients
and/or parents, 133, 134, 153
role of, 131–32
parents and parental counselling,
151–55
on changes in environment, 154
discussing feelings and emotions,
153–54
general counselling principles,
152–53
on helping with intervention
strategies, 154–55
prevention through early
intervention, 157–59
prevention techniques, 158–59
primary prevention, 157, 158
therapeutic approaches, 142–48
directive therapy, 143–45
nondirective therapy, 13–14,
145–48
work settings for, 132–42
hospital clinics and private
practice clinics, 138–39
public schools, 135–38
special intensive therapy
programs, 141–42
university training clinics, 140–41
Efficacy, clinical, 159–61
Egypt, occurrence of stuttering by
gender in, 119

Electroencephalographic (EEG) studies, 132

Electromyographic (EMG) studies, 132

Emotionally-based disfluencies, 38–39
illustrative case history of, 40–41

Emotional reaction, 84

Emotions
ethnic cultural values and, 123
fluency and emotional state, 201
of parents, discussing, 153–54

England, occurrence of stuttering in, 117

Environmental Manipulation and
Family Counselling, 229–30

Environmental manipulations,
counselling parents about,
154

Ethical issues
in genetic counselling, 156
in primary prevention, 158

Ethnic culture
effect on assessment and therapy,
121–24
occurrence of stuttering by, 117–18
speech behaviors and, 120

Evaluation. See Assessment techniques

Expectation(s)
behavioral, ethnic cultural values
and, 124
of fluency, 84
of stuttering, 84

Extended Length of Utterance (ELV),
217–18

Extinction, 178

Failures, explanations of clinical, 162–63

Feedback, auditory, 171–72
delayed (DAF), 19–20, 221, 240, 241

Feelings
of client during stuttering, 63
of parents, discussing, 153–54

Female-male interactions, culture and,
124–25

Fluency
aspects of communication affecting,
201–2
cognitive fluency program, 218–19
expectation of, 84
normalization of, prior to
termination, 205
reinforcement of, 179, 180

Fluency Assessment Instruments, 66, 86,
89–92

Fluency Baseline Record, 79, 80

Fluency enhancement theory, 19–21

Fluency-enhancing behaviors,
reinforcement of, 180, 181

Fluency failures. See Disfluency

Fluent speech rate, 101

Fluent stuttering, 18–19, 251

Four-factor definition of stuttering,
5–8

Freedom of Fluency, 222–23, 264, 266,
270

Freezing, 250

Frequency, measurements of, 74–75

Gender
effect on assessment and therapy,
124–25
fluency and, 201
occurrence of stuttering by, 118, 119

Generalization(s), 165, 195–202
activities, 201–2
combinations of stimulus and
response, 199
methods for enhancing, 199–201
response, 199, 200
stimulus, 197–98
structure of, 197–98
uses of, 195–97

Genetic counselling, 155–57
information to be conveyed, 156–57

Genetics, heredity model of stuttering
research and, 10–11

Gradual Increase in the Length and
Complexity of Utterance
(GILCU), 240, 241, 267

Guilt, parental, 58–59

Heredity model of stuttering research,
10–11

Historical perspective, definitions of
stuttering from, 3–5

Historical review of modern stuttering
research, 8–22
generalization and maintenance of
gains in therapy, 21–22
manipulable behavior model, 14–21
medical model, 9–11
psychological model, 11–14

Homosexuality, ethnic cultural values and, 125
Hospital clinics, 138–39

Ideal assessment situation for measuring disorder, 50–51
Incidence of stuttering, 113–19
  macroculture and, 113–15
  microculture and, 115–19
Incompetence, clinician, 163
Informed client
  cultural differences and procedures for conveying information, 128–29
  genetic counselling for, 155–57
  information to share with clients and/or parents, 133, 134, 153
  role of, 131–32
Initial interviews, guidelines for constructing, 53–54
Instructional rate control, 174–75, 176
Instrumentation, assessment, 77–78
  cultural differences and, 126
Integration of Approaches, 234–36
Interaction styles, 112, 123. *See also* Culture
Interpreters, using, 129
Interval schedule of reinforcement, 179
Intervention and transfer strategies. *See* PROLAM-GM; Treatment protocols
Intervention protocols, constructing, 259–73
  case history model, 262–72
    disfluency pattern that is not stuttering, 271–72
    selecting published protocols, 263–65
    selecting technique from various protocols, 265–67
    using all PROLAM strategies, 267–70
  decision-making process, 260–62
Interviews, guidelines for initial, 53–54. *See also* Diagnostic interview

Language disorders, 41–44
  illustrative case history, 43–44
Language groups

occurrence of stuttering and native, 119
  speech behaviors and, 120
Laryngeal dynamics, pairing stuttering behavior with, 10
Learned anxiety response, stuttering as, 15–16
Learning styles, ethnic cultural values and, 122–23
Legal issues, 156–57
Length of utterance
  controlling, in PROLAM-GM, 165, 186, 187, 188
  in Stuttering Assessment Protocol, 100, 101, 104
Linguistic revisions, 71
Listeners, fluency and number of, 201
Loose contacts, 102–3

Macroculture
  stuttering and, 113–15
  Of United States, ten values inherent in, 111–12
Maintenance programs, 21–22
Maintenance (PROLAM-GM), 165, 202–6
  enhancing activities for, 203
  relapse and, 203–6
Male-female interactions, culture and, 124–25
Malingering, 39–40
Malpractice suits, 157
Managing Stuttering, 237–38
Manipulable behavior model, 14–21
  diagnosogenic theory, 16
  fluency enhancement, 19–21
  stuttering as a learned anxiety response, 15–16
  stuttering modification, 16–19
Manipulative disfluency, 39
Mass therapy, 214
Mature adults, effective therapy for, 150–51
Measurement of stuttering disorder, 49–51. *See also* Assessment techniques
Measures of Disfluency of Speaking and Oral Reading, 79, 80
Medical model of stuttering research, 9–11
  heredity model, 10–11

laryngeal dynamics, 10
neurological functioning, 11
theory of cerebral dominance,
    9–10
Meta-analysis, 160
Microcultures, 112
    stuttering and, 115–19
Microstutterings, 204
Mixed disfluencies, 44–45
Modelling Approach to Stuttering
        Therapy for Children, 242–43
Modern stuttering research. *See*
        Historical review of modern
        stuttering research
Molecular analysis, 78
Monitoring
    in PROLAM-GM, 165, 193–95
    in Stuttering Assessment Protocol,
        100, 105
Monterey Fluency Program, 240–42
Motivation
    assessment of, 84
    lack of, as explanation for clinical
        failure, 162–63
Motor speech disfluencies, 36
    illustrative case history of, 37–38
Multiprocess Behavioral Approach,
        250–51

National origin, effect on assessment
        and therapy, 121–24. *See also*
        Ethnic culture
Negative practice, 17
Negative reinforcement, 177–78
Neurogenic disfluency, 34–38
    chemical reaction disfluencies, 36–37
    motor speech disfluencies, 36, 37–38
    neurolinguistic disfluencies, 36
Neurological functioning of stuttering,
        11
Neurotic behavior, stuttering as, 12–13
Nondirective (client-centered) therapy,
        13–14, 145–48
    advantages and disadvantages of,
        147–48
    clarification of perceptions, 145–47
    diagnosis, 147
    treatment, 147
Normal developmental disfluencies,
        25–26

Objective attitude (therapeutic
        technique), 16–17
Observable characteristics of stuttering,
        69, 70
Observations, client, 51–53
Occurrence of stuttering, 113–19
    macroculture and, 113–15
    microculture and, 115–19
Operant controls
    in PROLAM-GM, 165, 175–86
        basic concepts, 178–79
        basic terminology, 176–78
        punishment paradigm, 183–86, 188
        reinforcement protocols, 179–83
    in Stuttering Assessment Protocol,
        100, 103–4
Operational Approach to Stuttering
        Therapy, 232–33
Overt characteristics of stuttering, 69–82
    measurement procedures, 77–79
    overt assessment protocols, 79–82
    overt stuttering behaviors, 69–77
        linguistic revisions, 71
        measurements of duration, 71–74
        measurements of frequency, 74–75
        measures of speech rate, 75–76
        perceived severity of stuttering, 76–77
Overt communication behavior,
        stuttering as abnormal, 6–7

Parents of stutterer. *See also* Informed
        client
    belief system of, 57–58
    counselling for, 151–55
        on changes in environment, 154
        discussing feelings and emotions,
            153–54
        general counselling principles,
            152–53
        genetic counselling, 155–57
        on helping with intervention
            strategies, 154–55
        providing information, 133, 134,
            153
    guilt and defensiveness of, 58–59
    information from. *See under*
        Diagnostic interview
Past speech history, fluency and, 201
Perceived severity of stuttering, 76–77
Percentage of words stuttered, 101

Percent of syllables stuttered, 101
Perception
    clarification of client, 145–47
    of speech quality, 101
Perceptions of Stuttering Inventory
        (PSI), 66, 85–89, 90–92, 98
Personalized Fluency Control Therapy
        program, 92–95
*Personalized Fluency Control Therapy
        Revised*, 215–17, 269
Phonatory adjustment strategies, 167–68
Physiological adjustments
    in PROLAM-GM, 165, 166–73
        auditory feedback, 171–72
        drug therapies, 172–73
        phonatory adjustment strategies,
            167–68
        secondary characteristic
            elimination strategies, 173, 174
        stress-reducing techniques, 168–71
    in Stuttering Assessment Protocol,
        100, 102–3
Poland, occurrence of stuttering by
        gender in, 119
Positive reinforcement (RF+), 177,
        181–82, 188
Positron emission tomography (PET)
        scans of neurological
        functioning, 11
Practice
    for fluency, failure to, 204
    negative, 17
Precision Fluency Shaping Program,
        254–55
Preindustrial culture, stuttering in, 114–15
Preparatory-set (speech modification
        technique), 18
Preschool-aged children, effective
        therapy for, 148–49
Preschool Fluency Development
        Program, 220–21
Prevention of stuttering, 157–59
    prevention techniques, 158–59
    primary prevention, 157, 158
    secondary prevention, 157–58
    tertiary prevention, 158
Primary prevention, 157, 158
Primary school-aged children, effective
        therapy for, 149
Private practice clinics, 138–39

Program for the Initial Stages of Fluency
        Therapy, 218–19, 266, 270
Program to Establish Fluent Speech,
        233–34, 270
Progressive relaxation, 168–69
PROLAM-GM, 165–207. *See also*
        Intervention protocols,
        constructing; Treatment
        protocols
    attitude, 165, 189–93
        attitudes to be changed, 191–93
        clinician's decision to modify,
            189–91
    generalization, 165, 195–202
        activities, 201–2
        combination of stimulus and
            response, 199, 200
        methods for enhancing, 199–201
        response generalization, 199, 200
        stimulus, 197–98, 199
        structure of, 197–98
        uses of, 195–97
    length and complexity of utterance,
        165, 186–89
        complexity, 165, 186, 187–89
        length, 165, 186, 187, 188
    maintenance, 165, 202–6
        enhancing activities, 203
        relapse, 203–6
    monitoring, 165, 193–95
    operant controls, 165, 175–86
        basic concepts, 178–79
        basic terminology, 176–78
        punishment paradigm, 183–86, 188
        reinforcement protocols, 179–83
    physiological adjustments, 165,
        166–73
        auditory feedback, 171–72
        drug therapies, 172–73
        phonatory adjustment strategies,
            167–68
        secondary characteristics
            elimination strategies, 173, 174
        stress, 168–71
    rate of speech manipulations, 165,
        173–75
        combining rate reduction with
            continuous phonation, 174, 176
        instructional rate control, 174–75,
            176

prolongation, 174, 175
use in evaluation of case history
    models for intervention
    protocols, 267–70
Prolongation, 72
    continuous phonation and, 174,
        176
    as speech rate manipulation
        technique, 174, 175
Protocol for Differentiating the Incipient
    Stutterer, 26, 27–30
Protocols. *See* Treatment protocols
Psychogenic disfluency, 38–41
    emotionally-based disfluencies,
        38–39, 40–41
    malingering, 39–40
    manipulative disfluency, 39
Psychological model of stuttering
    research, 11–14
    nondirective (client-centered)
        therapy, 13–14, 145–48
    stuttering as neurotic behavior,
        12–13
Public schools, as setting for therapy,
    135–38
Pull-out (speech modification
    technique), 18
Punishment paradigms, 178, 183–86, 188
    basic issues and ethical concerns,
        183–84
    to reduce or eliminate secondary
        statements, 184, 186
    to reduce or eliminate stuttering, 184,
        185
    to reduce or eliminate undesirable
        statements, 185, 187

Questionnaires, 85
    written, 66

Rate of speech
    fluent, 101
    measures of, 75–76
    reducing, 250
Rate of speech manipulations
    in PROLAM-GM, 165, 173–75
        combining rate reduction with
            continuous phonation, 174, 176
        instructional rate control, 174–75,
            176

prolongation, 174, 175
    in Stuttering Assessment Protocol,
        100, 103
Ratio schedule of reinforcement, 179
Reciprocal inhibition therapy, 15–16
Recording information, cultural
    differences and methods of,
    128
Recording speech samples, guidelines
    for, 78–79
Referral patterns for children needing
    services, 112
Refresher programs, 203
Regular clinic contacts, 203
Reinforcement
    negative, 177–78
    positive (RF+), 177, 181–82, 188
Reinforcement protocols, 179–83
    fluency, 179, 180
    fluency-enhancing behaviors, 180,
        181
    speech devoid of secondary
        characteristics, 181–82
    types of statements, 182–83
Reinforcement schedules, 179
Relapse, 203–6
    attitude change and, 205
    client assumption of responsibility,
        205
    failure to practice and, 204
    genetic implications, 204–5
    normalization of speech fluency prior
        to termination of therapy, 205
    preparation for, 205–6
    slow decay due to similar stimuli, 204
Religion(s)
    effect on therapy, 124
    occurrence of stuttering within, 118
Repetitions, 72
Research. *See* Historical review of
    modern stuttering research
Resistive clients, 64–66
Response generalization, 199, 200
    combining stimulus generalization
        and, 199
Responsibility, client assumption of,
    205
Revisions, linguistic, 71
Rhythmic speech, 106
Role Therapy, 245–47

Samples, recording speech, 78–79
Scale for Rating Severity of Stuttering, 76, 77, 79, 80
School-based therapy, 135–38
Secondary characteristics
  eliminating, 252
    punishment for reducing or, 184, 186
    strategies for, 173, 174
  reinforcing speech devoid of, 181–82
Secondary prevention, 157–58
Self-help groups, 161
Self-monitoring activities, daily, 203
Self-perception, 85
Self-recording probe, 105
Severity of stuttering, perceived, 76–77
Severity Scale and Adjective Checklist, 66
Sex. See Gender
Shadowing, 106
Singing, 98
Social class, stuttering by, 116–17
South Dakota Indians, occurrence of stuttering among, 117
Special intensive therapy programs, 141–42
Speech behaviors, crosscultural studies of, 119–20
Speech-language clinicians, services for stuttering clients provided by, 135–38
Speech-language pathologist-initiated interviews, guidelines for, 54
Speech-language pathologists, ASHA certification of, 137
Speech rate. See Rate of speech
Status, fluency and, 201
Stimulus, discriminative, 177
Stimulus generalization, 197–98
  combining response generalization and, 199
Stress-reducing techniques, 168–71
  progressive relaxation, 168–69
  systematic desensitization, 169–70, 255
  visualization, 170–71
Stutterer's Self-Ratings of Reactions to Speech Situations, 85, 86, 87–89

Stutter-Free Speech, 196, 201, 244–45, 264, 266
Stuttering
  definitions of, 3–8
    comparison of definitions, 4
    four-factor definition, 5–8
    historical perspective, 3–5
  disfluency pattern of, 26–34
    developmental phases, 28, 31
    illustrative case history, 33–34
    schemata for development, 26–30
  fluent, 18–19, 251
  incidence and occurrence of, culture and, 113–19
    macroculture, 113–15
    microcultures, 115–19
Stuttering Assessment Protocol (SAP), 80, 82, 96, 98–106, 127, 260
  baseline data collection, 98–101
  other probes, 106
  probes of changeability, 99–106
Stuttering Attitudes Checklist, 66
Stuttering behaviors
  covert, 84–85
  overt, 69–77
Stuttering Diagnostic and Evaluative Checklist, 80, 82
Stuttering Frequency and Duration Estimate Record, 79, 80
Stuttering Intervention Program, 236–37
Stuttering modification techniques, 16–19
Stuttering Prediction Instrument (SPI), 239
Stuttering Problem Profile, 86, 89, 93–95
Stuttering Severity Instrument for Children and Adults (SSI), 80, 82, 83
Stuttering Severity Scale, 86, 89
Symptomatic therapy for stuttering, 18–19
Symptom Modification Therapy, 251–52, 269
Systematic desensitization, 169–70, 255
Systematic Fluency Training for Young Children, 80, 82, 247–49, 264

Techniques for Maintaining Fluency, 230–31
Tertiary prevention, 158

Test instruments, 77–78, 126
Therapy. *See also* Effective therapy,
  variables in; Treatment
  protocols
  cultural differences and, effect of,
    120–25
    ethnic or national origin,
      121–24
    gender/sex, 124–25
    religion, 124
  directive, 143–45
  drug, 172–73
  generalization
    as integrated part of therapy,
      196–97
    as stage in therapy, 196
  nondirective, 145–48
Time-out probes, 106
Timing, measurements of duration and,
  71–74
Translator, use of, 128
Treating the School-Aged Stutterer,
  223–25
Treatment protocols, 209–57
  Air Flow Therapy, 249–50
  Behavioral Cognitive Stuttering
    Therapy, 80, 82, 98, 226–28, 264,
    267, 270
  Clinical Management of Childhood
    Stuttering, 253–54
  Component Model for Treating
    Stuttering in Children,
    239–40
  Comprehensive Alberta Stuttering
    Program, 211–12
  Computer-Aided Fluency
    Establishment Trainer (CAFET),
    225–26, 270
  Conversational Rate Control Therapy,
    221–22, 270
  Cooper Personalized Fluency Control
    Therapy Revised, 215–17,
    269
  cultural differences and, 126
  Edinburgh Masker Device, 228
  Environmental Manipulation and
    Family Counselling, 229–30
  Extended Length of Utterance (ELV),
    217–18

format for each, 210
Freedom of Fluency, 222–23, 264, 266,
  270
Integration of Approaches, 234–36
Managing Stuttering, 237–38
Modelling Approach to Stuttering
  Therapy for Children, 242–43
Monterey Fluency Program, 240–42
Multiprocess Behavioral Approach,
  250–51
Operational Approach to Stuttering
  Therapy, 232–33
Precision Fluency Shaping Program,
  254–55
Preschool Fluency Development
  Program, 220–21
Program for the Initial Stages of
  Fluency Therapy, 218–19, 266,
  270
Program to Establish Fluent Speech,
  233–34, 270
Role Therapy, 245–47
Stutter-Free Speech, 196, 201, 244–45,
  264, 266
Stuttering Intervention Program,
  236–37
Symptom Modification Therapy,
  251–52, 269
Systematic Fluency Training for
  Young Children, 80, 82, 247–49,
  264
Techniques for Maintaining Fluency,
  230–31
Treating the School-Aged Stutterer,
  223–25
Two-Factor Behavior Therapy,
  213–15
use of inappropriate, as explanation
  for clinical failure, 163
Vocal Control Therapy, 255–57
Vocaltech Feedback Device, 243–44
Two-Factor Behavior Therapy, 213–15

United States
  occurrence of stuttering in, 117
    by gender, 119
  ten values inherent in macroculture
    of, 111–12
University training clinics, 140–41

Values, 111–12. *See also* Culture
Visualization, 170–71
Vocal Control Therapy, 255–57
Vocaltech Feedback Device,
    243–44
Voluntary stuttering (therapeutic
    technique), 16, 17

White Americans, occurrence of
    stuttering by gender in,
    119

Work settings for therapy interaction,
    132–42
    hospital clinics and private practice
        clinics, 138–39
    public schools, 135–38
    special intensive therapy programs,
        141–42
    university training clinics, 140–41
Written questionnaires, 66

Young adults, effective therapy for, 150

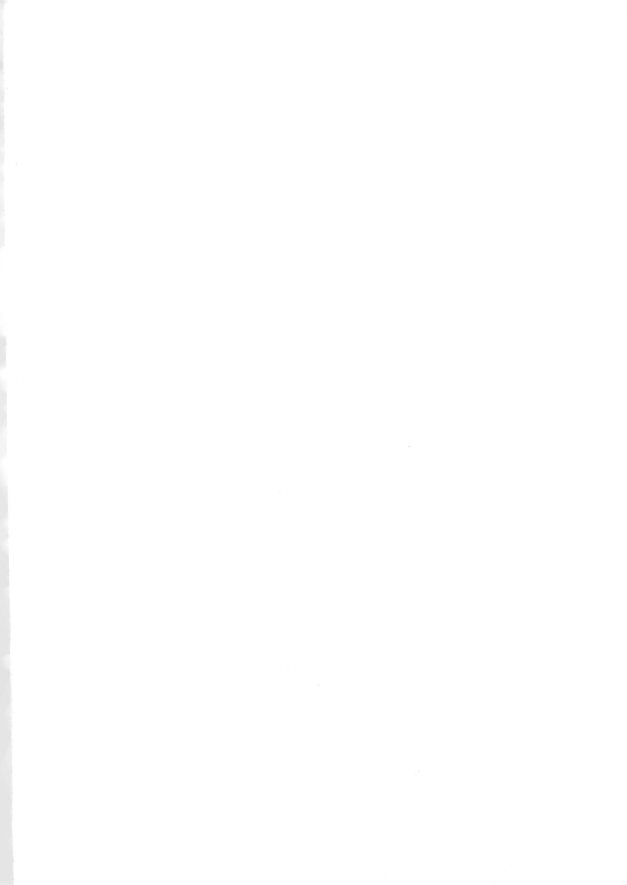